AMERICAN SOCIETY FOR PARENTERAL AND ENTERAL NUTRITION

The A.S.P.E.N. Nutrition Support Practice Manual

2nd Edition

EDITOR-IN-CHIEF

Russell Merritt, MD, PhD
Medical Director, Nutrition
Ross Products Division, Abbott Laboratories
Columbus, OH

SECTION EDITORS

Mark H. DeLegge, MD
Associate Professor of Medicine
Director, Section of Nutrition
Digestive Disease Center
Medical University of South Carolina
Charleston, SC

Beverly Holcombe, PharmD, BCNSP
Clinical Specialist
Department of Pharmacy
University of North Carolina Hospitals
Chapel Hill, NC

Charles Mueller, PhD, RD, CNSD
General Clinical Research Center
Department of Medicine
Weill/Cornell Medical College
New York, NY

Juan Ochoa, MD, FACS
Associate Professor of Surgery and Critical Care
University of Pittsburgh
Pittsburgh, PA

Karen Ringwald Smith, MS, RD, LDN
Clinical Coordinator/Research and Education Coordinator
Clinical Nutrition Services
St. Jude Children's Research Hospital
Memphis, TN

W. Frederick Schwenk II, MD
Professor of Pediatrics
Mayo Clinic College of Medicine
Rochester, MN

MANAGING EDITOR

Peggi Guenter, PhD, RN, CNSN
A.S.P.E.N. Managing Editor for Special Projects
Silver Spring, MD

A.S.P.E.N. is a scientific society whose members are health care professionals-physicians, dietitians, nurses, pharmacists, other allied health professionals, and researchers- dedicated to assuring that every patient receives optimal nutrition care.

A.S.P.E.N.'s mission is to serve as the preeminent, interdisciplinary, nutrition society dedicated to patient-centered clinical practice worldwide through advocacy, education and research in specialized nutrition support.

NOTE: This publication is designed to provide accurate authoritative information in regard to the subject matter covered. It is sold with the understanding that the publisher is not engaged in rendering medical or other professional advice. Trademarked commercial product names are used only for education purposes and do not constitute endorsement by A.S.P.E.N.

This publication does not constitute medical or professional advice, and should not be taken as such. To the extent the information published herein may be used to assist in the care of patients, this is the result of the sole professional judgment of the attending health professional whose judgment is the primary component of quality medical care. The information presented herein is not a substitute for the exercise of such judgment by the health professional.

 For information write: American Society for Parenteral and Enteral Nutrition (A.S.P.E.N.), 8630 Fenton Street, Suite 412, Silver Spring, MD 20910-3805; (301) 587-6315, www.nutritioncare.org, email:aspen@nutr.org.

ISBN #1-889622-06-0

American Society for Parenteral and Enteral Nutrition **aspen**

Contents

American Society for Parenteral and Enteral Nutrition

Contributors

Carolyn Abitbol, MD
Professor of Pediatrics
University of Miami
Division of Pediatric Nephrology
Miami, FL

Caroline M. Apovian, MD, FACN
Associate Professor of Medicine
Boston University School of Medicine
Director, Nutrition & Weight Management Center
Boston Medical Center
Boston, MA

Vince Armenti, MD, PhD
Professor of Surgery Temple University
Department of Surgery/Abdominal Organ Transplant Program
Philadelphia, PA

Stephen L. Barnes, MD
Major, United States Air Force
Center for Sustainment of Trauma and Readiness Skills
University Hospital
Cincinnati, OH

Eden Bateman MS, RD, LD
Wellness Institute, Northwestern Memorial Hospital
Chicago, IL

Sara L. Bergerson, MS, RD
Clinical Research Dietitian
National Institutes of Health
Clinical Center Nutrition Dept.
Bethesda, MD

Andrew C. Bernard, MD
Assistant Professor of Surgery
Division of General Surgery
University of Kentucky
Lexington, KY

Imad F. Btaiche, PharmD, BCNSP
Pharmacy Department
University of Michigan Hospitals
Ann Arbor, MI

Susan J Carlson, MMSc, RD, CSP, LD, CNSD
Neonatal Dietitian
Children's Hospital of Iowa at the University of Iowa Hospitals
Iowa City, IA

Paula M. Charuhas, MS, RD, FADA, CNSD
Clinical Dietitian/Pediatric Nutrition Specialist
Seattle Cancer Care Alliance
Seattle, WA

Glenn M. Chertow, MD, MPH
Division of Nephrology
Department of Medicine Research
University of California, San Francisco
San Francisco, CA

Mark R. Corkins, MD, CNSP, FAAP
Assistant Professor of Pediatrics
James Whitcomb Riley Hospital for Children/Indiana University School of Medicine
Indianapolis, IN

Mark H. Delegge, MD, FACG
Associate Professor of Medicine
Director, Section of Nutrition
Digestive Disease Center
Medical University of South Carolina
Charleston, SC

Donna DiVito, RD, CNSD
Department of Clinical Nutrition
Children's Hospital of Philadelphia
Philadelphia, PA

Charles E. Edmiston Jr., PhD
Associate Professor of Surgery
Department of Surgery
Medical College of Wisconsin
Milwaukee, WI

William Faubion, MD
Assistant Professor of Medicine Mayo Clinic College of Medicine
Division of Gastroenterology, Hepatology, Internal Medicine
Mayo Clinic
Rochester, MN

Erin Fennelly, RD, CNSD
Georgetown University Transplant Institute
Washington, DC

Cade Fields-Gardner, MS, RD, LD, CD
Director of Services
The Cutting Edge
Cary, IL

Maria Luisa Forchielli, MD
Pediatric Department
University of Bologna
Bologna, Italy

Charles Foulks, MD, FACP, FACN
Professor of Medicine, Texas A&M University System Health Science Center
Division Director of Nephrology-Hypertension
Vice Chairman of External Affairs
Department of Medicine
Scott & White Clinic & Hospital
Temple, TX

Eric H. Frankel, PharmD,MSE, BCNSP
Nutrition Support Coordinator
Covenant Health System
Lubbock, TX

David Frankenfield, MS, RD
Chief Clinical Dietitian
Milton S. Hershey Medical Center
Hershey, PA

Elizabeth Gleghorn, MD
Director, Division of Pediatric Gastroenterology, Hepatology, and Nutrition
Children's Hospital and Research Center
Oakland, CA

Michele M. Gottschlich, PhD, RD, CNSD
Director, Nutrition Services
Shriners Hospitals for Children
Cincinnati, OH

Jennifer C. Graf, MS, RD
Clinical Dietitian
National Institutes of Health
Clinical Center Nutrition Dept.
Bethesda, MD

Kathy Pesce-Hammond, MS, RD, LD, CNSD, RN, CNSN
Coordinator, Continuing Education
Clinical Nutrition Specialist
Chartwell Diversified Services, Inc.
Lilburn, GA

Lori Hards, BSc, RD
University of British Columbia
Vancouver, BC

Michelle Harrington, MS, RD, CSP, CNSD, LDN
Nutrition Information Specialist
McNeil Nutritionals
Fort Washington, PA

Jeanette Hasse, PhD, RD, LD, FADA, CNSD
Transplant Nutrition Specialist
Transplant Services
Baylor University Medical Center
Dallas, TX

Edmund M. Hayes, PharmD
Departments of Pharmacy and Medicine
University Medical Center
State University of New York at Stony Brook
Stony Brook, New York,

Angela K Iverson, RD, LMNT
Pediatric Dietitian
University Hospital
The Nebraska Medical Center
Omaha, NE

Deborah Johnson, RN, MSN
Meriter Hospital
Madison, WI

Stuart S. Kaufman, MD
Children's National Medical Center and
Georgetown University Transplant Institute
Washington, DC

Paul A Kearney, MD, FACS
Professor of Surgery
Section Head, Trauma and Surgical Critical Care
Division of General Surgery
University of Kentucky Medical Center
Lexington, KY

Darlene G Kelly, MD PhD
Associate Professor of Medicine
Mayo Clinic
Division of Gastroenterology/Hepatology/Internal Medicine
Rochester, MN

Donald F. Kirby, MD CNSP
Professor, Virginia Commonwealth University School of Medicine
Medical College of Virginia Hospitals
Section of Nutrition
Richmond, VA

Winston Koo, MB, BS, FRACP
Professor of Pediatrics
Wayne State University
Department of Pediatrics
Hutzel Hospital
Detroit, MI

Debra S. Kovacevich, RN, MPH
Home Care Services
University of Michigan Hospitals and Health Centers
Ann Arbor, MI

Rosemary Kozar, MD, PhD
Associate Professor
University of Texas Medical School
Houston, TX

Mary Kramlich, MS, RD, LD,CNSD
Transplant Nutrition Specialist
Transplant Services
Baylor University Medical Center
Dallas, TX

Elizabeth Krzywda, ANP, MSN
Adult Nurse Practitioner
Department of Surgery
Medical College of Wisconsin
Milwaukee, WI

Vanessa J. Kumpf, PharmD, BCNSP
Clinical Specialist
Nutrishare, Inc.
Elk Grove, CA

Robert F. Kushner, MD
Professor of Medicine, Northwestern University Feinberg School of Medicine
Medical Director, Wellness Institute, Northwestern Memorial Hospital
Chicago, IL

Polly Lenssen, MS, RD, FADA
Clinical Nutrition Manager
Childrens' Hospital & Regional Medical Center
Seattle, WA

Ann Connell Lipkin, MS, CNSD
Clinical Dietitian II
Childrens' Hospital & Regional Medical Center
Seattle, WA

Kathleen D. Liu, MD, PhD
University of California, San Francisco
San Francisco, CA

Linda M. Lord, NP, MS, CNSN
Nutrition Support Service
Strong Memorial Hospital
Rochester, NY

Julie O'Sullivan Maillet, PhD, RD, FADA
Professor and Associate Dean for Academic Affairs and Research
University of Medicine and Dentistry of New Jersey-School of Health Related Professions
Newark, NJ

Mary Marian, MS, RD
Clinical Nutrition Research Specialist
University of Arizona College of Medicine and Northwest Medical Center
Tucson, AZ

Paul E. Marik, MD, FCCM, FCCP
Chief of Pulmonary and Critical Care Medicine
Thomas Jefferson University School of Medicine
Philadelphia, PA

Robert G. Martindale, MD, PhD, FACS
Professor of Surgery
Chief, Gastrointestinal Surgery
Department of Surgery
Medical College of Georgia
Augusta, GA

Maria Mascarenhas, MBBS
Director, Nutrition Support Service
Children's Hospital of Philadelphia
Philadelphia, PA

Theresa Mayes, RD
Registered Dietitian
Shriners Hospitals for Children
Cincinnati, OH

Susan L Mayhew, PharmD, BCNSP
Nutrition Support Specialist
Coordinator, Pharmacy Education and Residency Programs
Columbus Regional Healthcare System
Columbus, OH

Stephen A. McClave, MD
Professor of Medicine
Division of Gastroenterology/Hepatology.
University of Louisville
Louisville, KY

Kathleen McLaughlin, MS, RNC, NNP
Neonatal Nurse Practitioner
Hutzel Hospital / Women's Hospital
Detroit, MI

M. Molly McMahon, MD
Associate Professor of Medicine
Division of Endocrinology, Diabetes, Metabolism,
Nutrition, and Internal Medicine
Mayo Clinic College of Medicine
Rochester, MN

Kerry McMillen, MS, RD
Clinical Dietitian
Seattle Cancer Care Alliance
Seattle, WA

Margaret M. McQuiggan, MS, RD, LD, CNSD
University of Texas Medical School Houston
Department of GI Nutrition
Houston, TX

Madeline Michael, MPH, RD
Chief, Clinical Nutrition Services
National Institutes of Health
Clinical Center Nutrition Dept.
Bethesda, MD

Stephanie Mighdoll, PharmD
Albany College of Pharmacy
Albany, NY

Sarah J Miller, PharmD
Professor, Dept. Pharmacy Practice
University of Montana
Missoula, MT

Jay Mirtallo, MS, RPh, BCNSP
The Ohio State University Medical Center
Dept. of Pharmacy
Columbus, OH

Frederick Moore, MD
James H. "Red" Duke Jr. Professor
and Vice Chairman, Department of Surgery
Medical Director, Trauma Services
University of Texas Medical School
Houston, TX

Michael S. Nyffeler, PharmD, BCNSP
Clinical Specialist Nutrition Support
Meriter Hospital
Madison, WI

Juan Ochoa, MD, FACS
Associate Professor of Surgery and Critical Care
University of Pittsburgh
Pittsburgh, PA

Marianne Opilla, RN, BSN, CNSN
Nutrition Support Nursing
Medical College of Virginia Hospitals
Richmond, VA

Marsha E. Orr, RN, MS
Faculty, Department of Nursing
California State University
Fullerton, CA

Craig Petersen, RD, CNSD
Pediatric Nutrition Support Specialist
University of California, Davis Med Center
Sacramento, CA

Mary Ellen Posthauer, RD, CD,LD
Corporate Consultant
Supreme Care West
Evansville, IN

Crystal Reil, RD, CD-N
Genetic Nutritionist
Department of Genetics
Yale University School of Medicine
Yale-New Haven Hospital
New Haven, CT

Mirta Rios, RD
Jackson Memorial Hospital
Miami, FL

Gretchen Robinson, MS, RD, LD, FADA
Consultant Dietitian
Ada, OH

Annette Stralovich-Romani, RD, CNSD
University of California, San Francisco
San Francisco, CA

Marie Rossique, PharmD
Jackson Memorial Hospital
Miami, FL

Julie L. Roth, MD
Assistant Professor of Medicine, Northwestern University
Feinberg School of Medicine
Wellness Institute, Northwestern Memorial Hospital
Chicago, IL

Mary Saba, PharmD, BCNSP
Clinical Coordinator
Wayne State University
Children's Hospital of Michigan
Department of Pharmacy Services
Detroit, MI

Gordon S Sacks, PharmD, BCNSP, FCCP
Clinical Associate Professor
University of Wisconsin, Madison
School of Pharmacy
Madison, WI

Jeffrey E. Salon, MD, FACP, FCCP, FCCM
Medical Director, Medical Nutrition
Ross Products Division, Abbott Laboratories
Columbus, OH

Margretta R. Seashore, MD, FAAP, FACMG
Professor, Genetics and Pediatrics
Director, Genetics Consultation Service
Department of Genetics
Yale University School of Medicine
Attending Physician
Yale-New Haven Hospital
New Haven, CT

Denise Baird Schwartz, MS, RD, FADA, CNSD
Nutrition Support Coordinator
Providence Health System
San Fernando Valley Service Area
Burbank, CA

James S. Scolapio, MD, CNSP
Associate Professor of Medicine
Director of Nutrition
Mayo Clinic
Jacksonville, FL

Karen Amorde-Spalding, MS, RD, CSP
Children's Hospital Oakland
Oakland, CA

Marjorie Swintosky, MS, RD
University of Kentucky Medical Center
Lexington, KY

Laura Sware, RD
University of British Columbia
Vancouver, BC

Elaine B. Trujillo, MS, RD
Nutritional Science Research Group
Division of Cancer Prevention
National Cancer Institute
National Institutes of Health
Rockville, MD

Jacqueline Wessel, MEd, RD, CSP, CNSD, CLE
Cincinnati Children's Hospital Medical Center
Cincinnati, OH

J. Scott Whittaker, MD
Clinical Professor, Gastroenterology
University of British Columbia
Vancouver, BC

Jennifer A. Wooley, MS, RD, CNSD
Nutrition Support Service
St. Joseph Mercy Health System
Ann Arbor, MI

American Society for Parenteral and Enteral Nutrition

Reviewers

Carolyn L. Abitbol, MD
Professor of Pediatrics
Division of Pediatric Nephrology
University of Miami School of Medicine
Miami, FL

Phyllis B. Acosta, MS,MPH, DrPH, RD
Director of Metabolic Diseases (retired)
Ross Products Division, Abbott Laboratories
Columbus, OH

Maria R. Andrews, MS, RD, FADA, CNSD, LDN
Chief, Nutrition & Food Service
New Mexico VA Health Care System
Albuquerque, NM

Deborah A. Andris, MSN, ANP
Nurse Practitioner; Bariatric Surgery Program
Medical College of Wisconsin
Milwaukee, WI

Caroline Apovian, MD
Director, Center for Nutrition and Weight Management
Associate Professor of Medicine
Boston University School of Medicine
Boston, MA

David A. August, MD
Associate Professor of Surgery, Chief, Division of Surgical Oncology
UMDNJ/ Robert Wood Johnson Medical School and The Cancer Institute of New Jersey
New Brunswick, NJ

Robin Bankhead, MS, CRNP, CNSN
Department of Surgery
Temple University Hospital
Philadelphia, PA

Jacqueline R. Barber, PharmD, FASHP, BCNSP
Clinical Associate Professor
University of Minnesota, Minneapolis, MN
Pharmacy Clinical Specialist
Methodist Hospital, Department of Pharmacy
St. Louis, MN

Randy Bechtel, PharmD, BS
Metabolic Support and Clinical Pharmacy Manager
Freeman Health System
Joplin, MO

Bruce Ryan Bistrian, MD, PhD
Professor of Medicine
Harvard Medical School
Beth Israel Deconess Medical Center
Boston, MA

Donna Zimmaro Bliss, PhD, RN, FAAN
Associate Professor and Professor in Long-Term Care of Elders
University of Minnesota School of Nursing
Minneapolis, MN

Carol Braunschweig, PhD
Associate Professor
University of Illinois at Chicago
Chicago, IL

Pamela Brown, MD, PhD
Clinical Assistant Professor of Pediatrics and Communicable Diseases
University of Michigan Medical Center
Ann Arbor, MI

Susan J Carlson MMSc, RD, CSP, LD, CNSD
Neonatal Dietitian
Children's Hospital of Iowa at the University of Iowa Hospitals
Iowa City, IA

David Charney, MD, FACP
Riverside Nephrology Association
Columbus, OH

Pamela Charney, MS,RD, LD, CNSD
PhD Candidate
School of Health Related Professions
University of Medicine and Dentistry of New Jersey
Newark, NJ

Ronni Chernoff, PhD, RD
Associate Director, GRECC; Professor of Geriatrics
CAVHS & University of Arkansas for Medical Sciences
Little Rock, AR

Kathy Clark, MS, RD, CNSD,LD
Metabolic Support Dietitian
Freeman Health System
Joplin, MO

Charlene Compher, PhD, RD, FADA, CNSD, LDN
Assistant Professor of Nutrition Science
University of Pennsylvania School of Nursing
Clinical Nutrition Support, Hospital of the University of Pennsylvania
Philadelphia, PA

Mark R. Corkins, MD, CNSP, FAAP
Assistant Professor of Pediatrics
James Whitcomb Riley Hospital for Children/Indiana University School of Medicine
Indianapolis, IN

Catherine M. Crill, PharmD, BCPS, BCNSP
Assistant Professor of Pharmacy and Pediatrics
University of Tennessee Health Science Center
Memphis, TN

Susan Curtas, RN, MSN
Clinical Nurse Specialist and Research Manager
Cleveland Clinic Foundation
Cleveland, OH

Joan Daniels, RD
Division of Pediatric Nephrology
Mott Children's Hospital
University of Michigan
Ann Arbor, MI

Roland Dickerson, PharmD
Professor of Pharmacy
University of Tennessee Health Science Center
Memphis, TN

Mark Fishbein, MD
Associate Professor
Southern Illinois University School of Medicine
Department of Pediatrics
Springfield, IL

Amy Andolina Fisher RN, MS, CNSN
Nutrition Support Nurse
Lucile Packard Childrens Hospital
Palo Alto, CA

M. Patricia Fuhrman, MS, RD, LD, FADA, CNSD
Area Clinical Nutrition Marketing Director
Coram Healthcare
St. Louis, MO

Susan T. Fussell, PhD, RD, CNSD
Pediatric Clinical Nutrition Specialist
Duke University Medical Center
Durham, NC

Debra K. Gardner, PharmD
Specialty Practice Pharmacist, Women and Infants
Ohio State University Medical Center
Columbus, OH

Donald E. George, MD
Chief, Division of GI/Nutrition
Nemours Children's Clinic
Jacksonville, FL

Kathleen Gura, PharmD, BCNSP, FASHP
Clinical Pharmacist GI/Nutrition
Team Leader, Surgical Program
Children's Hospital of Boston
Boston, MA

Gregory A. Hale, MD
Clinical Director, Division of Stem Cell Transplantation
St. Jude Children's Research Hospital
Memphis, TN

Michelle Harrington, MS, RD, CSP, CNSD, LDN
Nutrition Information Specialist
McNeil Nutritionals
Fort Washington, PA

Linda Heller, MS, RD, CSP
Childrens Hospital of Los Angeles
Los Angeles, CA

Kalman E. Holdy, MD, ABPNS
Medical Director of Clinical Nutrition
Sharp Memorial Hospital
San Diego, CA

Wanda H. Howell, PhD, RD
University Distinguished Professor
Nutritional Science Dept.
University of Arizona
Tucson, AZ

Deborah Johnson, RN, MSN
Clinical Nurse Specialist
Meriter Hospital
Madison, WI

Kimberly Joseph, MD, FACS, CNSP
Director, Trauma Intensive Care Unit
J.H. Stroger Hospital of Cook County
Department of Trauma
Chicago, IL

Kenneth A. Kudsk, MD, FACS
Professor of Surgery, Vice Chairman of Surgical Research
University of Wisconsin-Madison
Madison, WI

Jennifer Lefton, RD, LD/N, CNSD
Clinical Dietitian II
Jackson Memorial Hospital
Miami, FL

Neal S. LeLeiko, MD, PhD
Professor of Pediatrics Brown School of Medicine
Director of Pediatric Gastroenterology, Nutrition and Liver Diseases
Hasbro Children's Hospital and The Rhode Island Hospital
Providence, RI

Mary Marian, RD, MS
Clinical Nutrition Research Specialist
University of Arizona College of Medicine and Northwest Medical Center
Tucson, AZ

Ainsley M. Malone, MS, RD, LD, CNSD
Nutrition Support Team
Pharmacy Department
Mt. Carmel West Hospital
Columbus, OH

Todd W. Mattox, PharmD, BCNSP
Coordinator, Nutrition Support Team
H. Lee Moffitt Cancer Center and Research Institute
Tampa, FL

Carol McGinnis, RN, MS, CNSN
Clinical Nurse Specialist
Sioux Valley Hospital USD Medical Center
Sioux Falls, SD

Louise R. Merriman, MS, RD, CN/D
Corporate Manager, Clinical Nutrition
New York Presbyterian Hospital
New York, NY

Sarah J. Miller, PharmD, MS
Professor, University of Montana School of Pharmacy
Missoula, MT

Gayle Minard, MD
Professor of Surgery
The University of Tennessee Health Science Center
Memphis, TN

Ethel L. Mitty, EdD, RN
Adjunct Clinical Professor of Nursing
Research Associate
New York University
Division of Nursing
New York, NY

Barry Mizock, MD
Cook County Hospital
Chicago, IL

Joseph A. Molnar, MD, PhD
Assistant Professor of Plastic and Reconstructive Surgery
Wake Forest University School of Medicine
Winston-Salem, NC

Steve Montoya, MD
Medical Director
Angelo Dialysis Centers
San Angelo, TX

Charles Mueller, PhD, RD, CNSD
General Clinical Research Center
Department of Medicine
Weill/Cornell Medical College
New York, NY

Diane Olson, RD, CNSD
Registered Dietitian
Mayo Clinic
Rochester, MN

Adele K. Pattinson, RD, LD, CNSD
Nutrition Support Dietitian/ Home Enteral Coordinator
Mayo Clinic Medical Center
Rochester, MN

Marcia Kalista-Richards, MPH, RD, CNSD, LDN
Nutrition Support-Renal Dietitian
Easton Hospital/Sodexho Co.
Easton, PA

Carol J. Rollins, MS, RD, CNSD, PharmD, BCNSP
Coordinator, Nutrition Support Team and Clinical Associate Professor
University Medical Center and University of Arizona, College of Pharmacy
Tucson, AZ

Pamela Rothpletz-Puglia, EdD, RD
Nutrition Practitioner and Research Associate Francois-Xavier Bagnoud Center
University of Medicine and Dentistry of New Jersey
Newark, NJ

Mary Krystofiak Russell MS, RD
Director, Nutrition Services
Duke University Hospital
Durham, NC

Nancy Sacks, MS, RD
Research Coordinator
Division of Oncology
Children's Hospital of Philadelphia
Philadelphia, PA

Philip J. Schneider, RPh, MS, FASHP
Clinical Professor and Director
Latiolais Leadership Program
Division of Pharmacy Practice and Administration
College of Pharmacy
The Ohio State University
Columbus, OH

W. Frederick Schwenk II, MD
Professor of Pediatrics
Mayo Clinic College of Medicine
Rochester, MN

Douglas L. Seidner, MD
Director, Nutrition Support and Vascular Access Department
Program Director, Fellowship in Clinical Nutrition
Digestive Disease Center
The Cleveland Clinic Foundation
Cleveland, OH

David S. Seres, MD, CNSP
Assistant Professor
Albert Einstein College of Medicine
New York, NY

Marcia Silkroski RD
Executive Director
Nutrition Advantage
Chester Springs, PA

David L. Sigalet, MD, PhD, FRCSC, FACS
Director of Pediatric General Surgery
Professor, University of Calgary, Alberta Children's Hospital
Calgary, Alberta, CANADA

Edwin Simpser, MD
Chief Medical Officer
St. Mary's Hospital for Children
Bayside, NY

Joyce K Stechmiller, ARNP, PhD
Associate Professor
Department of Adult and Elderly Nursing
University of Florida
College of Nursing
Gainesville, FL

John A. Tayek, M.D.
Associate Professor of Medicine-In Residence
David Geffen School of Medicine at UCLA
Harbor-UCLA Medical Center
Department of Internal Medicine
Torrance, CA

Melody Thompson, MS, RD
Clinical Nutrition Specialist
Ross Products Division, Abbott Laboratories
Columbus, OH

Charles W. Van Way, III, MD
Ralph R. Coffey Professor and Chair of Surgery
School of Medicine, University of Missouri-Kansas City
Kansas City, MO

Susan J. Whitmire, RD, CNSD, LDN
Nutrition Support Dietitian
Geisinger Medical Center
Danville, PA

Marion Winkler, MS, RD, LDN, CNSD
Surgical Nutrition Specialist
Rhode Island Hospital and Brown University School of Medicine
Providence, RI

Patricia Worthington, RN, MSN, CNSN
Nutrition Support Clinical Nurse Specialist
Thomas Jefferson University Hospital
Philadelphia, PA

Jane Anne Yaworski, MSN, RN
Clinical Nurse Specialist for Nutrition Support and Intestinal Care
Children's Hospital of Pittsburgh
Pittsburgh, PA

Yi-Hao Yu, MD, PhD, CNSP
Director, Adult PN/Nutrition Service
Columbia-Presbyterian Hospital
Assistant Professor of Medicine
Columbia University College of Physicians and Surgeons
Department of Medicine, Division of Preventive Medicine and Nutrition
New York, NY

Gary P. Zaloga, MA, MD
Medical Director, Methodist Research Institute
Clinical Professor of Medicine
Indiana University School of Medicine
Indianapolis, IN

Russell Merritt, MD, PhD

Introduction

Background

The purpose of this manual is to help practitioners and healthcare organizations implement appropriate and up-to-date nutrition support practices based on the American Society for Parenteral and Enteral Nutrition (A.S.P.E.N.) Guidelines, Safe Practices, and Standards of Practice.[1-6] The goal of A.S.P.E.N. is to assure that every person receives optimal nutrition care.[7] In pursuing this vision, the Society establishes guidelines for the use of parenteral and enteral nutrition (which assess the strength of evidence behind each set of recommendations); actively promotes education related to nutritional support; and stresses the importance of interdisciplinary collaboration in clinical care, education and research. Among A.S.P.E.N.'s objectives is the development of clinical nutrition standards and programs for specialists and generalists working in integrated healthcare systems.[8]

The concept for the first edition of this manual emerged from discussions of the A.S.P.E.N. Publications Committee in 1994-1995 and was approved by the Board of Directors in 1995. The Committee recognized the need for A.S.P.E.N. to articulate methods of nutrition support useful for the implementation of clinical practice guidelines (CPG) in an era when medical practice is becoming increasingly interdisciplinary and protocol-driven. In 2002, the Board of Directors approved a second edition to update the content and offer a new CD format.

The editors have designed this manual to be useful to all practice disciplines within A.S.P.E.N. and to other healthcare professionals looking for guidance on the methods of providing nutrition support including practitioners, clinical administrators, and representatives of third-party payors seeking to identify appropriate nutrition support practices. This manual is a practical "how to" volume which provides focused information on the implementation of multidisciplinary nutrition support. It was developed using a "traditional" approach that is based on practices that have evolved from relevant clinical research and multidisciplinary clinical practices.[9] The volume draws from the relevant medical and nutrition literature, available textbooks, A.S.P.E.N.'s Core Curriculum,[10] and clinical expertise applied in a manner consistent with the A.S.P.E.N. Standards, Safe Practices, and Guidelines.[1-6,11-14.]

How To Use This Manual

The Compact Disc (CD) version of this manual is designed to create electronic portability and accessibility of this manual and to facilitate searches for specific information. There are two search functions. The first is a query-based searching function to find information specific to an inquiry. All paragraphs in the manual have been tagged for searching according to the categories listed below. A series of levels of categories are used in the search function. In the query mode the next level forces a choice of broad categories including:

Clinical Care
Health Care Management/Administration
Age Groups(s) of interest
Condition/Disease Specific Information

Depending on the categories chosen, the next query, subcategories of the above, appear and can be chosen to further specify the search. Using this approach, the information on the CD matching the selected criteria will be brought into a printable view on the screen in the order the material is contained in the Manual. Keywords can then be typed in to even further narrow the search of the material appearing on the screen. The other search function is to access whole chapters via the table of contents screen.

Contents of Manual

This manual describes methods for achieving safe and effective nutrition support. No attempt has been made to limit information to that derived exclusively from randomized clinical trials or meta-analyses as there are many clinical nutrition practices that remain to be comprehensively studied. At some future date, it may be possible to subject the practices described in this practice manual to more formal analysis[15] to develop more detailed CPG's which meet recommended criteria.[16] In its current form, we believe the Manual can be used to implement CPG's by virtue of its clinical applicability, clinical flexibility, clarity and multidisciplinary process.[16]

The manual does not specifically address indications for nutrition support as they have been addressed elsewhere.[1-3,5,17-19] With the downward pressure currently being exerted on the U.S. healthcare budget, there will inevitably be heavy scrutiny of nutrition support and evolution of the indications for nutrition support. In order to be effectively assessed, healthcare practices need to be well-delineated and, to some extent, standardized. This assures competence, safety and cost-predictability, even when cost-effectiveness is unknown or unaddressed. Well-delineated practices can be adapted to specific institutional needs and reassessed on an ongoing basis through randomized clinical trials and continuous quality improvement (CQI) programs. While the methods presented in this manual are state-of-the-art and consistent with the A.S.P.E.N. Guidelines and Safe Practices, they do not imply exclusion of other clinical approaches to specific situations. As with all clinical medicine, the professional judgment of the attending health care professional is the primary component of quality medical care and the propriety of a specific procedure must be assessed by the attending healthcare professional in light of all the circumstances presented by the individual patient and the resources particular to the locality of practice.[4]

General nutrition support practices relevant to most types of patients are presented in Chapters 1-9 and these are followed by Chapters 10-32 on specific conditions which are commonly managed at least in part by nutrition support. In these disease-specific chapters the authors describe the unique aspects of the conditions, including the pattern and mechanism of nutrition depletion, unique nutrition requirements and potential complications of nutrition support that require specific monitoring. Age-specific issues are included in each chapter. The remaining four chapters focus on practices relevant to specific sites of delivering nutrition care and the ethical issues important to nutrition support.

Integration of Nutrition Support into Patient Care

In the context of this volume, nutrition support refers to the use of foods and medical foods for specific conditions, enteral nutrition provided by tube-access to the gastrointestinal tract and parenteral nutrition. The delivery of nutrition support is a multidisciplinary, specialized practice which is utilized for almost all types of patients and extends beyond the hospital into alternative care sites such as long-term care facilities and homes. Differences in hospital size, patient population, healthcare delivery setting, local expertise, organizational structure and financial payment relationships dictate that there cannot be a single safe and effective system for providing nutrition support. Certain clinical activities are generally expected to reside in specific departments.

One well-established model for providing nutrition support is the Nutrition Support Team (NST).[20-21] In its Standards, A.S.P.E.N. defines the NST as, "A multi-disciplinary group of health care professionals with expertise in nutrition who aid in the provision of nutrition support." While all of the functions of a formal NST relative to patient care need to be performed, an NST is but one organizational approach to meet nutrition needs of patients. Wesley has previously summarized the role and the perceived cost-effective benefits of nutrition support teams[20]:

1. Recognition and treatment of malnutrition
2. Reduction of mechanical and metabolic complications of enteral and parenteral nutrition
3. Reduction of morbidity and mortality
4. Reduction in the cost of providing nutrition support by facilitating the appropriate use of enteral and parenteral therapies
5. Provision for more cost-effective selection of products
6. Reduction in costly wastage of formula
7. Selection of appropriate nutrition support equipment and devices
8. Reduction in length of stay and costs to the hospital
9. Reduction in liability exposure
10. Selection and monitoring of appropriate laboratory tests.

While other models may meet the needs of particular environments, the NST can be viewed as the *de facto* gold standard for delivering nutrition support. Some have justified personnel by using the projected cost savings from nutrition support teams resulting from decreased medical complications and decreased nutrition product wastage. For example, the Centers for Disease Control & Prevention have provisionally determined that "trained personnel designated with the responsibility to insert and maintain the intravascular devices provide a service that effectively reduce catheter-related infections and overall costs".[22] They further state, "As with vascular devices used for other purposes, the use of specially trained personnel to inspect and maintain the catheter appears to reduce the rate of infection in patients receiving TPN [total parenteral nutrition]."

Such teams may have either centralized, complete control over nutrition support or function in a consultative mode. Typical composition includes physician, nurse, dietitian, and pharmacist.[20] Other individuals may be included. A.S.P.E.N. has previously published standards of practice for the nutrition-support physician, pharmacist, nurse and dietitian.[11-14,23,24] An anthology of nutrition support team literature is available from A.S.P.E.N. While the roles of individuals on the nutrition support team have been well-described, the practice of nutrition support is becoming increasingly interdisciplinary at the bedside.[25] Some functions may be suitable for trained technicians under professional supervision. Important non-clinical roles of the NST include data collection for CQI related to nutrition support, analysis of the resultant data base, and implementation of indicated improvements in practices.

The structures and reporting relationships of agencies providing home nutrition support are potentially even more variable than those providing inpatient nutrition support, as the focus of the particular home agency may be predominately for infusion care, nutrition support, nursing care or oncology management. The management of such teams may be hospital-directed, nurse-agency directed, home-infusion company directed, or report directly to an insurer. While the organizational structures conducive to providing nutrition support vary with the type of organization, it is still possible to describe clinical procedures utilized for patient care independent of organizational framework.[5] This volume provides such information.

Certification

The National Board of Nutrition Support Certification offers credentialing for three of the major disciplines involved in nutrition support — physicians, dietitians, and nurses. Nutrition Support certification of pharmacists is offered by the Board of Pharmaceutical Specialties. The American Board of Physician Nutrition Specialists offers broad nutrition certification for Physician Nutrition Specialists.

Certification by professional organizations relevant to nutrition support can be used by hospitals as part of their process for defining clinical privileges.[26] Some hospitals also establish a local credentialing procedure for nutrition support such as passing a basic nutrition support examination or completing an orientation program. Such procedures are a part of the process of assuring quality nutrition support.

Accreditation

In 1986, the Joint Commission on Accreditation of Healthcare Organizations (JCAHO), initiated its Agenda for Change.[27] This culminated in the 1995 and later editions of its Accreditation Manual for Hospitals (AMH) and a new approach to assessing the adequacy of medical care, including nutrition.[21] The goal was to reformulate JCAHO standards, develop performance indicators and redesign the accreditation survey process to make the process patient-focused. Similar changes have been made in the JCAHO Accreditation Manuals for Home Care and Long-Term Care.[28]

JCAHO defines nutrition care as, "intervention and counseling of individuals to promote appropriate nutrition intake based on the nutritional assessment and information about food, other sources of nutrients, and meal preparation consistent with the patient's cultural background and socioeconomic status. Nutrition therapy, a component of medical treatment, includes enteral and parenteral nutrition".[4] The A.S.P.E.N. standards for nutrition support of hospitalized adult and pediatric patients are consistent with the JCAHO approach.[1,2,29,30]

Clinical Pathways

One mechanism by which clinical care standards, best management practices, cost-containment and CQI activities can be integrated and focused is by the use of Clinical Pathways. Clinical Pathways are most commonly and most effectively developed locally through the involvement of affected individuals and organizational entities to develop a standardized way of managing specific medical problems.[31,32] With the use of such algorithms, medical orders and nursing procedures are largely incorporated into protocols and expected outcomes are defined. Medical charting may be limited to describing variances from the pathway or from expected outcomes in contrast to traditional descriptive medical charting.[33] Such pathways can be applied to specific diagnoses (e.g. pneumonia) or to medical practices such as the provision of enteral or parenteral nutrition. Ideally, local clinical pathways are based on a thorough assessment of the relevant medical literature and consideration of guidelines and standards of care established by national professional societies or other experts who have developed guidelines for specific diagnoses or procedures.

Patient outcome data and variances from the CPG or clinical pathways can be analyzed to improve local practices or to benchmark local practices and outcomes versus historical performance or other data sets.[31,34] Such analyses can be restricted to medical issues, financial issues, or most commonly, a combination of these.[34] Since best practices develop in evolutionary fashion, such a process needs to become a major part of institutions' CQI activities. It is anticipated that the procedures and paradigms included in this manual can be used by local groups charged with the responsibility for developing clinical pathways, for assessing the efficacy or cost-effectiveness of local nutrition practices or for understanding the procedures involved in appropriate and safe utilization of nutrition support. A.S.P.E.N. has also developed a generic set of clinical pathways for the use of parenteral and enteral nutrition which may be helpful in this process.[4]

Acknowledgements

The editorial board expresses its appreciation to the authors for updating this manual and expanding its content and to the reviewers who worked with the authors to assure that the practices described are consistent with the best current scientific evidence and clinical judgment. Just as this manual has been developed for a multidisciplinary audience, the process of its development has involved the multiple professional disciplines of A.S.P.E.N. in an effective interdisciplinary collaboration. Acknowledgement of the first edition authors can be found following the text of each chapter and their chapter base for this second edition is appreciated. Special accolades are in order for Dr. Peggi Guenter whose tireless nurturing of the chapters and the editorial staff on behalf of the A.S.P.E.N. administration made final publication of the second edition possible.

REFERENCES

1. A.S.P.E.N. Board of Directors and Task Force on Standards for Specialized Nutrition Support for Hospitalized Adult Patients. Standards for specialized nutrition support: Adult hospitalized patients. *Nutr Clin Pract* 2002; 17:384-391.
2. A.S.P.E.N. Board of Directors and Task Force on Standards for Specialized Nutrition Support for Hospitalized Pediatric Patients. Standards for specialized nutrition support: Hospitalized pediatric patients. *Nutr Clin Pract* 2005; 29:103-116.
3. A.S.P.E.N. Board of Directors. Standards for nutrition support for adult residents of long-term care facilities. *Nutr Clin Pract* 1997; 12:284-293.
4. A.S.P.E.N. Board of Directors and The Clinical GuidelinesTask Force. Guidelines for the use of parenteral and enteral nutrition in adult and pediatric patients. *J Parenter Enteral Nutr* 2002; 26 (1 Suppl):1SA-138SA.
5. A.S.P.E.N. Board of Directors. Standards for home nutrition support. *Nutr Clin Pract* 1999; 14:151-162.
6. Task Force for the Revision of Safe Practices for Parenteral Nutrition. Safe practices for parenteral nutrition. *J Parenter Enteral Nutr* 2004;28:S39-S70.
7. A.S.P.E.N. Board of Directors. Itinerary for tomorrow. A.S.P.E.N.'s new strategic plan. *Nutr Clin Pract* 1995; 10:243-247.
8. Eddy DM. Practice policies: Where do they come from? *JAMA* 1990; 263(9):1265-1275.
9. Gottschlich MM, Matarese LE, Shronts EP. *Nutrition Support Dietetics Core Curriculum. 2 ed.* Silver Springs, MD: A.S.P.E.N., 1993.
10. Gottschlich MM.(ed). *The Science and Practice of Nutrition Spport: A Case-Based Core Curriculum.* A.S.P.E.N./Kendall Hunt Dubuque, IO. 2001.
11. A.S.P.E.N. Board of Directors. Standards of practice: Nutrition support pharmacist. *Nutr Clin Pract* 1999; 14:275-281.
12. A.S.P.E.N. Board of Directors. Standards of practice for nutrition support dietitians. *Nutr Clin Pract* 2000; 53:53-59.
13. A.S.P.E.N. Board of Directors. Standards of practice: Nutrition support nurse. *Nutr Clin Pract* 2001; 16:56-62.
14. A.S.P.E.N. Board of Directors. Standards of practice: Nutrition support physician. *Nutr Clin Pract* 2003;18:270-275.
15. Agency for Health Care Policy and Research. *Clinical Practice Guideline Development (AHCPR Publication No 93-0023).* 1993. Rockville, MD, U.S. Department of Health and Human Service.
16. *Clinical Practice Guidelines—Directions for a New Program.* Washington, DC: National Academy Press, 1990.
17. American College of Physicians. Parenteral nutrition in patients receiving cancer chemotherapy. *Ann Intern Med* 1989; 110(9): 734-736.
18. American Gastroenterological Association. Medical position statement: guidelines for the use of enteral nutrition. *Gastroenterology* 1995; 108:1280-1301.
19. Sitzmann JV, Pitt HA. Statement on guidelines for total parenteral nutrition. *Dig Dis Sci* 1989;(4):34-496.
20. Wesley JR. Nutrition support teams: past, present, and future. *Nutr Clin Pract* 1995; 10(6):219-228.
21. JCAHO. *2004 Comprehensive Accreditation Manual for Hospitals: The Official Handbook (CAMH).* Oakbrook Terrace, IL, 2004.
22. Department of Health and Human Services, Centers for Disease Control and Prevention. Draft guideline for prevention of intravascular device-related infections. *Fed Reg* 1995; 60:49978-50006.
23. Greer FR. Reimbursement for foods for special dietary use. *Pediatrics* 2003; 111(5 Pt 1):1117-1119.
24. Mattox TW. Drug use evaluation approach to monitoring use of total parenteral nutrition: a review of criteria for use in cancer patients. *Nutr Clin Pract* 1993; 8(5):233-237.
25. Vogel DP. Patient-focused care. *Am J Hosp Pharm* 1993; 50(11):2321-2329.
26. Davis AM, Baker SS, Leary RA. Advancing clinical privileges for nutrition support practitioners: The dietitian as a model. *Nutr Clin Pract* 1995; 10:98-103.
27. Dougherty D, Bankhead R, Kushner R, Mirtallo J, Winkler M. Nutrition care given new importance in JCAHO standards. *Nutr Clin Pract* 1995; 10:26-31.

28. JCAHO. *2004 Comprehensive Accreditation Manual for Long Term Care (CAMLTC).* Oakbrook Terrace, IL: Joint Commission Resources, 2004.
29. August DA, Kushner RF. A.S.P.E.N. Standards for Nutrition Support: Hospitalized Patients. *Nutr Clin Pract* 1995; 10(6):206-207.
30. JCAHO Standards: Environment of Care List of Standards TX.4. Retrieved 10/11/2004 from http://www.nyspi.org/jcho/jcahotx4.htm.
31. Flanel DF, Fairchild MM. Continuous quality improvement in inpatient clinical nutrition services. *J Am Diet Assoc* 1995; 95:65-74.
32. Lykins TC. Nutrition support clinical pathways. *Nutr Clin Pract* 1996; 11(1):16-20.
33. Hronek C. Redesigning documentation: clinical pathways, flowsheets, and variance notes. *MedSurg Nurs* 1995; 4(2):157-159.
34. Clare M, Sargent D, Moxley R, Forthman T. Reducing health care delivery costs using clinical paths: a case study on improving hospital profitability. *J Health Care Finance* 1995; 21(3):48-58.

SECTION EDITOR
Beverly Holcombe, PharmD, BCNSP

I

Fundamentals of Nutrition Support Practice and Management

Kathy Pesce-Hammond, MS, RD, LD, CNSD, RN, CNSN;
Jacqueline Wessel, MEd, RD, CSP, CNSD, CLE

1

Nutrition Assessment and Decision Making

In clinical practice, the nutrition assessment process focuses on parameters that are easy to obtain, cost-effective, age-appropriate, and clinically relevant. Nutrition assessment involves carefully selected objective parameters, in combination with a comprehensive physical exam and subjective parameters, to provide the best information for identifying those with preexisting malnutrition or those at risk.

In this chapter, discussion of pediatric and adult assessment has been combined. Much of pediatric and adult nutrition assessment is similar. Concepts unique to pediatrics are development of oral motor skills and growth. This chapter will also describe the nutrition care process.

I. Background: The Nutrition Care Process

A. Nutrition care process: Nutrition screening and assessment are part of the nutritional care process and comprise a series of steps with built-in feedback.[1,2]
B. Nutrition assessment is a systematic process of obtaining, verifying, and interpreting data to make decisions about the nature and cause of nutrition-related problems. The type of data collected depends on the practice setting.[1]
C. The nutrition assessment process includes screening and a more comprehensive assessment of nutritional status. Data from nutrition screening and the more comprehensive nutrition assessment are used to identify nutritional problems, including malnutrition, the risk for developing malnutrition, or specific nutrition-related problems. The nutrition assessment and diagnostic process is not static but continuous.
D. Nutrition interventions are specific to nutrition diagnoses. All interventions must be based on scientific principles and, when available, evidence-based practice.[2]
E. Nutrition monitoring involves periodic measurement and review of the individual's assessment data for the purpose of modifying interventions as needed to achieve desired clinical outcomes.[2] See Figure 1-1 for an illustration of the process.[2,3]

II. Nutrition Screening

A. Nutrition screening is the first step in the nutrition care process.[1] Screening identifies individuals who require a more comprehensive nutrition assessment and who are at nutritional risk.[4–8] Screening parameters should be simple, efficient, and able to be implemented by general hospital staff. An example of a simple screening tool is shown in Table 1-1.
B. Screening should be done within 24 hours of admission (for hospitalized patients) or at the outpatient visit.
C. Nutrition screening of the elderly should not be overlooked, in view of the prevalence of chronic illness and socioeconomic factors that are likely to place them at nutritional risk.[9,10]
D. Screening parameters unique to pediatric patients include gestational age (for neonates and infants), weight for age or length, and head circumference for children less than 2 years of age. Growth parameters are plotted on an appropriate growth chart such as the National Center for Health Statistics growth charts.[11,12]

III. Nutrition Assessment

A. Introduction
   1. The nutrition assessment process identifies patients who are at nutritional risk.
      a) Adults who are nutritionally-at-risk are those who have actual or potential for developing malnutrition. Factors indicative of malnutrition include involuntary loss or gain of ≥10% of usual body weight within 6 months or ≥5% of usual body weight in 1 month; body weight of 20% over or under ideal body weight, especially in the presence of chronic disease or increased metabolic requirements; and inadequate nutrition intake, including an impaired ability to ingest or absorb food adequately.[13]
      b) Neonates who are nutritionally-at-risk are those who are very low birth weight (<1500 gm) or low birth weight (<2500 gm) even in the absence of gastrointestinal, pulmonary, or cardiac disorders; have birth weight less than 2 standard deviations below the mean; or have acute weight loss of 10% or more.[3]
      c) Children are nutritionally-at-risk if they have a weight for length or weight for height less than the 10th percentile or greater than the 90th percentile, increased metabolic requirements, impaired ability to ingest or tolerate oral feedings, documented inadequate provision or tolerance of nutrients, or inadequate weight gain or a significant decrease in an individual's usual growth percentile.[3]
   2. Alterations in nutritional status occur because of altered nutritional intake, malabsorption, or altered metabolism.[14]
   3. Uncomplicated malnutrition is caused by an imbalance between nutrient intake and requirements in the absence of disease or trauma.[15]
   4. Historically, nutrition assessment has consisted of a combination of subjective and objective parameters. Subjective parameters include the medical and nutrition histories. Objective parameters

FIGURE 1-1. Adult Nutrition Screening and Assessment Algorithm

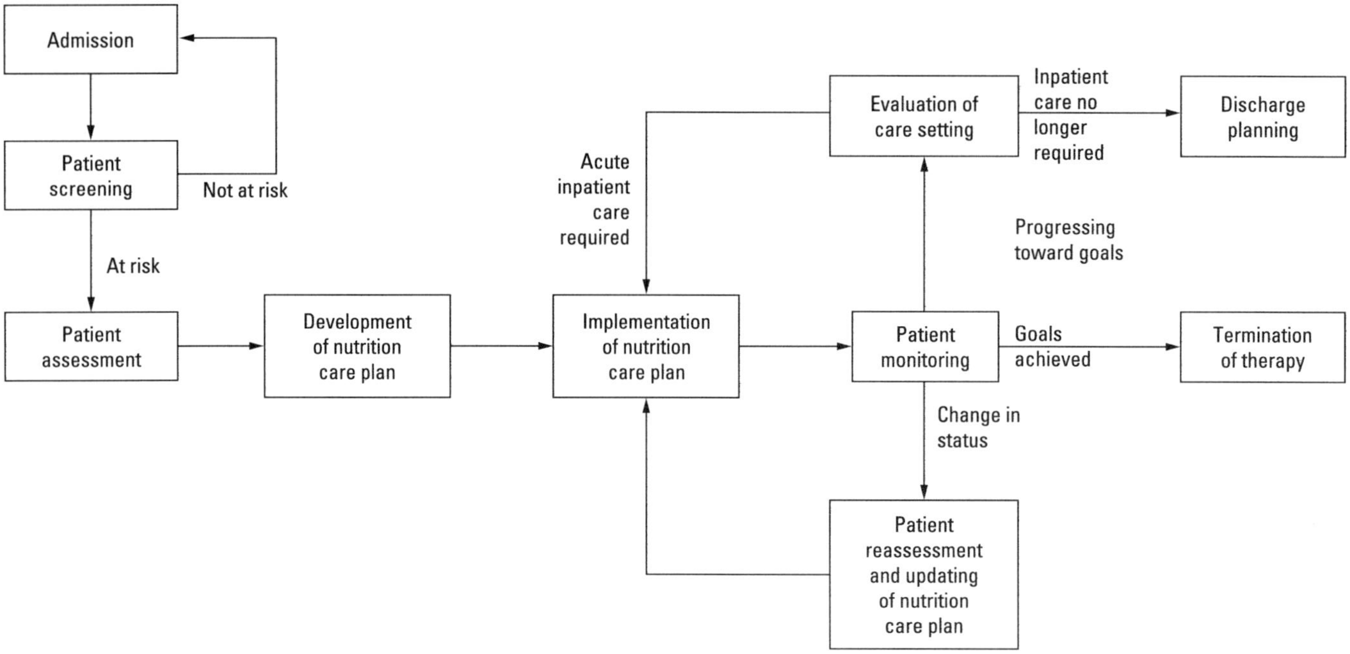

Reprinted with permission from the American Society of Parenteral and Enteral Nutrition.[2]

include the physical examination, anthropometric measurements, various body composition methodologies, laboratory tests, and clinically specific parameters.[16]

B. Medical and nutritional history

1. Medical history includes acute and chronic diseases, medications, diagnostic procedures, surgeries, and other therapies (ie, chemotherapeutics, immunosuppressives).[2,8,17] The review of medications should include prescription and nonprescription drugs, vitamin and mineral supplements, and other over-the-counter drugs. History also includes alternative medical treatments and socioeconomic status whenever possible. Medical history information specific to pediatrics includes maternal and prenatal health history; perinatal history; gestational age; history of prematurity; birth weight; whether small or large for gestational age; and growth patterns for weight, length, and head circumference. Growth records can typically be obtained with permission from the primary care physician. Other components of the history are developmental history including problems with hypotonia or hypertonia; and any problem with developmental milestones.
2. Nutritional history includes recent changes in appetite or weight, ability to eat, bowel habits, activity level, nutrient intake, use of diets, feeding skills, types of feeding equipment used, food allergies or intolerances, and use of oral supplements (Table 1-2). The history is important to set a baseline to assist in establishing the etiology of nutritional impairment, such as impediments to eating, absorbing, or both.[15]

   Nutritional history unique to pediatrics includes interest in feeding; feeding refusals; duration of feedings; frequency and times of feedings; whether getting up at night to feed; feeding jags; problems in acceptance of textures; suck and swallow quality; and symptoms of gastroesophageal reflux.
3. Subjective Global Assessment (SGA): The SGA is a nutritional assessment tool that relies on history of weight and dietary change, persistent gastrointestinal symptoms, functional capacity, effects of disease on nutritional requirements, and physical appearance. The SGA has been well tested and is widely accepted as a practical and reliable tool for nutrition assessment.[18,19] On the basis of these parameters, clinicians categorize patients' nutritional status as well nourished, moderate or suspected malnutrition, or severe malnutrition. See Table 1-3 for SGA features.

C. Physical examination

1. The physical examination is an excellent tool to help evaluate nutritional status.[20–22] A physical examination uses a systems approach and includes a logical assessment from head to toe. See Table 1-4 for full physical examination guidelines.
2. Specific to pediatrics is the assessment of sexual maturation using Tanner staging (Table 1-5). Tanner staging is based on the development of secondary sex characteristics. In adolescents, nutrition assessment findings may be altered depending on the stage of sexual maturity. In males the peak of the rapid height growth occurs in Tanner Stage 4. In females by the onset of menarche, the majority of linear growth has been completed. However, girls who enter puberty early may have more linear growth after menarche than girls who enter puberty later. The rate of weight gain approximates the velocity of linear growth, although in females, the peak weight gain velocity occurs 6 to 9 months before the height rate change.[23,24]

D. Anthropometric parameters

1. Body weight[25]
   a) Body weight measurement[26]
      (1) Standing weight: Use uniform clothing, equipment, and time of day and document these data with the weight

TABLE 1-1. Admission Nutrition Screening Tool

A. Diagnosis

If the patient has at least ONE of the following diagnoses, circle and proceed to section E to consider the patient AT NUTRITIONAL RISK and stop here.

Anorexia nervosa/bulimia nervosa
Malabsorption (celiac sprue, ulcerative colitis, Crohn's disease, short-bowel syndrome)
Multiple trauma (closed-head injury, penetrating trauma, multiple fractures)
Decubitus ulcers
Major gastrointestinal surgery within the last year
Cachexia (temporal wasting, muscle wasting, cancer, cardiac)
Coma
Diabetes
End-stage liver disease
End-stage renal disease
Nonhealing wounds

B. Nutrition intake history

If the patient has at least ONE of the following symptoms, circle and proceed to section E to consider the patient AT NUTRITIONAL RISK and stop here.

Diarrhea (>500 mL × 2 days)
Vomiting (>5 days)
Reduced intake (<½ normal intake for >5 days)

C. Ideal body weight standards

Compare the patient's current weight for height to the ideal body weight chart on the back of this form.

If at <80% of ideal body weight, proceed to section E to consider the patient AT NUTRITIONAL RISK and stop here.

D. Weight history

Any recent unplanned weight loss? No____ Yes ____

Amount (lbs or kg) ________________

If yes, within the past _________ wks or _________ mos

Current weight (lbs or kg) ________________

Usual weight (lbs or kg) ________________

Height (ft, in, or cm) ________________

Find percentage of weight loss: $\frac{\text{usual wt} - \text{current wt}}{\text{usual wt}} \times 100 =$ _____% wt loss

Compare the % wt loss with the chart values and circle the appropriate value

Length of time	Significant (%)	Severe (%)
1 wk	1–2	>2
2–3 wks	2–3	>3
1 mo	4–5	>5
3 mos	7–8	>8
5+ mos	10	>10

If the patient has experienced a significant or severe weight loss, proceed to section E and consider the patient AT NUTRITIONAL RISK.

E. Nurse assessment

Using the above criteria, what is this patient's nutritional risk? (check one)

____ LOW NUTRITIONAL RISK

____ AT NUTRITIONAL RISK

From Kovacevich DS, Boney AR, Braunschweig CL, et al. Nutrition risk classification: a reproducible and valid tool for nurses. *Nutr Clin Pract.* 1997;12:20–25 with permission.

measurement. Assess the patient's ability to stand. Balance or recalibrate the scale and position the patient on the center of the scale base. Obtain the measurement from the balance scale or digital readout.

(2) Bed or sling weight: Roll the patient to one side and place the sling under the patient. Position the sling under the patient evenly. Attach the sling to the scale and record the weight measurement.

(3) Wheelchair weight: Position the ramp for wheelchair access. Weigh the empty wheelchair and record the weight of the chair. Repeat the procedure with the patient in the chair and deduct the chair weight from the total weight.

(4) Pediatric weights are measured nude in infants and toddlers, and in underpants only for older children, using infant scales or a platform beam balance scale.

b) Ideal body weight (IBW)

(1) A commonly used method for determining IBW in clinical settings is the Hamwi rule of thumb method.[27] In this method, males are given 106 lbs (48 kg) for the first 5 ft (1.5 m) and an additional 6 lbs (2.7 kg) for each inch (2.54 cm) over 5 ft. Females are given 100 lbs (45 kg) for the first 5 ft and an additional 5 lbs (2.3 kg) for each inch over 5 ft. To account for a large frame, 10% of body weight is added; and for a small frame, 10% of body weight is subtracted from the initial calculated weight.

(2) Reference data on body weight are available from the National Health and Nutrition Examination Surveys (NHANES). These reference tables provide the most up-to-date weight available for the US population and reflect national diversity.[28,29] See Tables 1-6 and 1-7.

(3) Adjustments in IBW estimates are made for patients with amputations to account for the missing body part(s)

TABLE 1-2. Components of the Medical and Nutritional History

Diet	History (usual meal pattern), restrictions, alternative, complementary
Allergies	Food, intolerances, avoidances
Supplementation	Vitamin, mineral, oral nutritional drinks, other products
Weight	Recent changes—intentional, nonintentional
Dental/oral	Chewing, swallowing ability, salivation, dentition, pain
Mental status	Altered mental status, delirium, dementia
Gastrointestinal	Nausea, vomiting, heartburn, bloating, dyspepsia, gas, diarrhea, constipation, steatorrhea
Chronic disease	Long-term diseases affecting utilization of nutrients
Surgery	Surgical resection or disease of gastrointestinal tract
Medications	Prescription, over the counter, other
Drug/alcohol	Use, amount
Economic factors	Food procurement, preparation, physical limitations of food preparation, public aid assistance
Cultural factors	Religion, education, and customs and their influence on eating patterns
Physical activity	Occupation, exercise regimen, sleep/rest pattern

(Figure 1-2).[30] Estimated ideal weight = [(100 − percent of amputation)/100] × estimated ideal weight for original height.

c) Height/length/head circumference
   (1) Pediatrics: Recumbent lengths are measured with a length board for infants and toddlers and a stadiometer for children who are more than 3 years old (if they can stand). Heights are measured in stocking feet and with feet together, back straight, and arms hanging freely. Head circumference is measured until approximately 36 months. A flexible, narrow tape measure is used. Ideally, three measurements are done, and the results averaged. Arrested head growth (microcephaly) may indicate cranial defects or abnormal brain growth; accelerated growth may indicate catch-up growth or developmental defects (eg, hydrocephalus).
   (2) Height is measured directly or indirectly. Direct methods using a stadiometer or measuring rod require the patient to stand erect or lie flat. For those who cannot be moved and do not have musculoskeletal deformities, a recumbent bed length measurement can assist in determining height. Frame size can be determined by dividing the height in centimeters by the circumference of the wrist in centimeters.

2. Interpretation of weight data
   a) Comparison to ideal and usual weight: Weight comparisons in adults can indicate severity of malnutrition. Table 1-8 illustrates guidelines used to interpret weight data, including ideal, current, and usual weight and percentage of weight change. Of these, the change in recent weight most accurately predicts nutritional risk.[29] When obtainable, the weight history of the individual is more helpful than comparison to IBW. Cau-

TABLE 1-3. Features of Subjective Global Assessment (SGA)

(*Select appropriate category with a checkmark, or enter numerical value where indicated by "#".*)

A. History

1. Weight change
   Overall loss in past 6 mos: amount = # ___________ kg;
   % loss = # ___________
   Change in past 2 wks: ____ increase, ____ no change, ____ decrease

2. Dietary intake change (relative to normal)
   ____ No change
   ____ Change ____ duration = # __________ weeks
   ____ Type: ____ suboptimal solid diet
   ____ full liquid diet
   ____ hypocaloric liquids ____ starvation

3. Gastrointestinal symptoms (that persisted for >2 wks)
   ____ none ____ nausea ____ vomiting
   ____ diarrhea ____ anorexia

4. Functional capacity
   ____ No dysfunction (eg, full capacity)
   ____ Dysfunction ____ duration = # __________ wks
   ____ Type: ____ working suboptimally
   ____ ambulatory
   ____ bedridden

5. Disease and its relation to nutritional requirements
   Primary diagnosis (specify)
   Metabolic demand (stress): ____ no stress ____ low stress
   ____ moderate stress ____ high stress

B. Physical (for each trait specify 0 = normal, 1+ = mild, 2+ = moderate, 3+ = severe)
   # ____ loss of subcutaneous fat (triceps, chest)
   # ____ muscle wasting (quadriceps, deltoids)
   # ____ ankle edema
   # ____ sacral edema
   # ____ ascites

C. SGA rating (select one)
   ____ A = Well nourished
   ____ B = Moderately malnourished (or suspected of being malnourished)
   ____ C = Severely malnourished

Reprinted with permission from Detsky AJ, McLaughlin JR, Baker JP, et al. What is subjective global assessment of nutritional status? *J Parenter Enteral Nutr.* 1987;11:9.

TABLE 1-4. A Sample Outline for the Nutrition-Focused Physical Examination

This table is not intended to be a complete list of nutritional or non-nutritional causes for presenting physical signs and symptoms. This table serves only as an example and may need to be modified using clinical judgment.

System	Nutrition Physical Exam Focus	What Exam May Reveal in Regard to Nutritional/Metabolic Status	Non-Nutritional Examples of Similar Findings
General survey	*Using inspection:* Body weight for height, alertness, any general wasting of muscle or fat stores, coordination, speech, growth, body movements	Lack of calories and protein, ability to independently feed, or degree of vitamin, mineral, or trace element deficiency	Endocrine disorders, osteogenic disorders, menopausal changes
Vital signs	Temperature	Increased temperature—increase in energy and fluid requirements	Vital signs reflect major disease or illness factors and nutrition assists in preventing or decreasing severity
	Respiration	Increased rate, labor-intense—influences calorie and protein requirements along with quantity of food eaten at one time and type of food (eg, calorically dense)	Increases with hyperthyroidism, increased temperature, anxiety, pain, exercise, medication
	Pulse	Heart rate increases with anemia	Decreases with sleep/rest, organic heart disease, hypothyroidism, and medications
	Blood pressure	Diet modification such as calculated sodium used for high blood pressure	Blood loss, heart attack and heart failure, irregular heart rate, and certain medications lower blood pressure
		Dehydration lowers blood pressure	
Skin	*Inspect and palpate:* Color	Pallor—iron, folate, or B_{12} deficiency	Skin pigmentation disorders, disease of the bone marrow, hemorrhage, arsenic ingestion, steroids, low volume, low perfusion states
	Lesions, pigmentation	Dermatitis—essential fatty acid, zinc, niacin, or riboflavin deficiency	Hypersensitivity reactions, connective tissue disease, burns, Addison's disease
		Pellagrous dermatitis—niacin, tryptophan	Thermal, sun, or chemical burns; Addison's disease, psoriasis
		Flaky paint dermatitis—hyperpigmented areas on thighs, buttocks—protein	
	Petechiae, ecchymosis	Vitamin C deficiency, vitamin K deficiency	Hematologic disorder, trauma, liver disease, anticoagulant disorder, Cushing's disease
	Wound healing degree, pressure ulcers	Poor wound healing—zinc, vitamin C, protein deficiency	Diabetes, use of steroids, AIDS, malignancy
	Moisture, turgor	Poor skin turgor—poor fluid status	Heart failure, kidney disease, liver disease

(Continued)

TABLE 1-4. A Sample Outline for the Nutrition-Focused Physical Examination (*Continued*)

System	Nutrition Physical Exam Focus	What Exam May Reveal in Regard to Nutritional/Metabolic Status	Non-Nutritional Examples of Similar Findings
Skin (*Continued*)		Sweat may influence temperature and fluid status	
		Edema—generalized (anasarca) with accumulation of serum in connective tissue	
	Texture	Scaly, dry—vitamin A deficiency or essential fatty acid deficiency	Hypothyroidism, dermatitis, hygiene, uremia, psoriasis, environmental factors, aging
		Little lumps (or nodules) on elbows or eyelids present in those with high cholesterol levels	
	Temperature	Warmth will influence temperature status and hence fluid and energy	
		Cold will influence temperature status and energy demand	
Nails	*Inspect and palpate:*		
	Shape, color, angle contour, lesions	Spoon-shape (koilonychia)—iron deficiency	COPD, heart disease, aortic stenosis
		Lackluster, dull—protein	Infection, congenital systemic lupus erythematosus
		Mottled, pale, poor blanching—vitamin A, C	
Scalp/hair	*Inspect and palpate:*		
	Shape and symmetry of scalp, masses	Softening or craniotabes—vitamin D deficiency; open anterior fontanel (usually closes by ~18 mos of age)	Hydrocephalus
	Hair distribution, color, and texture	Dull, lackluster, thin, sparse—protein, iron, zinc, or essential fatty acid deficiency	Chemical effects, hypothyroidism, chemotherapy, psoriasis, color treatment
		Easily pluckable—protein deficiency	
		Alternating bands of light and dark hair in young children (flag sign)—protein deficiency	Chemically processed or bleached hair
Face (general)	*Inspect and palpate:*		
	Shape and symmetry	May influence ability to eat if masses are present	See skin assessment
		Moon face—protein-calorie deficiency	
		Bilateral temporal wasting—protein-calorie deficiency	
	Color, temperature, lesions, texture	Review skin assessment	Usually affected by a neuromotor dysfunction or disease
		Pallor—iron, folate, or B_{12} deficiency	

	Cranial nerves (really part of the neurological exam, but more practical at this point)		Cranial nerves are not usually a direct cause of nutrition deficiency but once injured affect nutritional status indirectly
	CN V (trigeminal)— assess muscles of mastication—test by clenching teeth and feeling masseter and temporal muscles	Control main muscles of chewing Note asymmetry in jaw movement or pain clenching teeth	Neuromuscular disorder, paralysis
	CN VII (facial)—test by raising eyebrows, frowning, smiling, showing upper and lower teeth	Weakness, asymmetry affect chewing and holding food	Bell's palsy, paralysis
	CN IX (glossopharyngeal)—gag reflex	Supplies nerve stimulation to muscle in throat, provides intervention to parotid glands that secrete saliva to assist with digestion, and stimulates the back one third of tongue with taste and touch	
	CN X (vagus)—tickle back of throat—gag reflex, phonate "ahh" and watch movement of soft palate and pharynx, voice quality	Provides impulses to throat to allow movement and swallowing, peristalsis motion of the gut in digesting food; note any dysphagia, fluids regurgitating through nose (important to note gag reflex if placing tube since postpyloric placement needed if absent to prevent aspiration)	Brain stem tumor, neck injury, lesion on cranial nerve, vocal cord weakness
	CN XI (accessory)—test by shrugging shoulders and moving chin to left and right against resistance	Moves trapezius and sternomastoid muscle	Neck injury, torticollis
	CN XII (hypoglossal)—test by sticking tongue out and wiggling side to side	Movement of tongue Improper alignment and movement may influence the ability to chew properly	Lower motor neuron lesions Bilateral upper motor neuron lesion
Eyes	*Inspect and palpate:* Adjustment to night	Night blindness—vitamin A deficiency	Tapetoretinal degeneration, status post panretinal photocoagulation, photic exhaustion (all day in bright sun; short-term effects), advanced glaucoma
	Any vision impairment	Affects ability to shop, cook, eat, etc	
	Skin color and texture, cracks, brows, lids	Cracked and reddened corners of eyes (angular palpebritis)—riboflavin, niacin deficiency Dry, grayish, yellow or white rings of whitish-yellow cholesterol deposits around edges of eye	Infection, foreign objects, allergic reaction, seborrheic dermatitis
	Sclerae	Foamy spots on eyes (Bitot's spots)—vitamin A deficiency Dull, dry rough appearance—vitamin A deficiency Pallor—iron, folate, or B_{12} deficiency	Pterygium, Gaucher's disease Chemical, environmental

(Continued)

TABLE 1-4. A Sample Outline for the Nutrition-Focused Physical Examination (*Continued*)

System	Nutrition Physical Exam Focus	What Exam May Reveal in Regard to Nutritional/Metabolic Status	Non-Nutritional Examples of Similar Findings
Eyes (*Continued*)	Conjunctiva	Dull, dry, rough appearance to inner lids (conjunctival xerosis) —vitamin A deficiency	Chemical, environmental
	Cornea	Dull, milky, or opaque (corneal xerosis)—vitamin A deficiency	Rule out cataracts
		Softening (keratomalacia)—vitamin A deficiency	
Nose	*Inspect and palpate external and internal structures:*		
	Shape, septum, nares, mucosa, discharge	Influences decision of nasal tube placement if polyps, obstruction, or prior surgery present. Redness of sinus tract should also be noted. Size of nare to use when inserting tube (may choose larger one).	
	Skin	Scaly, greasy, with gray or yellowish material around nares (nasolabial seborrhea)—riboflavin, niacin, pyridoxine deficiency	
	CN I (olfactory)	Identify smell that influences food eaten—favorable smells assist with enhancing appetite	
Oral cavity:			
Lips	*Inspect and palpate:*		
	Color, temperature, texture, cracking, lesions, symmetry	Bilateral cracks, redness of lips (angular stomatitis)—riboflavin, niacin, pyridoxine deficiency	Poor-fitting dentures, herpes, syphilis
		Vertical cracks of lips (cheilosis)—riboflavin, niacin deficiency	AIDS (Kaposi's sarcoma), environmental exposure
Mucosa	*Inspect and palpate:*		
	Color, texture, lesions, integrity, moisture	Pallor—iron, B_{12}, or folate deficiency	Side effects of medications
		Dryness—hydration status	
		Cracking—vitamin C deficiency	
		General inflammation—B complex, iron, C deficiency	Infection, trauma, dryness with aging, autoimmune disorders, cancer therapy, irritants, drug therapy
Tongue	*Inspect and palpate:*		
	Color	Magenta color—riboflavin deficiency	Crohn's disease, infection
		Beefy red color and atrophied taste—niacin, folate, riboflavin, iron, B_{12} deficiency	White overgrowth may be a sign of fungal infection

	Texture, moisture, lesions, symmetry	Smooth, slick, loss of papillae—folacin, niacin, iron, riboflavin, B_{12} deficiency	Cancer therapy, aging, dryness of mouth, influenza, multiple medications, diabetes mellitus
	Distorted taste (dysgeusia), Diminished taste (hypogeusia)	Zinc deficiency	
Teeth	*Inspect and palpate:* State of repair, missing, dentures, color	Influence ability to chew and texture of food able to handle	Trauma, syphilis, aging, poor dental hygiene, improper-fitting dentures
		Teeth vary in shades of white	
		Excess caries—excess sugar	Eating disorders, xerostomia, radiation, poor dental hygiene
		White or brownish patches (mottled)—fluoride excess	Enamel hypoplasia, erosion
Gums	*Inspect and palpate:* Lesions, integrity	Spongy, bleeding, receding—vitamin C deficiency	Phenytoin and other medication, poor hygiene, lymphoma, polycythemia, thrombocytopenia
	Moisture	Dry—fluid status	
	Color	Pale—iron deficiency	
Neck	*Inspect and palpate:* Vasculature appearance	Distended neck veins—fluid status (overload)	Disease or illness processes
	Range of motion	Influences ability to coordinate mechanics of eating	
	Symmetry, midline structures (trachea, thyroid)	Enlarged thyroid—iodine deficiency	Cancer, allergy, cold, infection
	Parotid gland	Located anterior to earlobe—bilateral enlargement—protein deficiency or bulimia	Cysts, tumor, hyperparathyroidism
Thorax and lungs: Thorax (general)	Inspect and palpate: Muscle and fat, accessory muscle usage (use of abdominal muscles, some of muscles between ribs, and some neck muscles besides the diaphragm)	Prominent bony skeleton with muscle and fat wasting—calorie and protein depletion Respiratory muscle mass and strength decrease with calorie protein depletion	
Lungs	While assessing this region also note any vascular access devices present	Assessment should be noted to ensure that access device is intact without redness or drainage or swelling so that nutrition therapy can be continued without risk of complications	

(*Continued*)

TABLE 1-4. A Sample Outline for the Nutrition-Focused Physical Examination (*Continued*)

System	Nutrition Physical Exam Focus	What Exam May Reveal in Regard to Nutritional/Metabolic Status	Non-Nutritional Examples of Similar Findings
Thorax and lungs: (*Continued*)	*Inspect and palpate:* Rate and depth of respiration	Increased and labor–intense uses more energy Fremitus (usually assessed by having patient say "99"; the vibration in examiner's hand is decreased when fluid has filled the space between lung and chest wall) Also influence acid-base status	Most causes are non-nutritional but influence nutrition therapy: Fluid status may influence fluid requirements and nutrition regimen such as parenteral nutrition fluid volume
	Percuss: Chest wall	Assess fluid collections	
	Auscultate: Breath sounds	Abnormal breath sounds such as rales (crackles) present with fluid overload Rhonchi also increase the work of breathing and present when fluid is in the airways	
Cardiovascular	*Inspect and palpate:* Neck vein distention edema	Neck vein distention, edema influences fluid status: Pitting edema—condition resulting from accumulation of interstitial fluid—may occur in protein malnutrition and is thought to result from decreased venous colloid pressure exerted from low serum albumin levels (<2.5 mg/dL)	Edema can be systemic or local in etiology: Systemic causes include heart failure, hypoalbuminemia, salt and water retention; local causes include venous stasis, lymphatic stasis, or prolonged dependency Heart failure, pregnancy, immobilization, and varicose veins
	Rhythm/rate	Irregular rhythm may be related to potassium excess or deficiency, calcium deficiency, magnesium deficiency or excess, phosphorus deficiency Increased rate (tachycardia)—thiamine, fluid (dehydration)	Cardiopulmonary conditions or influences Organic heart disease, severe chronic lung disease, respiratory insufficiency, drug toxicity, excess alcohol ingestion
	Auscultate: Rate, sounds	S3 presence (with edema, dyspnea, loud crackles that do not disappear with cough)—fluid excess	
Abdomen	Inspect: Color, contour	Scaphoid appearance—loss of subcutaneous fat—caloric deprivation	

		Rounded to protuberant—gas distention, obesity Rounded with tight, glistening skin, fine veins able to be seen, everted umbilicus (ascites)—fluid, sodium concerns	Pregnancy
	Muscle development	Poor muscle tone or wasting muscle—poor activity or nutritional depletion	Postpartum, neuromuscular decline, surgery
	Texture	See skin assessment	
	Wounds	Poor wound healing—protein or calorie inadequacy, vitamin C or zinc depletion	
	Feeding devices, ostomies	Feeding devices and ostomies should be assessed at this time—intact without drainage, erythema, swelling, or odor. Surrounding skin should also be pink without drainage, redness, or tenderness.	
	Auscultate: Bowel sounds	No sounds/hypoactive—influences the decision of what route of feeding should be used	Bowel obstruction after surgery, trauma injury, or diseases of the bowel peritonitis, paralytic ileus
	Percuss: For tympany	Hyperactive—influences what type of feeding route can be used and even the enteral substrate used if diarrhea is present	Gastroenteritis High-pitched tinkling—early obstruction
	Percuss: For tympany, dullness, density of abdominal contents, and liver span (takes practice to acquire this skill)	Tympany should be present since the air in the intestines rises when supine	Neoplastic disease, cirrhosis, infections, hematologic disorders, AIDS, megaloblastic anemia
		Check liver, which is a solid organ and sounds dull (combine with palpation to check for hepatomegaly)—protein deficiency	
	Palpate: Texture, temperature, specific organs such as liver	Warm to touch as with rest of body—temperature that increases calorie and fluid requirements	Note: From a nutritional standpoint, if the patient complains of any discomfort or pain, then palpation or percussion should be done only by a physician or physician-appointed attendee
Kidneys	*Inspect:* Color and clarity	Dark, concentrated urine—could be a sign of dehydration	Infection, sepsis, hematuria
		Light, dilute urine—could be a sign of overhydration	Diabetes insipidus

(*Continued*)

TABLE 1-4. A Sample Outline for the Nutrition-Focused Physical Examination (*Continued*)

System	Nutrition Physical Exam Focus	What Exam May Reveal in Regard to Nutritional/Metabolic Status	Non-Nutritional Examples of Similar Findings
Musculo-skeletal	*Inspect:* Size, shape, symmetry, deformity, involuntary movements	Craniotabes (<1 yr of age), softening of occipital, parietal area—vitamin D deficiency	
	Inspect and palpate: Head and neck movement, arms, fingers, wrists, elbows, and shoulders for strength, range of motion, and fluid, swelling, and pulses	Frontal or parietal bossing (infants), swelling or thickening of front and sides of head—vitamin D deficiency Open anterior fontanelle (persistent at >18 mos of age)—vitamin D deficiency	
		Inability to flex, extend, and rotate neck influences nutrition by interfering with ability to feed or make hand-to-mouth contact	
		Fat and muscle wasting in temporal regions, thorax, deltoid muscle, fine muscles of hand, decreased range of motion, swelling, impaired joint mobility- protein and calorie deprivation	Muscular dystrophy, deep vein thrombosis, arthritis, malignancy, paralysis, renal dysfunction, liver dysfunction, trauma, osteomalacia, hyperparathyroidism
		Swollen, painful joints—vitamin C deficiency	Connective tissue disease
		Epiphyses at wrist—vitamin C or D deficiency	Trauma, deformity, or congenital causes
		Assess range of motion of upper extremities so ability to feed independently and hand-to-mouth coordination can be evaluated	
		Assess finger manipulations for assistive devices for feeding	
	Inspect and palpate: Legs for hip strength and edema, hair distribution, pulses	Muscle wasting noted on buttocks, gastrocnemius muscle of legs, prominent body skeleton—calorie protein deficiency; also may be thiamine deficiency, vitamin C deficiency, phosphorus deficiency, calcium deficiency	Trauma, congenital deformity, renal disease, deep vein thrombosis, arthritis, chronic renal failure, pituitary tumor, idiopathic hypopituitarism, growth hormone deficiency
		Rickets, knock knees, bowleg—vitamin D, calcium, phosphorus epiphyseal enlargement—vitamin D (painless), vitamin C (painful)	
		Swollen, painful joints—vitamin C	
		Dwarfism—zinc	

Neurologic	*Inspect:* Alertness, orientation, gross and fine motor skills (in conjunction with musculoskeletal system), paresthesias, tremors, weakness, dementia, coordination, reflexes	Cranial nerves (see Face row) Motor weakness (lower extremities)—thiamine deficiency	Polyneuropathy of diabetes mellitus, weakness due to myogenic disorders
	Tests: Alertness: general conversation and asking basic questions such as time, date, year, name, family	Mental confusion, hyperirritability, apathy—protein peripheral neuropathy, thiamine, B_{12}, B_6 deficiency	Lyme disease, polyneuropathy of diabetes mellitus, collagen vascular disease
	Muscle tone: feeling muscle's resistance to passive stretch by, for example, taking patient's hand with yours and while supporting elbow flexing and extending patient's fingers, wrist, and elbow, and putting the shoulder through range of motion. For legs, support the patient's thigh with one hand, grasp foot with other, and flex and extend knees and ankles.		
	Muscle strength: have patient place hands (right then left) against yours and push as hard as he or she can and for lower extremities have the patient place right and then left foot in your hand and push against your hand		
	Coordination: observe patient touching finger to nose and mouth and even raising eating utensils to mouth		
	Reflexes: detect central nervous system disturbances using a reflex hammer with the pointed end to strike small areas and the larger, flatter end used in larger areas (patellar or brachioradialis)	Vibratory sense decrease, oss of position sense, loss of ankle or knee jerks bilaterally—thiamine, B_{12}	Hypothyroidism, sarcoidosis, amyloidosis, uremia, malignancy
		Hyperactive reflexes—hypocalcemia	Tetanus, upper motor neuron disease
	Reflexes usually tested—biceps, triceps, brachioradialis, abdominal, patellar, ankle, and plantar (graded 0–4+)	Hypoactive reflexes—hypokalemia	Neurologic disorders
		Hypoactive Achilles, patellar reflexes—thiamine, B_{12}	Neurologic disorders
		Tetany—lips, tongue, fingers, feet, generalized muscle aching, spasm—calcium, vitamin D, or magnesium deficiency	Neurologic disorders, respiratory alkalosis
		Calf tenderness bilaterally—thiamine deficiency	Deep vein thrombosis, peripheral neuropathy of other causes
		Dementia—niacin, B_{12}	Head trauma, cardiac arrest, cerebral hemorrhage, brain tumor, degenerative brain diseases

AIDS, acquired immunodeficiency syndrome; COPD, chronic obstructive pulmonary disease.
Reprinted from Hammond K. The nutritional dimension of physical assessment. *Nutrition.*1999;15:412-417 with permission from Elsevier Science.

TABLE 1-5. Tanner Stages of Development[23,24]

Stage	Girls	Boys
1	Prepubescent	Prepubescent
2	Pubic hair appears, breast buds, increased activity of sweat glands	Pubic hair appears, growth of genitalia, increased activity of sweat glands
3	Breast enlargement, axillary hair present	Continued enlargement of genitalia, changes in voice, faint moustache/facial hair begins, axillary hair present
4	Nipple and areola become more pronounced, menarche begins	Pubic hair thickens, voice deepens, facial hair increases, hair on legs becomes darker
5	Breasts fully mature	Genitalia fully mature

tion is recommended when using percent IBW.[31] Body shape and weight tend to vary across age and population groups.[29]

b) Growth charts: Various growth charts have been used for preterm infants,[32–42] term infants, children, and adolescents.[43] The Babson and Benda chart for premature infants[44] has been recently updated.[32] Postnatal growth parameters should be corrected for gestational age at birth for premature infants.[45–47] Weight, length, and head circumference are monitored for infants up to 36 months old.[48] Weight-for-length graphs are available for infants, children, and adolescents.[43] Specialized growth curves are available for children with diagnoses such as Trisomy 21; Turner, Williams, and Prader-Willi syndromes; and quadriplegic cerebral palsy.[49–53] Most commonly, a standard reference chart such as that from the Centers for Disease Control and Prevention (CDC) is used in conjunction with a specialized curve for evaluation.[11,48,54] Average weight gains per day according to gestational age from birth to 24 months are listed in Table 1-9. Table 1-10 lists growth rates for weight, length, and head circumference by birth weight group and sex. Table 1-11 gives general guidelines for weight gain, height, and head circumference from the age of 1 year to adolescence. Z scores can also be used as part of the evaluation process. Normal is accepted as lying between ±2 standard deviations from the mean. This range includes 95% of the reference population. Malnourished children have a weight or weight-for-height Z score of −2 or below. Serial Z scores can be used to evaluate the effects of dietary intervention, especially for populations.[55]

c) Weight changes: Recent weight changes in children can indicate acute nutrition issues. Significant weight losses for children are considered to be >2% in 1 week, >5% in 1 month, >7.5% in 3 months, and >10% in 6 months.[56] The National Center for Health Statistics data—or more recently, CDC growth charts—are used to determine the percentiles.[11,12,57] See Appendix 1-1 for CDC growth charts.

$$\text{Acute nutritional status} = \frac{\text{actual weight} \times 100}{\text{50th percentile weight/height}}$$

$$\text{Chronic nutritional status} = \frac{\text{actual weight} \times 100}{\text{50th percentile height/age}}$$

d) Weight comparisons in adults can indicate severity of malnutrition (Table 1-8). In adults, developing malnutrition is evidenced by an involuntary loss or gain of ≥10% of usual body weight within 6 months or ≥5% of usual body weight in 1 month, or a weight 20% over or under IBW.[58]

e) Factors that influence interpretation of weight measurements
   (1) Edema, ascites, diuretic therapy, and other fluid alterations can significantly alter body weight within short time periods.
   (2) Fluid shifts from the intravascular space to the extravascular space and the intracellular space to the extracellular space with a concurrent decline in lean body mass occur in malnutrition. Therefore, loss of lean body mass may be masked, with little obvious change in weight.

3. Body mass index (BMI): BMI is a measure of weight for height.

   a) BMI is calculated as follows: $\text{BMI} = \dfrac{\text{Weight}(\text{kg})}{\text{Height}^2(\text{m})}$

   b) In adults, a BMI of less than 15 kg/m^2 is associated with a significant increase in morbidity,[59] while a BMI of less than 18.5 kg/m^2 is considered underweight. A healthy weight is considered a BMI between 18.5 and 24.9 kg/m^2.[2,4,60] According to the National Institutes of Health, a BMI between 25 and 29.9 kg/m^2 is considered overweight and a BMI ≥ 30 is obese.[60] For the elder healthy adult, the BMI range is between 22 and 27 kg/m.[2,61]

   c) The CDC growth charts with BMI for age,[11] male or female, are recommended to assess weight in relation to height for children 2 to 20 years of age. A BMI in the 85th to 95th percentile means that a child is considered to be at risk for being overweight. Some athletic children who are not overweight may fall into these categories due to increased muscle mass.[40,41] See Appendix 1-1 for CDC growth charts.

4. In adults, abdominal girth measurement is commonly used to indicate risk of coronary artery disease and other morbidity.[62,63] The waist circumference is measured by obtaining the distance around the smallest area right below the rib cage and above the umbilicus. The measurement is used to determine excess abdominal fat. Waist girth circumference is not very useful for those with a BMI ≥ 35 kg/m^2 since at this level the incremental predictive power is lost.

5. Mid-arm circumference (MAC), mid-arm muscle circumference (MAMC), and skinfold thickness (ST) estimate lean and fat mass.[64,65] The techniques and standards have been widely published elsewhere.[28]

   a) MAC, MAMC, and ST measurements are appropriate for assessing change over time in individual patients. Single measurements are less useful than serial measurements over time.

   b) Major limitations to these measurements include fluid shifts, changes in hydration status, and interobserver variability.

E. Creatinine height index (CHI)[64–68]: CHI has traditionally been mentioned as part of the nutritional assessment but is seldom used clinically. Creatinine is the metabolic end-product of muscle and dietary protein creatine. Endogenous muscle creatine is released at a constant rate. Creatinine excretion correlates with lean body mass and body

TABLE 1-6. Weight in Pounds for Males 20 years and Over-number of Examined Persons, Mean, Standard Error of the Mean, and Selected Percentiles, by Race-ethnicity and Age: United States, 1988-1994[28]

Race-ethnicity and age	Number of examined persons	Mean	Standard error of the mean	Selected percentile 5th	10th	15th	25th	50th	75th	85th	90th	95th
All race/ethnicity groups[1]												
20 years and over	7,942	180.7	0.83	131.3	140.1	145.5	155.9	175.9	199.2	214.3	226.1	243.8
20–29 years	1,630	172.1	1.37	126.9	134.0	138.7	147.5	164.9	187.6	205.2	217.7	236.8
30–39 years	1,481	182.5	1.49	136.1	142.1	148.1	158.2	175.9	200.9	217.4	226.4	247.9
40–49 years	1,226	187.3	1.67	135.4	145.1	150.9	163.6	180.7	206.5	223.3	232.5	256.4
50–59 years	855	189.2	1.76	139.6	150.1	158.4	166.7	184.7	206.8	221.6	231.5	251.3
60–69 years	1,175	182.8	1.44	134.5	141.9	148.8	160.1	181.1	203.3	216.4	224.4	236.2
70–79 years	875	173.6	1.57	128.7	136.3	141.2	151.4	171.3	191.2	205.7	211.4	227.1
80 years and over	700	157.8	1.63	114.3	123.5	128.5	140.1	155.8	173.1	185.2	193.4	204.7
Non-Hispanic white												
20 years and over	3,287	183.1	0.97	135.1	142.9	149.1	159.1	178.0	201.9	216.5	227.2	245.6
20–29 years	393	173.7	1.99	130.6	137.3	142.8	149.6	166.2	188.5	206.2	219.5	234.6
30–39 years	454	185.6	1.96	138.7	145.3	152.2	162.1	179.6	204.5	220.4	226.6	250.9
40–49 years	428	189.5	2.04	139.9	148.6	155.0	166.2	181.9	206.8	224.6	233.1	259.4
50–59 years	418	191.5	1.80	145.3	155.1	161.7	169.5	187.3	209.5	224.6	232.9	252.8
60–69 years	510	185.4	1.56	137.6	143.7	151.9	163.6	183.9	205.3	217.4	225.7	236.7
70–79 years	524	175.1	1.45	132.0	139.0	144.1	153.6	172.5	192.6	206.0	211.6	227.3
80 years and over	560	159.0	1.31	114.6	124.6	131.7	141.2	157.1	173.8	185.7	193.5	205.3
Non-Hispanic black												
20 years and over	2,113	181.5	1.09	129.3	136.7	143.0	153.0	176.0	201.1	217.7	231.1	255.1
20–29 years	488	181.6	2.14	130.1	136.2	140.7	151.9	173.9	197.5	219.6	238.6	269.1
30–39 years	497	182.4	2.00	131.7	141.1	146.4	153.1	176.6	199.4	215.7	230.0	261.6
40–49 years	370	185.4	2.11	131.7	139.9	145.6	156.3	179.1	207.7	222.2	234.7	254.1
50–59 years	217	186.0	3.09	128.9	135.2	144.8	158.4	182.3	207.8	223.6	232.4	265.9
60–69 years	295	176.9	2.25	124.2	133.6	141.3	152.6	172.0	199.1	216.4	226.1	241.1
70–79 years	187	169.9	2.63	130.1	132.1	144.0	167.7	190.6	202.1	213.1	*	
80 years and over	59	155.4	4.48	*	*	*	133.1	157.9	173	*	*	*
Mexican American												
20 years and over	2,256	170.5	1.01	125.8	134.4	139.9	148.1	166.4	188.1	202.6	212.2	228.3
20–29 years	674	162.3	1.46	123.4	129.1	134.9	141.7	157.5	175.9	191.6	201.0	220.1
30–39 years	474	173.0	1.83	126.8	136.7	143.1	153.0	169.3	189.9	204.1	210.2	234.5
40–49 years	381	181.4	2.13	139.5	144.4	149.9	160.2	175.1	202.5	214.3	223.5	240.8
50–59 years	178	182.2	3.08	144.6	150.2	158.5	179.2	199.4	213.4	221.2	*	
60–69 years	337	172.3	1.91	134.8	139.2	142.2	150.2	170.1	191.6	202.2	213.1	223.5
70–79 years	149	160.7	2.89	126.9	131.9	139.9	164.5	178.7	186.8	193.6	*	
80 years and over	63	145.7	3.56	*	*	*	129.6	146.8	154.5	*	*	*

* Figure does not meet standard of reliability or precision.
[1] Includes all other race-ethnicity groups not listed separately.

weight. It has been estimated that 18 to 20 kg of muscle is needed to yield 1 g of urinary creatinine per day.

1. CHI is calculated by comparing the actual measured creatinine excretion value with an expected value from reference values for the same height and gender as follows:

$$\text{CHI} = \frac{(\text{actual 24-hour creatinine excretion})}{(\text{expected creatinine excretion})}$$

2. Expected creatinine excretion is calculated as follows: IBW (kg) multiplied by 23 mg/kg for males and by 18 mg/kg for females.

TABLE 1-7. Weight in Pounds for Females 20 Years and Over—Number of Examined Persons, Mean, Standard Error of the Mean, and Selected Percentiles, by Race-Ethnicity and Age: United States, 1988-1994[28]

Race-Ethnicity and Age	Number of Examined Persons	Mean	Standard Error of the Mean	Selected Percentile								
				5th	10th	15th	25th	50th	75th	85th	90th	95th
All race/ethnicity groups[1]												
20 years and over	8,764	152.3	0.81	105.5	112.0	117.1	125.5	144.4	171.3	190.5	202.7	225.6
20–29 years	1,665	141.7	1.25	102.9	108.0	111.2	118.3	133.2	157.3	175.2	188.9	216.5
30–39 years	1,775	154.2	1.46	106.2	112.5	117.4	125.4	144.0	172.7	195.7	211.9	232.9
40–49 years	1,368	157.4	1.58	109.2	116.9	122.6	130.0	150.6	175.6	193.8	209.4	230.3
50–59 years	1,006	163.7	1.85	114.0	120.2	125.7	135.1	157.2	185.8	201.6	213.3	239.9
60–69 years	1,172	155.9	1.57	109.0	115.6	121.9	130.3	151.4	174.7	191.1	202.2	220.7
70–79 years	988	148.2	1.66	100.5	110.5	116.3	125.0	142.4	166.8	180.6	189.5	213.8
80 years and over	790	133.2	1.50	92.0	100.0	105.4	114.1	131.4	149.4	159.1	168.7	186.3
Non-Hispanic white												
20 years and over	3,758	150.7	0.91	105.6	112.1	117.0	125.0	143.0	169.3	187.5	200.2	221.2
20–29 years	452	140.1	1.92	102.9	108.7	111.2	118.1	130.4	153.0	171.1	185.6	218.8
30–39 years	579	151.4	2.06	105.4	112.1	116.6	123.6	141.6	170.0	192.6	207.5	227.7
40–49 years	477	155.1	2.10	109.7	117.2	122.8	129.2	147.7	172.1	191.6	202.7	227.1
50–59 years	484	163.5	2.17	115.0	120.6	125.8	135.2	157.1	185.4	200.2	211.2	239.8
60–69 years	501	155.4	1.91	110.0	115.9	122.1	130.9	151.5	172.7	190.9	201.2	219.5
70–79 years	644	147.0	1.64	100.8	111.1	116.3	124.4	141.6	164.5	178.1	187.3	206.2
80 years and over	621	132.9	1.39	92.1	100.1	105.5	114.2	131.3	149.1	158.9	167.1	185.9
Non-Hispanic black												
20 years and over	2,495	168.2	1.07	110.7	118.9	125.6	137.4	161.1	191.1	211.8	226.8	250.8
20–29 years	563	155.6	1.83	106.7	112.1	118.1	128.0	146.9	177.4	193.1	208.1	224.0
30–39 years	626	169.0	2.03	114.8	120.7	127.0	136.6	159.9	192.1	215.1	230.7	251.7
40–49 years	456	180.2	2.53	116.5	124.0	134.4	146.4	171.7	204.7	227.5	245.7	276.4
50–59 years	275	177.6	2.94	112.6	123.8	137.4	148.1	174.4	203.7	220.2	236.0	250.2
60–69 years	300	173.4	2.84	114.0	125.6	135.2	145.0	168.1	193.3	209.1	219.9	253.1
70–79 years	182	166.0	3.45	124.1	127.5	138.1	159.7	185.2	205.4	228.6		
80 years and over	93	138.7	3.65	111.0	117.0	136.1	151.0	176.5				
Mexican American												
20 years and over	2,135	151.6	1.12	105.6	112.9	118.3	127.1	145.4	171.2	185.9	196.6	217.1
20–29 years	575	142.5	1.68	101.4	105.7	110.5	119.0	136.9	157.3	177.6	188.3	205.7
30–39 years	493	154.6	2.05	107.1	114.6	120.1	129.9	145.7	174.2	191.2	208.0	229.6
40–49 years	367	163.0	2.13	117.1	125.4	130.9	139.7	157.8	180.0	194.0	204.6	225.9
50–59 years	193	156.0	2.64	121.5	123.2	134.8	153.8	175.7	182.7	192.2		
60–69 years	321	154.4	2.19	114.5	118.6	125.1	133.2	148.3	171.1	181.1	193.4	214.2
70–79 years	127	140.2	3.04	113.7	121.7	135.5	153.2	163.8				
80 years and over	59	118.4	3.83	*	*	*	96.7	116.0	135.2	*	*	*

* Figure does not meet standard of reliability or precision.
[1] Includes all other race-ethnicity groups not listed separately.
NOTE: Pregnant women are excluded.

FIGURE 1-2. Percent of Body Weight Contributed by Individual Body Parts

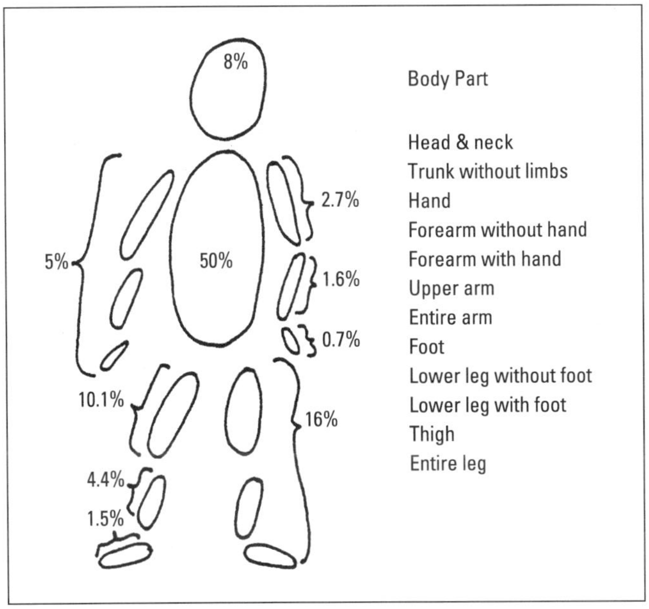

Reprinted from the Journal of the American Dietetic Association, 95, Osterkamp LK, Current perspective on assessment of human body proportions of relevance to amputees, 215–218, 1995, with permission from American Dietetic Association.

TABLE 1-8. Evaluation of Body Weight Data

$$\% \text{ of IBW} = \frac{\text{weight}}{\text{IBW}} \times 100$$

80% to 90% = mild malnutrition
70% to 79% = moderate malnutrition
0% to 69% = severe malnutrition

$$\% \text{ of UBW} = \frac{\text{current weight}}{\text{usual weight}} \times 100$$

85% to 95% = mild malnutrition
75% to 84% = moderate malnutrition
0% to 74% = severe malnutrition

$$\% \text{ of recent weight} = \frac{\text{usual weight—curent weight}}{\text{usual weight}} \times 100$$

Time	Significant weight loss (%)	Severe weight loss (%)
1 wk	1–2	>2
1 mo	5	>5
3 mos	7.5	>7.5
6 mos	10	>10

IBW, ideal body weight; UBW, usual body weight
Adapted with permission from Blackburn GL, Bistrian BR. Nutritional and metabolic assessment of the hospitalized patient. J Parenter Enteral Nutr. 1977;1(1):11–22.

3. Dietary protein may contribute up to 20% of the excreted creatinine.
4. Interpretation of CHI: 90–80%, mild depletion; 60% to 80%, moderate depletion; <60%, severe depletion.
5. Several factors affect the measurement of CHI: addition of meat to a previously meat-free diet, strenuous exercise, second half of menstrual cycle, lean tissue loss with aging, renal impairment, rhabdomyolysis, bed rest, and catabolic states; an incomplete 24-hour urine collection will invalidate creatinine excretion results but may be recognized.
6. Creatinine excretion can also assist in verifying the accuracy of 24-hour urine collections for nitrogen balance determinations, as daily creatinine excretion should vary little over the short term.

F. Bioelectrical impedance analysis (BIA)[63,64,69,70]
1. BIA is a body composition measurement technique based on the principle that lean tissue has higher electrical conduction and lower impedance than fat. It uses resistance and reactance to estimate fat-free and fat mass.
2. An imperceptible, low electric current (900 A; frequency, 50 kHz) is passed through electrodes attached to the extremities of a patient to measure resistance and reactance.
3. Factors that affect reliable BIA measurements include hydration, electrolyte abnormalities, and lack of standards for specific body sizes.

G. Hepatic transport proteins[68,71,72]
1. Serum hepatic transport protein concentrations have historically been thought to be markers for malnutrition. Those used to assess malnutrition are albumin, transferrin, prealbumin, and retinol-binding protein, which are synthesized in the liver.
2. These proteins have been referred to as negative acute-phase proteins because they decrease in serum concentration (due to decreased hepatic synthesis) at least 25% in response to chronic or acute inflammation. Proteins that increase in concentration at least 25% (due to inflammation) by virtue of increased hepatic synthesis are referred to as positive acute-phase proteins (Table 1-12).[73] Of these proteins, C-reactive protein is the most frequently cited as an indicator of inflammation. Altered hepatic synthesis of positive and negative acute-phase proteins during inflammatory metabolism presumably facilitates immune function and tissue repair.
3. In addition to inflammation, serum concentrations are affected by liver and renal function, hydration, pregnancy, iron deficiency, and blood loss. Substantial published reports correlating hepatic protein concentrations with morbidity and mortality have replaced previously published conclusions that low concentrations are associated primarily with malnutrition. The earlier reports did not account for or consider the variable of inflammation.[74] As such, serum hepatic protein levels assist in the identification of patients who are the most morbid and, thus, at risk for developing nutritional deficits and in need of carefully monitored nutrition support interventions.

H. Nitrogen balance[65,72,75,76]
1. Nitrogen balance evaluates adequacy of protein intake relative to need. Nitrogen metabolism is dependent on both energy and protein intake. Increasing energy intake often improves nitrogen balance.
2. Nitrogen balance is calculated as follows:

Nitrogen balance (g/d) = (Protein intake/6.25) – (urinary nitrogen{mostly urea} + fecal losses + obligatory losses)

TABLE 1-9. Infant Weight Gain (g/d) According to Gestational Age

		Age								
		Gestational Age (wks)			Postterm Age (mos)					
Age at Birth (wks)	Sex	28–32	32–36	36–40	Term to 3 mos	3–6	6–9	9–12	12–18	18–24
28–32	M*	32 ± 7	32 ± 7	32 ± 7	26 ± 7	16 ± 6	12 ± 4	6 ± 1	6 ± 1	5 ± 1
	F*	27 ± 6	27 ± 6	27 ± 6	23 ± 4	16 ± 3	13 ± 4	7 ± 1	7 ± 1	6 ± 2
	M + F**	30 ± 5	32 ± 6	26 ± 5	29 ± 6	19 ± 3	13 ± 4	9 ± 3		
33–36	M*		32 ± 7	32 ± 7	28 ± 6	20 ± 5	14 ± 4	11 ± 4	8 ± 3	6 ± 2
	F*		30 ± 6	30 ± 6	27 ± 6	20 ± 5	14 ± 4	10 ± 4	8 ± 3	7 ± 2
	M + F**		32 ± 6	26 ± 5	29 ± 6	19 ± 3	13 ± 4	9 ± 3		
37–42 (term)	M*				31 ± 7	21 ± 6	16 ± 4	12 ± 6		
	F*				27 ± 6	21 ± 6	16 ± 6	11 ± 4		
	M + F**				29 ± 6	19 ± 3	13 ± 4	9 ± 4		
	M***				30 (21–36)	21 (20–22)	15 (15–16)	11 (12–12)	7 (6–8)	6 (5–7)
	F***				24 (20–33)	20 (18–22)	15 (13–16)	11 (9–12)	7 (6–8)	6 (5–7)

F, female; M, male; SD, standard deviation
*From Fomon SJ, ed. *Infant Nutrition.* 2nd ed. Philadelphia, PA: WB Saunders; 1973. Values given are mean ± 1 SD.
**From Babson and Benda.44 Values were calculated from growth chart and are mean ± 2 SD.
***From Hamill PVV, Drizd RA, Johnson CL, et al. Physical growth: National Center for Health Statistics percentiles. *Am J Clin Nutr.* 1979;32:607–615. Values represent the mean. Values in parentheses include the 5th to 95th percentiles.
Reprinted with permission from the Ohio Neonatal Nutritionists. *Nutritional Care for High Risk Newborns.* Philadelphia, PA: George F. Stickley; 1985:207.

3. Nitrogen intake, assuming usual protein and amino acid sources, is calculated by dividing grams of protein intake by 6.25 to obtain grams of nitrogen intake. Specialized enteral or parenteral formulations may have a slightly different conversion factor.
4. Total nitrogen output is determined by measuring 24-hour urinary nitrogen and adding fecal and other obligatory losses (generally an additional 2–4 g/d).
5. For clinical purposes, nitrogen balance calculations using urinary urea nitrogen instead of total urinary nitrogen are more practical and generally suffice.
6. The goal for nitrogen balance is zero (or equilibrium) for maintenance or 2 to 4 g for repletion. A positive nitrogen balance reflects that nitrogen intake exceeds nitrogen losses; however, it does not reveal which tissues are being repleted and may not correlate with changes in hepatic transport proteins that are affected as much by stress and hepatic diseases as by protein status.
7. The validity of nitrogen balance is affected by severe nitrogen retention disorders (eg, creatinine clearance) < 50 units or severe hepatic failure), completeness of the 24-hour urine collection, and completeness of the record of protein or amino acid intake.

I. Immunocompetence[77–79]
1. Malnutrition is associated with immunosuppression.
2. Delayed hypersensitivity reactivity (DHR) and total lymphocyte count (TLC) have been used to detect malnutrition-related immunosuppression in uncomplicated malnutrition.
3. DHR is a measure of cell-mediated immunity. This involves intradermal injection of an antigen to which the individual has probably been exposed. An appropriate induration response in a healthy person indicates immunocompetence. Anergy is associated with malnutrition. DHR testing is not a useful parameter in individuals with infection, cancer, immunosuppressive disease or medications, renal failure, liver disease, or trauma.[77]
4. TLC is an indicator of immune function that reflects the status of B cells or T cells. TLC is calculated by multiplying the white blood cell count by the percentage of lymphocytes.
5. TLC is not necessarily a specific indicator of nutritional status since it decreases with age, acquired immunodeficiency syndromes, and radiotherapy. Other non-nutritional factors that affect TLC include hypoalbuminemia, metabolic stress, infection, cancer, and long-term diseases.

J. Vitamin and trace mineral abnormalities[16,25,65]
1. The clinical evaluation (medical history, nutritional history, physical exam) provides the basis for evaluating patients for potential vitamin and trace mineral deficits.
2. Laboratory assessment is usually required to confirm clinically suspicious signs and symptoms.
3. Patients with malnutrition generally exhibit symptoms associated with multiple micronutrient deficiencies rather than a single nutrient deficiency. See Tables 1-13 and 1-14 for assessment of vitamin and trace mineral status.

TABLE 1-10. Toddler Growth Rates of Weight, Length, and Head Circumference by Birth Weight Group and Sex

	Group I*		Group II**		Group III***	
	Male	Female	Male	Female	Male	Female
	n = 65	*n* = 67	*n* = 200	*n* = 226	*n* = 168	*n* = 155
Growth rate (g/d)						
12 mos	9.3 ± 1.6	8.9 ± 1.8	9.0 ± 1.6	9.0 ± 1.7	9.1 ± 1.6	8.9 ± 1.9
24 mos	5.7 ± 1.3	5.6 ± 1.4	5.6 ± 1.3	5.9 ± 1.6	5.9 ± 1.5	6.0 ± 2.0
36 mos	4.2 ± 1.2	4.3 ± 1.3	4.2 ± 1.2	4.6 ± 1.5	4.6 ± 1.5	4.7 ± 2.2
	n = 64	*n* = 67	*n* = 200	*n* = 224	*n* = 168	*n* = 154
Growth rate (mm/mo)						
12 mos	13.0 ± 1.1	13.0 ± 1.3	12.3 ± 1.1	12.4 ± 1.1	12.0 ± 1.0****	12.0 ± 1.0****
24 mos	8.0 ± 1.0	8.4 ± 1.0	8.0 ± 0.9	8.4 ± 1.0	8.0 ± 0.9	8.2 ± 0.9
36 mos	6.0 ± 1.0	6.5 ± 0.9	6.1 ± 0.8	6.6 ± 1.0	6.3 ± 0.9	6.6 ± 0.9
Head circumference						
	n = 65	*n* = 66	*n* = 198	*n* = 226	*n* = 169	*n* = 155
Growth rate (mm/mo)						
12 mos	3.1 ± 0.3	3.0 ± 0.4	3.0 ± 0.4	3.0 ± 0.4	3.0 ± 0.3	3.0 ± 0.3
24 mos	1.3 ± 0.2	1.3 ± 0.2	1.4 ± 0.3	1.4 ± 0.3	1.5 ± 0.2****	1.5 ± 0.2****
36 mos	0.7 ± 0.1	0.8 ± 0.2	0.9 ± 0.2	0.9 ± 0.2	0.9 ± 0.2****	0.9 ± 0.2****

Values (except n) are expressed as mean ± standard deviation.
*Birth weight < 1250 g.
**Birth weight > 1251 g but < 2000 g.
***Birth weight > 2001 g but < 2500 g.
****$p < 0.001$
Reprinted with permission from Casey PH, Kraemer HC, Bernbaum J, et al. Growth patterns of low birth weight preterm infants: longitudinal analysis of a large, varied sample. *J Pediatr.* 1990;117:298–307; and Casey PH, Kraemer HC, Bernbaum J, et al. Growth status and growth rates of a varied sample of low birth weight preterm infants: longitudinal cohort from birth to three years of age. *J Pediatr.* 1991;119:599–605.

TABLE 1-11. General Growth Guidelines for Children and Adolescents[55]

	Age (yrs)	Weight gain	Height (cm/yr)	Circumference (cm/yr)
Preschool	1–2	3.5 kg/yr	12	5
	4	2–4 kg/yr	6–8	<1
Middle childhood	7	2 kg/yr	5–6	
	10	4 kg/yr	5–6	
Adolescent boys	14–18	13 kg over 4 yrs	9.5–10.3	
Adolescent girls	13–16	11 kg over 3 yrs	8.4–9.0	

IV. Nutrition Support Decision Making

Increased morbidity and mortality are associated with malnutrition.[80–82] Malnutrition results in loss of lean body mass and subsequent loss of structure or function. Impaired respiratory function, reduced cardiac contractility, impaired renal function, altered immune function, and poor wound healing are known consequences of malnutrition.[58,80,81] Based on data gathered from the comprehensive nutritional assessment, a nutrition diagnosis is made and a plan of care set forth. Nutritional intervention decisions include timing, nutrient needs, route of therapy, and whether specialized nutritional formulations are needed. See Figure 1-3 for a decision-making algorithm.

A. Nutrition diagnosis
   1. Malnutrition is often diagnosed as mild, moderate, or severe, as seen in Table 1-8. This model is based on weight loss, while other models are a combination of nutritional assessment parameters. An example of the latter is the Nutrition Risk Index, which stratifies nutritional status based on serum albumin and percentage of usual body weight.[83]
   2. Marasmus and kwashiorkor are other diagnostic terms used to describe malnutrition. While these terms traditionally labeled

TABLE 1-12. Acute-Phase Protein Classification and Function

Positive	Negative	Function
Fibrinogen		Clotting process
Prothrombin		Clotting process
Antihemophilic		Clotting process
Plasminogen		Clotting process
Complement proteins (C1s, C1, C2, B, C3, C4, C5, C56, 1NH)		Complement cascade, including cell lysis, opsonic action, and target roles in immune response
Pancreatic secretory trypsin inhibitor α_1-Antitrypsin α-Antichymotrypsin		Protease enzyme inhibitor that prevents damage to healthy tissue
Haptoglobulin		Binding of free hemoglobin, inhibition of prostaglandin synthesis
Ceruloplasmin		Binding of copper, antioxidant
C-reactive protein		Complement activation, opsonization of DNA and cell membrane debris for subsequent scavenging
	Albumin	Binding of multiple molecules, antioxidant, plasma oncotic pressure
	Prealbumin	Thyroxine transport and formation of a complex with retinol binding protein
	Retinol-binding	Retinol transport protein
	Transferrin	Iron absorption and transport
	Fibronectin	Opsonization of noxious agents, enhancing immune clearance
	Insulin-like growth factor	Promotion of protein synthesis in liver and muscle and inhibition of lipolysis

Reprinted with permission from Mueller C. True or false: serum hepatic protein concentrations measure nutritional status. *Support Line.* 2004;26(1):8–16.

marasmus malnutrition as depleted fat and muscle stores and the kwashiorkor type as pure protein malnutrition, these terms are controversial. Both refer to states of uncomplicated malnutrition, which is a rare occurrence in acute care settings. Further, kwashiorkor, first described in malnourished children in the 1930s, may actually be a condition of undernutrition and inflammation rather than uncomplicated protein deficiency.[84]

3. Coding for malnutrition diagnoses can be found in Chapter 33.

B. Timing of nutritional intervention

1. A well-nourished adult patient without excessive metabolic stress can be expected to tolerate little or no nutrition for up to 7 days.[2] In adults, it is reasonable to initiate specialized nutrition support (provision of nutrients orally, enterally, or parenterally with therapeutic intent) within 7 to 14 days of inadequate oral intake or if inadequate oral intake is expected over a period of at least 7 to 14 days.[2,8]
2. Pediatric patients have increased metabolic rate nutrient needs for growth, and lower nutrient reserves. Surgery or a short-term illness can alter a child's nutritional status rapidly.[85] Early introduction of nutrition support is thought to be indicated for children at high risk of malnutrition or those who are malnourished. For example, initiation of parenteral nutrition on the first or second day of life in premature infants has been shown to be beneficial for improving early growth[86,87] and establishing positive nitrogen balance.[88] For those under 2 years with malnutrition prior to admission, initiation of trophic feedings within 8 hours has been suggested, along with advancing to the nutrition goal within 48 hours if tolerated.[89] For older children, it is suggested that nutrition support start within the first 18 hours and be advanced as tolerated within 24 to 36 hours to goal.

C. Mode of nutrition intervention. Integral to the process of nutrition care and the administration of specialized nutrition support is the decision on route of administration (Figure 1-3).[2]

1. Indications for enteral nutrition. Enteral nutrition should generally be given in preference to parenteral nutrition when nutritional requirements are not met by oral intake and there is a functional gastrointestinal tract of sufficient length and condition to allow adequate nutrient absorption.[2] See Chapter 5 for further indications and enteral nutrition management.
2. Indications for parenteral nutrition. Parenteral nutrition should be used when the gastrointestinal tract is not functional or cannot be accessed and in patients who cannot be adequately nourished by oral diets or enteral nutrition.[2] See Chapter 8 for parenteral nutrition indications and management.
3. Specialized nutrition support may be needed for management of specific conditions such as renal failure, liver failure, or critical illness.

D. Nutrition monitoring and evaluation

1. Once the nutrition assessment is complete and nutrition intervention begins, continuous reassessment (otherwise known as monitoring) is needed. Many of the assessment parameters used initially are repeated serially to assess the efficacy of therapy related to desired outcomes and for potential complications associated with the therapy.
2. The data collected also determine the need for continued nutrition care or discharge from nutrition care.[1,2]

(Nutrition assessment chapters from the 1st edition were contributed by Eva Politzer Shronts, Judith Fish, Kathy Pesce-Hammond, Kimberly A. Klotz, Jacqueline Wessel, and Geraldine A. Hennies.)

TABLE 1-13. Assessment of Vitamin Status[64,72]

Vitamin	Laboratory assay	Normal values	Signs of deficiency	Signs of toxicity
Niacin	Urinary niacin Metabolites	>1.6 mg per g of creatinine	Pellegra, dermatitis, dementia, death, loss of memory, headaches, glossitis	Liver damage, vascular dilation, flushing, and irritation
Folate (B_9)	Serum folate	>6.0 ng/mL	Macrocytic anemia, diarrhea, glossitis, lethargy, and stomatitis	None known
Cyanocobalamin (B_{12})	Serum B_{12}	>150 pg/mL	Pernicious anemia, glossitis, spinal cord degeneration, and peripheral neuropathy	None known
Thiamine (B_1)	Urinary thiamine	>60 mcg per g of creatinine	Beriberi, paresthesias, nystagmus, impaired memory, congestive heart failure, lactic acidosis, and Wernicke-Korsakoff syndrome	(Rare) irritability, headache, insomnia, and interference with B_2 and B_6
Riboflavin (B_2)	Urinary riboflavin	>80 mcg per g of creatinine	Mucositis, dermatitis, cheilosis, vascularization of cornea, photophobia, lacrimation, decreased vision, impaired wound healing, and normocytic anemia	None known
Pyridoxine (B_6)	Plasma B_6	>50 ng/mL	Dermatitis, neuritis, convulsions, and microcytic anemia	None known
Pantothenic acid (B_3)	Urinary pantothenic acid	>1 mg/d	Fatigue, malaise, headache, insomnia, vomiting, and abdominal cramps	Diarrhea
Biotin	Serum biotin	0.5–2.7 ng/mL	Dermatitis, depression, alopecia, lassitude, somnolence, anorexia, and paresthesias	None known
Ascorbic acid (C)	Serum ascorbic acid	>0.30 mg/dL	Enlargement and keratosis of hair follicles, impaired wound healing, anemia, lethargy, depression, bleeding, and ecchymosis	Osmotic diarrhea, oxalate kidney stones, and interference with anticoagulation therapy
A	Plasma vitamin A	>20 mcg/dL	Dermatitis, night blindness, keratomalacia, and xerophthalmia	Acute: nausea, vomiting, headache, dizziness; chronic: peeling skin, gingivitis, and alopecia
D	Plasma 25-hydroxyvitamin D	29.4 ± 15.7 ng/mL	Rickets, osteomalacia, and muscle weakness	Excess bone and soft tissue calcification, kidney stones, and hypercalcemia
E	Plasma alpha-tocopherol	>0.5 mg/dL	Hemolysis, anemia, neuronal axonopathy, and myopathy	Prolonged clotting time
K	Prothrombin time	Clotting with 1 s of laboratory control	Bleeding, purpura, and bruising	Jaundice

TABLE 1-14. Assessment of Trace Mineral Status[64,72]

Trace Mineral	Laboratory Assay	Normal Serum Values	Signs of Deficiency	Signs of Toxicity
Zinc	Serum value	50–150 mcg/dL	Dermatitis, hypogeusia, diarrhea, apathy, depression, impaired wound healing, immunosuppression	Nausea, vomiting, metallic taste, chills, headache
Copper	Serum value	70–150 mcg/dL	Neutropenia, microcytic anemia, osteoporosis, decreased hair and skin pigmentation, dermatitis, hypotonia	Nausea, vomiting, epigastric pain, diarrhea
Chromium	Serum value	1–3 mg/mL	Glucose intolerance, peripheral neuropathy, increased serum cholesterol and triglyceride, insulin resistance	None known
Manganese	Serum value	2–3 mcg/dL	Nausea, vomiting, dermatitis, color changes in hair, hypocholesterolemia, growth retardation	Extrapyramidal symptoms, encephalitis like symptoms
Selenium	Serum value	0.01–0.34 mcg/dL	Muscle weakness and pain, cardiomyopathy	Hair loss, dermatitis, garlic odor, brittle nails
Molybdenum	Neutron	0.4–0.5 mg/mL	Tachycardia, tachypnea, altered mental status, vision changes, headache, nausea, vomiting	Increased copper excretion

FIGURE 1-3. Routes to Deliver Nutrition Support to Adults: Clinical Decision Algorithm

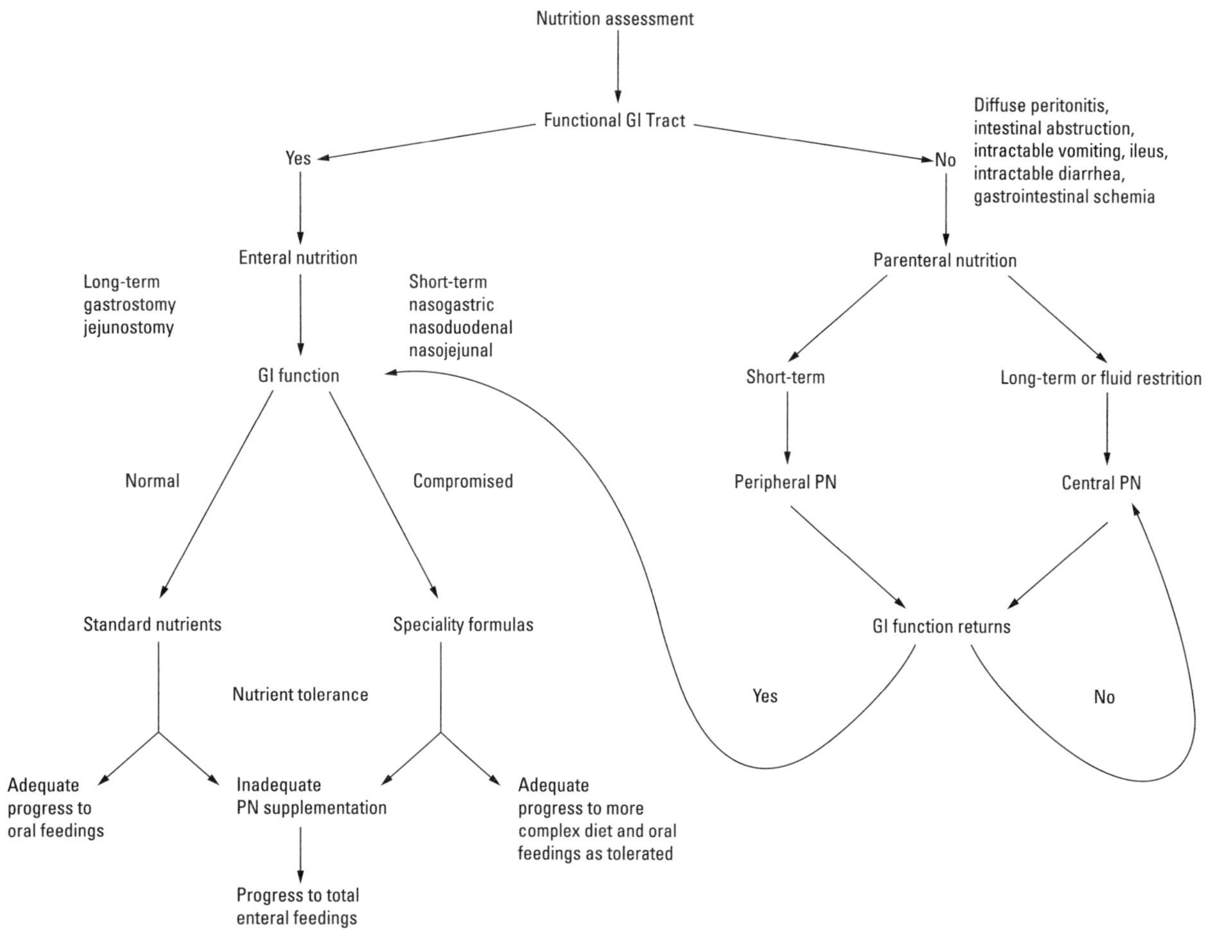

Reprinted with permission from American Society for Parenteral and Enteral Nutrition.[2]

REFERENCES

1. Lacey K, Pritchett E. Nutrition care process and model: ADA adopts road map to quality care and outcomes management. *J Am Diet Assoc.* 2003;103:1061–1072.
2. A.S.P.E.N. Board of Directors. Guidelines for the use of parenteral and enteral nutrition in adult and pediatric patients, III: nutrition assessment—adults. *J Parenter Enteral Nutr.* 2002;26:(1 suppl):9SA–12SA.
3. A.S.P.E.N. Board of Directors. Standards for specialized nutrition support: hospitalized pediatric patients. *Nutr Clin Pract.* 2005:103–16.
4. ADA's definition for nutrition screening and assessment. *J Am Diet Assoc.* 1994;94:838–839.
5. Nutrition Interventions Manual for Professionals Caring for Older Americans: Project of the American Academy of Family Physicians, the American Dietetic Association, and National Council on Aging. Washington, DC: Nutrition Screening Initiative; 1994.
6. American Society for Parenteral and Enteral Nutrition Board of Directors. *Clinical Pathways and Algorithms for Delivery of Parenteral and Enteral Nutrition Support in Adults.* Silver Spring, MD: A.S.P.E.N.; 1998.
7. A.S.P.E.N. Board of Directors. Standards for home nutrition support. *Nutr Clin Pract.* 1999;14(3):151–162.
8. A.S.P.E.N. Board of Directors. Standards for specialized nutrition support; adult hospitalized patients. *Nutr Clin Pract.* 2002;17(6):384–391.
9. Bates CW. What does it mean to be "at nutritional risk"? Seeking clarity on behalf of the elderly. *Am J Clin Nutr.* 2001;74(2):155–156.
10. Jensen GL, Friedmann JM, Doleman CD, Smiciklas-Wright H. Screening for hospitalization and nutritional risks among community-dwelling older persons. *Am J Clin Nutr.* 2001;74(2):201–205.
11. Centers for Disease Control and Prevention, National Center for Health Statistics in collaboration with the National Center for Chronic Disease Prevention and Health Promotion. Growth charts. 2000. Available at: http://www.cdc.gov/growth charts. Accessed November 23, 2004.
12. Kuczmarski RJ, Ogden CL, Guo SS, et al. 2000 CDC growth charts for the United States: methods and development. *Vital Health Stat.* 2002;11(246):1–190.
13. A.S.P.E.N. Board of Directors. Definition of terms used in A.S.P.E.N. guidelines and standards. *J Parenter Enteral Nutr.* 1995;19:1–2.
14. Shronts EP, Cerra FB. The rational use of applied nutrition in the surgical setting. In: Paparella M, ed. *Otolaryngology.* Philadelphia, PA: WB Saunders; 1990.
15. Jeejeebhoy KN. Nutritional assessment. *Gastroenterol Clin North Am.* 1998;27(2):347–369.
16. Teasley-Strausburg KM, Anderson JD. Assessment, prevalence and clinical significance of malnutrition. In: DiPiro JT, ed. *Pharmacotherapy: A Pathophysiologic Approach.* 2nd ed. Norwalk, CT: Appleton & Lange; 1993.
17. Ireton-Jones CS, Hasse JM. Comprehensive nutritional assessment: the dietitians' contribution to the team effort. *Nutrition.* 1992;8(2):75–81.
18. Detsky AS, McLaughlin JR, Baker JP, et al. What is subjective global assessment of nutritional status? *J Parenter Enteral Nutr.* 1987;11:8–14.
19. Baker JP, Detsky AS, Wesson DL, et al. Nutritional assessment: a comparison of clinical judgment and objective measurements. *N Engl J Med.* 1988;306:969–973.
20. Hammond K. The history and physical exam. In: Matarese L, Gottschlich M, eds. *Contemporary Nutrition Support Practice.* 2nd ed. Philadelphia, PA: WB Saunders; 2003:14–30.
21. Ignatavicius D, Workman L, Mishler M. *Medical-Surgical Nursing.* 2nd ed. Philadelphia, PA: WB Saunders; 1995.
22. Hammond KA, Hillhouse J. *Nutrition-Focused Physical Assessment Skills for Dietitians.* Chicago, IL: Dietitians in Nutrition Support, American Dietetic Association; 2000.
23. Tanner JM. *Growth in Adolescents.* 2nd ed. Boston, MA: Blackwell Scientific Publications; 1962.
24. Krug-Wispe S. Nutritional assessment. In: Queen PM, Lang CE, eds. *Handbook of Pediatric Nutrition.* Gaithersburg, MD: Aspen Publishers; 1993:26–76.
25. Hopkins B. Assessment of nutritional status. In: Gottschlich MM, ed. *Nutrition Support Dietetics Core Curriculum.* 2nd ed. Silver Spring, MD: A.S.P.E.N.; 1993.
26. Guenter PA, Smithgall JM, Williamson JM, Rombeau JL. Body weight. In: Rombeau JL, Caldwell MD, Forlaw L, Guenter PA, eds. *Atlas of Nutrition Support Techniques.* Boston, MA: Little, Brown; 1989:1–12.
27. Hamwi GJ. Changing dietary concepts. In: Danowski TS, ed. *Diabetes Mellitus: Diagnosis & Treatment.* Vol. 1. New York, NY: American Diabetes Association; 1964:73–78.
28. US Department of Health and Human Services, Centers for Disease Control and Prevention, National Center for Health Statistics. National Health and Nutrition Examination Survey. Available at: http://www.cdc.gov/nchs/about/major/nhanes/survey. Accessed September 22, 2004.
29. Howell WH. Anthropometry and body composition analysis. In: Matarese LE, Gottschlich MM, eds. *Contemporary Nutrition Support Practice.* Philadelphia, PA: WB Saunders; 2003:31–44.
30. Osterkamp LK. Current perspective on assessment of human body proportions of relevance to amputees. *J Am Diet Assoc.* 1995;95(2):215–218.
31. Grant JP. Nutritional assessment by body composition analysis. In: Grant JP, ed. *Handbook of Parenteral Nutrition.* 2nd ed. Philadelphia, PA: WB Saunders; 1992:15–47.
32. Fenton TR. A new growth chart for preterm babies: Babson and Benda's chart updated with recent data and a new format. *BMC Pediatr.* 2003;3:13–28.
33. Shaffer SG, Quimiro CL, Anderson JV, et al. Postnatal weight changes for low-birth-weight infants. *Pediatrics.* 1987;79:702–706.
34. Wright K, Dawson JP, Fallis D, et al. New postnatal growth grids for very-low-birth- weight infants. *Pediatrics.* 1993;91:922–926.
35. Guo SS, Roche AF, Chumlea WC, et al. Growth in weight, recumbent length, and head circumference for preterm low birthweight infants during the first three years of life—using gestational adjusted ages. *Early Hum Dev.* 1997;47:305–325.
36. Guo SS, Wholihan K, Roche AF, et al. Weight for length reference data for preterm low birth weight infants. *Arch Pediatr Adolesc Med.* 1996;150:964–970.
37. Brandt I. Growth dynamics of low birth weight infants with emphasis on the perinatal period. In: Falkner F, Tanner JM, eds. *Human Growth: 2. Postnatal Growth.* New York, NY: Plenum Press; 1978:557–617.
38. Casey PH, Kraemer HC, Bernbaum J, et al. Growth patterns of low birth weight preterm infants: longitudinal analysis of a large, varied sample. *J Pediatr.* 1990;117:298–307.
39. Casey PH, Kraemer HC, Bernbaum J, et al. Growth status and growth rates of a varied sample of low birth weight preterm infants: longitudinal cohort from birth to three years of age. *J Pediatr.* 1991;119:599–605.
40. Ehrenkranz RA, Younes N, Lemons JA, et al. Longitudinal growth of hospitalized very low birth weight infants. *Pediatrics.* 1999;104:280–289.
41. Gairdner D, Pearson J. A growth chart for premature and other infants. *Arch Dis Child.* 1971;46:783–787.
42. Lubchenco LO, Hansman C, Boyd E. Intrauterine growth in length and head circumference as estimated from live births at gestational ages from 26–42 weeks. *Pediatrics.* 1966;37:403–408.
43. Klawitter B. Nutrition assessment of infants and children. In: Nevin-Folino N, ed. *Pediatric Manual of Clinical Dietetics.* Chicago, IL: American Dietetic Association; 2003:148–162.
44. Babson SG, Benda GJ. Growth graphs for the clinical assessment of infants of varying age. *J Pediatr.* 1976;89:814–820.
45. Sherry B, Mei Z, Grummer-Stawn L, et al. Evaluation and recommendations for growth references for very low birth weight (<1500 grams) infants in the United States. *Pediatrics.* 2003;111:750–757.
46. Wang Z, Sauve RS. Assessment of postnatal growth in VLBW infants: selection of growth references and age adjustment for prematurity. *Can J Public Health.* 1998;89:109–114.
47. Elliman AM, Bryan EM, Harvey DR. Gestational age correction for height in preterm children to seven years of age. *Acta Paediatr.* 1992; 81:836–839.
48. Cox JH. Growth assessment. In: Cox JH, ed. *Nutrition Manual for At-Risk Infants and Toddlers.* Chicago, IL: Precept Press; 1997:43–58.
49. Cronk C, Crocker AC, Pueschel SM, et al. Growth charts for children with Down syndrome. *Pediatrics.* 1988;81:102–110.
50. Lyon AJ, Preece MA, Grant DB. Growth curve for girls with Turner syndrome. *Arch Dis Child.* 1985;60:932–935.

51. Morris CA, Demsey MS, Leonard CL, et al. Height and weight of males and females with Williams syndrome. *Williams Syndrome Assoc Newsletter.* summer 1991:29–30.
52. Butler MG, Meany FJ. Standards for selected anthropometric measurements in Prader-Willi syndrome. *Pediatrics.* 1991;88:853–858.
53. Krick J, Murphy-Miller P, Zeger S, et al. Pattern of growth in children with cerebral palsy. *J Am Diet Assoc.* 1996;96:680–685.
54. Bonnema S. Neurological compromise. In: Cox JH, ed. *Nutrition Manual for At-Risk Infants and Toddlers.* Chicago, IL: Precept Press; 1997:113–133.
55. Hendricks K. Nutritional assessment. In: Baker SB, Baker RD, Davis A, eds. *Pediatric Enteral Nutrition.* New York, NY: Chapman and Hall; 1994:105–118.
56. Ekvall SW. Nutrition assessment and early intervention. In: Ekvall SW, ed. *Pediatric Nutrition in Chronic Diseases and Developmental Disorders: Prevention, Assessment and Treatment.* New York, NY: Oxford University Press; 1993:41.
57. Waterlow JC. Classification and definition of protein energy malnutrition. *BMJ.* 1972:3:566–569.
58. Blackburn GL, Bistrian BR. Nutritional and metabolic assessment of the hospitalized patient. *J Parenter Enteral Nutr.* 1977;1(1):11–22.
59. Charney DE, Meguid MM. Current concepts in nutritional assessment. *Arch Surg.* 2002;137(1):42–45.
60. Centers for Disease Control and Prevention, National Center for Health Statistics. *Prevalence of Overweight and Obesity Among Adults: United States, 1999–2000.* Washington, DC: US Department of Health and Human Services; 2002.
61. American Academy of Family Physicians, American Dietetic Association, and National Council on Aging. *Nutrition Interventions Manual for Professionals Caring for Older Americans.* Washington, DC: Nutrition Screening Initiative; 1992.
62. National Heart, Lung, and Blood Institute. Clinical Guidelines on the Identification, Evaluation, and Treatment of Overweight and Obesity in Adults: Executive Summary. Washington, DC: National Institutes of Health; 2002.
63. Hammond KA. Dietary and clinical assessment. In: Mahan LK, Escott-Stump S, eds. *Krause's Food, Nutrition, and Diet Therapy.* 11th ed. Philadelphia, PA: WB Saunders; 2004:407–435.
64. Strausburg KT. Nutrition/metabolic assessment. In: Teasley-Strausburg K, ed. *Nutrition Support Handbook.* Cincinnati, OH: Harvey Whitney; 1992.
65. Shronts EP. Nutritional assessment in hepatic failure. *Nutr Clin Pract.* 1988;3(3):113–119.
66. Forbes GB, Bruining GJ. Urinary creatinine excretion and lean body mass. *Am J Clin Nutr.* 1976;29:1359–1366.
67. Bistrian BR, Blackburn GL, Sherman M, et al. Therapeutic index of nutritional depletion in hospitalized patients. *Surg Gynecol Obstet.* 1975;141:512–516.
68. Russell MK. Laboratory monitoring. In: Matarese LE, Gottschlich MM, eds. *Contemporary Nutrition Support Practice.* Philadelphia, PA: WB Saunders; 2003:45–62.
69. Zarowitz BJ, Pilla AM. Bioelectrical impedance in clinical practice. *Annals Pharmacother.* 1989;23:548–555.
70. Chumlea WC, Guo S. Bioelectrical impedance and body composition: present status and future directions. *Nutr Rev.* 1994;52(4):123–131.
71. Daley BJ, Bistrian BR. Nutritional assessment. In: Zaloga GP, ed. *Nutrition in Critical Care.* St Louis, MO: Mosby; 1994.
72. Shopbell JM, Hopkins B, Shronts EP. Nutrition screening and assessment. In: Gottschlich MM, Fuhrman MO, Hammond KA, Holcombe BJ, Seidner DL, eds. *The Science and Practice of Nutrition Support.* Dubuque, IA: American Society for Parenteral and Enteral Nutrition/Kendall Hunt; 2001:107–140.
73. Gabay C, Kishner I. Acute-phase proteins and other systemic responses to inflammation. *N Engl J Med.* 1999;340:448–454.
74. Fuhrman MP, Charney P, Mueller CM. Hepatic proteins and nutrition assessment. *J Am Diet Assoc.* 2004;104:1258–1264.
75. Kopple JD. Uses and limitations of the balance technique. *J Parenter Enteral Nutr.* 1987;11(5):173–179.
76. Evans-Stoner N. Nutrition assessment: a practical approach. *Nurs Clin North Am.* 1997;32(4):637–650.
77. Twomey P, Ziegler D, Rombeau J. Utility of skin testing in nutritional assessment: a critical review. *J Parenter Enteral Nutr.* 1982;6(1):50–58.
78. Chandra RK. Interactions of nutrition, infection and immunity: immunocompetence in nutritional deficiency, methodological considerations, and intervention strategies. *Acta Paediatr Scand.* 1979;68:137–144.
79. Langkamp-Henken B, Wood SM. Evaluating immunocompetence. In: Matarese LE, Gottschlich MM, eds. *Contemporary Nutrition Support Practice.* Philadelphia, PA: Saunders; 2003:63–76.
80. Black DR, Sciacca JP, Coster DC. Extremes in body mass index: probability of health care expenditures. *Prev Med.* 1994;23:385–393.
81. Reinhardt GF, Myscofski JW, Wilkens DB, et al. Incidence and mortality of hypoalbuminemic patients in hospitalized veterans. *J Parenter Enteral Nutr.* 1980;4:357–359.
82. Seres DS. Nutritional assessment: current concepts and guidelines for the busy physician. *Practical Gastroenterology.* August 2003;Series 8:30–39.
83. The Veterans Affairs Total Parenteral Nutrition Cooperative Study Group. Perioperative total parenteral nutrition in surgical patients. *N Engl J Med.* 1991;325:525–532.
84. Seres DS, Resurreccion LB. Kwashiorkor: dysmetabolism versus malnutrition. *Nutr Clin Pract.* 2003;18:297–301.
85. Cresci G. Nutritional care of surgery patients. In: Williams SR, Schlenker ED, eds. *Essentials of Nutrition and Diet Therapy.* St Louis, MO: Mosby; 2003:550–567.
86. Marian M. Pediatric nutrition support. *Nutr Clin Pract.* 1993;8:199–209.
87. Ho MY, Nsieh MC, Chen NT, et al. Early versus late nutrition support in premature neonates with respiratory distress syndrome. *Nutrition.* 2003; 19:1257–1260.
88. Clark RH, Wagner CL, Merritt RJ, et al. Nutrition in the neonatal intensive care unit: how do we reduce the incidence of extrauterine growth restriction? *J Perinatol.* 2003;23:337–344.
89. Thureen P. Early aggressive nutrtion support. *Pediatr Rev.* 1999;20:e45–e55.

APPENDIX 1-1

Pediatric Growth Charts

Centers for Disease Control and Prevention, National Center for Health Statistics in collaboration with the National Center for Chronic Disease Prevention and Health Promotion. Growth charts. 2000. Available at: http://www.cdc.gov/growth charts. Accessed November 23, 2004.

Birth to 36 months: Boys
Length-for-age and Weight-for-age percentiles

NAME ____________________

RECORD # ____________

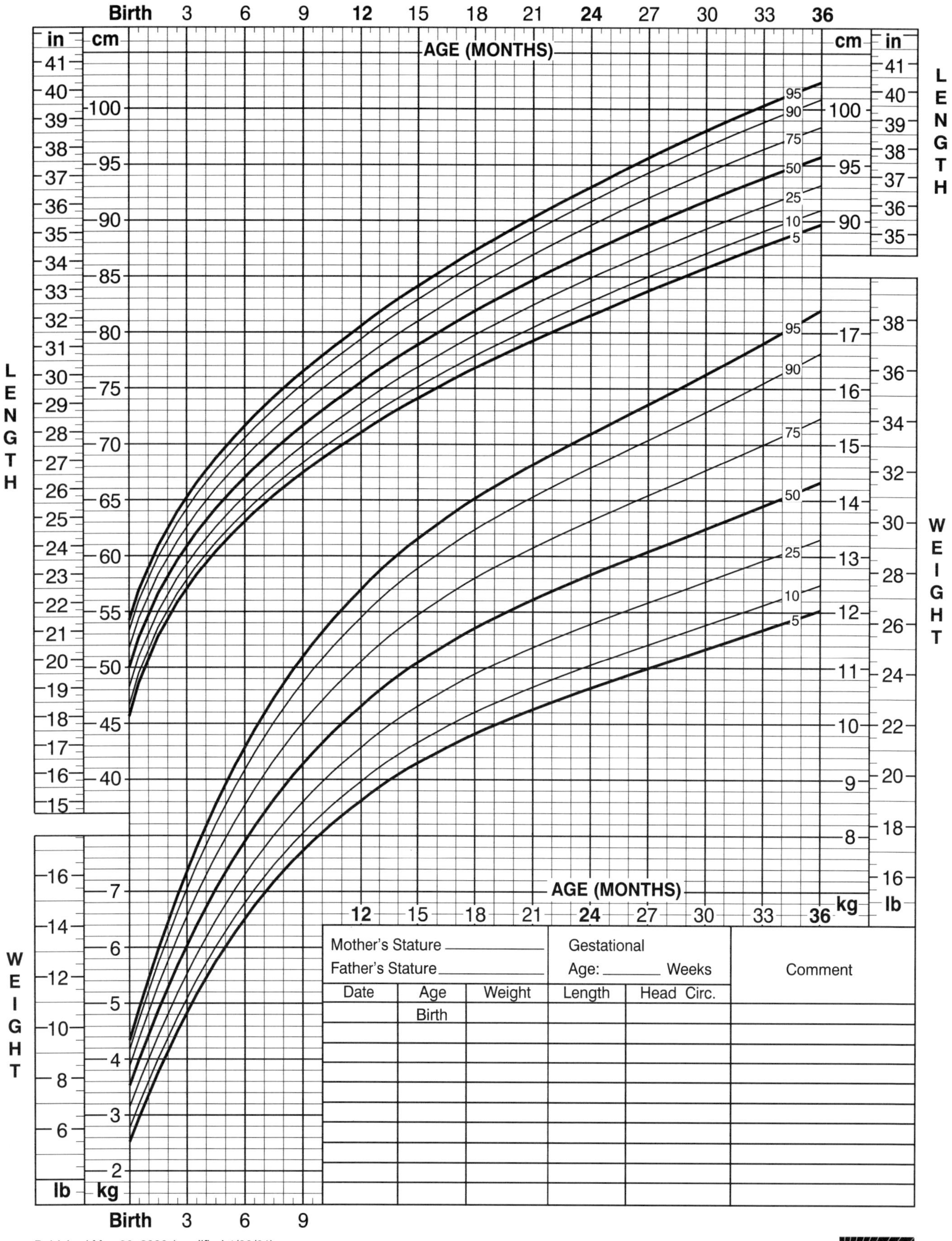

Mother's Stature ____________

Father's Stature ____________

Gestational Age: ________ Weeks

Date	Age	Weight	Length	Head Circ.	Comment
	Birth				

Pubished May 30, 2000 (modified 4/20/01).
SOURCE: Developed by the National Center for Health Statistics in collaboration with the National Center for Chronic Disease Prevention and Health Promotion (2000).
http://www.cdc.gov/growthcharts

Birth to 36 months: Girls
Length-for-age and Weight-for-age percentiles

NAME ______________________

RECORD # ____________

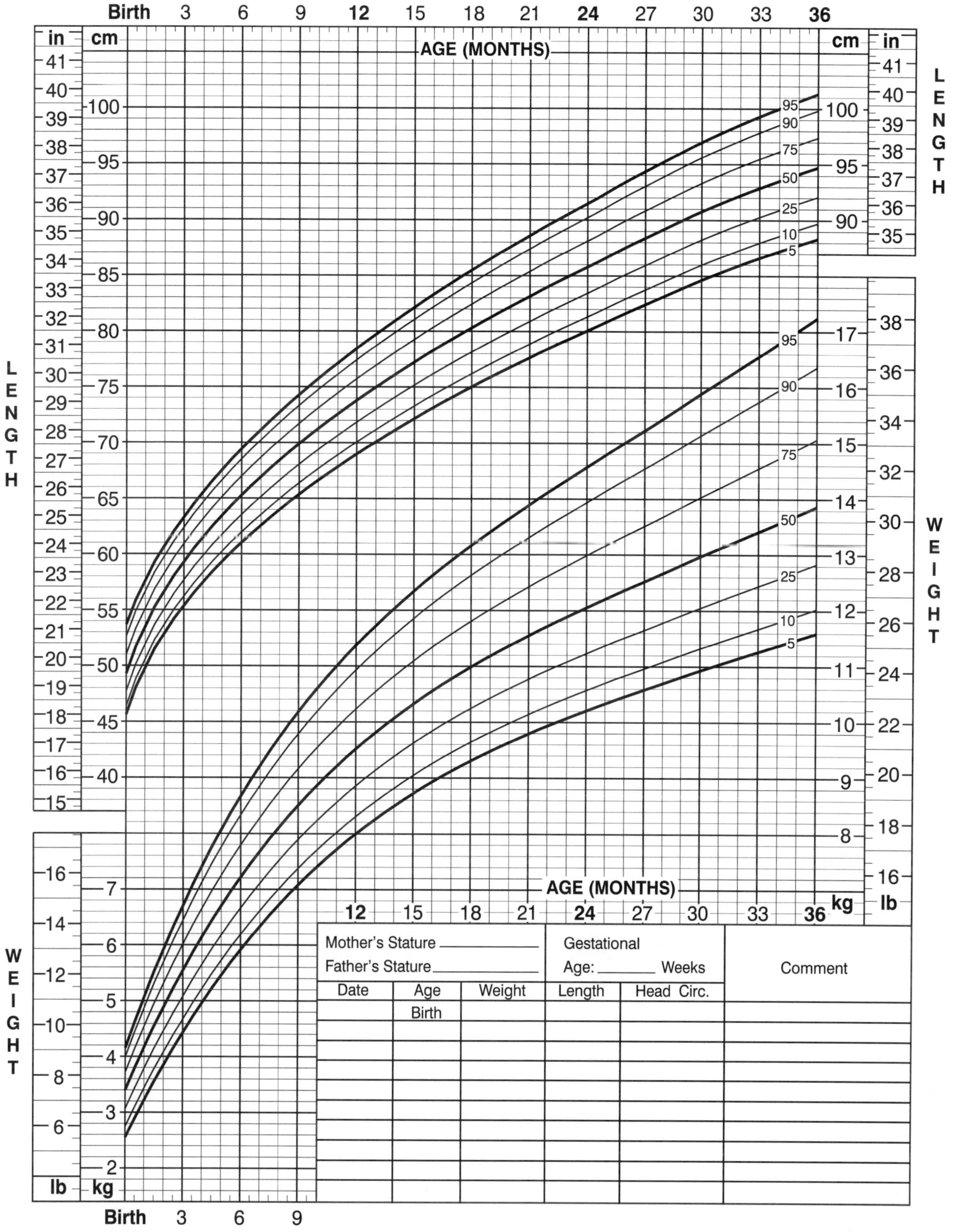

Mother's Stature ______ Father's Stature ______			Gestational Age: ______ Weeks		Comment
Date	Age	Weight	Length	Head Circ.	
	Birth				

Published May 30, 2000 (modified 4/20/01).
SOURCE: Developed by the National Center for Health Statistics in collaboration with the National Center for Chronic Disease Prevention and Health Promotion (2000).
http://www.cdc.gov/growthcharts

SAFER • HEALTHIER • PEOPLE™

Birth to 36 months: Boys
Head circumference-for-age and
Weight-for-length percentiles

NAME ______________________

RECORD # __________

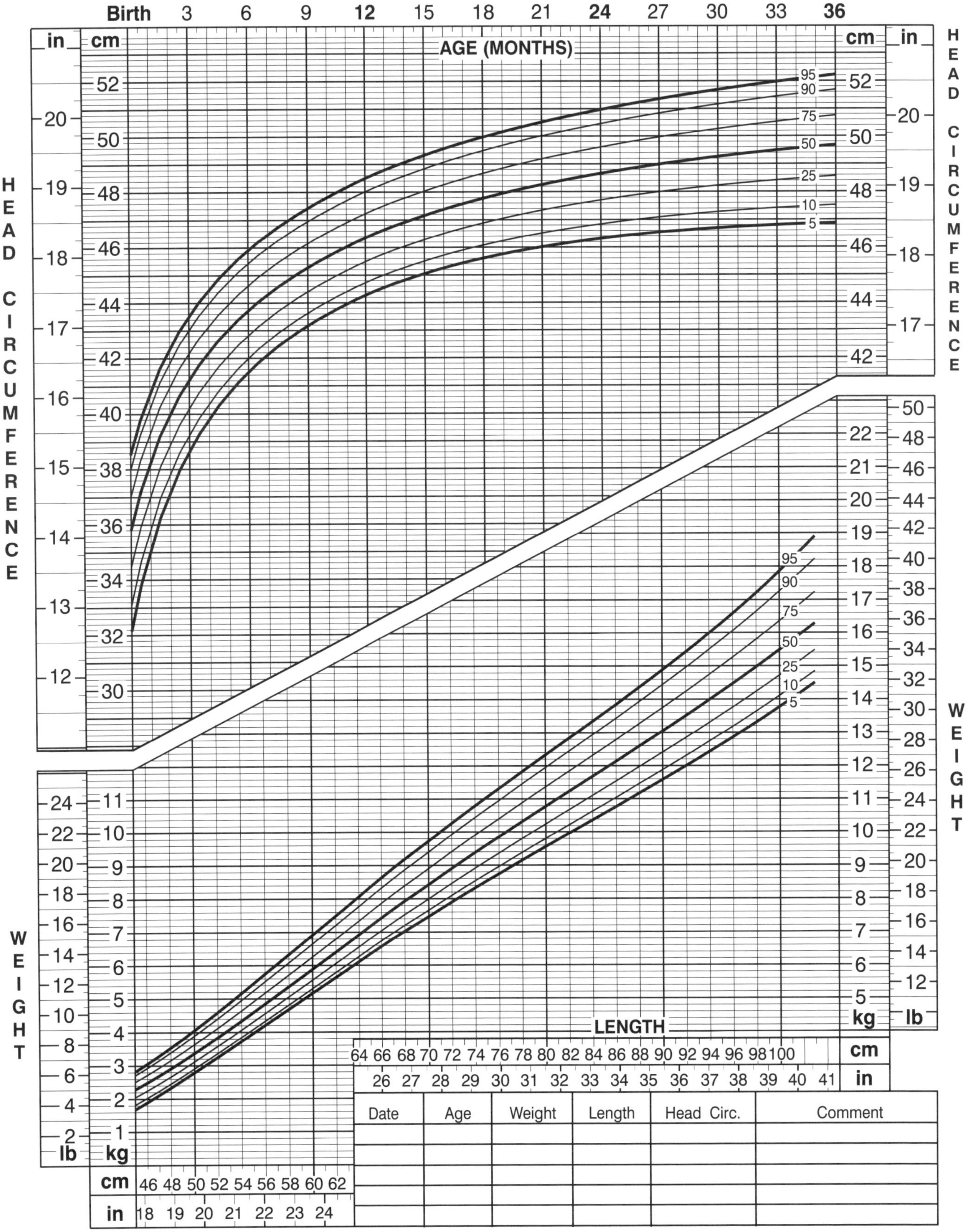

Published May 30, 2000 (modified 10/16/00).
SOURCE: Developed by the National Center for Health Statistics in collaboration with the National Center for Chronic Disease Prevention and Health Promotion (2000).
http://www.cdc.gov/growthcharts

CDC
SAFER • HEALTHIER • PEOPLE™

Birth to 36 months: Girls
Head circumference-for-age and Weight-for-length percentiles

NAME ______________________________

RECORD # ______________

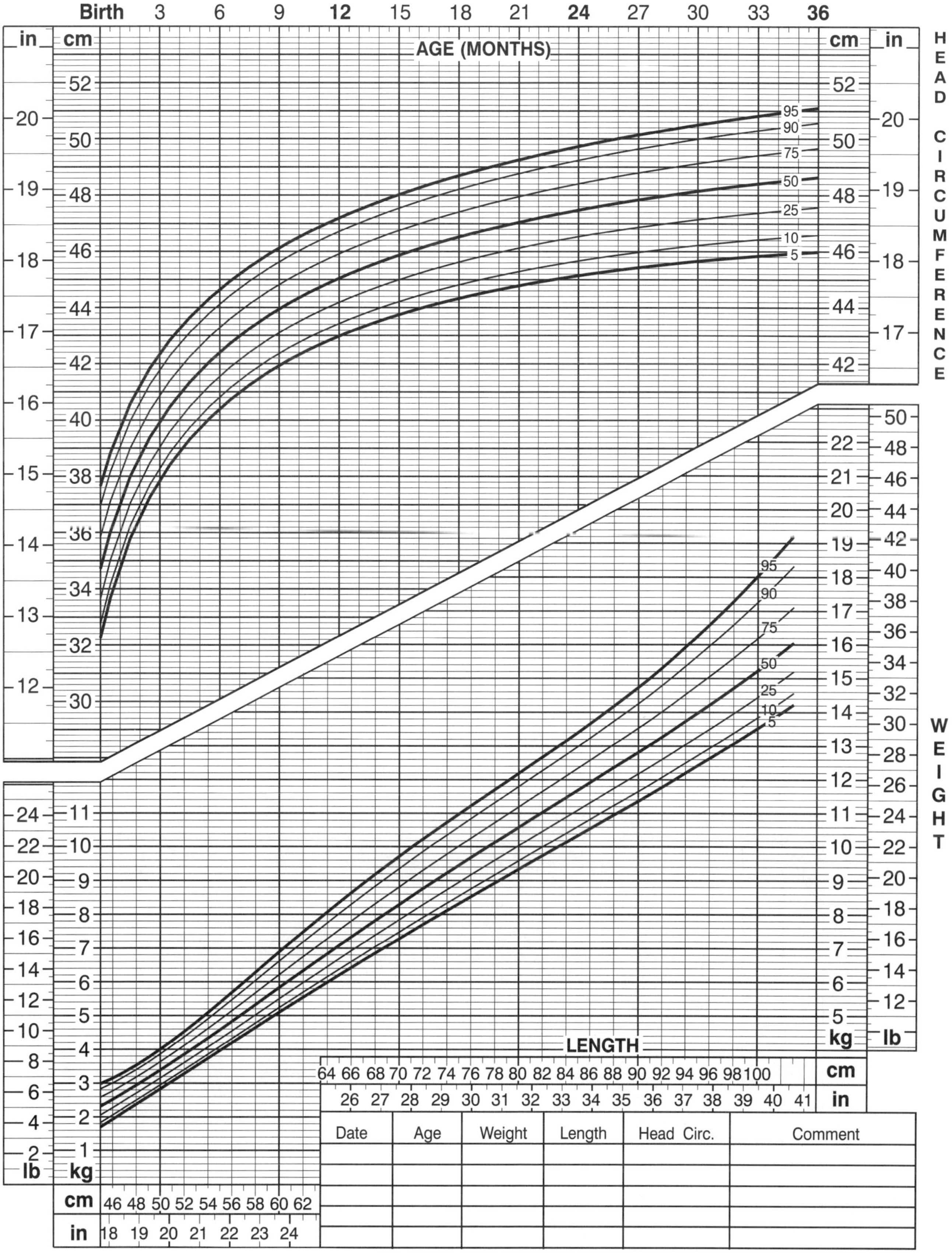

Date	Age	Weight	Length	Head Circ.	Comment

Published May 30, 2000 (modified 10/16/00).
SOURCE: Developed by the National Center for Health Statistics in collaboration with the National Center for Chronic Disease Prevention and Health Promotion (2000).
http://www.cdc.gov/growthcharts

CDC
SAFER • HEALTHIER • PEOPLE™

2 to 20 years: Boys
Stature-for-age and Weight-for-age percentiles

NAME ______________________

RECORD # ____________

Mother's Stature ____________ Father's Stature ____________

Date	Age	Weight	Stature	BMI*

***To Calculate BMI**: Weight (kg) ÷ Stature (cm) ÷ Stature (cm) x 10,000
or Weight (lb) ÷ Stature (in) ÷ Stature (in) x 703

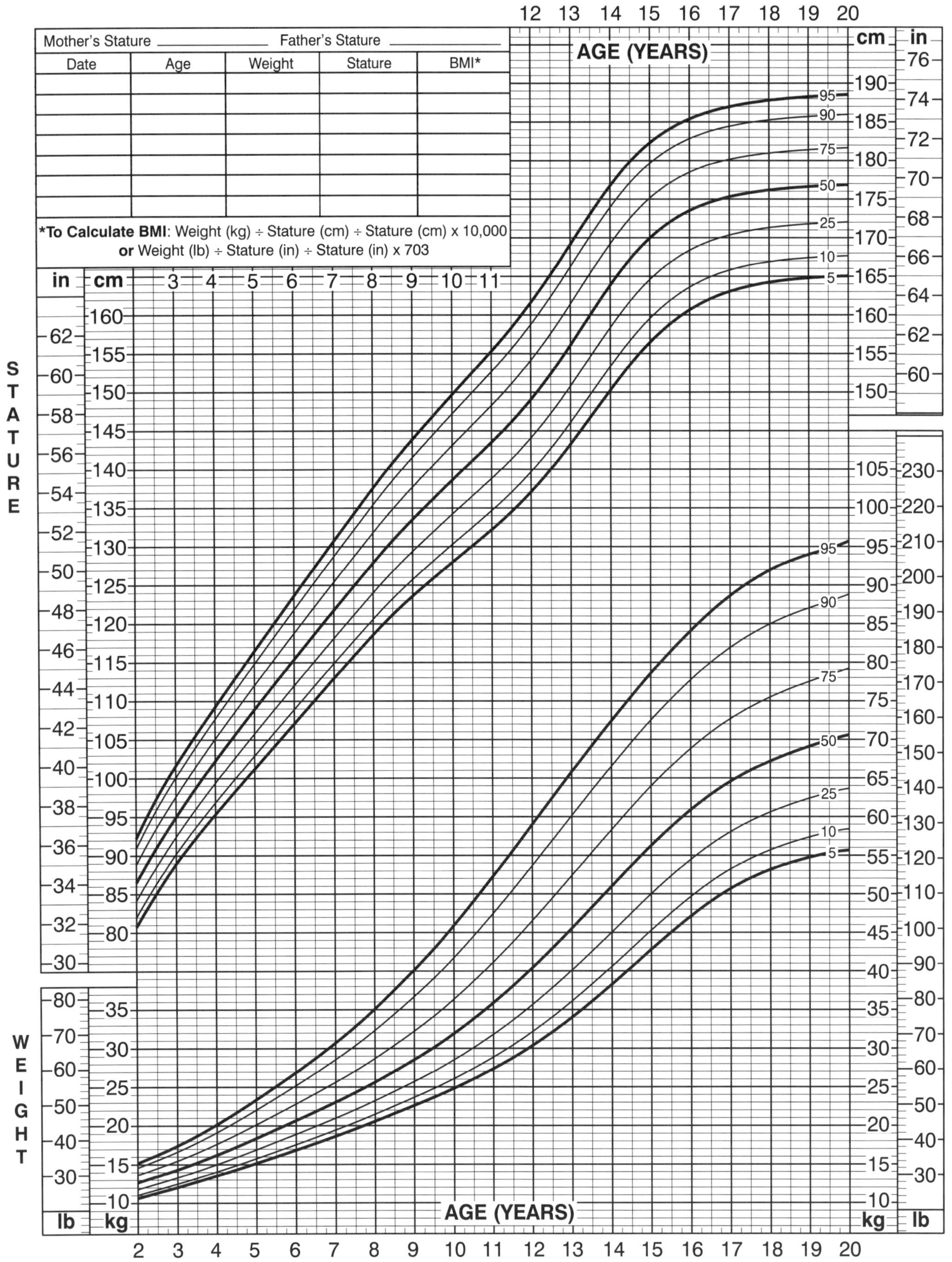

Published May 30, 2000 (modified 11/21/00).
SOURCE: Developed by the National Center for Health Statistics in collaboration with the National Center for Chronic Disease Prevention and Health Promotion (2000).
http://www.cdc.gov/growthcharts

CDC
SAFER • HEALTHIER • PEOPLE™

2 to 20 years: Girls
Stature-for-age and Weight-for-age percentiles

NAME ____________________

RECORD # ____________

Mother's Stature ____________ Father's Stature ____________

Date	Age	Weight	Stature	BMI*

***To Calculate BMI**: Weight (kg) ÷ Stature (cm) ÷ Stature (cm) x 10,000
or Weight (lb) ÷ Stature (in) ÷ Stature (in) x 703

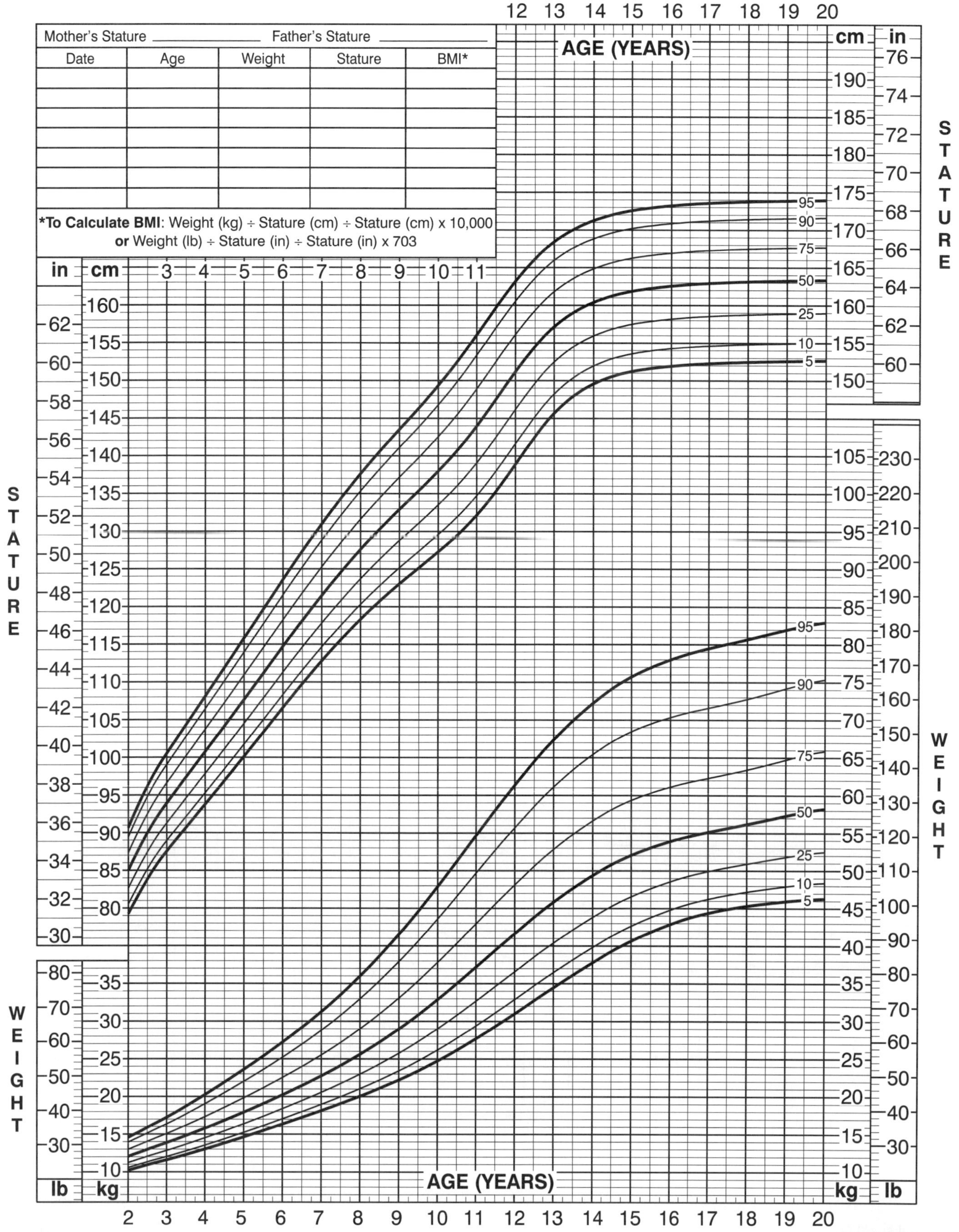

Published May 30, 2000 (modified 11/21/00).
SOURCE: Developed by the National Center for Health Statistics in collaboration with the National Center for Chronic Disease Prevention and Health Promotion (2000).
http://www.cdc.gov/growthcharts

CDC
SAFER • HEALTHIER • PEOPLE™

2 to 20 years: Boys
Body mass index-for-age percentiles

NAME ____________________

RECORD # ____________

Date	Age	Weight	Stature	BMI*	Comments

***To Calculate BMI**: Weight (kg) ÷ Stature (cm) ÷ Stature (cm) x 10,000
or Weight (lb) ÷ Stature (in) ÷ Stature (in) x 703

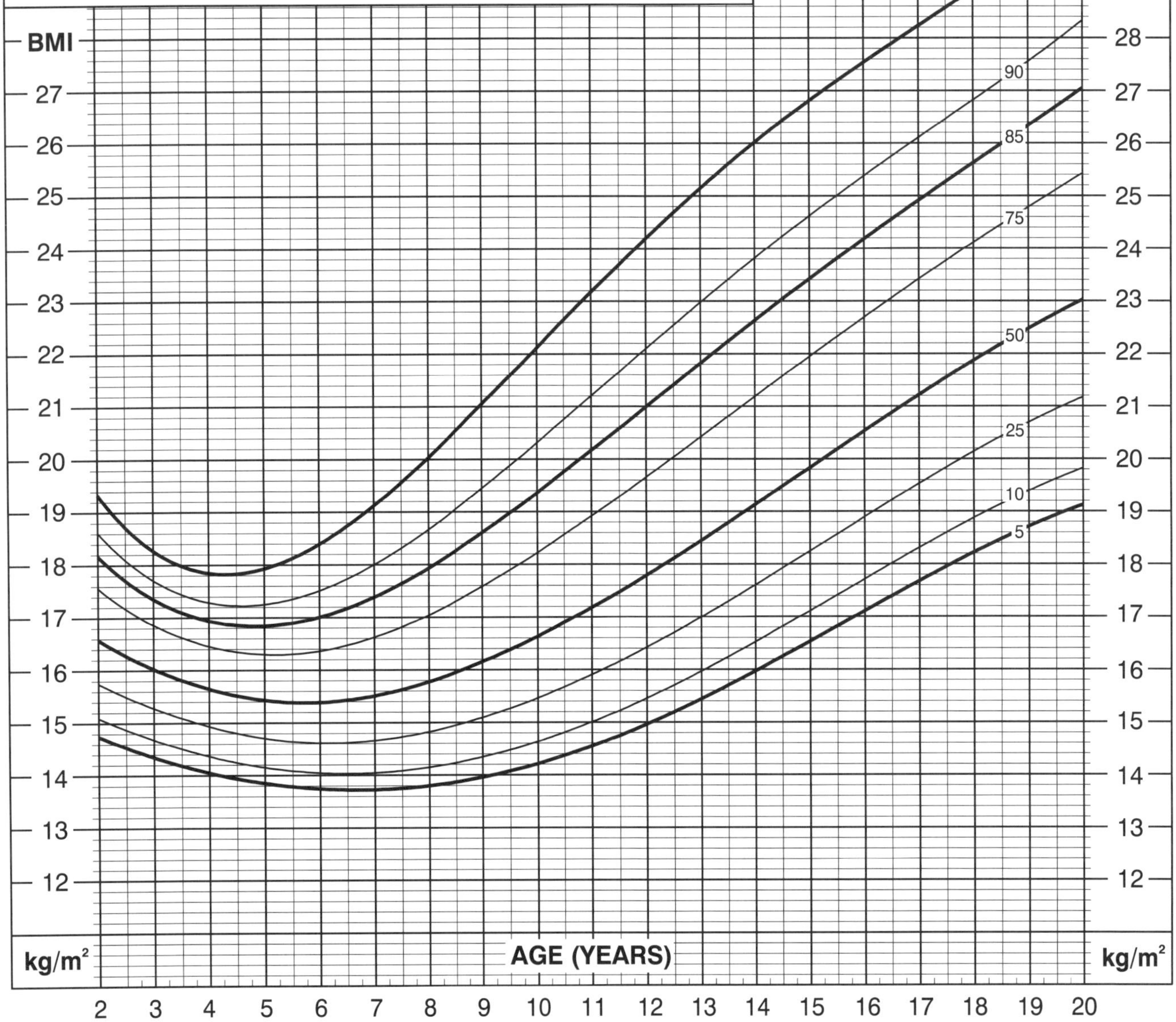

Published May 30, 2000 (modified 10/16/00).
SOURCE: Developed by the National Center for Health Statistics in collaboration with the National Center for Chronic Disease Prevention and Health Promotion (2000).
http://www.cdc.gov/growthcharts

CDC
SAFER • HEALTHIER • PEOPLE™

2 to 20 years: Girls
Body mass index-for-age percentiles

NAME ____________________

RECORD # ____________

Date	Age	Weight	Stature	BMI*	Comments

***To Calculate BMI**: Weight (kg) ÷ Stature (cm) ÷ Stature (cm) x 10,000
or Weight (lb) ÷ Stature (in) ÷ Stature (in) x 703

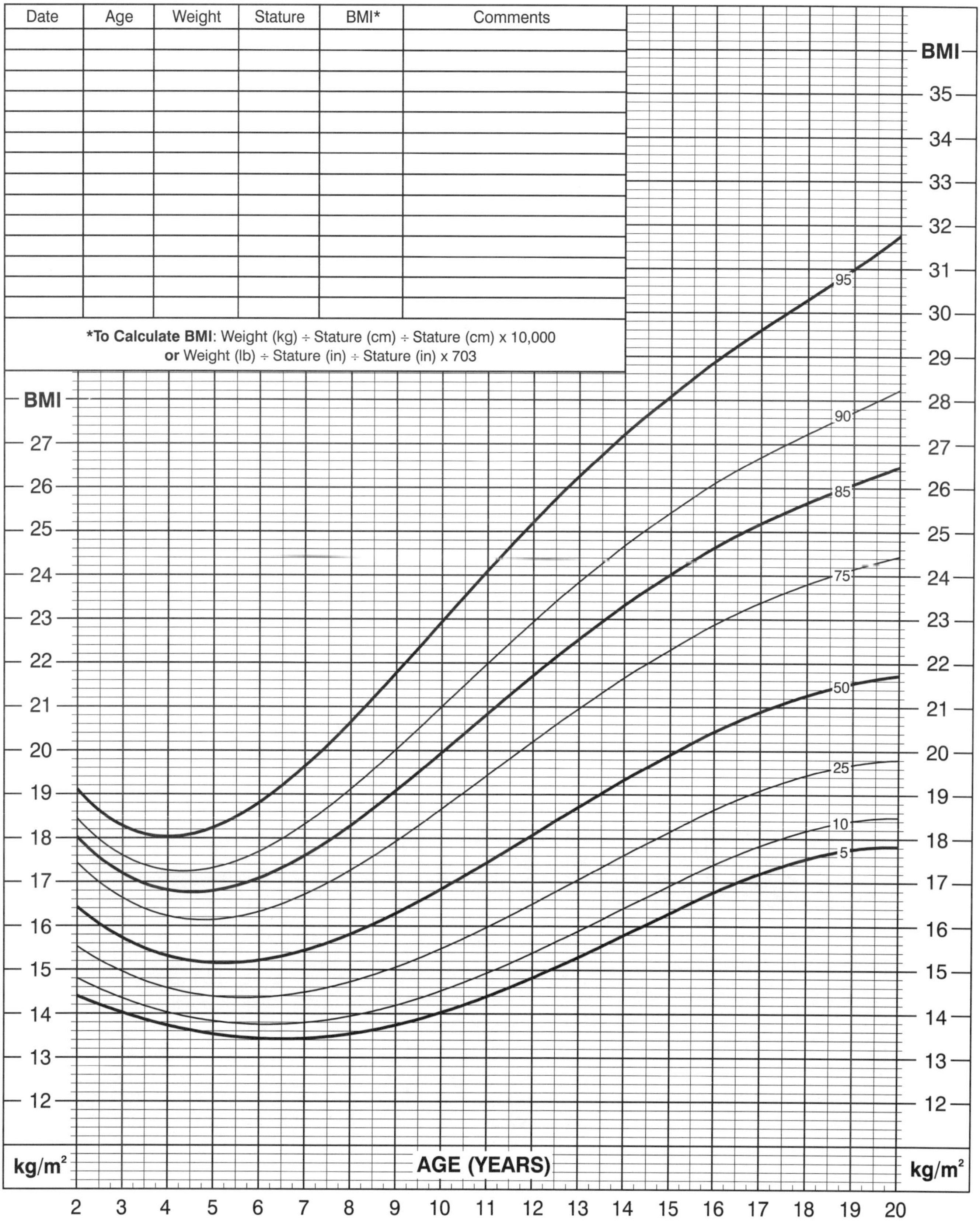

Published May 30, 2000 (modified 10/16/00).
SOURCE: Developed by the National Center for Health Statistics in collaboration with the National Center for Chronic Disease Prevention and Health Promotion (2000).
http://www.cdc.gov/growthcharts

SAFER • HEALTHIER • PEOPLE™

NAME ____________________

Weight-for-stature percentiles: Boys

RECORD # ____________

Date	Age	Weight	Stature	Comments

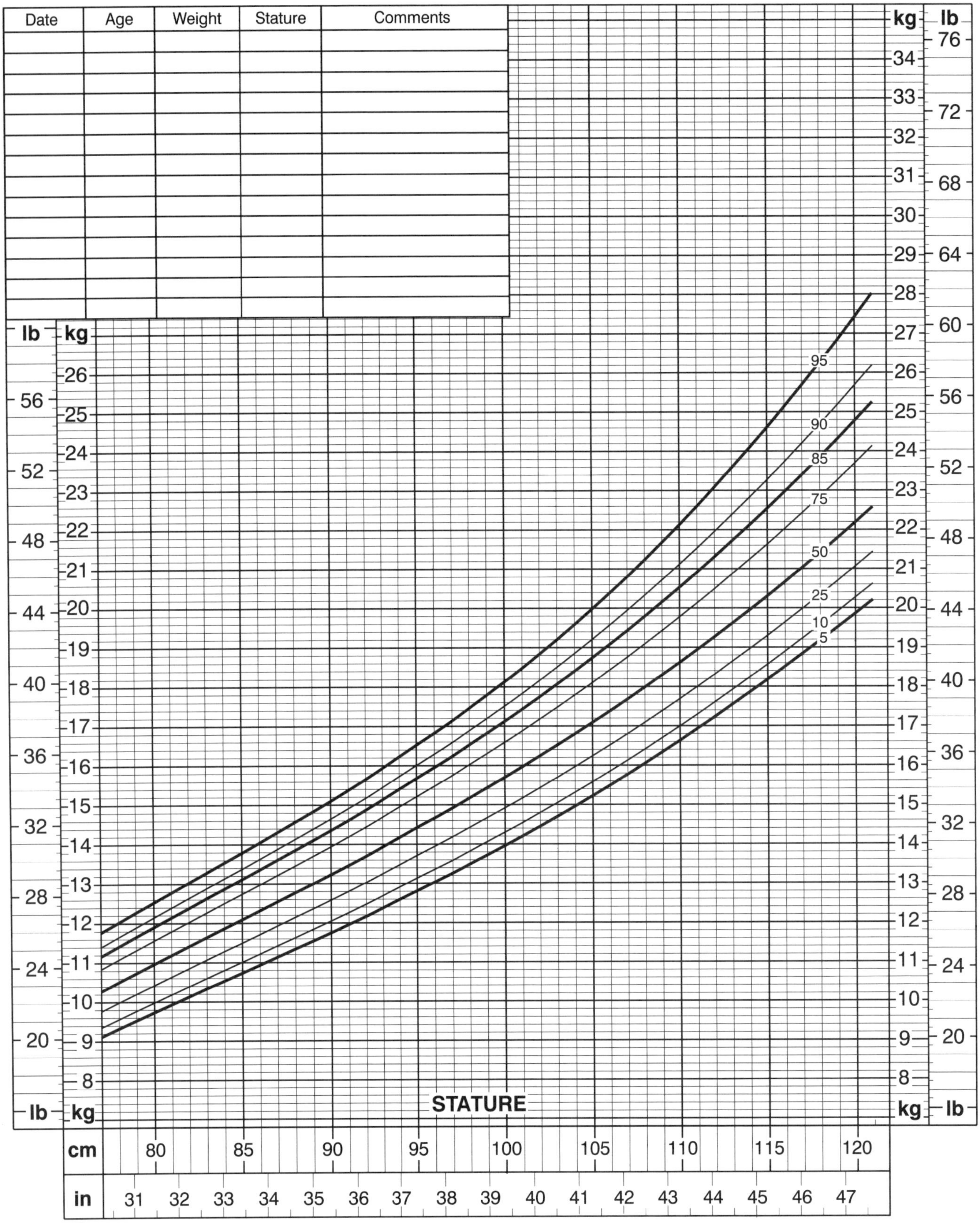

Published May 30, 2000 (modified 10/16/00).
SOURCE: Developed by the National Center for Health Statistics in collaboration with the National Center for Chronic Disease Prevention and Health Promotion (2000).
http://www.cdc.gov/growthcharts

CDC
SAFER • HEALTHIER • PEOPLE™

NAME ____________________

Weight-for-stature percentiles: Girls

RECORD # ____________

Date	Age	Weight	Stature	Comments

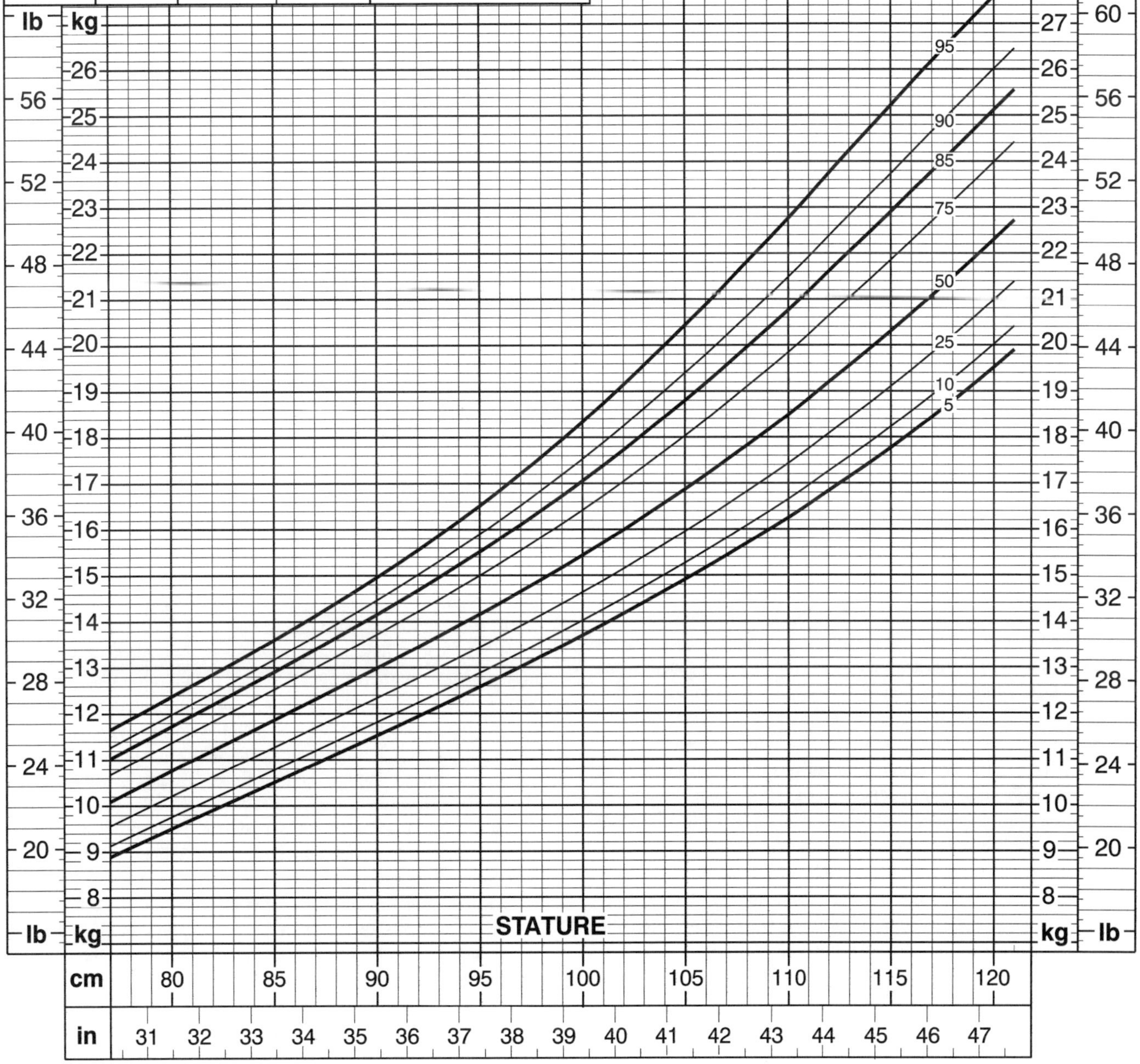

Published May 30, 2000 (modified 10/16/00).
SOURCE: Developed by the National Center for Health Statistics in collaboration with the National Center for Chronic Disease Prevention and Health Promotion (2000).
http://www.cdc.gov/growthcharts

SAFER • HEALTHIER • PEOPLE™

Maria Luisa Forchielli, MD;
Sarah J. Miller, PharmD

2

Nutritional Goals and Requirements

Introduction

Due to nutrition's direct impact on health and disease, nutritional goals and requirements for patients under medical care should be set as clearly as possible. These goals and requirements are constantly revised, following the progressive understanding of the quantitative and qualitative role of nutrients in biological pathways and clinical outcomes. This chapter describes current nutritional goals and requirements in health and disease.

I. Nutritional Goals

A. Nutritional goals are different for different interventional applications. For example, goals of nutrition support for therapeutic aims are often different from goals for prevention of nutrient deficiency, which, in turn, may be different from goals for prevention of chronic disease.

B. Nutrition plays an important role in disease evolution and significantly affects patient response to disease, and consequently outcomes. With regard to the role of nutrition in disease evolution, it is well recognized that

1. Malnutrition and malabsorption of macro- and/or micronutrients contribute to many disease outcomes (malnutrition: cancer, acute and chronic infections, etc; malabsorption: gastrointestinal diseases such as celiac disease or inflammatory bowel disease, hereditary diseases such as cystic fibrosis, etc). For example, survival is typically shorter in cancer patients who have already lost weight prior to beginning chemotherapy.[1] Another example of how malnutrition affects disease outcome is provided by children with Crohn's disease.[2] Malnutrition in these children can contribute to growth failure and delayed sexual maturation.
2. Malnutrition increases both morbidity and mortality. Hospitalized patients are at risk (up to 65%) of developing malnutrition. No major changes in this percentage have been detected over the years.[3,4] The vicious circle of malnutrition and infections has been well documented.

C. Reversal or alteration of disease outcomes is possible through appropriate nutrition support[3,4]:

1. The clinical course of disease may be improved through avoiding or correcting macro- and micronutrient deficiencies. Improvements involve anthropometric parameters and body metabolism.
2. Morbidity and mortality are less likely and the need for hospitalization and further treatments may be reduced, which has implications for cost containment.

D. Benefits from nutritional therapy have been detected in both "healthy" children and children receiving treatments for various diseases either in the hospital or at home. Overall pediatric nutritional goals can be summarized as follows:

1. To avoid limitations in the rate of growth and reverse weight loss or extreme conditions such as failure to thrive. In the presence of a disease, ponderal and/or statural growth are usually affected—the former in acute conditions, both in chronic ones. Proper nutritional intervention allows catch-up growth.[5–7]
2. To maintain positive nitrogen balance, necessary for growth, tissue repair, and subsequent multiorgan functioning. Children are at greater risk than adults of protein wasting because of a proportionally higher basal metabolic rate and protein turnover.[8,9] Children can lose as much as one third of their lean body mass in 3 to 5 days after caloric stores are depleted.[10] Malnutrition can lead to progressive muscle weakness, altered respiratory function, impaired immune response, and other hazards of debilitation, including cellular and mitochondrial impairments.
3. To reduce short- and long-term morbidity (eg, infectious episodes of various origins such as respiratory and intravenous [IV] catheter-related infections or postoperative complications) and mortality. Evidence in this regard exists for both in- and outpatients suffering from different diseases (eg, human immunodeficiency virus, cancer requiring bone marrow transplant).[11,12]
4. To avoid or diminish the rate of long-term disabilities. Cognitive and behavioral development is influenced by adequate nutrition. For instance, extreme situations such as failure to thrive—as well as singular deficiencies regarding iron, iodine, zinc, and so forth—have been associated with poor cognitive and behavioral performances in children of different ages. Energy and nutrients such as polyunsaturated fatty acids (PUFA) are also implicated in cognitive and behavioral performance.[13–15]
5. To reduce costs for the patient and for the health care system. With the advent of home-based nutrition support and the reduction in complication rates, patients tend to have briefer hospitalizations. The choice of nutrition intervention has a profound impact on costs. A report on home nutrition support showed enteral nutrition (EN) to cost, on average, one sixth of home parenteral nutrition (PN) and to halve the hospital admissions/year/patient rate.[16]
6. To improve quality of life. Although difficult to assess and quantify, quality of life appears to be enhanced, especially during home nutrition support. Happiness, activity, sense of freedom, and willingness to socialize were reported to be improved in children on both home EN and PN.[17,18]

E. Goals of nutrition support in adults
   1. The primary goal of nutrition support in adults should be to improve clinical outcome. To achieve this goal, provision of nutrition support is based on two different rationales:
      a) To prevent starvation-induced complications (eg, death, infection). This rationale is indisputable and includes patients who, without nutrition support, would eventually die from starvation because they cannot eat.
      b) To alter favorably the natural history or treatment of a specific disease process.
         (1) This goal is based on correcting nutritional or metabolic deficiencies that arise from a disease or treatment so that outcome will improve.
         (2) The role of nutrition support in this scenario is controversial because improvements in prognostic markers such as serum protein concentrations, nitrogen balance, and weight gain have not consistently been accompanied by clinical benefits.[19–21]
   2. Nutrition therapy should be directed toward a specific objective, with the intent of improving outcome. Depending on the patient's nutritional status and clinical condition, this objective may be as follows:
      a) To diminish the rate of weight loss and body protein turnover. This is the goal in markedly catabolic patients (eg, severely injured patients).
      b) To maintain body weight and lean body mass. This is the goal in patients who cannot eat for indefinite or long periods: patients with certain intestinal disorders (eg, short-bowel syndrome, long-term obstruction), permanent neurologic impairment, or oropharyngeal dysfunction.
      c) To achieve weight gain and anabolism. This is the goal in depleted patients.

II. Overall Nutritional Requirements

A. The human body requires the daily provision of macronutrients (carbohydrates, fats, and proteins) and micronutrients (vitamins and trace elements) along with water and electrolytes. Macronutrients have an energetic and structural-functional role, while micronutrients are vital regulators of cellular, metabolic, or structural components. Nutrient requirements have been established according to age, gender, weight, and/or height.

B. For patients under medical care, nutrients can be delivered enterally and/or parenterally. The enteral route includes the physiological route of ingestion of food by mouth as well as the introduction of nutrients directly into the stomach or duodenum/jejunum by enteric tubes or stoma. Nutritional requirements depend on the patient's health status. Nutritional requirements for healthy people refer specifically to food ingested orally. Those for people using PN are set for people with acute or chronic illness that renders their gastrointestinal tract either nonfunctional or inaccessible. The requirements for healthy people or for people using PN can indirectly be applied to EN, but only partially and with adjustments. Recommendations for the enteral and the parenteral requirements can overlap.

C. Given extreme inter- and intrapersonal variability and difficulties in assessing nutrient requirements in studies on healthy subjects, suggested intakes are reference standards and are continuously revised to reflect advances in knowledge. Requirements have been extensively investigated for energy, protein, and some micronutrients. The list is growing, however, and other nutrients such as specific lipids and fibers are now included. For each nutrient, specific indicators are used to set the requirements.

D. Energy is measured in calories (in the United States) with specific respect to its individual components:
   1. Basal metabolic rate (BMR): the energy necessary to allow normal function at the cellular, organ, and systemic levels, and to maintain homeostasis, body temperature, and heart and respiratory rate when the body is in a fasted state for 12 hours, awake, and in a thermoneutral environment. BMR decreases proportionally with age.[22] Approximately two thirds of BMR is used by the fat-free mass in both adults and children.[23] More specifically, BMR is directly proportional to metabolically active organ mass such as heart, central nervous system, liver, and kidneys in infants and children, and to metabolically active muscle mass in adults.[24] BMR at rest, but not fasted, is called resting energy expenditure (REE). REE and BMR are often used interchangeably, even though the former can be approximately 10% higher than the latter. In young infants, growth may account for as much as 25% to 33% of total energy expenditure.
   2. Thermic effect of food (TEF): the energy required to allow digestion, absorption, and storage of nutrients. TEF is influenced by energy intake, time of delivery, and meal composition for both EN and PN.[25] The highest thermic effect is seen for proteins (protein synthesis from amino acids requires 25% to 57% of their energy content), followed by carbohydrates (glycogen from glucose requires 4%) and lipids (lipids from lipids or glucose require 2% and 28%, respectively).[26] Metabolic response to food (TEF) may account for 5% to 10% of energy expenditure.
   3. Losses: the energy lost in stool and urine.
   4. Activity: the energy required for physical activity. Activity requirements are expressed as percentage increases over BMR requirements. With regard to activity, percentage increases over BMR requirements can range from 5% to 10% of the daily energy expenditure in premature neonates and up to 50% in 8- to 12-year-old children. These values decrease with illnesses and hospitalization. Activity typically represents about a 5% increase over BMR in hospitalized adults but can be much higher.[27]
   5. Growth: the energy cost for new tissue to be generated. It is approximately 5 kcal/g of body weight, ranging from 3 to 6 kcal/g according to type of tissue. Except in young infants, growth represents a very small part of the total energy requirement.[28]
   6. Illness/stress: any amount of energy to overcome other nonphysiologic or "stress" conditions, usually expressed by a BMR correction factor.
   7. The sum of the first five energy components above is called total energy expenditure (TEE). Each component should not be seen as a separate contributor to TEE, as they are all intertwined and subject to wide variability.
   8. The minimum level of energy compatible with health is termed *maintenance energy requirement.*

E. Proteins (nitrogen) are critical for body homeostasis. Appropriate nitrogen and energy intakes along with body metabolism help maintain nitrogen balance. In disease states, due to higher turnover and catabolism of endogenous proteins, this balance may become negative. Although proteins are not one of the two major macronutrients for supplying energy, they can be used for energy when energy intake is insufficient.

F. Lipids are energy dense, facilitate the absorption of fat-soluble vitamins and their precursors, and are structural components of cell membranes and some hormones. They consist of saturated and unsaturated (mono- and polyunsaturated) fatty acids, phospholipids, and cholesterol. Among these, only the PUFA (omega-3 and omega-6) are essential components of the diet, as humans cannot synthesize them. For this reason, dietary reference intakes have been set only for PUFA. For the others, only limitations of daily intakes are available. The recent attention to PUFA is due to their immunomodulatory effects: anti-inflammatory effects in the omega-3 series and pro-inflammatory effects in the omega-6 series, through modulation of different prostaglandins, thromboxanes, leukotrienes, and lipoxins.[29] Other PUFA functions include alteration in membrane fluidity, additional immunomodulatory effects through intracellular signal transduction and changes in gene expression, and modifications of the intestinal bacterial ecosystem due to a hypothesized disruption of the wall membrane.[29] They are also important for development and maintenance of the eye and brain.

G. Fiber requirements have been set because of the recently recognized importance of functional fibers. All fibers are nondigestible carbohydrates, but functional fibers are defined as those that have beneficial physiological effects in humans. These beneficial effects include laxation, improvement in blood lipid concentrations, and reduction in glycemic response. Different functional fibers demonstrate differing effects on these physiological responses.

H. Micronutrient requirements remain largely empirical due to assessment problems and lack of knowledge. Vitamin requirements are better characterized than those of trace elements.

III. Nutritional Requirements for Health and Disease (Enteral and Parenteral Nutrition)

A. Premature infants

1. The goal is to achieve a postnatal growth rate approximating normal fetal intrauterine growth rates (weight, length, and head circumference). This is not usually possible in the first 1 to 2 weeks of life. Growth parameters are routinely plotted on Babson-Benda or Lubchenco growth grids to determine trends. Weight gain should approximate 10–20 g/kg/day for preterm infants After reaching 2.5 kg, daily weight gain is around 20 to 30 g/day. Length and head circumference gains are expected to be between 0.7 and 1 cm/week.[30] The goal is accretion of protein, fat, and minerals approximating normal fetal intrauterine accretion rates.

2. EN and PN requirements are shown in Table 2-1.[31–39]

a) Energy. Actual energy needs are affected by weight, gestational age, postnatal age, gender, environment, feeding regimen and composition, activity, rate of growth, and development. Energy needs increase with fever, cardiac failure, major surgery, severe sepsis, long-term growth failure, protein-calorie malnutrition, and chronic lung disease (bronchopulmonary dysplasia [BPD]). Energy intake below or above requirements may lead to growth retardation or excessive fat accumulation, respectively.

(1) EN. The energy requirement for premature infants is approximately 120 kcal/kg/day (50 kcal/kg for maintenance plus 70 kcal/kg for a daily weight gain of 15 g/kg), with a range of 105 to 130 kcal/kg/day. Most energy components are extrapolated from the norm to provide adequate energy for catch-up growth, high energy costs of thermoregulation and body functions, and inefficient utilization of ingested nutrients.

(2) PN. Because energy is not required for digestion, there are no absorptive losses, activity is limited, and cold stress is reduced, energy requirements for PN are lower than for EN. After the first 2 weeks of life, energy intake of 90 to 120 kcal/kg/day promotes weight gains approximating the intrauterine growth rate. Greater weight gains associated with greater energy intakes are thought to reflect fat deposition.[35] In conditions such as BPD, 150 kcal/kg/day may be required. Both carbohydrate and fat are provided as energy sources to provide a balanced PN formulation. Provision of fat in addition to carbohydrate for energy decreases the volume needed for the PN formulation, decreases the respiratory quotient, may help avoid fatty infiltration of the liver, and prevents deficiency of essential fatty acids.

b) Protein. The protein requirement varies according to body weight and is highest in the most immature infants. Provision of amino acids is necessary to reverse the 1% daily loss of endogenous protein stores by premature infants. The protein loss begins the first day after birth. Clinical conditions including surgery, necrotizing enterocolitis, sepsis, and BPD may increase protein requirements.

(1) Net protein utilization depends on energy intake. Protein utilization ensures growth and minimizes complications. High rates of protein utilization (protein not used exclusively as an energy source) are achieved with 150 to 200 nonprotein kcal per g of nitrogen (24–32 nonnitrogen kcal per g of protein). If energy intake is deficient (<150 nonprotein kcal per g of nitrogen), endogenous proteins are oxidized to produce the needed energy and nitrogen balance becomes negative. If protein intake is suboptimal, increasing energy intake will spare protein for lean tissue gain, but only up to a certain level. Above this level, protein gain plateaus.

(2) Conditionally essential amino acids for preterm infants include tyrosine, cysteine, and taurine in addition to the other amino acids essential for term infants.

(3) EN. The protein requirement for appropriate growth in premature infants is estimated at 2.5 to 4 g/kg/day, which is primarily devoted to preserving or depositing lean body mass. Excessive protein administration (>6 g/kg/day) has been associated with adverse effects, including azotemia, pyrexia, and lower IQ scores. Inadequate (<2.5 g/kg/day) protein intake is associated with slow growth and decreased nitrogen retention.[31]

(a) Human milk varies with stage of lactation. Early milk is 60% to 90% whey protein and 10% to 40% casein. Within 1 to 2 weeks, the ratio becomes closer to 50:50.

(b) Formulas designed for premature infants or fortified human milk are required to provide adequate protein. Standard infant formulas do not provide adequate protein.

(4) PN. The protein requirement to approximate intrauterine nitrogen accretion is estimated at 3 to 4 g/kg/day, with a minimum concomitant delivery of 60 to 90 nonprotein kcal/kg/day. Azotemia may result from administration of >4 g/kg/day in low birth weight infants. Current practice is to initiate amino acids just after birth at variable doses of 1 to 3 g/kg/day. Doing so could decrease subsequent protein requirements for catch-up growth. The target for normalization of plasma amino acids during PN is generally set at the postprandial amino acid concentrations for the term breast-fed infant. For this reason, specific amino acid formulations have been designed with the addition of taurine, glutamate, aspartate, and cysteine; the reduction

TABLE 2-1. Guidelines for Daily Nutrient Intakes of Enterally or Parenterally Fed Preterm Infants[31–39]

Nutrient	Unit measurement	Suggested enteral intake	Suggested parenteral intake
Fluid	mL/kg/day	120–200	100–150
Energy	kcal/kg/day	105–130	90–120
Protein	g/kg/day	2.5–4	3–4
Carbohydrate		40%–50% total energy	6–15 mg/kg/minute
Fat		40%–55% total energy	
	g/kg/day	5–7	1–3
Minerals			
Calcium	mg/kg/day	100–220	40-80
Phosphorus	mg/kg/day	60–140	31-62
Magnesium	mg/kg/day	8–15	3.6-6
Iron	mg/kg/day	2–4	—
Sodium	mEq/kg/day	2–7	2–5
Potassium	mEq/kg/day	2–3	2–4
Chloride	mEq/kg/day	2–7	As needed to maintain acid-base balance
Zinc	mcg/kg/day	600–3000	400
Copper	mcg/kg/day	110–160	20
Iodine	mcg/kg/day	30–60	1
Selenium	mcg/kg/day	1.3–4.5	1.5-2
Chromium	mcg/kg/day	0.1–2.25	0.05-0.2
Molybdenum	mcg/kg/day	0.3	0.25
Manganese	mcg/kg/day	0.75–7.5	1
Vitamins			
Vitamin A*	IU/kg/day	700–1500	1643; max 2300 IU/day (500 mcg/kg/day, max 700 mcg/day)
Vitamin D**	IU/day	400	160; max 400 IU/day (4 mcg/day; max 10 mcg/day
Vitamin E***	IU/day	6–12	2.8; max 7 IU/day (2.8 mg; max 7 mg/day)
Vitamin K	mcg/kg/day	8–10	80; max 200 mcg/day
Thiamine	mcg/kg/day	180–240	350; max 1200 mcg/day
Riboflavin	mcg/kg/day	250–360	150; max 1400 mcg/day
Niacin	mg/kg/day	3.6–4.8	6.8; max 17 mg/day
B_6	mcg/kg/day	150–210	180; max 1000/day
B_{12}	mcg/kg/day	0.30	300; max 1000/day
Folic acid	mcg/kg/day	25–50	56; max 140/day
Biotin	mcg/kg/day	3.6–6	6; max 20/day
Pantothenic acid	mg/kg/day	1.2–1.7	2; max 5/day
Vitamin C	mg/kg/day	18–24	25; max 80/day
Carnitine	mg/kg/day	—	10–30

*Vitamin A (retinol) 0.3 mcg = 1 IU.
**Vitamin D 0.025 mcg = 1 IU.
***Vitamin E 1 mg = 1 IU.
The following conversion factors apply to: Ca 40 mg=1 mmol=2 mEq; P 31 mg=1 mmol; Mg 24 mg=1 mmol=2 mEq; Na 23 mg=1 mmol= 1 mEq; K 39 mg=1 mmol= 1 mEq; Cl 35 mg=1 mmol= 1 mEq.

of methionine, glycine, and alanine; and an increase of arginine and leucine. The N-acetyl-L-tyrosine salt is a more soluble form of tyrosine. Cysteine, along with glutamine and glycine, is a precursor of glutathione. These formulations have been demonstrated to improve weight gain, nitrogen balance, and mineral solubility.

c) Carbohydrate. Carbohydrate delivery is recommended to be 40% to 50% of the total caloric intake. Infants with chronic lung diseases benefit from as little as 35% of energy as carbohydrates.
   (1) EN. The carbohydrate composition of preterm infant formulas is generally equally divided between lactose and glucose polymers.
      (a) Glucose polymers may be digested more effectively than lactose by premature infants early in life.
      (b) Glucose polymers contribute fewer osmotic particles to formula than do individual glucose molecules.
      (c) Lactose appears to lower intestinal pH, facilitating absorption of some minerals (eg, calcium) and development of normal flora.
      (d) Functional fibers or prebiotics such as galactooligosaccharide and oligofructose may improve the intestinal ecosystem (development of beneficial flora such as *Lactobacillus* and *Bifidobacterium,* change in pH, enterocyte and immune system maturation). Oligosaccharides are present in breast milk but not current North American formulas.
   (2) PN. Carbohydrate is provided as dextrose (D-glucose) in the monohydrate form at 3.4 kcal/g. Dextrose is the major contributor to the osmolarity of the PN formulation.
      (a) Current practice is to initiate glucose approximating the rate of endogenous glucose production (6 mg/kg/minute for infants weighing <1000 g; 8 mg/kg/minute for infants weighing >1000 g) with stepwise advancements of 1 to 2 mg/kg/minute to a maximum of 15 mg/kg/minute to optimize glucose tolerance. Serum and urine glucose monitoring provides an indication of acute intolerance reflected as hyperosmolarity and osmotic diuresis. Glucose delivery of >26 mg/kg/minute may result in fatty infiltration of the liver.
      (b) Nonprotein calories need to be balanced between glucose and fat. Glucose without fat increases water retention and may thereby worsen existing respiratory compromise. Glucose alone may exacerbate fatty infiltration of the liver.

d) Lipids. Fat delivery is recommended to be at 40% to 55% of total calories. The essential fatty acid requirement is estimated at approximately 3–12% of total calories.
   (1) EN. The lipid requirement is 4.5 to 6 g/100 kcal, or 5 to 7 g/kg/day.
      (a) The recommended omega-6 (C18:2ω-6) to omega-3 (C18:3ω-3) ratio ranges from 5:1 to 15:1, while the ratio of their derivatives, docosahexaenoic acid (DHA) (C22:6ω-3) to arachidonic acid (ARA)(C20:4ω-6), ranges from 1:1 to 1:2.7. Inclusion of one international unit of vitamin E per g of linoleic acid will prevent peroxidation of unsaturated lipids in food and tissues. PUFA content has been revised in some formulas to include DHA and ARA.
      (b) Premature infants (especially if <34 weeks of gestational age) may absorb and use medium-chain triglycerides (MCT) more effectively than long-chain ones, because their concentration of bile salts is low. Formulas for premature infants include both MCT and long-chain triglycerides in various concentrations. The European Society for Pediatric Gastroenterology, Hepatology and Nutrition (ESPGHAN) has recommended limiting the amounts of MCT to <40% of total calories in preterm formula.[40] MCT do not provide essential fatty acids and do not promote the absorption of minerals. Therefore, essential fatty acids and fat-soluble vitamins have to be supplied when formulas with high MCT content (>80%) are used.
   (2) PN. Lipids are provided as IV fat emulsions (IVFE) (see Chapter 7) at a dose of 1 to 3 g/kg/day (30%–60% of nonprotein calories when full calories are administered). Lipids should be provided from the first day of life, because premature infants do not have essential fatty acid stores. Serum triglycerides should be monitored, with values <200 mg/dL considered acceptable. A continuous infusion and 20% IVFE promote optimal metabolic tolerance. No adverse effects have been observed in terms of lung dysfunction.

e) Fluids. Fluid requirements are generally higher for EN than PN and should take into account the following points:
   (1) Diuresis during the first 1 to 2 weeks of life results in a 5% to 15% weight loss in premature infants. Fluids must be adjusted accordingly, based on urine parameters (maintenance of specific gravity between 1.010 and 1.016 g/mL, flow 2–3 mL/kg/hour by day 3 and up to 6 mL/kg/hour later, osmolality 200–400 mOsm/kg of water) and normal serum sodium values.
   (2) Higher fluid intake may be required to meet energy needs after 2 weeks of life. Tolerance to increased fluids depends on the clinical condition (eg, BPD and patent ductus arteriosus are exacerbated by excessive fluid intake). Premature infants are susceptible to both dehydration and fluid overload.
   (3) The infant's environment and other factors directly affect fluid requirements. Examples that increase requirements are exposure to radiant warmers, phototherapy, fluid losses (diarrhea, glycosuria), or respiratory distress. Examples that decrease requirements are oliguria and conditions of neutral thermal range or high ambient humidity.
   (4) EN. Ranges are 120 to 200 mL/kg/day or 100 to 160 mL/100 kcal. Infants weighing <1000 g preferably require 150 to 200 mL/kg/day. Infants weighing >1000 g require 120 to 150 mL/kg/day.
   (5) PN. Infants weighing <1000 g require 150 mL/kg/day; infants weighing >1000 g require 100 to 150 mL/kg/day. Some infants require >150 mL/kg/day, depending on their environmental situation.

f) Vitamin, mineral, and trace element recommendations for EN and PN have been developed for premature infants (Table 2-1).[31–39] PN requirements are generally lower than EN requirements.
   (1) Vitamins. Preterm infants do not have fat-soluble vitamin reserves at birth. Requirements may change based on the quality and quantity of nutrient intake.
      (a) EN. In general, specific formulas and fortified breast milk supply adequate amounts. Most water-soluble

vitamins are affected by macronutrient intake and exposure to environmental factors. For instance, exposure to light or phototherapy destroys riboflavin.

(b) PN. A preterm parenteral multivitamin preparation has not yet been developed. Current practice is to use 2 mL/kg/day of a pediatric multivitamin to a maximum of 5 mL/day. The American Society for Clinical Nutrition recommends intakes of 500 mcg/kg/day vitamin A and approximately 3 mg/kg/day of vitamin E, and these should be started just after birth.[37] When other intakes are compared with estimates, at the current doses, water-soluble vitamins largely cover the recommended needs. Ascorbic acid and riboflavin are given in excess.

(2) Minerals. Premature infants require higher calcium, phosphorus, and magnesium intakes than do term infants to promote intrauterine accretion rates and to prevent osteopenia. An infant in utero accrues 75% of its total body calcium from gestation weeks 24 to 40. Drugs such as corticosteroids, furosemide, theophylline, and caffeine cause calcium loss. Due to high urinary sodium losses during the first 3 weeks of life, premature infants require more sodium. Therefore, 5 to 7 mEq/kg/day of sodium are recommended in infants <32 weeks gestational age, while 3 to 5 mEq/kg/day are more appropriate for less premature infants. After that critical time and upon stabilization and growth, premature infants require 2 to 4 mEq/kg/day of sodium along with equal amounts of chloride and potassium. Some of the anion is commonly provided as acetate to decrease the likelihood of metabolic acidosis.

(a) EN. The following points are emphasized:

i) Mineral bioavailability averages 60% for calcium, 70% for phosphorus, and 50% for magnesium. Mineral absorption is improved with the addition of MCT, lactose, enrichment with vitamin D and minerals, and appropriate quantity of calcium and phosphorus.

ii) Standard infant formulas and unfortified human milk do not provide enough calcium and phosphorus to meet the mineral needs of preterm infants. Fortified human milk or formulas specifically designed for premature infants provide higher calcium and phosphorus delivery and appropriate amounts of sodium, potassium, and chloride (see Chapter 4).

iii) Preterm infants require more iron. Iron requirements are between 2 and 4 mg/kg/day, to be started within 2 months of age or at doubling of weight. Iron absorption is enhanced in premature infants. Formulas specifically for premature infants are iron fortified (see Chapter 4).

(b) PN. Specific IV recommendations are as follows: A calcium-phosphorus ratio of 1.3:1 (≥1:1 molar) replicates the fetal mineral accretion ratio and allows for the highest retention of both minerals, provided they are supplied together and daily. Addition of calcium and phosphorus to PN is limited by solubility (see Chapter 7). Cysteine HCl increases calcium/phosphorus solubility. It is frequently impossible to provide adequate amounts of these minerals for prevention of osteopenia in infants requiring long-term PN. Long-term diuretic use or aluminum contamination of the components of PN formulations may further deplete calcium reserves. At birth, the magnesium level is elevated and, upon its normalization, IV supplementation can start.

(3) Trace elements. Zinc and copper are required for growth. Deficiencies of zinc (alteration of the intestine, skin, immunity, and growth) and copper (hypochromic anemia, osteoporosis, and neutropenia) can occur. Zinc requirements may increase in infants with high stool output, gastrointestinal fluid losses, or renal failure.

(a) EN. Zinc and copper have a limited absorption rate: 36% and 60% from fortified human milk and preterm formula for zinc, and 10% to 30% for copper. They exhibit competition for absorption and may be involved in drug-nutrient interactions. Recommendations for zinc are 600 to 1500 (up to 3000) mcg/kg/day and for copper 110 to 160 mcg/kg/day.

(b) PN. Copper and manganese need to be omitted in the presence of cholestasis as indicated by direct bilirubin > 2 mg/dL. Selenium, chromium, and molybdenum need to be omitted in infants with renal dysfunction.

g) Other. Carnitine: Premature infants receiving exclusively PN need carnitine to allow fat oxidation at the mitochondria. Estimates range from 10 and 20, with supplementation up to 30 mg/kg/day without risk of side effects.

B. From infancy to adolescence

1. The child's age-specific regular growth and development are the final tests of nutritional needs. Appetite and self-selection usually result in adequate nutrient intake for the normal, healthy child. When illness or physical disability prevent adequate nutrient intake, requirements must be artificially determined considering the disease factor involved. In this case, ongoing reassessments of many nutrients are essential, especially for energy expenditure. For healthy children and adults, a joint committee of the governments of Canada and the United States, after reassessing the previous recommended dietary allowances (RDAs) plus the qualities of subsequent studies, has developed dietary reference intakes (DRI) (full reports are available at www.nap.edu). DRI define the levels of nutrient intake that are necessary to achieve good health and avoid adverse effects. These levels, obtained after selecting specific indicators, are age-specific and identify first and second semesters (0–6 months and 7–12 months) of life, infants, toddlers, children, and adolescents. No similar age-specific nutritional recommendations are available for sick children nourished either enterally or parenterally. DRI include the RDA plus three other reference values[41,42]:

a) Adequate intake (AI): the usual intake at or above which there is a low probability of inadequacy (replaces RDA when RDA cannot be determined)

b) Tolerable upper level (UL): the average daily nutrient intake level above which adverse effects may arise

c) Estimated average requirement (EAR): the average daily nutrient intake level that meets the requirements of half the healthy individuals of a specific age and gender

2. Energy needs. Pediatric energy needs originate from maintenance, activity, and growth. Each component is subject to age variability because maintenance progressively declines from birth to adolescence, activity increases during childhood, and growth has two major spikes during infancy and adolescence.

TABLE 2-2. Criteria and Dietary Reference Intake Values for Energy by Active Individuals by Life Stage Group*[43]

Life stage group	Active PAL EER (kcal/day) Criterion	Male	Female
0–6 mos	Energy expenditure plus energy deposition	570	520 (3 mos)
7–12 mos	"	743	676 (9 mos)
1–2 yrs	"	1046	992 (24mos)
3–8 yrs	"	1742	1642 (6 yrs)
9–13 yrs	"	2279	2071 (11 yrs)
14–18 yrs	"	3152	2368 (16 yrs)

EER = estimated energy requirement; PAL = physical activity level.
*For healthy, moderately active Americans and Canadians.
Printed with permission from the Institute of Medicine. *Dietary Reference Intakes for Energy, Carbohydrate, Fiber, Fat, Fatty Acids, Cholesterol, Protein, and Amino Acids (Macronutrients).* Washington, DC: National Academy Press; 2002.

TABLE 2-3. Equations for Predicting REE from Body Weight[45]

Sex and age range (yrs)	Equation to derive REE (kcal/day)
Male	
0–< 3	(60.9 x wt) – 54
3–<10	(22.7 x wt) + 495
10–18	(17.5 x wt) + 651
Female	
0–< 3	(61 x wt) – 51
3–<10	(22.5 x wt) + 499
10–18	(12.2 x wt) + 746

REE, resting energy expenditure; wt = weight in kilograms.
Printed with permission from World Health Organization. Energy and Protein Requirements Technical Report Series, No 724. Geneva, Switzerland: World Health Organization; 1985.

a) EN
(1) Energy needs for healthy infants/children/adolescents. The estimated requirement is defined as the average dietary energy intake that is predicted to maintain energy balance in healthy individuals of a defined age, gender, weight, height, level of physical activity, and deposition of new tissues. Physical activity is classified into four levels (sedentary, low active, active, and very active) with different coefficients. The activity-level coefficient is approximately 1.25 to 1.4. Estimates have been extrapolated from reported energy intakes and body mass index data, factorial approaches, and measurements of energy expenditure by double-labeled water. Table 2-2 summarizes the recommended energy intake.[43]
(2) Energy needs for stressed infants/children/adolescents. See PN section.

b) PN
(1) In the presence of illness or disability, DRI may not apply secondary to decrease in activity or growth or change in thermic effect of food. Energy expenditure may shift from growth to the needs of acute illness.[44]
(2) The starting point for the estimation of an individual's energy expenditure is the BMR or the REE. Approaches for estimating BMR or REE differ according to the number of variables included (eg, age, sex, weight, height.) The World Health Organization equations are two examples of energy expenditure estimates based on weight, age, and/or sex (see Tables 2-3 and 2-4).[45–47]

TABLE 2-4. Basal Metabolic Rate Requirement in kcal/Day Based on Body Weight[46,47]

Kg	Male	Female	Kg	Male	Female	Kg	Male	Female	Kg	Male	Female
3	150 (120*)	136 (144*)	16	750	747	38	1305	1207	62	1660	1572
4	210 (191*)	205 (191*)	17	780	775	40	1340	1241	64	1690	1599
5	270	274	18	810	802	42	1370	1274	66	1725	1626
6	330	336	19	840	827	44	1400	1306	68	1765	1653
7	390	395	20	870	852	46	1430	1338	70	1785	1679
8	445	448	22	910	898	48	1460	1369	72	1815	1705
9	495	496	24	980	942	50	1485	1399	74	1845	1731
10	545	541	26	1070	984	52	1505	1429	76	1870	1756
11	590	582	28	1100	1025	54	1555	1458	78	1900	1781
12	625	620	30	1140	1063	56	1580	1487	80	1935	1805
13	665	655	32	1190	1101	58	1600	1516	82	1970	1830
14	700	687	34	1230	1137	60	1630	1544	84	2000	1855
15	725	718	36	1270	1173						

*From reference 46. These values differ from those in reference 47. Printed with permission from World Health Organization. Energy and Protein Requirements Technical Report Series, No 522. Geneva, Switzerland: World Health Organization; 1973.

TABLE 2-5. Daily Energy Requirements for Pediatric Patients on Parenteral Nutrition[38]

Age	kcal/kg
<6 mos	85–105
6–12 mos	80–100
>1–7 yrs	75–90
>7–12 yrs	50–75
>12–18 yrs	30–50

Reprinted from Task Force for the Revision of Safe Practices for Parenteral Nutrition. Safe practices for parenteral nutrition. J Parenter Enteral Nutr. 2004;28:S39–S70, with permission from A.S.P.E.N.

(3) Illness tends to decrease activity but may increase energy expenditure. Therefore, estimates of BMR or REE (Tables 2-3 and 2-4) must be corrected by a factor of 0.7 for starvation, 1 to 1.2 for minimal stress, 1.2 to 1.5 for moderate stress, and 1.5 to 2 for severe stress.

(4) Indirect calorimetry may be used to determine the actual energy expenditure of a specific child with greater accuracy. Measurements of resting metabolic expenditure can be adjusted for activity and other factors as needed. This determination may help to reduce the likelihood of under- or overfeeding. See Chapter 22.

(5) Energy estimates for pediatric patients on PN are provided by A.S.P.E.N. (Table 2-5).[38] Regardless of the energy recommendations used, calorie distribution among lipids, carbohydrates, and proteins should be carefully prescribed.

3. Protein needs
   a) EN
      (1) Healthy infants/children/adolescents. DRI values may be used to determine protein needs. Acceptable protein intake should range between 10% and 20% of total calories. These values are based on a combination of intake, growth, nitrogen accretion, and nitrogen balance data. AI (or RDA) and EAR are also provided (Table 2-6).[43]
      (2) Stressed infants/children/adolescents. See PN section.
   b) PN
      (1) In the stressed child, protein requirements are increased. Rates of catabolism and synthesis of proteins are higher. Protein recommendations are listed in Table 2-7.[38]
      (2) Provision of approximately 12% to 16% of calories as protein minimizes negative nitrogen balance.
      (3) To maximize protein utilization and avoid gluconeogenesis, appropriate calorie distribution and intake are essential. A nonprotein calorie-to-nitrogen ratio of 150:1 to 300:1 is most likely to achieve positive nitrogen balance. The ratio should be determined based on age, metabolic stress, nutritional intake and status, and ongoing losses.
      (4) 1 g/kg/day daily advances in protein intake are suggested, after starting at an initial rate of 0.5 g/kg/day.
      (5) All formulations contain crystalline amino acids.
         (a) Children under 1 year of age have special amino acid requirements, and therefore the IV formulations used are as discussed under the PN section for premature infants. In patients older than 1 year, adult formulations can be used. These formulations are designed to

TABLE 2-6. Criteria and Dietary Reference Intake Values for Protein by Life Stage Group[43]

		AI or RDA for Reference Individual (g/day)		EAR (g/kg/day)		RDA (g/kg/day)			
Life stage group	Criteria	Male	Female	Male	Female	Male	Female	AI (g/kg/day)	AMDR %
0–6 mos	Average consumption of protein from human milk	9.1 (AI)	9.1 (AI)					1.52	ND
7–12 mos	Nitrogen equilibrium + protein deposition	13.5 (AI)	13.5 (AI)	1.10	1.10	1.50	1.50		ND
1–3 yrs	"	13.0	13.0	0.88	0.88	1.10	1.10		5–20
4–8 yrs	"	19.0	19.0	0.76	0.76	0.95	0.95		10–30
9–13 yrs	"	34.0	34.0	0.76	0.76	0.95	0.95		10–30
14–18 yrs	"	52.0	46.0	0.73	0.71	0.85	0.85		10–30
>18 yrs	Nitrogen equilibrium	56.0	46.0	0.66	0.66	0.80	0.80		10–35

AI, adequate intake (the observed average or experimentally determined intake by a defined population or subgroup that appears to sustain a defined nutritional status, such as growth rate, normal circulatory nutrient values, or other functional indicators of health; used if sufficient scientific evidence is not available to derive an EAR; for healthy infants receiving human milk, the AI is the mean intake; not equivalent to an RDA); AMDR, acceptable macronutrient distribution range (the intake for a particular energy source associated with a reduced risk of chronic disease while providing intakes of essential nutrients); EAR, estimated average requirement (the intake that meets the estimated nutrient needs of half of the individuals in a group); ND, not determinable; RDA, recommended dietary allowance (the intake that meets the nutrient need of almost all [97%–98%] individuals in a group).

Printed with permission from Institute of Medicine. *Dietary Reference Intakes for Energy, Carbohydrate, Fiber, Fat, Fatty Acids, Cholesterol, Protein, and Amino Acids (Macronutrients).* Washington, DC: National Academy Press; 2002.

TABLE 2-7. Daily Protein Requirements for Children on Parenteral Nutrition with Normal Organ Function[38]

Age	g/kg
Neonates	3–4
Infants (1-12 months)	2–3
Children (above 10 kg or 1 through 10 years)	1–2
Adolescents (11 through 17 years)	0.8–1.5

Reprinted from Task Force for the Revision of Safe Practices for Parenteral Nutrition. Safe practices for parenteral nutrition. *J Parenter Enteral Nutr.* 2004;28:S39–S70 with permission from A.S.P.E.N.

meet the amino acid requirements of orally fed adults and contain high levels of methionine, glycine, and phenylalanine and low levels of branched-chain amino acids, cysteine, and tyrosine.

(b) Glutamine, a primary fuel for intestinal mucosa and immune cells and precursor for nucleotide synthesis and the antioxidant glutathione, seems to improve nitrogen balance, gut barrier functions, and mortality and morbidity in selected patients. Limited stability in PN still limits its use in the United States.

4. Carbohydrate. Without carbohydrate in the diet, lipolysis, limited ketone accumulation, and transient protein breakdown may occur. Fifty to 100 g per day of carbohydrate usually prevents or minimizes these effects.
   a) EN. The subcommittee on the 10th edition of the RDA recommended that beyond infancy, greater than 50% of energy needs be given as carbohydrate to limit fat and possibly protein intake in the diet.[41] The acceptable carbohydrate intake as a percentage of energy should be 45% to 65% of total calories in all age groups. EAR for carbohydrates has been established only for older adolescents and adults, based on the average amount of glucose used by the brain. Pediatric data have been extrapolated from adults (Table 2-8).[43]
   b) PN. Carbohydrates should comprise 40% to 60% of the total caloric intake. Dextrose monohydrate is used as the major source of energy in PN and contributes to PN osmolality. Glucose infusion rates of 5 to 13 mg/kg/minute are generally tolerated. Above 14 mg/kg/minute, complications such as liver fatty infiltration, hypertriglyceridemia, hyperglycemia, and excessive carbon dioxide production may occur. In general, the infusion rate usually starts at 5 to 7 mg/kg/minute and advances daily by 2 to 4 mg/kg/minute.
5. Fat. Fat requirements range from 25% to 55% of total calories, with a minimum requirement of 3% to 4% of calories as essential fatty acids (1%–3% as linoleic and close to 1% as linolenic acid).
   a) EN. Fat does not have DRI values, with few exceptions (AI for infants of 31 g/day in the age range 0–6 months and 30 g/day from 7–12 months, obtained from average consumption data of total fat from human milk). More detailed recommendations are available for the essential PUFA (Table 2-9).[43] The American Academy of Pediatrics Committee on Nutrition and the National Cholesterol Education Program have agreed that fat and cholesterol should not be restricted in children less than 2 years of age. In children over 2 years of age, the American Academy of Pediatrics recommends 30% of calories from fat, with less than 10% from saturated fat, and less than 300 mg of cholesterol daily. Acceptable enteral fat intake as a percentage of energy is 25% to 30% (up to 55% in infants).

TABLE 2-8. Criteria and Dietary Reference Intake Values for Carbohydrate by Life Stage Group[43]

		EAR (g/day)		RDA (g/day)			
Life stage group	Criteria	Male	Female	Male	Female	AI (g/day)	AMDR %
0–6 mos	Average content of human milk					60	ND
7–12 mos	Average intake from human milk plus complementary foods					95	ND
1–3 yrs	Extrapolation from adult data	100	100	130	130		45–65
4–8 yrs	Extrapolation from adult data	100	100	130	130		45–65
9–13 yrs	Extrapolation from adult data	100	100	130	130		45–65
14–18 yrs	Extrapolation from adult data	100	100	130	130		45–65
>18 yrs	Brain glucose use	100	100	130	130		45–65

AI, adequate intake (the observed average or experimentally determined intake by a defined population or subgroup that appears to sustain a defined nutritional status, such as growth rate, normal circulatory nutrient values, or other functional indicators of health; used if sufficient scientific evidence is not available to derive an EAR; for healthy infants receiving human milk, the AI is the mean intake; not equivalent to an RDA); AMDR, acceptable macronutrient distribution range (the intake for a particular energy source associated with a reduced risk of chronic disease while providing intakes of essential nutrients; reflects the source of kcal to maintain body weight); EAR, estimated average requirement (the intake that meets the estimated nutrient needs of half of the individuals in a group); ND, not determinable; RDA, recommended dietary allowance (the intake that meets the nutrient need of almost all [97%–98%] individuals in a group).

Printed with permission from Institute of Medicine. *Dietary Reference Intakes for Energy, Carbohydrate, Fiber, Fat, Fatty Acids, Cholesterol, Protein, and Amino Acids (Macronutrients).* Washington, DC: National Academy Press; 2002.

TABLE 2-9. Criteria and Dietary Reference Intake Values for PUFA by Life Stage Group[43]

		Linoleic Acid			Linolenic Acid		
		AI (g/day)		AMDR	AI (g/day)		AMDR
Life stage group	Criteria	Male	Female	%	Male	Female	%
0–6 mos	Average consumption of total fat from human milk	4.4	4.4	ND	0.5	0.5	ND
7–12 mos	Average consumption of total fat from human milk and complementary foods	4.6	4.6	ND	0.5	0.5	ND
1–3 yrs	Median intake of specific PUFA from CSFII	7.0	7.0	5–10	0.7	0.7	0.6–1.2
4–8 yrs	Median intake of specific PUFA from CSFII	10.0	10.0	5–10	0.9	0.9	0.6–1.2
9–13 yrs	Median intake of specific PUFA from CSFII	12.0	10.0	5–10	1.2	1.0	0.6–1.2
14–18 yrs	Median intake of specific PUFA from CSFII	16.0	11.0	5–10	1.6	1.1	0.6–1.2

AI, adequate intake (the observed average or experimentally determined intake by a defined population or subgroup that appears to sustain a defined nutritional status, such as growth rate, normal circulatory nutrient values, or other functional indicators of health; used if sufficient scientific evidence is not available to derive an EAR; for healthy infants receiving human milk, the AI is the mean intake; not equivalent to an RDA); AMDR, acceptable macronutrient distribution range (the intake for a particular energy source associated with a reduced risk of chronic disease while providing intakes of essential nutrients; reflects the source of kcal to maintain body weight); CSFII, Continuing Survey of Food Intake by Individuals; ND, not determinable; PUFA, polyunsaturated fatty acids.

Printed with permission from Institute of Medicine. *Dietary Reference Intakes for Energy, Carbohydrate, Fiber, Fat, Fatty Acids, Cholesterol, Protein, and Amino Acids (Macronutrients).* Washington, DC: National Academy Press; 2002.

b) PN

(1) High glucose loads expose the patient to fatty liver infiltration and possibly metabolic and respiratory stresses. The minimum fat requirement is determined by essential fatty acid need, and the daily maximum is 50% to 60% of energy. Fats provide concentrated energy and decrease IV osmolality. Fat emulsion infusion rate starts at 1 g/kg/day with increments of 0.5 to 1 g/kg/day. A 20% fat emulsion supplies 2 kcal/mL. Continuous infusions are better tolerated.

(2) Fat emulsion formulations come from soybean oil, safflower oil, or both, with different long-chain fatty acid (LCFA) content. The combination of MCT with LCFA formulations are under investigation. MCT are better hydrolyzed, with less storage in the body.

6. Fiber. AI estimates are available exclusively for EN. Recommendations are shown in Table 2-10.[43]

7. Vitamins and minerals

a) EN

(1) The DRI provide recommendations based on dietary intakes, a factorial approach of nutrient retention, and estimates of physiological needs extrapolated from previous studies in adults or children (see Tables 2-11 and 2-12).[42,48–50] Upper Levels are also available for most vitamins and minerals. Requirements are usually met by eating a variety of foods. The nutrient content of enteral formulations mirrors these recommendations.

(2) Administration of vitamin K to newborn infants is recommended for the prevention of hemorrhagic disease. Breastfed or formula-fed infants receive one intramuscular dose of 0.5 to 1.0 mg at birth or later, or multiple oral doses of 1.0 to 2.0 mg.

TABLE 2-10. Criteria and Dietary Reference Intake Values for Total Fiber by Life Stage Group[43]

		AI (g/day)	
Life stage group	Criteria	Male	Female
0–6 mos	—	ND	ND
7–12 mos	—	ND	ND
1–3 yrs	Intake level shown to provide the greatest protection against coronary heart disease (14 g/1000 kcal of required energy) ? median energy intake level (kcal/1000 kcal/day)	19	19
4–8 yrs	"	25	25
9–13 yrs	"	31	26
14–18 yrs	"	38	26
19–50 yrs	"	38	25
>51 yrs	"	30	21

AI, adequate intake (the observed average or experimentally determined intake by a defined population or subgroup that appears to sustain a defined nutritional status, such as growth rate, normal circulatory nutrient values, or other functional indicators of health; used if sufficient scientific evidence is not available to derive an EAR; for healthy infants receiving human milk, the AI is the mean intake; not equivalent to an RDA); ND, not determinable.

Printed with permission from Institute of Medicine. *Dietary Reference Intakes for Energy, Carbohydrate, Fiber, Fat, Fatty Acids, Cholesterol, Protein, and Amino Acids (Macronutrients).* Washington, DC: National Academy Press; 2002.

TABLE 2-11. Dietary Reference Intakes (DRIs): Recommended Intakes for Individuals, Vitamins
Food and Nutrition Board, Institute of Medicine, National Academies

Life stage group	Vit A (μg/d)[a]	Vit C (mg/d)	Vit D (μg/d)[b,c]	Vit E (mg/d)[d]	Vit K (μg/d)	Thia- (mg/d)	Ribo- (mg/d)	Niacin (mg/d)[e]	Vit B_6 (mg/d)	Folate (μg/d)[f]	Vit B_{12} (μg/d)	Panto-thenic acid (mg/d)	Biotin (μg/d)	Choline (mg/d)[g]
Infants														
0–6 mo	400*	40*	5*	4*	2.0*	0.2*	0.3*	2*	0.1*	65*	0.4*	1.7*	5*	125*
7–12 mo	500*	50*	5*	5*	2.5*	0.3*	0.4*	4*	0.3*	80*	0.5*	1.8*	6*	150*
Children														
1–3 y	**300**	**15**	5*	**6**	30.0*	**0.5**	**0.5**	**6**	**0.5**	**150**	**0.9**	2*	8*	200*
4–8 y	**400**	**25**	5*	**7**	55.0*	**0.6**	**0.6**	**8**	**0.6**	**200**	**1.2**	3*	12*	250*
Males														
9–13 y	**600**	**45**	5*	**11**	60.0*	**0.9**	**0.9**	**12**	**1.0**	**300**	**1.8**	4*	20*	375*
14–18 y	**900**	**75**	5*	**15**	75.0*	**1.2**	**1.3**	**16**	**1.3**	**400**	**2.4**	5*	25*	550*
19–30 y	**900**	**90**	5*	**15**	120.0*	**1.2**	**1.3**	**16**	**1.3**	**400**	**2.4**	5*	30*	550*
31–50 y	**900**	**90**	5*	**15**	120.0*	**1.2**	**1.3**	**16**	**1.3**	**400**	**2.4**	5*	30*	550*
51–70 y	**900**	**90**	10*	**15**	120.0*	**1.2**	**1.3**	**16**	**1.7**	**400**	**2.4**[h]	5*	30*	550*
> 70 y	**900**	**90**	15*	**15**	120.0*	**1.2**	**1.3**	**16**	**1.7**	**400**	**2.4**[h]	5*	30*	550*
Females														
9–13 y	**600**	**45**	5*	**11**	60.0*	**0.9**	**0.9**	**12**	**1.0**	**300**	**1.8**	4*	20*	375*
14–18 y	**700**	**65**	5*	**15**	75.0*	**1.0**	**1.0**	**14**	**1.2**	**400**[i]	**2.4**	5*	25*	400*
19–30 y	**700**	**75**	5*	**15**	90.0*	**1.1**	**1.1**	**14**	**1.3**	**400**[i]	**2.4**	5*	30*	425*
31–50 y	**700**	**75**	5*	**15**	90.0*	**1.1**	**1.1**	**14**	**1.3**	**400**[i]	**2.4**	5*	30*	425*
51–70 y	**700**	**75**	10*	**15**	90.0*	**1.1**	**1.1**	**14**	**1.5**	**400**	**2.4**[h]	5*	30*	425*
> 70 y	**700**	**75**	15*	**15**	90.0*	**1.1**	**1.1**	**14**	**1.5**	**400**	**2.4**[h]	5*	30*	425*
Pregnancy														
14–18 y	**750**	**80**	5*	**15**	75.0*	**1.4**	**1.4**	**18**	**1.9**	**600**[j]	**2.6**	6*	30*	450*
19–30 y	**770**	**85**	5*	**15**	90.0*	**1.4**	**1.4**	**18**	**1.9**	**600**[j]	**2.6**	6*	30*	450*
31–50 y	**770**	**85**	5*	**15**	90.0*	**1.4**	**1.4**	**18**	**1.9**	**600**[j]	**2.6**	6*	30*	450*
Lactation														
14–18 y	**1,200**	**115**	5*	**19**	75.0*	**1.4**	**1.6**	**17**	**2.0**	**500**	**2.8**	7*	35*	550*
19–30 y	**1,300**	**120**	5*	**19**	90.0*	**1.4**	**1.6**	**17**	**2.0**	**500**	**2.8**	7*	35*	550*
31–50 y	**1,300**	**120**	5*	**19**	90.0*	**1.4**	**1.6**	**17**	**2.0**	**500**	**2.8**	7*	35*	550*

Note: This table (taken from the DRI reports, see www.nap.edu) presents Recommended Dietary Allowances (RDAs) in **bold type** and Adequate Intakes (AIs) in ordinary type followed by an asterisk (*). RDAs and AIs may both be used as goals for individual intake. RDAs are set to meet the needs of almost all (97 to 98 percent) individuals in a group. For healthy breastfed infants, the AI is the mean intake. The AI for other life stage and gender groups is believed to cover needs of all individuals in the group, but lack of data or uncertainty in the data prevent being able to specify with confidence the percentage of individuals covered by this intake.

[a] As retinol activity equivalents (RAEs). 1 RAE = 1 μg retinol, 12 μg β-carotene, 24 μg β-carotene, or 24 μg β-cryptoxanthin. The RAE for dietary provitamin A carotenoids is twofold greater than retinol equivalents (RE), whereas the RAE for preformed vitamin A is the same as RE.

[b] As cholecalciferol. 1 μg cholecalciferol = 40 IU vitamin D.

[c] In the absence of adequate exposure to sunlight.

[d] As α-tocopherol. α-Tocopherol includes *RRR*-α-tocopherol, the only form of α-tocopherol that occurs naturally in foods, and the *2R*-stereoisomeric forms of α-tocopherol (*RRR-*, *RSR-*, *RRS-*, and RSS-α-tocopherol) that occur in fortified foods and supplements. It does not include the *2S*-stereoisomeric forms of α-tocopherol (*SRR-*, *SSR-*, *SRS-*, and *SSS*-α-tocopherol), also found in fortified foods and supplements.

[e] As niacin equivalents (NE). 1 mg of niacin = 60 mg of tryptophan; 0–6 months = preformed niacin (not NE).

[f] As dietary folate equivalents (DFE). 1 DFE = 1 μg food folate = 0.6 μg of folic acid from fortified food or as a supplement consumed with food = 0.5 μg of a supplement taken on an empty stomach.

[g] Although AIs have been set for choline, there are few data to assess whether a dietary supply of choline is needed at all stages of the life cycle, and it may be that the choline requirement can be met by endogenous synthesis at some of these stages.

[h] Because 10 to 30 percent of older people may malabsorb food-bound B12, it is advisable for those older than 50 years to meet their RDA mainly by consuming foods fortified with B12 or a supplement containing B12.

[i] In view of evidence linking folate intake with neural tube defects in the fetus, it is recommended that all women capable of becoming pregnant consume 400 μg from supplements or fortified foods in addition to intake of food folate from a varied diet.

[j] It is assumed that women will continue consuming 400 μg from supplements or fortified food until their pregnancy is confirmed and they enter prenatal care, which ordinarily occurs after the end of the periconceptional period—the critical time for formation of the neural tube.

TABLE 2-12. Dietary Reference Intakes (DRIs): Recommended Intakes for Individuals, Elements
Food and Nutrition Board, Institute of Medicine, National Academies

Life stage group	Calcium (mg/d)	Chromium (μg/d)	Copper (μg/d)	Fluoride (mg/d)	Iodine (μg/d)	Iron (mg/d)	Magnesium (mg/d)	Manganese (mg/d)	Molybdenum (μg/d)	Phosphorus (mg/d)	Selenium (μg/d)	Zinc (mg/d)	Potassium (g/d)	Sodium (g/d)	Chloride (g/d)
Infants															
0–6 mo	210*	0.2*	200*	0.01*	110*	0.27*	30*	0.003*	2*	100*	15*	2*	0.4*	0.12*	0.18*
7–12 mo	270*	5.5*	220*	0.5*	130*	**11.0**	75*	0.6*	3*	275*	20*	**3**	0.7*	0.37*	0.57*
Children															
1–3 y	500*	11.0*	**340**	0.7*	**90**	**7.0**	**80**	1.2*	**17**	**460**	**20**	**3**	3.0*	1.0*	1.5*
4–8 y	800*	15.0*	**440**	1.0*	**90**	**10.0**	**130**	1.5*	**22**	**500**	**30**	**5**	3.8*	1.2*	1.9*
Males															
9–13 y	1,300*	25.0*	**700**	2.0*	**120**	**8.0**	**240**	1.9*	**34**	**1,250**	**40**	**8**	4.5*	1.5*	2.3*
14–18 y	1,300*	35.0*	**890**	3.0*	**150**	**11.0**	**410**	2.2*	**43**	**1,250**	**55**	**11**	4.7*	1.5*	2.3*
19–30 y	1,000*	35.0*	**900**	4.0*	**150**	**8.0**	**400**	2.3*	**45**	**700**	**55**	**11**	4.7*	1.5*	2.3*
31–50 y	1,000*	35.0*	**900**	4.0*	**150**	**8.0**	**420**	2.3*	**45**	**700**	**55**	**11**	4.7*	1.5*	2.3*
51–70 y	1,200*	30.0*	**900**	4.0*	**150**	**8.0**	**420**	2.3*	**45**	**700**	**55**	**11**	4.7*	1.3*	2.0*
> 70 y	1,200*	30.0*	**900**	4.0*	**150**	**8.0**	**420**	2.3*	**45**	**700**	**55**	**11**	4.7*	1.2*	1.8*
Females															
9–13 y	1,300*	21.0*	**700**	2.0*	**120**	**8.0**	**240**	1.6*	**34**	**1,250**	**40**	**8**	4.5*	1.5*	2.3*
14–18 y	1,300*	24.0*	**890**	3.0*	**150**	**15.0**	**360**	1.6*	**43**	**1,250**	**55**	**9**	4.7*	1.5*	2.3*
19–30 y	1,000*	25.0*	**900**	3.0*	**150**	**18.0**	**310**	1.8*	**45**	**700**	**55**	**8**	4.7*	1.5*	2.3*
31–50 y	1,000*	25.0*	**900**	3.0*	**150**	**18.0**	**320**	1.8*	**45**	**700**	**55**	**8**	4.7*	1.5*	2.3*
51–70 y	1,200*	20.0*	**900**	3.0*	**150**	**8.0**	**320**	1.8*	**45**	**700**	**55**	**8**	4.7*	1.3*	2.0*
> 70 y	1,200*	20.0*	900	3.0*	**150**	**8.0**	**320**	1.8*	**45**	**700**	**55**	**8**	4.7*	1.2*	1.8*
Pregnancy															
14–18 y	1,300*	29.0*	**1,000**	3.0*	**220**	**27.0**	**400**	2.0*	**50**	**1,250**	**60**	**13**	4.7*	1.5*	2.3*
19–30 y	1,000*	30.0*	**1,000**	3.0*	**220**	**27.0**	**350**	2.0*	**50**	**700**	**60**	**11**	4.7*	1.5*	2.3*
31–50 y	1,000*	30.0*	**1,000**	3.0*	**220**	**27.0**	**360**	2.0*	**50**	**700**	**60**	**11**	**4.7***	**1.5***	**2.3***
Lactation															
14–18 y	1,300*	44.0*	**1,300**	3.0*	**290**	**10.0**	**360**	2.6*	**50**	**1,250**	**70**	**14**	5.1*	1.5*	2.3*
19–30 y	1,000*	45.0*	**1,300**	3.0*	**290**	**9.0**	**310**	2.6*	**50**	**700**	**70**	**12**	5.1*	1.5*	2.3*
31–50 y	1,000*	45.0*	**1,300**	3.0*	**290**	**9.0**	**320**	2.6*	**50**	**700**	**70**	**12**	5.1*	1.5*	2.3*

Note: This table presents Recommended Dietary Allowances (RDAs) in bold type and Adequate Intakes (AIs) in ordinary type followed by an asterisk (*). RDAs and AIs may both be used as goals for individual intake. RDAs are set to meet the needs of almost all (97 to 98 percent) individuals in a group. For healthy breastfed infants, the AI is the mean intake. The AI for other life stage and gender groups is believed to cover needs of all individuals in the group, but lack of data or uncertainty in the data prevent being able to specify with confidence the percentage of individuals covered by this intake.

Sources: Dietary Reference Intakes for Calcium, Phosphorous, Magnesium, Vitamin D, and Fluoride (1997); Dietary Reference Intakes for Thiamin, Riboflavin, Niacin, Vitamin B6, Folate, Vitamin B12, Pantothenic Acid, Biotin, and Choline (1998); Dietary Reference Intakes for Vitamin C, Vitamin E, Selenium, and Carotenoids (2000); Dietary Reference Intakes for Vitamin A, Vitamin K, Arsenic, Boron, Chromium, Copper, Iodine, Iron, Manganese, Molybdenum, Nickel, Silicon, Vanadium, and Zinc (2001); and Dietary Reference Intakes for Water, Potassium, Sodium, Chloride, and Sulfate (2004). These reports may be accessed via http://www.nap.edu.

(3) Vitamin D supplementation (200–400 international units/d) is recommended for breast-fed infants and older infants (>6 months), especially those with limited exposure to sunlight.

(4) Iron-fortified formula should be provided to infants who are not breast-fed. The breast-fed infant should be provided with an additional source of iron such as iron-fortified cereal by 4 to 6 months of age. Other sources of iron in addition to cereal may be beneficial after 6 months of age.

b) PN

(1) Guidelines for the provision of IV vitamins and trace elements in pediatrics follow the indications of the

Subcommittee on Pediatric Parenteral Nutrient Requirements from the Committee on Clinical Practice Issues of the American Society for Clinical Nutrition and A.S.P.E.N.[36–38]

(2) The multivitamin needs of term infants are commonly met by a pediatric multivitamin at 2 mL/kg up to a maximum of 5 mL/day (dose used in children up to 11 years old). For children over 11 years of age, the adult version of multivitamins will meet estimated requirements plus the addition of vitamin K (2–4 mg/week or 1 mg/day).[51] See Chapter 8, Table 8-6, for PN multivitamins.

(3) The trace element needs are described in Chapter 8, Table 8-7.

(4) If the patient is to be on PN for >1 month, supplemental selenium and possibly molybdenum should be added. Selenium should be provided at 2 to 3 mcg/kg/day (maximum: 40–60 mcg/day), while molybdenum requirements may be met by providing 0.25 mcg/kg/day (maximum: 5 mcg/day). Also, carnitine can become deficient in long-term PN patients receiving all their calories from PN. The recommended IV intake is 10 to 30 mg/kg/day (maximum 100 mg/day).

(5) If liver or renal complications occur, some trace element regimens have to be reformulated for PN patients (see Section III.A.2.f).(3).(b)).

8. Fluids and electrolytes. Body homeostasis is maintained by fluids, which are the bulk of body weight in children (60%–70%) and especially in neonates (up to 80%). To maintain water and electrolyte homeostasis and to allow metabolic processes (including the effects of insensible and sweat losses), a certain amount of fluid has to be introduced daily regardless of health conditions. Maintenance is mainly dependent on TEE and environmental temperature, whereas deficit replacements seem to be directly related to the size of the deficit and the body mass. Factors such as losses and organ dysfunction may require volume individualization. New DRI for some electrolytes can be found in Table 2-12.[52]

a) Fluid maintenance requirements can be computed following the A.S.P.E.N. recommendations based on the Holliday-Segar method. The Holliday-Segar formula estimates fluid needs by calculating energy expenditure and relating this to water losses and water of metabolism. The formula is based on energy expenditure for bed rest and therefore may not be adequate for highly active children:

(1) 2 to 10 kg, 100 mL/kg

(2) 10 to 20 kg, 1000 mL + 50 mL/kg for each kg over 10

(3) 20 kg and up, 1500 mL + 20 mL/kg for each kg over 20[38]

b) Another method, based on body surface area, can be accurate for children of abnormal height for weight: 1500 to 1700 mL/m^2/day.[53]

c) Based on caloric intake, infant and child fluid needs are, respectively, 1.5 and 1 mL/kcal of energy expenditure.

d) PN electrolyte recommendations are outlined in Chapter 8, Table 8-2.[38,54] Addition of calcium and phosphorus to PN is limited by solubility.

C. Adults

1. Energy requirements

a) Estimated energy requirement (EER) as defined by the Institute of Medicine (IOM) for healthy adults is the dietary energy intake predicted to maintain energy balance in a healthy adult of a defined age, gender, weight, height, and level of physical activity consistent with good health.[43] EER equations for men and women are given in Table 2-13.[43]

TABLE 2-13. EER for Healthy Adults[43]

Men age 19 years and older:

EER = 662 − 9.53 (age in yrs) + PA (15.91 × weight in kg) + 539.6(height in m)
- PA = 1.00 for sedentary men
- PA = 1.11 for low-activity men
- PA = 1.25 for moderate-activity men
- PA = 1.49 for high-activity men

Women age 19 years and older:

EER = 354 − 6.91 (age in yrs) + PA (9.36 × weight in kg) + 726 (height in m)
- PA = 1.00 for sedentary women
- PA = 1.12 for low-activity women
- PA = 1.27 for moderate-activity women
- PA = 1.45 for high-activity women

Harris-Benedict equations

Men	66.42 + 13.75 (weight in kg) + 5.00 (height in cm) − 6.78 (age in yrs)
Women	655.1 + 9.65 (weight in kg) + 1.85 (height in cm) − 4.68 (age in yrs)

EER, estimated energy requirements; PA = physical activity coefficient. Printed with permission from Institute of Medicine. *Dietary Reference Intakes for Energy, Carbohydrate, Fiber, Fat, Fatty Acids, Cholesterol, Protein, and Amino Acids (Macronutrients).* Washington, DC: National Academy Press; 2002.

b) Energy requirement may be measured by indirect calorimetry if equipment is available; this measurement may be particularly valuable in the critically ill patient. The value derived is REE, which is the energy expended at rest (not necessarily fasting). Then appropriate factors can be applied to account for physical activity.

c) In the absence of indirect calorimetry capability, various methods are used to estimate energy requirements of sick patients.[55,56]

(1) Harris-Benedict equations (Table 2-13) derived from healthy adults, adjusted for activity and stress, have been widely applied to sick patients to predict REE.

(2) Alternatively, more recently, regression equations based on sick populations have been derived; two of the more commonly used are the Ireton-Jones equations (Table 2-14).[57] These equations already factor in the stress level of the patient.

(3) Also frequently used is the simple calculation of energy requirement based on kcal per kg body weight. The typical range is 20 to 35 total kcal per kg body weight per day.[36]

(4) With most of these methods, the question of what body weight to use in a patient who is significantly above ideal body weight must be addressed. See Chapter 28 for a discussion of this topic.

(5) Another source of confusion when applying these equations is whether to express energy requirements in terms of total kcal or nonprotein kcal. In the early days of PN,

TABLE 2-14. Ireton-Jones Equations for Estimation of Energy Requirements of Hospitalized Patients[57]

Spontaneously breathing patients:

kcal/day = 629 – 11 (age in yrs) + 25 (weight in kg) – 609(O)*

Ventilator-dependent patients:

kcal/day = 1784 – 11 (age in yrs) + 5 (weight in kg) + 244(S)** + 239(T)*** + 804(B)****

*O stands for obesity (>30% above initial weight from 1959 Metropolitan Life Insurance tables or body mass index > 27 kg/m²): use 1 if present and 0 if absent.
**S stands for sex: use 1 for male and 0 for female.
***T stands for diagnosis of trauma: use 1 if present and 0 if absent.
****B stands for diagnosis of burn: use 1 if present and 0 if absent.
Reprinted from Ireton-Jones C, Jones JD. Improved equations for predicting energy expenditure in patients: the Ireton-Jones equations. *Nutr Clin Pract.* 2002;17:29–31 with permission from A.S.P.E.N.

kcal requirements were often referred to in terms of nonprotein kcal, since it was felt that the protein supplied by the nutrient solution was being given not to act as an energy source for the body but rather as a substrate for synthesis of lean body mass. The recent trend is to express energy requirements in terms of total kcal, since the body does not distinguish that infused protein is not to be used as a fuel source.

d) Energy requirements of patients requiring nutritional support should generally be met through provision of a mixed fuel system, that is, one providing substantial kcal from both carbohydrate and fat. Carbohydrate should generally be provided at a rate not to exceed 7 g/kg/day (about 5 mg/kg/minute).[36] Fat should generally be provided at a rate not to exceed 2.5 g/kg/day; at least 1% to 2% of kcal should be derived from linoleic and 0.5% from alpha-linolenic acid to prevent essential fatty acid deficiency.[36] Many clinicians would limit fat infusion to closer to 1 g/kg/day, especially in critically ill and immunocompromised adults. The typical distribution of carbohydrate and fat in PN solutions is about 70% to 85% nonprotein kcal as carbohydrate and 15% to 30% nonprotein kcal as fat. Corresponding distributions for EN would be about 65% to 80% nonprotein kcal as carbohydrate and 20% to 35% nonprotein kcal as fat.
e) Carbohydrate in PN is provided exclusively as dextrose in the United States. Carbohydrate sources for EN are more varied. Starch or glucose polymers found in standard formulas require digestion to be absorbed. The formulas that require less digestive function typically contain oligosaccharides as the carbohydrate source.
f) Commercially available lipid for IV infusion in the United States is derived from soybean oil or a combination of soybean and safflower oils. These emulsions contain LCFAs. Use of MCT as an IV fat source remains investigational in the United States, although commercial products containing a blend of MCT and long-chain triglycerides for IV use are available in several other countries. Fat sources in standard adult EN formulas include vegetable oils such as soy or corn oil rich in PUFA. Canola oil is another common source of fat in enteral feeding products. MCT are a source of some of the fat in many enteral formulas and serve as a readily utilizable energy source.
g) Special considerations in the elderly. Both REE and physical activity decrease with age; the decrease in REE is primarily due to decrease in lean body mass and increase in fat mass with age. Individual differences in the elderly make estimation of energy requirements challenging.

2. Protein requirements
   a) The RDA for protein for healthy adults is 0.8 g/kg/day (Table 2-6).[43]
   b) Protein requirements for catabolic patients are generally higher, in the range of 1.2 to 2.0 g/kg/day.[36,38] About 25% to 30% of protein intake should typically be provided by essential amino acids.[36]
   c) Adequate kcal must be provided along with protein to ensure the proper utilization of protein.
   d) Patients with certain disease states such as renal failure and end-stage liver disease may require protein restriction (see disease-specific chapters 17, 23, 24 and 29).
   e) Provision of individual amino acids for specific situations may be beneficial, although general recommendations cannot yet be made.[36]
   f) Although there has been some suggestion that protein requirements may be increased in the elderly, the RDA for adults 50 years and older was set at the same level as for younger adults (0.8 g/kg/day).[43]
3. Fluid requirements
   a) Typical fluid requirements for adults are 20 to 40 mL/kg/day or 1 to 1.5 mL/kcal of energy expended.[36,38,41,52] Fluid supplied by nutritional support should be individualized on the basis of patient inputs and outputs and estimates of insensible losses.
   b) Fluid requirements of the elderly are similar to those quoted above. However, many elderly persons are underhydrated, due to impaired thirst mechanisms and inability to obtain or consume liquids by themselves, thus making attention to intake and output data critical in this population.[58] On the other hand, fluid may sometimes need to be restricted in the ill elderly due to underlying conditions such as congestive heart failure.
4. Electrolyte requirements
   a) Daily electrolyte requirements for generally healthy people receiving PN or EN as published by A.S.P.E.N. are shown in Table 2-15.[36,38] Note that some of these values for enteral electrolytes are slightly different from the AI and RDA values recently published by the IOM and presented in Table 2-12.
   b) The requirements of ill patients receiving these therapies can be much different, especially in the presence of organ dysfunction, thus necessitating close clinical and laboratory monitoring of these patients.
5. Vitamin requirements
   a) Vitamin requirements for patients receiving enteral feedings are based on the RDA or, if no RDA has been set for a particular vitamin, the AI.[42,48–50] See Table 2-11 for vitamin recommendations for healthy persons on oral diets; these recommendations can be extrapolated with caution to patients on enteral feedings.[36]
   b) Parenteral vitamin requirements are poorly defined. Current parenteral recommendations are largely based on guidelines adopted by the American Medical Association Department of Foods and Nutrition, which were approved by the Food and Drug Administration (FDA) in 1979.[59] Amendments to these

TABLE 2-15. Daily Adult Enteral and Parenteral Electrolyte Requirements Assuming Normal Age-Related Organ Function[36]

	Enteral	Parenteral
Sodium	500 mg (22 mEq)	1–2 mEq/kg
Potassium	2 g (51 mEq)	1–2 mEq/kg
Chloride	750 mg (21 mEq)	As needed to maintain acid-base balance
Acetate	—	As needed to maintain acid-base balance
Calcium	1200 mg (60 mEq)	10–15 mEq
Magnesium	420 mg (35 mEq)	8–20 mEq
Phosphorus	700 mg (23 mmol)	20–40 mmol

Reprinted from A.S.P.E.N. Board of Directors and the Clinical Guidelines Task Force. Guidelines for the use of parenteral and enteral nutrition in adult and pediatric patients. *J Parenter Enteral Nutr.* 2002;26(1 suppl): 1SA–138SA with permission from A.S.P.E.N.

recommendations were published by the FDA in 2000.[60] See Chapter 8, Table 8-4, for parenteral vitamin recommendations. Note that the parenteral vitamin recommendations are generally higher than the corresponding enteral recommendations, since the parenteral recommendations were intended for patients with increased requirements due to illness, although this assumption would lead to the question of whether the RDA and AI values for healthy adults (as in Table 2-11) are truly appropriate for extrapolation to very sick patients who receive tube feedings.

c) Measurement of serum vitamin concentrations or other biochemical markers of vitamin status may be useful in patients receiving long-term nutrition support or occasionally in patients receiving shorter-term therapies if the clinical condition suggests the possibility of a deficiency or excess.

d) Currently, US nutrient recommendations are being established for older adults in 51- to 70-year and over-70-year age categories. In the future, these categories may be further substratified.[61] Under the current scheme, requirements for vitamin D and vitamin B_6 are higher for adults 51 years old and over than for adults 19 to 50 years old.[42,48,50]

6. Trace elements
   a) As with vitamin requirements, requirements for trace elements in patients receiving EN are generally set in accord with RDA or AI amounts. (see table 2-12)
   b) Recommendations for parenteral chromium, copper, manganese, and zinc were set by the Nutrition Advisory Group of the Department of Foods and Nutrition, American Medical Association, in 1979 (Chapter 8, table 8-5).[62] The American Medical Association has not published updates to these recommendations; however, other definitive guidelines have set copper and manganese recommendations at levels significantly lower than those originally recommended and have also set a recommendation for the parenteral requirement for selenium.[36,38] Note that parenteral requirements for iodine and molybdenum are not well defined, and therefore these minerals are not routinely added to PN solutions. However, some commercially available multiple–trace element solutions contain these minerals. Many patients on long-term PN will require parenteral iron supplementation; many clinicians wait until laboratory abnormalities consistent with iron insufficiency develop before supplementing with parenteral iron.
   c) Trace element RDAs and AIs are generally identical for older adults and younger adults. The two exceptions are the AI values for chromium, which are lower for adults 51 years old and older than for younger adults, and the RDA for iron, which is lower for postmenopausal women than for premenopausal women.

(Nutritional Requirements chapters from the 1st edition were contributed by Harry C. Sax, Wiley W. Souba, Nancy Baugh, Marilyn A. Recupero, and John A. Kerner Jr)

REFERENCES

1. Dewys WD, Begg C, Lavin PT, et al. Prognostic effect of weight loss prior to chemotherapy in cancer patients. *Am J Med.* 1980;69:491–497.
2. Kirshner BS, Voinchet O, Rosenberg IH. Growth retardation in inflammatory bowel disease. *Gastroenterology.* 1978;75:504–511.
3. Sermet-Gaudelus I, Poisson-Salomon AS, Colomb V, et al. Simple pediatric nutritional risk score to identify children at risk of malnutrition. *Am J Clin Nutr.* 2000;72:64–70.
4. Naber TH, Schermer T, deBree A, et al. Prevalence of malnutrition in nonsurgical hospitalized patients and its association with disease complications. *Am J Clin Nutr.* 1997;66:1232–1239.
5. Parekh RS, Flynn JT, Smoyer WE, et al. Improved growth in young children with severe chronic renal insufficiency who use specified nutritional therapy. *J Am Soc Nephrol.* 2001;12:2418–2426.
6. Savage MO, Beattie RM, Camacho-Hubner C, et al. Growth in Crohn's disease. *Acta Paediatr.* 1999;88(suppl):S89–S92.
7. Miller TL, Awnetwant EL, Evans S, et al. Gastrostomy tube supplementation for HIV-infected children. *Pediatrics.* 1995;96:696–702.
8. Lees MH, Bristow JD, Griswold HE, et al. Relative hypermetabolism in infants with congenital heart disease and undernutrition. *Pediatrics.* 1965;36:183–191.
9. Owen OE, Morgan AP, Kemp HG, et al. Brain metabolism during fasting. *J Clin Invest.* 1967;46:1589–1595.
10. Seashore JH. Nutritional support in the intensive care unit. *Yale J Biol Med.* 1984;57:111–134.
11. Fawzi WW, Mbise RL, Hertmark E, et al. A randomized trial of vitamin A supplements in relation to mortality among human immunodeficiency virus-infected and uninfected children in Tanzania. *Pediatr Infect Dis J.* 1999;18:127–133.
12. Weisdorf SA, Lysne J, Wind D, et al. Positive effect of prophylactic total parenteral nutrition on long term outcome of bone marrow transplantation. *Transplantation.* 1987;43:833–838.
13. Pollitt E, Jahari A, Walka H. A development view of the effect of an energy and micronutrient supplement in undernourished children in Indonesia. *Eur J Clin Nutr.* 2000;54(suppl 2):S107–S113.
14. Heird WC. The role of polyunsaturated fatty acids in term and preterm infants and breastfeeding mothers. *Pediatr Clin North Am.* 2001;48:173–188.
15. Lucas A. Does early diet program future outcome? *Acta Paediatr.* 1990;365(suppl):S58–S67.
16. Reddy P, Malone M. Cost and outcome analysis of home parenteral and enteral nutrition. *J Parenter Enteral Nutr.* 1998;22:302–310.
17. Holden CE, Puntis JWL, Charlton CPL, et al. Nasogastric feeding at home: acceptability and safety. *Arch Dis Child.* 1991;66:148–151.
18. De Potter S, Goulet O, Lamor M, et al. Two hundred sixty-three patient-years of home parenteral nutrition in children. *Transplant Proc.* 1992; 24:1056–1057.

19. DeCicco M, Panarello G, Fantin D, et al. Parenteral nutrition in cancer patients receiving chemotherapy: effects on toxicity and nutritional status. *J Parenter Enteral Nutr.* 1993;17:513–518.
20. Sax HC, Warner BW, Talamini MA, et al. Early total parenteral nutrition in acute pancreatitis: lack of beneficial effects. *Am J Surg.* 1987;153: 117–124.
21. Valdivieso M, Frankmann C, Murphy WK, et al. Long-term effects of intravenous hyperalimentation administered during intensive chemotherapy for small cell bronchogenic carcinoma. *Cancer.* 1987;59:362–369.
22. Ferraro R, Lillioja S, Fontvieille AM, et al. Lower sedentary metabolic rate in women compared with men. *J Clin Invest.* 1992;90:780–784.
23. Holliday MA. Metabolic rate and organ size during growth from infancy to maturity and during late gestation and early infancy. *Pediatrics.* 1971; 47(suppl 2):169–179.
24. Weinsier RL, Schutz Y, Bracco D. Reexamination of the relationship of resting metabolic rate to fat-free mass and to metabolically active components of fat-free mass in humans. *Am J Clin Nutr.* 1992;55:790–794.
25. Tai MM, Castillo P, Pi-Sunyer FX. Meal size and frequency: effect on the thermic effect of food. *Am J Clin Nutr.* 1991;54:783–787.
26. Flatt JP. The biochemistry of energy expenditure. In: Bray G, ed. *Recent Advances in Obesity Research.* Volume 2. London, UK: Newman Publ; 1978:211–228.
27. Payne PR, Waterlow JC. Relative energy requirement for maintenance, growth, and physical activity. *Lancet.* 1971;2:210–211.
28. Frankenfield DC, Wiles CE 3rd, Bagley S, et al. Relationships between resting and total energy expenditure in injured and septic patients. *Crit Care Med.* 1994;22:1796–1804.
29. Teitelbaum J, Walker WA. Review: the role of omega 3 fatty acids in intestinal inflammation. *J Nutr Biochem.* 2001;12:21–32.
30. Usher R, McLean F. Intrauterine growth of live-born Caucasian infants at sea level: standards obtained from measurements in 7 dimensions of infants born between 25 and 44 weeks of gestation. *Pediatrics.* 1969;74:901–910.
31. Groh-Wargo S. Recommended enteral nutrient intakes. In: Groh-Wargo S, Thompson M, Cox T, eds. *Nutritional Care for High-Risk Newborns.* Rev 3rd ed. Chicago, IL: Precept Press; 2000:231–263.
32. Aggett PJ. Trace elements of the micropremie. *Clin Perinatol.* 2000;27: 119–129.
33. Herin P, Zetterstrom R. Sodium, potassium and chloride needs in low-birth-weight infants. *Acta Paediatr.* 1994;405(suppl):43–48.
34. American Academy of Pediatrics, Committee on Nutrition. Nutritional needs of preterm infants. In: American Academy of Pediatrics, Committee on Nutrition. *Pediatric Nutrition Handbook.* 4th ed. Elk Grove, IL: American Academy of Pediatrics; 1998:55–87.
35. Schanler RJ. The low birth weight infant. In: Walker WA, Watkins JB, Duggan C., eds. *Nutrition in Pediatrics.* 3rd ed. Hamilton, Ontario: BC Decker; 2003:491–514.
36. A.S.P.E.N. Board of Directors and the Clinical Guidelines Task Force. Guidelines for the use of parenteral and enteral nutrition in adult and pediatric patients. *J Parenter Enteral Nutr.* 2002;26(1 suppl):1SA–138SA.
37. Greene HL, Hambridge KM, Schanler R, et al. Guidelines for the use of vitamins, trace elements, calcium, magnesium, and phosphorus in infants and children receiving total parenteral nutrition: report of the Subcommittee on Pediatric Parenteral Nutrient Requirements for the Committee on Clinical Practice Issues of the American Society for Clinical Nutrition. *Am J Clin Nutr.* 1998;48:1324–1342.
38. Task Force for the Revision of Safe Practices for Parenteral Nutrition. Safe practices for parenteral nutrition. *J Parenter Enteral Nutr.* 2004;28: S39–S70.
39. Denne SC, Clark SE, Poindexter BB. Nutrition and metabolism in the high-risk neonate. In: Fanaroff AA, Martin RJ, eds. *Neonatal-Perinatal Medicine. Diseases of the Fetus and Infant.* St Louis, MO: Mosby; 1997:562–621.
40. Aggett PJ, Haschke F, Heine W, et al. Comment on the content and composition of lipids in infant formulas. ESPGHAN Committee on Nutrition. *Acta Paediatr Scand.* 1991;80:887–896.
41. Food and Nutrition Board, National Academy of Sciences, National Research Council. *Recommended Dietary Allowances.* 10th ed. Washington, DC: National Academy Press; 1989.
42. Institute of Medicine. *Dietary Reference Intakes for Calcium, Phosphorus, Magnesium, Vitamin D, and Fluoride.* Washington, DC: National Academy Press; 1997.
43. Institute of Medicine. *Dietary Reference Intakes for Energy, Carbohydrate, Fiber, Fat, Fatty Acids, Cholesterol, Protein, and Amino Acids (Macronutrients).* Washington, DC: National Academy Press; 2002.
44. Ford G. Nutrition in newborn and pediatric patients. In: Torosian M, ed. *Nutrition for the Hospitalized Patient. Basic Science and Principles of Practice.* New York, NY: Marcel Dekker; 1995:509–535.
45. World Health Organization. *Energy and Protein Requirements. Technical Report Series, No 724.* Geneva, Switzerland: World Health Organization; 1985.
46. Schofield W. Predicting basal metabolic rate, new standards and review of previous work. *Hum Nutr Clin Nutr.* 1985;39C(S1):5–41.
47. World Health Organization. *Energy and Protein Requirements Technical Report Series, No 522.* Geneva, Switzerland: World Health Organization; 1973.
48. Institute of Medicine. *Dietary Reference Intakes for Thiamin, Riboflavin, Niacin, Vitamin B6, Folate, Vitamin B12, Pantothenic Acid, Biotin, and Choline.* Washington, DC: National Academy Press; 1998.
49. Institute of Medicine. *Dietary Reference Intakes for Vitamin C, Vitamin E, Selenium, and Carotenoids.* Washington, DC: National Academy Press; 2000.
50. Institute of Medicine. *Dietary Reference Intakes for Vitamin A, Vitamin K, Arsenic, Boron, Chromium, Copper, Iodine, Iron, Manganese, Molybdenum, Nickel, Silicon, Vanadium, and Zinc.* Washington, DC: National Academy Press; 2001.
51. Kerner JA. Parenteral nutrition. In: Walker WA, Watkins JB, Duggan C, eds. *Nutrition in Pediatrics.* 3rd ed. Hamilton, Ontario: BC Decker; 2003: 957–985.
52. Institute of Medicine. *Dietary Reference Intakes for Water, Potassium, Sodium, Chloride, and Sulfate.* Washington, DC: National Academy Press; 2004.
53. Udall JN Jr, Noel RA. Fluids and electrolytes. In: Baker RD, Baker SS, Davis AM, eds. *Pediatric Parenteral Nutrition.* New York, NY: Chapman & Hall; 1997:85–98.
54. American Academy of Pediatrics Committee on Nutrition. Parenteral nutrition. In: Kleinman RE, ed. *Pediatric Nutrition Handbook.* 4th ed. Elk Grove, IL: American Academy of Pediatrics; 1998:282–305.
55. Malone AM. Methods of assessing energy expenditure in the intensive care unit. *Nutr Clin Pract.* 2002;17:21–28.
56. Barak N, Wall-Alonso E, Sitrin MD. Evaluation of stress factors and body weight adjustments currently used to estimate energy expenditure in hospitalized patients. *J Parenter Enteral Nutr.* 2002;26:231–238.
57. Ireton-Jones C, Jones JD. Improved equations for predicting energy expenditure in patients: the Ireton-Jones equations. *Nutr Clin Pract.* 2002;17: 29–31.
58. Castellanos VH, Silver HJ, Gallagher-Allred C, et al. Nutrition issues in the home, community, and long-term care setting. *Nutr Clin Pract.* 2003;18: 21–36.
59. American Medical Association, Department of Foods and Nutrition. Multivitamin preparations for parenteral use. A statement by the Nutrition Advisory Group. *J Parent Enteral Nutr.* 1979;3:258–261.
60. Food and Drug Administration. Parenteral multivitamin products: drugs for human use: drug efficacy study implementation: amendment. *Federal Register.* April 20, 2000;65(77):21200–21201.
61. Chernoff R. Normal aging, nutrition assessment, and clinical practice. *Nutr Clin Pract.* 2003;18:12–20.
62. American Medical Association. Guidelines for essential trace element preparations for parenteral use. A statement by the Nutrition Advisory Group. *J Parenter Enteral Nutr.* 1979;3:263–267.

Donald F. Kirby, MD, CNSP;
Marianne Opilla, RN, BSN, CNSN

3

Enteral Access and Infusion Equipment

Introduction

Patients who are unable to meet their nutritional requirements with oral intake frequently need supplementation, either enterally or parenterally. The enteral route is preferred whenever possible because it is associated with lower costs, fewer complications, and improved outcome. In this chapter, we discuss how to choose among the multiple enteral access routes and tubes that are available. We also address how to care for the tubes and administration devices.

I. Background. To choose the proper access device after determining that enteral feeding can be used, the clinician needs to ask several questions:

A. How long will feeding be required?
B. Can the patient tolerate gastric feeding, or is postpyloric (or ideally, post–ligament of Treitz) access required?
C. Who is available with the expertise to place the access (ie, nurse, dietitian, surgeon, endoscopist, or radiologist)? After the access tube has been placed, further decisions about infusion equipment are necessary. These decisions are somewhat dictated by the route and type of tube selected as well as by the availability of personnel and resources.

II. Selection of Enteral Feeding Route (Figure 3-1)

A. The estimated length of time that tube feeding will be required is an important issue that should be addressed before access placement. If feeds are needed for only a short time, tubes that are easily placed with low-risk procedures are usually recommended; however, occlusion and displacement rates are higher with these tubes. More complex, higher-risk procedures (ie, surgery) may be required to secure permanent tubes. Children's growth will need to be monitored so that feeding tube shaft lengths can be changed as needed and complications prevented.
   1. Short—term feeding tubes (<3 weeks)
      a) Patients not undergoing laparotomy—nasogastric or orogastric, nasoenteric or oroenteric: Orogastric tube feedings may be better tolerated in premature and small infants, as they are obligatory nasal breathers. Orogastric feedings are also indicated for children with choanal atresia or basilar skull fracture who cannot feed orally.
      b) Patients undergoing laparotomy for another indication: Gastrostomy, jejunostomy (standard), needle catheter jejunostomy (NCJ), or a nasoenteric tube can be placed during surgery.
   2. Long-term feeding tubes adults >4–8 weeks; pediatrics >4–6 weeks)
      a) Patients not undergoing laparotomy: percutaneous endoscopic gastrostomy (PEG), percutaneous endoscopic jejunostomy (PEJ), percutaneous radiologic gastrostomy, percutaneous radiologic jejunostomy, laparoscopic gastrostomy or jejunostomy, or cervical pharyngostomy/esophagostomy (not commonly done)
      b) Patients undergoing laparotomy for feeding tube placement: gastrostomy, transgastric jejunostomy, jejunostomy

B. Does the patient need pre- or postpyloric access? Technically, prepyloric tubes are the easiest to insert, and they have the advantage of delivering feeds in a more "standard" physiologic manner into the stomach. However, some patients may have severe reflux or delayed gastric emptying, necessitating postpyloric access to prevent tube feeding–related aspiration (TFRA). The more distal to the stomach the location of feeding delivery, the less likely TFRA is to occur.[1–3] Thus, the optimal postpyloric tube placement is in the fourth portion of the duodenum or past the ligament of Treitz.

C. Who has the interest and expertise to place tubes? Choices include gastroenterologists, surgeons, dietitians, nurses, and radiologists. Most specialists favor specific tubes and access methods, so the route of insertion varies among them. Methods of access insertion include blind passage, operative, endoscopic, laparoscopic, and radiologic placement.

D. In children, a gastrostomy tube is the most common method for long-term enteral access. Gastrostomy avoids nasopharyngeal irritation and the psychosocial issue of the nasoenteric tube. Gastrostomy tubes have larger diameters than jejunostomy tubes and are less likely to clog.

III. Short-Term Nonsurgical Prepyloric Tubes

A. Nasogastric tubes (NGTs). Commonly used, traditional NGTs (eg, Salem sumps) may perform many functions in addition to feeding, such as decompression of the stomach, administration of medication, and measurement of gastric pH or residuals. NGTs are made in various sizes (5F–18F), but, to avoid clogging, at least a 10F tube

FIGURE 3-1. Enteral access feeding options. Artwork by Mary Beatty, McGuire Veteran's Affairs Medical Center Media Department, Richmond, VA.

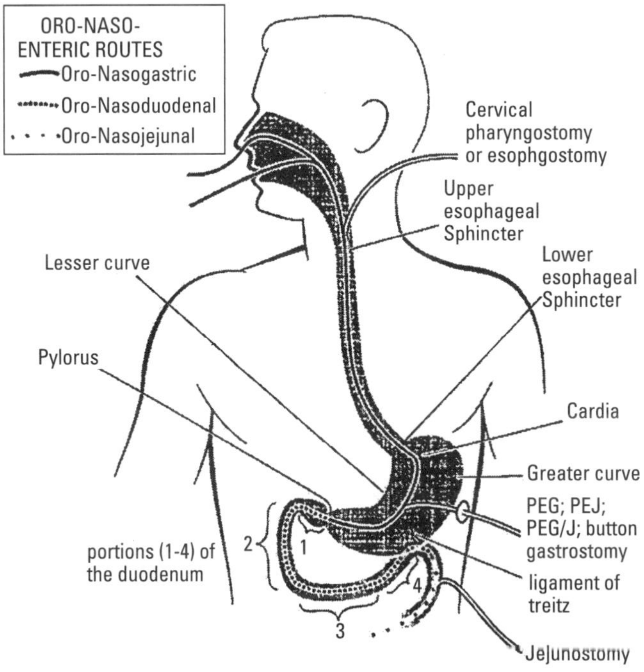

is required for commercially available enteral formulations. For improved patient comfort, some institutions use small-caliber tubes (8F–12F) for short-term nasogastric feedings.

1. Insertion: uncomplicated
   a) If the tube is to be inserted through the nose, it is important to obtain a history of sinus problems, deviated septum, frequent nosebleeds, known platelet or bleeding disorders, recent head or facial trauma, or difficulty with a previous nasal tube passage. Before tube passage, the nasal passages should be inspected. If the patient already has a tube (nasotracheal) in one nostril, the NGT is best placed in the other nostril. Hanson's formula[4] has been used to estimate the length of tube needed to pass 1 to 10 cm beyond the gastric cardia in adults: $[(NEX - 50)/2] + 50$ cm, where N = tip of nose, E = earlobe, and X = xiphoid process.
   b) The tube is marked 50 cm from its tip and, with the patient's head in a neutral position, is placed along the shortest course with the end of the tube at the tip of the nose (N) passing to the earlobe (E) and then to the xiphoid process (X). A second mark is made on the tube at the point where the tube meets the xiphoid process. The length of tube insertion should be halfway between the xiphoid process mark and the 50-cm mark. A simplified method is also used, whereby the tube is measured from the tip of the patient's nose to the earlobe and from the earlobe to the xiphoid process. Some commercially available feeding tubes have markings to denote length.
   c) Lubrication of the tube with a water-soluble lubricant facilitates passage; use of local anesthetic jelly (eg, 2% lidocaine jelly) may promote comfort and improve success in an alert patient. To decrease the risk of aspiration, the head of the bed should be raised or the patient should sit up. In comatose or anesthetized patients, the left lateral decubitus position may decrease this risk. The tube is carefully directed back through the nares to the hypopharynx. When the tip is in the posterior pharynx, the patient should be asked to take small sips of water or initiate dry swallows to facilitate passage of the tube past the upper esophageal sphincter (UES). If the patient begins to cough or cannot speak, the tube should be retracted because it may be in the trachea. Once the tube has passed the UES, it is important to be aware of any intrinsic esophageal disease (esophageal stricture, tumor, or diverticulum) that may impede safe passage to the lower esophageal sphincter (LES). Disorders of the LES, such as achalasia, may also hinder tube passage into the stomach. If significant resistance is met, the procedure should be terminated and the reason for the resistance should be assessed. Another method of placement may need to be used.
2. Insertion: complicated. A stethotube is a feeding tube that is adapted to a stethoscope.[5] If the feeding tube is passed incorrectly into the trachea, there will be a very loud noise, indicating that the tube should be removed and redirected. In comatose or anesthetized patients, a laryngoscope may be used to help guide the tube past the UES into the esophagus and beyond. A physician who is comfortable with the technique generally performs this procedure.
3. Documentation of placement. Auscultation of air insufflation over the midepigastrium has been used to document passage of the tube into the stomach. Caution is needed because inadvertent pulmonary placement can result in bronchial sounds being transmitted through the diaphragm, simulating gastric placement.[6] Auscultation alone should not be used to confirm tube placement. However, a positive air insufflation test combined with aspiration of gastric contents is a fairly reliable predictor of successful placement. X-ray verification of tube placement remains the gold standard; it also shows whether the tube is in the preferred antral position or is curled.
4. Pros. Nasogastric tubes are available in a variety of sizes and tube materials, making it possible to select the smallest size that will allow the appropriate enteral formulation to be infused by the administration method intended. Placement is generally easy, especially in an alert, cooperative patient. Larger-caliber tubes and ease of replacement permit bolus feeding and administration of medication.
5. Cons. Nasogastric tubes are contraindicated if severe coagulopathy, severe thrombocytopenia, some nasal and facial fractures, or esophageal obstruction is present. In addition, intrinsic problems of the esophagus (masses, diverticula, or strictures) or disorders of the LES (hypertensive LES or achalasia) can increase the risk of complications, such as bleeding, perforation, or coiling of the tube in the esophagus, and result in aspiration of feeding.
6. Complications (Table 3-1)

B. Orogastric tubes. The oral route may be preferred when nasal or facial trauma, head injury, sinusitis, or other factors prevent a tube from being placed nasally. In addition, the oral route may be a good option in patients who are sedated, paralyzed, or mechanically ventilated. Orogastric tubes are used for premature infants, as they are obligatory nasal breathers.

1. Pros. The incidence of sinusitis is lower than with nasoenteric tubes.
2. Cons. Orogastric tubes are not tolerated for prolonged periods in alert patients; tubes may be damaged by teeth.
3. Complications. Except for nasal-related events, the complications are similar to those for nasogastric tubes (Table 3-1).

TABLE 3-1. Potential Complications of Nasogastric and Nasoenteric Tubes

Nasal mucosal ulceration	Gastrointestinal bleeding
Clogging	Epistaxis
Esophageal perforation	Otitis media
Pneumothorax	Pulmonary aspiration
Pulmonary intubation	Pyriform sinus perforation

Adapted with permission from Kirby DF, DeLegge MH. Enteral nutrition: the challenge of access. In: Kirby DF, Dudrick SJ, eds. *Practical Handbook of Nutrition in Clinical Practice.* Boca Raton, FL: CRC Press; 1994:87–117.

IV. Short-Term Nonsurgical Postpyloric Tubes

A. Nasoenteric. These tubes are ideal if short-term feeds are required but the patient is at high risk of aspiration, esophageal reflux, or delayed gastric emptying. It is assumed that if the tip of the tube is placed past the pyloric sphincter, the risk of TFRA is reduced. However, duodenogastric reflux is limited only if the tube is in the distal third of the duodenum and preferably past the ligament of Treitz.[7] Newer tubes have a separate gastric port for gastric suction, decompression, or medication delivery, with a second lumen for simultaneous small-bowel feeding. These tubes are generally more difficult to place and may require pharmacologic, endoscopic, intraoperative, or radiologic assistance.[8,9]

1. Nasoenteric tube insertion methods
   a) pH sensors. Small-bowel tubes with pH sensors are available. It is assumed that an increase in pH over the presumed gastric reading is consistent with the end of the tube entering the duodenum. In one study, the pH profile and radiograph were in agreement in 87% of the cases, but small-bowel tube location was not discussed.[10]
   b) Pharmacologic measures. Medications with promotility properties have been used to facilitate passage of feeding tubes into the small intestine. Metoclopramide (10 mg intravenously) has been studied the most and appears to be most effective when given about 15 minutes before tube insertion. Only diabetic patients appear to benefit from a dose of metoclopramide given after tube placement.[11] When used in low doses, the antibiotic erythromycin also has promotility properties and can be useful for tube placement. In adults, an intravenous (IV) dose of 500 mg administered prior to tube insertion has been reported to facilitate tube placement.[11,12] In children, a dose of 3 mg/kg given intravenously 1 hour prior to tube insertion has been reported.[13] (Note that this is an off-label use for erythromycin.)
   c) Fluoroscopy. Radiologic techniques can be very useful for placing nasoenteric tubes. Passage into the third portion of the duodenum or beyond was successful in 86% of attempts in one study.[14] Procedures can be performed in the radiology department or at the bedside if portable fluoroscopy is available.
   d) Endoscopy. Endoscopy can facilitate feeding-tube placement into the small bowel; however, in adults, tubes of sufficient length (>105 cm) need to be used.[15] Friction from the endoscope may drag tubes back as the endoscope is removed, so postprocedure radiographs are recommended. Success rates of 90% to 95% have been reported with this technique.
2. Pros. Postpyloric feeding tubes are usually of smaller diameter than standard NGTs and cause less patient discomfort. Delayed gastric emptying does not preclude feeding.
3. Cons. It may be difficult to achieve postpyloric or post–ligament of Treitz positioning. Small-caliber tubes may preclude administration of some medications. Infusion pumps are usually required for infusion of enteral formulations.
4. Complications (Table 3-1)

B. Oroenteric. There are the same indications for oral placement as for orogastric tubes, and there are similar complications as for nasoenteric tubes except for nasal-related events.

V. Short-Term Surgical Pre- and Postpyloric Tubes

A. Gastrostomy. If a patient is already undergoing laparotomy, a gastrostomy or jejunostomy tube can easily be placed even for short-term use. For example, someone undergoing a partial gastrectomy may have a gastrostomy and jejunostomy tube placed. The gastrostomy would initially be used for decompression; the jejunostomy would be used for immediate postoperative feedings. See Section VI.A.3.

B. Jejunostomy (standard). See above and Section VII.A.3.

C. NCJ These are small-caliber jejunal tubes that can be easily placed at surgery. Older models were 5F, which predisposed them to clogging. Newer versions are 7F or 8F, which allows administration of enteral formulations with extra protein or fiber.

1. Pros. These are easily placed, with a low risk of enteric leak if inadvertently dislodged.
2. Cons. They require diligent nursing care because they are easily occluded. Infusion pumps are required for administration of enteral formulations. Medications can rarely be infused through NCJs.
3. Complications (Table 3-2)

D. Surgical nasoenteric. Some surgeons provide short-term enteral access postoperatively by manually guiding a nasoenteric tube through the stomach, then through the duodenum, and into the small bowel during laparotomy. The frequency and success of this practice are not known.

VI. Long-Term Prepyloric Tubes.

Gastrostomy. Although surgical gastrostomy has been performed for over 150 years, technical advances and procedural improvements have made PEG a preferred method of gastrostomy placement if the patient is not undergoing laparotomy for another reason.[16] Gastrostomies can also be placed radiologically or laparoscopically. There are no significant differences

TABLE 3-2. Potential Complications of Jejunostomy (All Methods)

Pneumatosis intestinalis	Bowel obstruction
Bleeding	Tube occlusion
Dislodgment	Stomal leakage
Tube deterioration	Wound infection
Volvulus	

Adapted with permission from Kirby DF, DeLegge MH. Enteral nutrition: the challenge of access. In: Kirby DF, Dudrick SJ, eds. *Practical Handbook of Nutrition in Clinical Practice.* Boca Raton, FL: CRC Press; 1994:87–117.

in complication rates among the different methods of gastrostomy insertion; however, nonoperative access is less costly.[17] Local expertise is an important deciding factor for determining how a gastrostomy is placed.

A. Gastrostomy insertion methods.

1. PEG. Prior to an attempt to place a PEG, a screening upper endoscopy is performed to make sure that there are no contraindications to the procedure such as a large ulcer (higher risk of ulcer perforation) or a gastric or duodenal mass or obstruction. Conscious sedation is usually sufficient to perform the procedure, but occasionally deep sedation with propofol or even general anesthesia may be required.

   After the initial endoscopy, the patient is placed supine and an area of transillumination in the left upper quadrant is identified. When a proposed site is located, palpation with a finger is used to indent the insufflated stomach. The site is then prepped with iodine swabs and infiltrated with 1% lidocaine solution. A 1-cm skin incision is made, and a catheter is placed through the incision into the stomach. A suture or guidewire is placed through the catheter and grasped with a snare. The endoscope, snare, and suture are removed from the patient. The PEG tube is tied onto the suture coming from the mouth and then pulled through the mouth, esophagus, and stomach to reach the anterior abdominal wall. The endoscope is reinserted and the intragastric position of the PEG bumper is visualized. The endoscope is removed from the patient, and the external bumper and a feeding adapter are placed.

   Kits are commercially available with tube sizes from 14F to 28F. Adults commonly have 20F tubes placed. Larger tubes may be required to insert a smaller feeding tube into the small intestine if small bowel feedings are desired. Infants and children often have 14F tubes placed, but later 18F to 20F tubes are necessary to facilitate flow rates commensurate with growth.

2. Radiologic. Gastrostomy tubes may be placed with radiologic guidance, which avoids passage of the endoscope through a bacteria-laden oral cavity. This reduces the risk of contamination of the subcutaneous tissues and avoids general anesthesia that may be required for surgical placement. In patients with head and neck cancer, there is a very small but real risk of causing PEG stoma site metastases when pulling a tube through the oropharynx. This risk can be obviated by doing the procedure radiologically or endoscopically by the introducer technique.[18,19] Fluoroscopy is the most commonly used imaging modality; however, ultrasonography or computed tomography can provide additional information about intra-abdominal structures that may be overlying the stomach or provide a safe tract when endoscopic transillumination fails. The size of feeding tubes varies from 10F to 28F. The two most common complications associated with radiologic placement are tube clogging and displacement; these complications often lead to catheter replacement. If stabilizing sutures are used, larger tubes with a lower rate of dislodgment or clogging can be inserted.

3. Surgical. Most operative gastrostomies are performed under general anesthesia in an operating room, but doing so can escalate costs. Surgical gastrostomies have been performed under conscious sedation. Operative gastrostomies are very cost-effective when done during another intra-abdominal procedure. An operative alternative to laparotomy is laparoscopic insertion.[20]

   Surgical placement in pediatric patients is most commonly achieved with a Stamm gastrostomy procedure. This is technically a temporary gastrostomy because the tract closes spontaneously after the tube is removed. A gastropexy is performed in which the stomach is sutured to the abdominal wall. Once postprocedure healing is complete, a reliable, established tract for replacing tubes exists. Gastrostomy tube placement itself may alter the contour of the stomach enough to cause some gastroesophageal reflux. Children with documented gastroesophageal reflux or gastric aspiration may need a fundoplication procedure performed with the surgical gastrostomy, which may obviate the need for postpyloric feedings. A pyloroplasty may be performed also if delayed gastric emptying has been documented.

B. Pros. These tubes allow long-term access and are easily cared for and replaceable. Bolus feeding and administration of medication are possible because of the large caliber of the tube.

C. Cons. Compared with the oral or nasal route, this technique is more invasive.

D. Complications (Table 3-3)

VII. Long-Term Postpyloric Tubes. Jejunostomy.

As with gastrostomy, many methods of jejunostomy insertion are now possible, including operative, percutaneous endoscopic, radiologic, and laparoscopic placement. Indications for jejunal access include reflux esophagitis, gastric aspiration, gastroparesis, insufficient stomach remnant because of previous resection, and establishment of access for postoperative feeding after major surgical procedures and of feeding access in patients who have unresectable gastric or pancreatic cancers. During urgent abdominal surgery, jejunostomy placement to facilitate early postoperative feeding should be considered.

A. Methods of insertion[21–23]

1. Percutaneous gastrojejunostomy—also called a JET-PEG or jejunal extension through a PEG. This jejunal feeding tube is a small 9F to 12F tube that is dragged or passed over a guidewire into the small bowel through a previously placed PEG. Initial versions of this tube were unsatisfactory in their design, were difficult to place past the proximal duodenum, and often migrated back into the stomach. Devices now available are easier to place in the distal duodenum or jejunum and are more reliable because the likelihood of migration is greatly decreased. To decrease the incidence of TFRA, the feeding port must be located in the distal duodenum or jejunum. Although placement of a primary Percutaneous Endoscopic Jejunostomy (PEJ) tube (tube placed with the PEG technique directly into the small intestine) as the initial procedure is not as common as the PEG procedure, it is becoming more widely practiced. It has been performed in patients with normal anatomy and in those who have had gastric resection.[24–27] There are also commercially available dual-lumen tubes that have both a gastric and a jejunal port. These are usually placed

TABLE 3-3. Potential Complications of Gastrostomy (All Methods)

Aspiration	Bleeding	Tube occlusion
Dislodgment	Pneumoperitoneum	Stomal leakage
Tube deterioration	Wound infection	

Adapted with permission from Kirby DF, DeLegge MH. Enteral nutrition: the challenge of access. In: Kirby DF, Dudrick SJ, eds. *Practical Handbook of Nutrition in Clinical Practice.* Boca Raton, FL: CRC Press; 1994:87–117.

through mature gastrostomy tracts and can be placed radiologically or endoscopically. The fact that the internal retention device is a balloon often limits these devices' use. When the balloon fails (usually within 3 months), the entire tube must be replaced. These tubes are too large to be used in infants and small pediatric patients.

2. Radiologic jejunostomy. Radiologists can insert a small feeding tube through the stomach and fluoroscopically guide it through the pylorus to the duodenojejunal flexure. This provides small-bowel feeding with a reduced risk of TFRA, but because smaller catheters (10F) are placed by this technique, a higher obstruction rate is expected. One series retrospectively compared surgical gastrostomy with radiologic percutaneous jejunostomy transgastric, in which ultrasound and fluoroscopy were used to insert a feeding tube through the stomach wall and then a 10F catheter was passed to the duodenojejunal junction.[28] Complications were fewer in the nonsurgical jejunostomy group, despite the fact that the stomach wall was not fixed to the anterior abdominal wall. However, radiologic techniques do not allow for placement of feeding tubes of sufficient size to provide both gastric and small-bowel access. Some centers are now performing dual-lumen gastrojejunostomies. The gastric port is 16F with a 10F jejunal port. While this may allow for decompression of the stomach or medication administration and feeding into the jejunum, the tube sizes may be associated with a higher rate of occlusion. More long-term data are needed. Direct percutaneous access to the jejunum has been performed under radiologic control; however, this is technically more difficult.
3. Open surgery. Surgical placement of jejunostomy tubes has been performed for over 100 years. A variety of techniques are available, including Witzel jejunostomy (probably the most common), Roux—en-Y jejunostomy, serosal tunnel jejunostomy, button jejunostomy, and laparoscopic jejunostomy.[29,30] Numerous tubes have been used, including red rubber catheters, biliary T tubes, and dialysis catheters. Surgical gastrojejunostomy tubes, which allow gastric decompression or medication administration in addition to jejunal feeding, are also available. The common belief that only elemental diets should be given through jejunostomy tubes has been shown to be untrue.[31] Standard polymeric diets containing fiber can be used; however, the catheter must be flushed routinely to maintain tube patency.

B. Pros. These tubes decrease the risk of TFRA. Early postoperative feeding is possible in most patients except those who are hemodynamically unstable, have peritonitis, or have a bowel obstruction.

C. Cons. An infusion pump is required. Administration of medication is precluded in some instances but is dependent on the size of the T-tube. Invasive procedures are required for access. Outside connectors are prone to break and may require replacement of the entire T-tube. The tubes are difficult if not impossible to replace unless a mature tract has developed.

D. Complications: similar to PEG (Table 3-2)

VIII. Selection of Access Device Features.

When a particular enteral access device is being selected, the tube's composition, intended use, estimated length of time required, cost-effectiveness, and features (eg, stylet, weighted tip, length of tube) should be considered.

A. Tube composition

1. In the presence of gastric secretions, polyvinyl chloride tubes harden and become brittle with time, which may cause tissue irritation or necrosis. Thus, these tubes should be used only for short periods for gastric drainage, decompression, lavage, or diagnostic procedures.[32]
2. Polyurethane or silicone tubes are better for long-term use because they are more flexible and less irritating to tissue. Most small-bowel feeding tubes are made of polyurethane or silicone. Polyurethane tubes may have improved longevity, but this concept needs further investigation.[33] Silicone tubes are flexible and may collapse when assessing gastric residuals. Fungal colonization has been associated with silicone rubber PEG tubes and may contribute to tube failure over time.[34]
3. Latex tubes are still available but should not be used in patients who are allergic to or at high risk of developing an allergy to latex. In addition, latex tubes need to be replaced more frequently because of susceptibility to degradation by microbes and gastric acid.
4. Red rubber catheters are soft and pliable, which makes them easy to place at the time of surgery. Although the tubes are generally large enough to infuse enteral formulations and medications, they are subject to gastric acid degradation and are used mostly for gastric gavage feeding or jejunostomies. If long-term feeding is required, another feeding tube material should be considered after the short-term problem has been addressed.

B. Weighted versus nonweighted. It is commonly believed that weighted tubes are easier to pass into the small bowel when they are being placed blindly; however, nonweighted tubes have actually been shown to pass at a higher rate.[35] In theory, weight may help keep the tube in place, but this concept has not been proven.

C. Use of a stylet. A stylet may facilitate passage of a small, very pliable tube. Reinsertion of the stylet after removal is not recommended because it may pass through the wall of the tube and perforate the gastrointestinal tract. Stylets may need to be lubricated before the tube is used. Obtain information about any product before using it, especially for the first time; do not assume that all tubes are alike.

D. Tube length. The length of a nasoenteric tube may influence its ability to pass the duodenojejunal junction. In adults, tubes longer than 105 cm are preferred if passage past the ligament of Treitz is desired.[11]

E. Low-profile device (LPD) versus standard gastrostomy

1. LPDs are cosmetically appealing to patients and may decrease the possibility of pyloric obstruction from inward migration of the feeding tube. LPDs are composed of an internal stabilizer, a shaft, an external stabilizer, a connecting tube, and an antireflux valve to keep gastric contents from leaking onto the skin. It is important to choose the appropriate shaft length. If the shaft is too short, the patient may develop pressure necrosis of the skin or the internal stabilizer may become embedded in the wall of the stomach. If the adult patient gains or loses 10 pounds, the shaft length should be reevaluated.[36] In infants and children, the size must be reevaluated routinely and the shaft replaced to accommodate growth. One design allows the physician to customize the shaft length, as the tube resembles a standard PEG tube. The shaft length is determined and then a valve-and-collar assembly is put into place. This obviates the need for multiple LPDs with various shaft lengths in inventory.
2. Initial placement of an LPD should be performed by a physician. Contraindications to switching to an LPD are gastrostomies placed by the Witzel and Janeway surgical techniques or patients who require gastric decompression. LPDs may not be a good choice for patients with tracheostomies, neurology patients with spastic posturing, or other patients with increased abdominal pressure. In these patients, forceful coughing or movement can

damage or expel the device or cause leakage of gastric contents and lead to maceration of the abdominal wall.[37,38]

IX. Care of Feeding Tubes. Feeding tubes require regular assessment and monitoring to ensure continued correct placement and to avoid complications such as skin breakdown or infection. When problems arise, early intervention is key to maintaining enteral access. This section reviews significant care issues for each type of feeding tube, with special emphasis on routine tube care, skin care, and replacement.

A. Oro- or nasogastric and oro- or nasoenteric tubes. Care of orally or nasally inserted tubes requires vigilance in checking placement, protecting the mucosal surfaces, and flushing routinely.

1. Checking placement. Placement of the tube should be checked every 8 hours during continuous feedings and before each intermittent feeding. Verification methods include x-ray, marking the tube where it exits the patient and measuring it, checking the pH of the aspirate, observing the color of the aspirate, and auscultation.[39] Any time tube misplacement or displacement is suspected, a roentgenogram should be taken.
2. Protecting the mucosal surfaces.[40] Mucosal irritation of the nasopharynx may occur anywhere along the path of the feeding tube.
   a) Inspect the nares, mouth, and pharynx daily for skin irritation, ulceration, pressure necrosis, and lesions.
   b) Clean the nares daily with warm water or saline and keep mucous membranes moist with petroleum jelly. If the nares are crusty, clean them with dilute hydrogen peroxide and then moisturize.
   c) Change the fixator device or tape on the nose or mouth as needed if loose or soiled and at least every 3 to 5 days. Incorrect taping can lead to pressure necrosis.
   d) Maintain good oral hygiene. Even when patients are not eating, their teeth should be brushed at least twice a day. If gum inflammation is present, the patient may benefit from an oral antiseptic rinse (eg chlorhexidene gluconate). Tube-fed patients receiving antibiotics may benefit from an oral antifungal formulation (eg, nystatin 500, 000 units applied to the oral cavity 4 times a day) to help prevent overgrowth of fungus.
3. Flushing routinely. Tubes should be flushed with water every 6 hours during continuous feeds, between and after medications, after intermittent feeds, after residuals are checked, and if feeds need to be turned off for more than 4 to 6 hours.
   In children, the flushing volume should be scaled down to the size of the child.
4. Replacement. Orally or nasally placed tubes should be replaced only when necessary (eg, tube occlusion, problems at the insertion site). Any time a tube is replaced, placement should be verified (see Section III.A.3). Some parents/caregivers learn to place and remove their infant's or child's orogastric or nasogastric feeding tube and do so routinely at home. The American Academy of Pediatrics recommends that NGTs be changed from one nostril to the other every 1 to 3 weeks to decrease sinus and ear infections.

B. Gastrostomy and jejunostomy tubes. The care of these tubes includes maintaining patency, protecting the skin at the exit site, and preserving proper placement and integrity of the tube.[37,40–42]

1. Checking placement
   a) For traditional gastrostomy and jejunostomy tubes, measure the length of the tube protruding from the abdomen and document the external length in the medical record daily. If no external markings are on the tube, an indelible mark can be made on the tube and used to monitor position.[34] Gastrostomy tubes with internal bumpers should be pushed in several centimeters and the tube rotated 360°. In pediatric patients, the tube is rotated 360° but not pushed in. If this is not possible, a buried bumper may be developing, and the patient will need to be referred to an experienced health care provider for further care and ultimate replacement.[1,43]
   b) LPDs should also be monitored daily. The tube should have some movement (ie, you should be able to slide the tube in and out about 0.5 inch). An LPD should be gently pushed in approximately 0.5 inch and rotated 360° daily to prevent the balloon or internal bumper from adhering to the gastric wall. For infants and small children, the LPD should be pushed in approximately one-eighth inch and rotated.
2. Care of exit site and tube
   a) Exit site assessment. Check for erythema (initially, a small amount of serosanguineous drainage can be expected), edema, warmth, and exudate. Foul-smelling drainage is a sign of infection. Also monitor for skin breakdown, pressure necrosis, hypergranulation (keep site dry), gastric leakage (identify the cause; do not just try to repair), displacement (tube movement >1 inch for adults and >0.25 inches for infants and small children), and enlargement of the stoma tract (stabilize tube; avoid excessive tube movement.
   b) Skin care. When the tube tract is new and has drainage or crusting, clean the exit site with diluted hydrogen peroxide. After the tract is healed, clean the site daily with soap and water. Clean carefully under external bumpers or disks to keep dry and clean and to check for excessive pressure. External bumpers and disks should be just above skin level and not taut against the skin.
   c) Dressings. Dressings are commonly used for 48 hours after initial placement when the tract is considered an open wound, when the tract is soiled, or when the patient is at high risk for inadvertent tube removal.
3. Tube stabilization. Stabilizing a tube can reduce the risk of tube displacement, pain, and enlargement of the tract.
   a) Sutures or T- fasteners may be present to secure gastrostomy or jejunostomy tubes. If a gastrostomy tube has anchoring sutures or T- fasteners, check with the physician about possible removal when the tract is healed. Most jejunostomy tubes require a secure suture at all times.
   b) Anchoring devices can secure the tube and protect the skin from the effects of frequent dressing changes.[44,45] Anchoring devices typically last twice as long as tape. Examples of anchoring devices are Hollister Drain/Tube Attachment Device (Hollister, Libertyville, IL), Cath-Secure (MC Johnson, Naples, FL), and Flexi-Trak (ConvaTec, Skillman, NJ). If adhesive tube holders are used, the exit site must be cleaned around the tube daily and as needed to prevent accumulation of tissue debris.
   c) If the tube has a balloon, check the water in the balloon at least once a week.
   d) Patients with enteral devices or tubes may shower or bathe according to the directions of their health care provider. If a bumper or disk is present, the skin underneath it should be dried carefully to prevent maceration from trapped moisture.[36,37]
4. Irrigation (see Section IX.A.3)
5. Replacement of gastrostomy tubes

a) Maturation of the tract generally occurs in 2 to 3 weeks in the adult patient and 6 weeks in the pediatric patient. This process takes longer if the patient is immunocompromised, diabetic, or severely malnourished.[41] If the tract is disturbed during this time, the stomach may separate from the abdominal wall. During the maturation process, only a physician should change the gastrostomy tube; a radiologic procedure (eg, fluoroscopy, contrast study) may be indicated to confirm proper tube replacement. Once the tract is fully mature, nurses may replace tubes—depending on their knowledge and experience, facility policies, and state regulations—if a health care provider orders it. Some parents/caregivers become comfortable enough to replace their child's gastrostomy tube through a mature tract.

b) If the tube is inadvertently removed, it should be replaced as soon as possible; the tract can close within hours of the incident. The patient can be instructed to take the tube (so caregivers know what type and size tube is being used) to an acute-care facility for replacement, taught how to replace the tube in an emergency situation, or instructed to call a home-care nurse.

c) Gastrostomy tubes should be replaced when they show signs of degradation, balloon breakage, malfunction, or irreversible occlusion. Removal of any tube requires knowledge of the tube type and initial placement procedure. For example, some endoscopically placed tubes require endoscopy for tube removal.

d) Replacement gastrostomy tubes are usually inserted when the tract is well formed and further endoscopy is not necessary.[41] Many replacement tubes are made of silicone. If a latex tube (eg, Foley catheter) is selected as a replacement tube, providers should be aware of possible latex sensitivities. There are a variety of replacement gastrostomy tubes and LPDs on the market with balloons or solid bolsters.

e) Jejunostomy tubes are almost always replaced or changed by a health care provider with specialized education, training, and experience in the procedure. They are replaced surgically, endoscopically, or via fluoroscopy in radiology.[46]

C. Problem skin care. The most crucial step in preventing or minimizing skin problems is early identification and removal of the problem.

1. Hypergranulation (everted mucosa) typically develops when the exit site remains moist or the tube is not stabilized and moves in the stoma. Keeping the site dry and stabilizing the tube may help prevent this problem. Excessive growth (>0.25 inch for adults; >2 mm for pediatric patients) of granulation tissue can be eliminated around the tube by carefully cauterizing with silver nitrate sticks.[37,47]

2. For other skin problems, the cause should be identified and removed, if possible. Certain liquid or solid barriers can be used to protect the skin as it heals.[48,49]

a) Minor skin breakdown. If there is slight irritation, a protective skin barrier (eg, zinc oxide).

b) Skin that is already denuded. Dry the skin well and dust with a powder (eg, Stomadhesive [ConvaTec, Skillman, NJ]). Then apply a waterproof ointment (eg, Critic Aid Skin Paste [Coloplast, Marietta, GA]). If the patient is not receiving an acid-suppressing medication (eg, histamine-2 receptor antagonist [eg, ranitidine, famotidine] or a proton pump inhibitor [eg, omeprazole]), then this may be necessary to decrease the risk of acid damage to the skin.

c) Hydrocolloids and pectin wafers (eg, Stomadhesive, DuoDERM [ConvaTec, Skillman, NJ]) can also be used to prevent skin breakdown at the exit site and at sites distant from the exit site. These should be placed on clean, dry skin and changed when soiled to prevent trapped moisture.

X. Selection of Infusion Equipment[50,51]

A. Times to use an infusion pump

1. Enteral infusion pumps are designed and used exclusively for delivery of tube feedings. A pump should be considered when a controlled volume or infusion rate is desired. Continuous drip feedings via pump may improve gastrointestinal tolerance and reduce the risk of aspiration associated with reflux.[52] Generally, postpyloric feedings require a pump.

2. Intravenous infusion pumps should not be used for enteral formulation delivery because of the risk of inadvertent connection of tube feeding to an IV site. In addition, IV pumps have unnecessary alarms and are more costly than enteral pumps.

B. Pump selection. Issues to consider when selecting a pump include how easy the product is to use and who will be operating the pump (nurse, patient, or caregiver), the patient's size and overall condition (which can affect the ability to lift or move a pump), and the patient's ambulation status.

C. Pumps for the outpatient

1. Pump requirements. Some special considerations with regard to pump selection are necessary for patients who receive feeds in the home setting.

a) Most pumps come with a built-in carrying handle and pole clamp. In the home setting, pumps should be portable or attached to a mobile pole. Some pumps are designed with shoulder straps or a carrying case for ease of transport, which is ideal for school or work.

b) All pumps have rechargeable batteries and run on AC power. Pumps should have a battery life of at least 8 to 12 hours; some pumps have 24-hour batteries.

2. Reimbursement in the home-care setting varies greatly among payers. Most payers have very rigid criteria, and the necessity of a pump must be documented before reimbursement is approved.

D. Infusion pump mechanics

1. Fluid delivery mechanisms[53]

a) Rotary peristaltic devices. The pump insert is looped around the pump rotor. The pressure of the rotary mechanism against the tubing pulls the fluid out of the bag and through the administration set. The infusion rate is determined by the speed of the rotor. For the infusion rate to remain accurate, the rotor assembly must be installed and operating correctly, and the pump insert must be placed in accordance with the manufacturer's instructions.

b) Cassette devices. These pump sets incorporate a measured-volume cassette that works with the pumping mechanism to deliver enteral fluid to the patient. These sets tend to be less susceptible to alarm conditions than rotary peristaltic devices. Cassette devices may not deliver reconstituted powdered formulations accurately; manufacturers' recommendations should be followed.

2. Infusion rates. All pump manufacturers claim an accuracy rate of ±10% of the selected flow rate. Formulation viscosity affects the accuracy of the flow rate. Adding a powdered protein supplement to a ready-to-feed formulation may also reduce the expected infusion rate.[54] Institutions should evaluate the delivery accuracy of the

pump and follow manufacturers' instructions for their selection of enteral formulations. Administration sets and tubing should have a safety feature preventing free flow of the formulation.

3. Automatic flush systems. Some manufacturers provide pumps with automatic flush systems. These pumps combine infusion of the enteral formulation with programmable water flushes. The flush feature can be turned off if manual flushing is desired.[55]
4. Pump alarms. Most pumps come with an adjustable alarm control. Troubleshooting guidelines are usually located on the side of the pump.
   a) Low battery power. When this alarm sounds, battery operation should be stopped. Ideally, the pump should be plugged in to an electrical outlet whenever feasible, not only to provide electricity to run the pump but also to recharge the battery. The battery is primarily a backup system in case of a power outage and for use when transporting the patient.
   b) Flow obstruction alarm. An alarm sounds when fluid is not being administered because of an empty bag, kinked tubing, an occluded feeding tube, or an overfilled drip chamber.
   c) Dose-delivered feature. An alarm sounds when a preset dose has been delivered.
   d) Free-flow alarm or runaway alarm. An alarm sounds when the measured rate exceeds the set rate by some percentage.
   e) Set out alarm. An alarm alerts the user if the pump set has not been seated correctly in the set slot.

E. Cleaning and maintenance. The pump should be of a simple design and have as few crevices as possible, because residue and dirt may build up, creating an environment for microbial growth. Pumps should be unplugged and cleaned weekly with a mild soap and warm water. When spills occur, the pump should not be immersed in water.

F. Pump servicing. With use, the rotor mechanism may wear and no longer exert correct pressure, resulting in inaccurate volume delivery. The pump should be serviced on a schedule recommended by the manufacturer.

G. Administration sets. Enteral pumps should have dedicated administration sets that are incompatible with the patient's IV infusion line. Some manufacturers have developed tubing that prevents free flow of the formulation when the set is disconnected from the pump. To minimize microbial contamination of the enteral formulation, the tubing set is usually changed every 24 hours.

(Enteral Access and Infusion Equipment chapter in the 1st edition was contributed by Donald F. Kirby, Gayle Minard, and Carol Kohn-Keeth)

REFERENCES

1. Kirby DF, DeLegge MH, Fleming CR. American Gastroenterological Association technical review of tube feeding for enteral nutrition. *Gastroenterology.* 1995;108:1282–1301.
2. DeLegge MH, Duckworth PF Jr, McHenry L, Foxx-Orenstein A, Craig RM, Kirby DF. Percutaneous endoscopic gastrojejunostomy: a dual center safety and efficacy trial. *J Parenter Enteral Nutr.* 1995;19:239–243.
3. Duckworth PF Jr, Kirby DF, McHenry L, DeLegge MH, Foxx-Orenstein A. Percutaneous endoscopic gastrojejunostomy (PEG/J) made easy: a new over-the-wire technique. *Gastrointest Endosc.* 1994;40:350–353.
4. Hanson RL. Predictive criteria for length of naso/gastric tube insertion for tube feeding. *J Parenter Enteral Nutr.* 1979;3:160–163.
5. Haddad N, Nawaz T, Potter L, Lipman T. Avoidance of naso-pulmonary intubation by feeding tubes with stethoscopic guidance: the "stethotube" [abstract]. *Gastroenterology.* 1993;104:A623.
6. Metheny N, McSweeney M, Wehrle MA, Wiesema L. Effectiveness of the auscultatory method in predicting feeding tube location. *Nurs Res.* 1990;39:262–267.
7. Gutske RF, Varma RR, Soergel KH. Gastric reflux during perfusion of the proximal small bowel. *Gastroenterology.* 1970;59:890–895.
8. Patrick PG, Kirby DF, DeLegge MH. Outcome study on nasojejunal feeding in critically ill patients [abstract]. *Gastrointest Endosc.* 1995;41:370.
9. Baskin WN, Johanson JF. An improved approach to the delivery of enteral nutrition in the intensive care unit. *Gastrointest Endosc.* 1995;42:161–165.
10. Heiselman DR, Vidovich RR, Milkovich G, Black LD. Nasointestinal tube placement with a pH sensor feeding tube. *J Parenter Enteral Nutr.* 1993;17:562–565.
11. Booth CM, Heyland DK, Paterson WG. Gastrointestinal promotility drugs in the critical care setting: a systematic review of the evidence. *Crit Care Med.* 2002;30:1429–1435.
12. Griffith DP, McNally AT, Battey CH, et al. Intravenous erythromycin facilitates bedside placement of postpyloric feeding tubes in critically ill adults: a double-blind, randomized, placebo-controlled study. *Crit Care Med.* 2003;31:315–316.
13. Di Lorenzo C, Lachman R, Hyman PE. Intravenous erythromycin for postpyloric intubation. *J Pediatr Gastroenterol Nutr.* 1990;11:45–47.
14. Gutierrez ED, Balfe DM. Fluoroscopically guided nasoenteric feeding tube placement: results of a 1-year study. *Radiology.* 1991;178:759–762.
15. Mathus-Vliegen EMH, Tytgat GNJ, Merkus MP. Feeding tubes in endoscopic and clinical practice: the longer the better? *Gastrointest Endosc.* 1993;39:537–542.
16. Gauderer MWL, Ponsky JL, Izant RJ Jr. Gastrostomy without laparotomy: a percutaneous endoscopic technique. *J Pediatr Surg.* 1980;15:872–875.
17. Stiegmann GV, Goff JS, Silas D, et al. Endoscopic versus operative gastrostomy: final results of a prospective randomized trial. *Gastrointest Endosc* 1990;36:1–5.
18. Thakore JN, Mustafa M, Suryaprasad S, Agrawal S. Percutaneous endoscopic associated gastric metastasis. *J Clin Gastroenterol.* 2003;37:307–311.
19. Hunter JG. Tumor implantation at PEG exit sites in head and neck cancer patients: how much evidence is enough? [editorial]. *J Clin Gastroenterol.* 2003;37:280.
20. Edelman DS, Unger SW. Laparoscopic gastrostomy and jejunostomy: review of 22 cases. *Surg Laparosc Endosc.* 1994;4:297–300.
21. Kirby DF, DeLegge MH. Enteral nutrition: the challenge of access. In: Kirby DF, Dudrick SJ, eds. *Practical Handbook of Nutrition in Clinical Practice.* Boca Raton, FL: CRC Press; 1994:87–117.
22. Parasher VK, Abramowicz CJ, Bell C, et al. Successful placement of percutaneous gastrojejunostomy using steerable guidewire: modified controlled push technique. *Gastrointest Endosc.* 1995;41:52–55.
23. Baskin WN. Enteral access techniques. *Gastroenterologist.* 1996; 4(suppl 1):S40–67.
24. Shike M, Schroy P, Ritchie MA, et al. Percutaneous endoscopic jejunostomy in cancer patients with previous gastric resection. *Gastrointest Endosc.* 1987;33:372–374.
25. Mellert JK, Fischer H, Grund KE. Direct endoscopic percutaneous jejunostomy (EPJ): an alternative for operative catheter-jejunostomy [abstract]. *Gastrointest Endosc.* 1993;39:254.
26. Duckworth PF Jr, Kirby DF, McHenry L, et al. Percutaneous endoscopic gastrojejunostomy (PEG/J) made easy: a new over-the-wire technique. *Gastrointest Endosc.* 1994;40:350–353.
27. Patrick PG, Kirby DF, DeLegge MH. Evaluation of percutaneous endoscopic gastrojejunostomy tubes as a long-term feeding option [abstract]. *Gastroenterology.* 1996;110:A830.
28. Ho C-S, Yee ACN, McPherson R. Complications of surgical and percutaneous nonendoscopic gastrostomy: review of 233 patients. *Gastroenterology.* 1998;95:1206–1220.
29. Gorman RC, Morris JB, Metz CA, Mullen JL. The button jejunostomy for long-term jejunal feeding: results of a prospective randomized trial. *J Parenter Enteral Nutr.* 1993;17:428–431.
30. Reed DN. Percutaneous peritoneoscopic jejunostomy. *Surg Gynecol Obstet.* 1992;174:527–529.
31. Collier P, Kudsk KA, Glezer J, Brown RO. Fiber-containing formula and needle catheter jejunostomy: a clinical evaluation. *Nutr Clin Pract.* 1994;9:101–103.

32. Petrosino BM, Christian BJ, Wolfe J, Becker H. Implications of selected problems with naso-enteral tube feedings. *Crit Care Nurs Q.* 1989; 12:1–18.
33. Grant JP. Percutaneous endoscopic gastrostomy: initial placement by single endoscopic technique and long-term follow-up. *Ann Surg.* 1993; 217:168–174.
34. Iber FL, Livak A, Patel M. Importance of fungus colonization in failure of silicone rubber percutaneous gastrostomy tubes (PEGs). *Dig Dis Sci.* 1996; 41:226–231.
35. Lord LM, Weiser-Maimone A, Pulhamus M, Sax HC. Comparison of weighted vs unweighted enteral feeding tubes for efficacy of transpyloric intubation. *J Parenter Enteral Nutr.* 1993;17:271–273.
36. Faller NA, Lawrence KG, Ferraro CB. Gastrostomy replacement feeding tube: the long and short of it. *Ostomy Wound Management.* 1993;39:26–33.
37. Townsend LC. Practical considerations of the gastrostomy button. *Gastroenterol Nurs.* 1991;14:18–26.
38. Lehmann S. Parenteral and enteral access devices. In: Teasley-Strausburg KM, Cerra FB, Lehmann S, Shronts EP, eds. *Nutrition Support Handbook: A Compendium of Products with Guidelines for Usage.* Cincinnati, OH: Harvey Whitney Books; 1992:228–257.
39. Metheny N. Verification of feeding tube placement. In: Silver E, Gussler JD, eds. *Current Issues in Enteral Nutrition Support: Report of the First Ross Conference on Enteral Devices.* Columbus, OH: Ross Products Division, Abbott Laboratories; 1996:34–41.
40. Teasley-Strausburg KM, Lehmann S. Guidelines for administration of nutrition support and nutrition support service forms. In: Teasley-Strausburg KM, Cerra FB, Lehmann S, Shronts EP, eds. *Nutrition Support Handbook: A Compendium of Products with Guidelines for Usage.* Cincinnati, OH: Harvey Whitney Books; 1992:321–330.
41. Eisenberg PG. Gastrostomy and jejunostomy tubes. *RN.* 1994;57:54–59.
42. Broscious SK. Preventing complications of PEG tubes. *Dimens Crit Care Nurs.* 1995;14:37–41.
43. Boyd JW, DeLegge MH, Shamburek RD, Kirby DF. The buried bumper syndrome: a review of the literature and a new technique for safe, endoscopic PEG removal. *Gastrointest Endosc.* 1995;41:508–511.
44. Blaylock B, Clayton G, Milnes M, Foster C. A catheter anchoring device. *Ostomy Wound Management.* 1993;39:36–43.
45. Wilson RE. Case study: a system for stabilizing percutaneous tubes. *Ostomy Wound Management.* 1994;40:44–49.
46. Stogdill BJ, Page CP, Pestana C. Nonoperative replacement of a jejunostomy feeding catheter. *Am J Surg.* 1984;147:280–282.
47. Kaufman MW, Faller NA, Lawrence KG. Low profile gastrostomy devices. *Gastroenterol Nurs.* 1995;18:171–176.
48. Maklebust J. Using wound care products to promote a healing environment. *Crit Care Nurs Clin N Am.* 1996;8:141–158.
49. Hagelgans NA, Janusz HB. Pediatric skin care issues for the home care nurse: part 2. *Pediatr Nurs.* 1994;20:69–75.
50. Lehmann S. Nutrient infusion devices. In: Teasley-Strausburg KM, Cerra FB, Lehmann S, Shronts EP, eds. *Nutrition Support Handbook: A Compendium of Products with Guidelines for Usage.* Cincinnati, OH: Harvey Whitney Books; 1992:259–272.
51. Saladow J. Making sense of the options: enteral infusion pumps. *Infusion.* 1995;2:22–27
52. Minard G, Lysen LK. Enteral access devices. In: Gottschlich MM, ed. *The Science and Practice of Nutrition Support.* Dubuque, IA: Kendall/Hunt; 2001:178–181.
53. Goff K. The nuts and bolts of enteral infusion pumps. *MedSurg Nurs.* 1997;6:9–15.
54. Dietscher JE, Foulks CJ, Watts M. Accuracy of enteral pumps: in vitro performance. *J Parenter Enteral Nutr.* 1994;18:359–361.
55. Guenter P. Tube feeding administration. In: Guenter P, Silkroski M, eds. *Tube Feeding Practical Guidelines and Nursing Protocols.* Gaithersburg, MD: Aspen Publishers; 2001:81–94.

SUGGESTED READINGS

Ireton-Jones C, Hennessy K. Care of patients receiving home enteral nutrition. *Infusion.* 1996;2:30–43.

Marks JM, Ponsky JL. Access routes for enteral nutrition. *Gastroenterologist.* 1995:3:130–140.

Payne KM, King TM, Eisenach JB. The technique of percutaneous endoscopic gastrostomy: a safe and cost-effective alternative to operative gastrostomy. *J Crit Ill.* 1991;6:611–619.

Vanek V. Ins and outs of enteral access, I: short-term enteral access. *Nutr Clin Pract.* 2002;17:275–283.

Vanek V. Ins and outs of enteral access, II: long-term enteral access—esophagostomy and gastrostomy. *Nutr Clin Pract.* 2003;18:50–74.

Vanek V. Ins and outs of enteral access, III: long-term access—jejunostomy. *Nutr Clin Pract.* 2003;18:201–220.

Young M, McClure E, Thimsen-Whitaker K. Management of percutaneous tubes. In: Bryant RA, ed. *Acute and Chronic Wounds and Nursing Management.* St Louis, MO: Mosby Year Book; 1992:213–247.

Mary Marian, MS, RD;
Susan J. Carlson, MMSc, RD, CSP, LD, CNSD

4

Enteral Formulations

Introduction

Numerous commercially prepared enteral formulations are available and include standard formulations and specialty products designed to provide nutrition support for specific disease states. It is important to choose formulations that deliver the most beneficial and cost-effective enteral nutrition support. The formulations can be grouped by composition to facilitate formula selection. Once a formulation has been chosen, the compounding (if necessary) and delivery must be undertaken in a manner that will avoid potential infectious complications.

I. Composition and Characteristics of Enteral Formulations

A. Carbohydrate

1. Commonly used carbohydrate sources include maltodextrin, modified cornstarch, and corn syrup. Each of these carbohydrate sources is derived from cornstarch. Other carbohydrate sources often used in infant formulas are lactose and sucrose. The size of individual carbohydrate polymers is defined by dextrose equivalents (DEs). A low DE value indicates a complex carbohydrate source (unaltered cornstarch, DE = 1), whereas a high DE value indicates a simpler source (dextrose, DE = 100).[1]
   a) Maltodextrin, with a DE of <20, is the most complex carbohydrate source commonly added to enteral formulas. Important characteristics of maltodextrin include ease of digestion and relatively low osmotic contribution to an enteral formulation.[1]
   b) Modified cornstarch is variable and cannot be characterized by a specific DE. Modified cornstarch is used to reduce osmolalities in products with otherwise high osmolalities.
   c) Corn syrup, with a DE value ranging from 20 to 65, is a simpler form of carbohydrate than maltodextrin. Like maltodextrin, it is a product of cornstarch hydrolysis.[1]
   d) Monosaccharides and disaccharides, such as lactose and sucrose, have a high DE value and osmolality.
      (1) Lactose is routinely used in standard infant formulations to mimic the carbohydrate found in human milk. Lactose may also enhance the absorption of calcium from these formulations.[2] Most adult medical nutritional products are lactose-free because of the prevalence of lactose intolerance in many populations and because lactase production may be decreased during illness.
      (2) Sucrose is added to some infant formulations in conjunction with maltodextrin to provide carbohydrate, requiring different enzyme systems for digestion and absorption. It also increases the sweetness of the formula.
2. The percentage of energy in products contributed by carbohydrate varies from <30% to >90% depending on the condition for which the product was formulated (see pulmonary disease and glucose intolerance formulations). In pediatric products, the percentage of calories from carbohydrate ranges from 42% to 58%, while in infant formulations it ranges from 40% to 54%.
3. Modular carbohydrate products are available in liquid or powder for use in modifying the carbohydrate content of an existing product. The carbohydrate content ranges from 50 to 95 g of carbohydrate per 100 g of product.

B. Fat

1. Commonly used fat sources include the following:
   a) Vegetable oils such as corn, canola, soybean, sunflower, and safflower. Vegetable oils, which contain long-chain triglycerides (LCTs), contribute essential fatty acids, moderate osmolality, and enhance palatability.
   b) Medium-chain triglyceride (MCT) oil. MCT oil (Mead Johnson, Evansville, IN) does not require bile salts or pancreatic lipase for absorption into portal circulation. It also stimulates the pancreas less than LCTs. MCT oil is useful as an alternative calorie source for patients with malabsorption disorders.[3]
   c) Long-chain polyunsaturated fatty acids including arachidonic acid (ARA), an omega-6 fatty acid, and docosahexaenoic acid (DHA), an omega-3 fatty acid, are supplied from fungal and algae sources.[4] These fatty acids are considered by some to be essential in infancy, particularly in the very lowbirthweight infant, because of their role in visual and neural development.[5,6]
2. The percentage of energy from fat ranges from approximately 1% to 55% in adult formulations according to the formulation's intended use. For example, products designed for patients with pulmonary disease and glucose intolerance are high in fat, whereas products designed for patients with intestinal malabsorption are lower in total fat and LCTs. Pediatric formulations contain 25% to 46% of the calories from fat, while infant formulations range from 35% to 50%. The higher fat content of infant formulations reduces the osmolality of the feeding and provides the necessary fat intake for growth.
3. Modular fat products can be used to increase the fat content of an enteral formulation. MCT oil may be added to a product to increase its caloric density and provide a readily absorbable source of calories. Vegetable oils available for purchase in the grocery store can be used as a source of fat. Microlipid (Novartis Medical Nutrition,

Minneapolis, MN) contains emulsified safflower oil (50% fat emulsion) and may be used to increase the caloric and linoleic acid content of an enteral feeding regimen. In general, emulsified lipid products are better choices for tube feedings, because unemulsified oils separate out of the feeding formulation over time and cling to enteral feeding tubes and administration containers.[7]

C. Protein. Products traditionally are broadly characterized according to their protein type.
   1. Commonly used protein sources include the following:
      a) Cow milk protein, whey protein isolates, caseinates, soy protein isolates, milk protein concentrate, or beef. Intact protein or polymeric formulations contain these types of protein.
      b) Enzymatically hydrolyzed casein, whey, lactalbumin, wheat, and soy or meat protein. Oligomeric or semielemental formulations contain protein sources that have undergone enzymatic hydrolysis (these formulations are often termed *peptide based*). Peptide chain length may vary from product to product depending on the degree of hydrolysis.
      c) Free amino acids. Monomeric or elemental formulations contain free amino acids. Use of free amino acids enables manipulation of the amino acid composition of a product and avoidance of allergens in certain populations.
      d) Other amino acids that may be added to enteral formulations include methionine (soy infant formulas). branched-chain amino acids (BCAAs), glutamine, and arginine. These nutrients are added to certain formulations because of their proposed roles in nutrition support of critically ill patients. (See immunomodulating formulations and formulations for gastrointestinal impairment and liver disease.)
         (1) BCAAs (valine, leucine, and isoleucine) are metabolized by skeletal muscle instead of liver. These amino acids act as a key nitrogen source for synthesis of protein and the amino acids alanine and glutamine during periods of stress. In addition, BCAAs have been promoted for use in liver disease when disorders of aromatic amino acid (AAA) metabolism occur.[8,9]
         (2) L-glutamine appears to be a conditionally essential amino acid during stress-induced conditions. Although glutamine is the most abundant free amino acid in the body, during times of stress and infection, glutamine levels throughout the body fall as production through transamination of α-ketoglutarate or glutamate is unable to meet the increased demands.[10] Glutamine is the preferred energy source for rapidly replicating cells in both the small intestinal mucosa and the immune system. Feeding enteral formulations supplemented with glutamine has been associated with improved microbial colonization patterns, reduced bacterial overgrowth, and improved clinical outcome.[11]
         (3) Like L-glutamine, L-arginine is considered an essential amino acid under certain conditions, including metabolic stress and infection. It also serves as a substrate for the production of nitric oxide. Arginine has been shown to convey potential benefits, including improving cell-mediated immunity following injury, enhancing proliferation of fibroblasts and collagen (thus promoting wound healing), and improving nitrogen balance in critically ill patients.[11]
   2. The protein content in adult formulations ranges from approximately 6% to 32% of calories. Products designed for renal disease can contain very low amounts of protein, whereas stress and immune-enhancing formulations contain up to 94 g/L. Pediatric formulations have little variation in protein content, with approximately 12% of calories from protein. Infant formulations contain 8% to 13% of calories from protein.
   3. Modular protein products are indicated when the protein content of an enteral nutrition regimen needs to be increased without greatly increasing the caloric content or volume of the regimen. Most protein modules contain polymeric protein such as calcium caseinate, whey protein, or egg albumin (eg, ProMod, Ross Products, Columbus, OH).

D. Water content
   1. The energy density of a formulation is dictated largely by the amount of water in the formulation.
   2. Infant formulations providing energy densities of 20 to 24 kcal/fluid ounce (0.67–0.8 kcal/mL) have the highest water content, ranging from 88% to 90%.
   3. Formulations that provide 1 kcal/mL are approximately 75% to 85% water.
   4. Formulations that provide 2 kcal/mL are approximately 70% water. These concentrated formulations are often indicated in adult patients who require fluid restriction.

E. Fiber
   1. Common types of fiber added to enteral formulations include the following:
      a) Soy polysaccharide. This predominantly insoluble fiber is the most prevalent fiber source in fiber-containing enteral formulations. Soy polysaccharide may prevent constipation, increase stool volume, and decrease gastrointestinal (GI) transit time in critically ill patients.[1] In infants, soy polysaccharide can be used to firm stools in the case of diarrhea.
      b) Gum arabic, guar gum, and pectin. These fibers are categorized as soluble fibers. Products that contain soluble fibers may improve glucose tolerance, lower serum cholesterol (if used over the long term), and maintain the ileal and colonic mucosal production of short-chain fatty acids, which are trophic to those mucosal surfaces.[1] Partially hydrolyzed guar gum reportedly also decreases the incidence of enteral nutrition–related diarrhea in non–critically ill and critically ill patients with sepsis.[12]
      c) Fructooligosaccharides (FOSs) have recently been added to some enteral formulations. FOSs are naturally occurring, nondigestible sugars that are selectively used by bifidobacteria in the human intestinal tract. FOS has been demonstrated to improve intestinal flora, relieve constipation, improve blood lipids, and suppress production of putrefactive substances. Excess FOS (more than approximately 45 g for adults) causes diarrhea in humans.[13] Lower doses (eg, 30 g/day) may cause flatulence.
   2. Fiber-containing formulations can create complications in patients who are fluid restricted or have delayed GI transit. Patients receiving fiber-containing formulations should be monitored for symptoms of GI intolerance (eg, abdominal distention, gas, cramping, impaction, or bezoar formation).[14]
   3. The fiber content of adult formulations ranges from 0–22 g/L. Pediatric formulas contain 0–8 g/L. Infant formulations do not routinely contain fiber.

F. Micronutrients
   1. Adult formulations
      a) When provided in adequate volume, nutritionally complete products meet 100% of the US recommended Dietary Reference Intakes (DRI). The volume required to provide the RDI varies greatly among products (≤1–4 L).
      b) Patients who do not receive volumes of formulations adequate to provide the RDI should receive a multivitamin and mineral supplement unless contraindicated.

c) Some disease-specific enteral formulations are not nutritionally complete. Decisions to supplement patients must be made on the basis of an individual patient's condition and severity of organ dysfunction. (See disease-specific chapters.)

2. Pediatric and infant formulations
   a) Most pediatric formulations meet 100% of the US RDI in 1000 mL for children from 1 to 8 years of age and in 1500 mL for children from 9 to 13 years of age.
   b) Infant formulations
      (1) Most infant formulations are designed to meet vitamin and mineral requirements as outlined by the Infant Formula Act. Products for infants with certain diseases (eg, inborn errors of metabolism) are exempt from some of the nutrient requirements in the Infant Formula Act.
      (2) Infants and children with very low energy needs may be unable to meet micronutrient needs with formula alone if fed to their energy need. Nutrients at highest risk for insufficient intake include calcium and phosphorus. A multivitamin and mineral supplement should be provided to meet nutrient goals for these nutrients.

II. Adult Enteral Formulations

A. General-purpose formulations
1. These formulations are generally palatable, easily absorbed, economical, and useful for most patients except those with special metabolic needs or intolerance. These formulations may be the sole source of nutrition, or they may be used to supplement inadequate oral intake.
2. Formulation characteristics
   a) The osmolality for oral formulations generally ranges from isotonic to hypertonic (ie, about 300–700 mOsm per kg of water).
   b) Energy density ranges from 1 to 2 kcal/mL.
   c) Protein content is between 35 and 62 g/L. The protein is high quality and is commonly provided as milk protein concentrate, casein, or soy protein. These intact proteins are readily broken down to peptides and amino acids in most clinical scenarios, with the possible exception of conditions where the bowel absorptive surface is severely eroded.
   d) To minimize osmolality, carbohydrates are provided in complex forms.
   e) Fats are provided as MCTs and LCTs, usually providing 29% to 38% of calories.

B. Nutrient-dense formulations
1. These formulations are designed for use in patients who require fluid restriction (eg, patients with cardiac, renal, pulmonary, or hepatic failure).
2. Formulation characteristics
   a) These formulations are generally hypertonic, as the osmolality ranges from 640 to 950 mOsm per kg of water.
   b) Energy density ranges from 2 to 2.25 kcal/mL.
   c) Protein sources include sodium and calcium caseinates, soy and milk protein isolates, and milk protein concentrate at 57 to 84 g/L.
   d) Carbohydrate is supplied by corn syrup, maltodextrin, hydrolyzed cornstarch, and/or sucrose as 39% to 45% of total calories.
   e) Fat content includes various combinations of soy, corn, safflower, MCT, and canola oils in amounts ranging from 30% to 55% of total calories.

B. Cancer
1. Weight loss and loss of functional tissue (lean body mass) is a common problem in patients with advanced cancer despite aggressive nutritional interventions. Continued deterioration of nutritional status is thought to result from changes mediated by proinflammatory cytokines, hormones, and other tumor-derived metabolites. Enteral formulations enriched with fish oils (omega-3 fatty acids) and other immune-promoting substrates have been used in patients with GI cancers. The results of their use as revealed in clinical studies have been promising.[15–20]
2. Formulation characteristics
   a) Osmolality is 635 mOsm per kg of water.
   b) Energy density is 1.27 kcal/mL.
   c) The protein provided is approximately 64 g/L (21% of total energy).
   d) Carbohydrate sources include corn syrup solids, maltodextrin, sugar, fructooligosaccharides, gum arabic, and soy fiber.
   e) Omega-3 fatty acids are provided through a unique blend of sardine oil and canola oil. Additionally, MCT oil, soybean oil, and lecithin are included as fat sources (18% of total calories).
3. Clinical studies comparing the use of immune-enhancing formulations with standard formulations when enteral support is required for patients undergoing surgery for GI cancer have yielded mixed results.[14–18] The contrasts in study results are likely due to differences in study design and the insufficient number of patients enrolled in each of the studies. Despite the flaws in study design, subanalysis of many of these studies suggests a role for immune-enhancing formulations for malnourished patients undergoing surgery for upper GI cancer (both pre- and postoperatively).[18] To obtain the maximal benefits associated with using these formulations, patients should be fed for at least 5 to 7 days.[19]
4. Consumption of a nutritional supplement enriched with fish oil (providing 2 g/day of eicosapentaenoic acid [EPA]) for at least 3 weeks was associated with gains in weight and lean body mass and reduced levels of several inflammatory biomarkers in severely cachectic patients with pancreatic cancer cachexia.[20] However, further research is needed to determine specifically which patients with cancer cachexia are likely to benefit from consumption of this supplement.

D. Critical care/immunomodulating
1. Patients with trauma, sepsis, burns, or postsurgical stress are in a relative state of immunosuppression. When these patients must undergo surgical procedures, they have high rates of infectious complications such as pneumonia, intra-abdominal abscess, and wound infections. Commercially prepared enteral formulations have been developed through fortifying standard enteral formulations with omega-3 fatty acids, nucleotides, arginine, and glutamine. Unfortunately, it is still unclear which of these substrates is responsible for the immune-enhancing benefits associated with these formulations. The results from clinical studies and meta-analyses suggest that the use of immune-enhancing formulations for patients posttrauma and perioperative patients may reduce the number of overall infectious complications. Furthermore, clinical trials investigating immunomodulating formulations have demonstrated decreased antibiotic use, fewer days on mechanical ventilation, decreased length of hospitalization, and, ultimately, reduced health care costs.[21–25]
2. Critically ill patients have been found to have reduced levels of antioxidants (vitamins C and E, retinol, beta-carotene, and selenium). Whether supplementation with therapeutic levels of these

micronutrients results in positive clinical outcomes has yet to be determined. Excess supplementation may be undesirable.

3. Formulation characteristics
   a) Osmolality is moderate, at a range of 375 to 630 mOsm per kg of water.
   b) Energy density ranges from 1 to 1.5 kcal/mL.
   c) The high protein content (55–84 g/L) is uniquely formulated to include the following:
      (1) Arginine and glutamine, which, as previously discussed, may be conditionally essential during stress and are supplemented in some of the stress formulations
      (2) BCAAs, which are essential amino acids mobilized from skeletal muscle during stress. Supplemental BCAAs may preserve muscle in metabolically stressed patients; however, studies have not consistently shown improved clinical outcomes.[26,27]
      (3) Nucleotides, which are required by rapidly proliferating tissues such as the intestinal epithelium. Nucleotides also enhance lymphocyte proliferation and responsiveness.
      (4) Carbohydrate sources, which include maltodextrin or hydrolyzed cornstarch. Fiber may also be provided as hydrolyzed guar gum or soy fiber.
      (5) Fat sources, which contribute between 20% and 55% of total calories. Long-chain omega-3 fatty acid content is one of the defining characteristics of this category of formulations. Inflammatory mediators normally produced during critical illness may be minimized with administration of omega-3 fatty acids because their metabolism produces prostaglandins and thromboxanes of a less inflammatory and less immunosuppressive nature than the products of omega-6 fatty acid metabolism. Supplementation with omega-3 fatty acids has been shown to attenuate the inflammatory response, stabilize the nuclear factor-K-B complex, possess antithrombotic properties, reduce platelet adhesion, enhance neutrophil function, and support membrane stability and microvasculature profusion.[11]
      (6) Structured lipids, which are also added to some of the immunomodulating formulations. Structured lipids are chemical combinations of long-, medium-, and short-chain fatty acids on a single glycerol backbone. The resultant product has improved absorption (compared with LCT), minimizes immune dysfunction,[11] and can provide essential fatty acids.
   d) A variety of commercially prepared formulations are available with various substrates added that may modulate the immune system. According to the recommendations of the US Summit on Immune-Enhancing Enteral Therapy[25] held in 2000, immune-enhancing formulations may be beneficial for the following:
      (1) Patients undergoing major elective GI surgery, especially malnourished patients
      (2) Patients with blunt and penetrating torso trauma
      (3) Malnourished patients undergoing surgery for head and neck cancer
      (4) Patients with severe head injury
      (5) Burn patients
      (6) Ventilator-dependent non-septic patients at risk for infection
      (7) Patients needing formulations for a minimum of 5 days
      (8) Patients with preexisting severe sepsis. Two studies suggest that patients with preexisting severe sepsis may have an increased mortality rate when fed an immune-enhancing diet. A third study reported a decreased incidence of mortality. Therefore, the use of immune-enhancing diets in this patient population requires further study.

E. Diabetes/glucose intolerance
1. Patients with diabetes mellitus or stress-induced glucose intolerance have difficulty tolerating the carbohydrate content of general-purpose enteral formulations. Hyperglycemia is associated with an increased risk for infectious complications, so promoting glycemic control is important when providing nutrition support. In addition to pharmacotherapeutic interventions, a number of commercially prepared fiber-containing, reduced carbohydrate, modified fat formulations are now available for enteral feeding for patients with poor glucose control.[28]
2. Formulation characteristics
   a) These formulations are essentially isotonic.
   b) Energy density is 1 to 1.2 kcal/mL.
   c) An intact protein source provides 42 to 63 g/L.
   d) Carbohydrate is primarily polysaccharide, with fructose for flavor, and provides 31% to 40% of total calories.
   e) Fiber content ranges from 8 to 21 g/L. Fiber sources vary but generally are derived from hydrolyzed guar gum, soy fiber, acacia, cellulose, soy polysaccharides, pectin, gum arabic, or fruit and vegetable fiber.
   f) Fat provides 40% to 50% of calories; the ratio of omega-6 to omega-3 fats is variable. There is generally a greater proportion of fat calories than is recommended by the American Diabetes Association for healthy patients with diabetes.[29,30]
   g) There is limited published evidence that the use of these specialty formulations results in improved glucose control in hospitalized patients, especially the critically ill. Patients with glucose intolerance should be carefully evaluated for concomitant morbidities (eg, gastroparesis, renal impairment) when selecting the appropriatc formula. Improved glycemic control can reduce diabetic gastroparesis. Important goals of nutrition therapy should include avoiding overfeeding and controlling glucose through administration of insulin, if needed.

F. Hepatic disease
1. Patients with decompensated liver disease are typically malnourished and benefit from nutritional supplementation. Some patients who have worsening encephalopathy when they receive standard enteral formulations may improve when given a formulation containing a higher BCAA-to-AAA ratio. Hepatic disease formulations should not be used in patients with nonencephalopathic manifestations of liver disease.[31]
2. Formulation characteristics
   a) These formulas are hypertonic, with osmolalities of >450 mOsm per kg of water.
   b) Energy density ranges from 1.2 to 1.5 kcal/mL.
   c) To minimize ammonia production, protein content is low (40–46 g/L). BCAAs are provided in greater amounts than AAAs because of the increased quantities of AAAs in patients with liver failure. This abnormal AAA-to-BCAA ratio, which results in AAAs acting as false neurotransmitters, is one of the theoretical etiologies of hepatic encephalopathy.[31]
   d) Carbohydrate is supplied as maltodextrin and sucrose.
   e) Hepatic formulations are low in fat because absorption can be impaired as a result of cholestasis.
3. Clinical studies have not demonstrated improved outcomes in patients who received formulations high in BCAAs.[31,32] Use of

these formulations should be restricted to patients who present with grade II or greater encephalopathy or whose grade of encephalopathy worsens as nutrition support with a standard enteral formulation is advanced.

G. Impaired GI digestion or absorption
   1. In certain disease states, there may be impaired absorption of nutrients. Absorption may be enhanced with the use of a chemically defined formulation. Also, because they are less viscous, chemically defined formulations are commonly used in patients with needle catheter jejunostomies to minimize catheter clogging. Conditions that can benefit from the use of a chemically defined formulation include the following:
      a) Diffuse diseases of the intestinal mucosa, such as celiac disease, inflammatory bowel disease, and enterokinase deficiency
      b) Critical illness, especially after shock, trauma, sepsis, or surgery
      c) Pancreatic or bile salt deficiencies
      d) Intestinal atrophy or loss of absorptive surface, as with prolonged nothing-by-mouth status, profound malnutrition, and short-bowel syndrome
   2. Formulation characteristics
      a) Semi-elemental or peptide-based formulations have a lower osmolality than elemental formulations but a higher osmolality than polymeric formulations.
      b) Energy density ranges from 1 to 1.5 kcal/mL.
      c) Protein is supplied as crystalline amino acids (elemental formulations) or as hydrolyzed whey, casein, wheat protein, soy, or lactalbumin or a mixture of free amino acids and hydrolyzed protein.
      d) The fat content ranges from very low fat (1% of total calories) to 30% of total calories.
      e) Peptides may be better absorbed than free amino acids by both healthy and diseased guts.[33] Individual amino acids are absorbed by a less efficient, passive diffusion mechanism. However, tolerance and clinical outcomes with peptide-based formulations have not been demonstrated to be superior to the outcomes of polymeric formulation use.[34,35] Additional concerns of using these products include increased cost, evidence that less complex products are less trophic to the GI tract and may increase the risk of bacterial translocation, and deleterious effects on immunocompetence.[36,37] To summarize, these products should be reserved for use in patients with disease states that lead to malabsorption of conventional polymeric formulations and in patients who have demonstrated intolerance to polymeric feedings.

H. Pancreatitis
   1. Traditionally, parenteral nutrition was the preferred method of providing specialized nutrition support to patients with severe pancreatitis because it was thought that not using the GI tract would result in less stimulation of and more rest for the pancreas. However, evidence has accumulated that favors the use of enteral nutrition support for patients with pancreatitis when specialized nutrition support is warranted. (See Chapter 15.)
   2. Formulation characteristics
      a) Elemental and peptide-based formulations generally range in osmolality from 270 to 650 mOsm per kg of water.
      b) Energy density ranges from 1 to 1.5 kcal/mL.
      c) Protein content ranges from 21 to 94 g/L.
      d) Carbohydrate sources include maltodextrin, and hydrolyzed cornstarch, sucrose, and soy fiber; carbohydrates generally contribute 36% to 91% of total calories.
      e) Fat content ranges from approximately 1% to 39% of total calories.
      f) These products are nutritionally complete and provide 100% of the RDI in approximately 950 mL to 2 L.
   3. Studies show that jejunal administration of specialized enteral nutrition support not only is well tolerated but also attenuates the inflammatory response, reduces hyperglycemia and infectious complications, and hastens recovery from the pancreatic insult compared with parenteral nutrition.[38–40] While the "ideal" enteral formulation for patients with pancreatitis has not been agreed upon, clinical studies where enteral nutrition has been successfully employed have generally used peptide-based formulations with good tolerance.

I. Pulmonary disease
   1. Formulations for use in patients with long- or short-term pulmonary disease are designed based on the theory that, when more energy is provided from fat and less from carbohydrate, a patient's carbon dioxide production will be lowered and thereby the amount of carbon dioxide retention will be reduced. Additionally, some investigators have demonstrated significantly reduced time on mechanical ventilation for patients who receive these formulations.[41,42]
   2. Formulation characteristics
      a) These formulas are moderately hypertonic (330–650 mOsm per kg of water).
      b) Energy density is 1.5 kcal/mL.
      c) Protein content ranges from 63 to 75 g/L.
      d) Carbohydrate sources include sucrose, maltodextrin, and hydrolyzed cornstarch, which contribute between 28% and 40% of total calories. Some pulmonary formulations also contain fiber (8 g/L) from sources including hydrolyzed guar gum and soy fiber.
      e) Fat content ranges from approximately 38% to 55% of total calories.
      f) These products are nutritionally complete and provide 100% of the RDI in ≤1 L.
      g) Formulations designed for patients with Acute Respiratory Distress Syndrome (ARDS) also contain borage and sardine oils.
   3. In general, studies demonstrating the benefits of pulmonary formulations over general-purpose formulations have been criticized for having a small sample size.[41,42] Recent studies suggest that avoiding overfeeding of energy is as effective in reducing PCO_2, as is a low-carbohydrate feeding regimen.[43] Thus, pulmonary formulations may not provide clinically significant benefits above those of a nutrition support regimen that provides adequate (instead of excessive) energy regardless of the carbohydrate-to-fat ratio.
   4. Conversely, a recent clinical study reported positive clinical outcomes with the use of an enteral formulation specifically designed for patients with ARDS. Although this product provides a high fat content, the fat composition has been altered to provide greater amounts of EPA and gamma-linolenic acid. This combination has been shown to alter membrane phospholipid makeup, subsequently resulting in the synthesis of the less inflammation-producing eicosanoids.[44] Improved clinical outcomes included decreased length of stay and fewer ventilator days.
   5. Ambulatory patients with long-term pulmonary disease often need an oral supplement because these patients have high energy needs, fatigue easily, and often have trouble eating and breathing simultaneously, which makes it difficult to consume adequate energy and protein from common foods. Energy-dense products allow

such patients to consume a large amount of energy and protein in a small volume and with little effort.

J. Renal disease
 1. Enteral formulations for patients with renal disease must provide adequate nutrients and minimize complications such as fluid overload, uremia, and elevated serum electrolyte and mineral concentrations. To achieve these goals, renal formulations typically are energy dense, low in electrolyte and mineral contents, and moderate in protein content.
 2. Formulation characteristics
   a) These formulations are very hypertonic, with osmolalities ranging from 570 to 700 mOsm per kg of water.
   b) Energy density is 2 kcal/mL.
   c) Protein content ranges from 30 to 75 g/L. Protein sources include sodium, calcium and magnesium caseinates, milk protein isolate, whey protein, and free amino acids.
   d) Carbohydrate sources include maltodextrin, sucrose, fructose, corn syrup, and hydrolyzed cornstarch.
   e) Fat sources include safflower, soy, canola, corn, and MCT oil and contribute 35% to 46% of calories.
   f) Some formulations are not nutritionally complete; some are essentially vitamin- and mineral-free, and others contain some water-soluble vitamins and no fat-soluble vitamins or minerals
 3. Historically, enteral renal formulations with protein sources derived chiefly from essential amino acids were used for patients with short-term renal failure who could not tolerate dialysis, or for whom dialysis was being postponed or avoided. However, today most patients with acute renal failure are dialyzed; therefore, the use of these formulations is rarely warranted. A variety of formulations designed for patients with impaired renal function are available with modified electrolyte and micronutrient compositions. These formulations may be appropriate for patients whose serum electrolyte and mineral levels are difficult to control.

K. Wound healing
 1. Obesity, poor oxygenation, infection, aging, impaired immune function, vascular insufficiency, and some medications can impair wound healing.[45] Poor nutrition can also contribute to delayed and impaired wound healing. Reportedly, enteral nutrition is associated with improvements in wound healing when compared with parenteral support.[46] The optimal provision of both macro- and micronutrients is required for cellular, collagen, and connective tissue synthesis. Of the micronutrients, vitamins A, E, K, and C, thiamine, riboflavin, and zinc have been identified with improved wound healing.[46] The conditionally essential amino acid arginine may also enhance wound repair.[46]
 2. Formulation characteristics
   a) Osmolality is moderate, at a range of 300 to 630 mOsm per kg of water.
   b) Energy density ranges from 1 to 1.5 kcal/mL.
   c) The high protein content (55–84 g/L) generally is provided by protein sources similar to those discussed in the immune-modulating formulation section; it typically includes sodium and calcium caseinates, L-arginine, whey and wheat protein hydrolysates, soy protein isolate, and free amino acids. Some formulations are supplemented with L-arginine and L-glutamine.
   d) L-arginine may be a conditionally essential amino acid to promote wound healing. Arginine supplementation has been found not only to improve nitrogen balance but also to enhance immune function and increase hydroxyproline accumulation in healthy people supplemented with arginine for 2 weeks.[46] However, the optimal amount of arginine needed to promote wound healing is unknown. As previously discussed, several formulations are available that contain not only arginine but other substrates associated with wound healing.
   e) Carbohydrate sources include hydrolyzed cornstarch, sucrose, maltodextrin, and corn syrup solids. Many formulations also offer fiber supplementation with hydrolyzed guar gum, soy fiber, or soy polysaccharides.
   f) Fat generally comprises 25% to 40% of total calories. Sources include palm kernel, sunflower, canola, safflower, and MCT oil; soy lecithin; and menhaden fish oil.
   g) Nutrition is one of many factors that influence wound healing. A variety of commercially prepared enteral formulations are now available that contain greater levels of vitamins A, C, and E as well as zinc. While clinical studies have found these micronutrients to play an important role in wound healing, supplementation beyond the RDI has not been shown to improve wound healing when no clinical deficiency exists. In some cases, excess supplementation may be detrimental.
 3. Poor nutritional status has been linked with the development of pressure ulcers. Provision of adequate nutrition is key in prevention and treatment. To promote positive patient outcomes as well as wound healing, the choice of the "optimal" enteral formulation should be dictated by both the patient's clinical status and nutritional requirements.
 4. Arginine, glutamine, omega-3 fatty acids, vitamins A and C, and zinc are specific substrates frequently associated with stimulating immunocompetence and enhanced wound healing postburn. The results of clinical trials using commercially prepared enteral formulations to alter clinical outcomes are mixed.[45,47] In one study, burn patients receiving a formulation high in protein and low in fat but fortified with omega-3 fatty acids, arginine, cysteine, histidine, vitamins A and C, and zinc experienced fewer overall infections and had a shortened length of hospitalization.[47] Another study found that an immune-enhancing formulation fortified with omega-3 fatty acids, nucleotides, and arginine provided no significant benefits.[45] The A.S.P.E.N. Clinical Guidelines for the Use of Parenteral and Enteral Nutrition in Adult and Pediatric Patients state that "there is no current role for the routine use of specific nutrients in burn patients."[48]

III. Pediatric Enteral Formulations

A. General-purpose formulations
 1. General-purpose formulations are designed for children from 1 to 10 years of age who require tube feedings or oral formula supplements to meet nutrient needs. These formulations are available in two forms, one for tube feeding and the other for use as an oral supplement.
 2. Formulation characteristics
   a) The enteral tube-feeding products are isotonic, with osmolalities of 335 to 380 mOsm per kg of water. The osmolalities of the oral formulations are higher, ranging from 430 to 520 mOsm per kg of water.
   b) Energy density is 30 kcal/fluid ounce (1 kcal/mL).
   c) Protein sources are typically sodium and calcium caseinates, milk protein, and/or whey protein concentrate. A blenderized formulation also contains beef as a protein source. All products contain at least one source of cow milk protein. The protein content of these formulations ranges from 30 to 38 g/L, with most formulas containing 30 g/L.

d) Carbohydrate sources are typically maltodextrin and sucrose. Other carbohydrate sources include fructose, apple juice, fruits, and vegetables. The sucrose content is higher in oral supplements (30%–70% of carbohydrate) than in tube-feeding products (13% of carbohydrate) to enhance flavor. The carbohydrate content of these formulations ranges from 110 to 138 g/L. Products are available with and without fiber. Fiber sources include soy fiber, pea fiber, gum arabic, oat fiber, carboxymethylcellulose, oligofructose, fruits, and vegetables. The fiber content of the fiber-containing products ranges from 4.4 to 8 g/L.

e) Fat sources include high oleic sunflower and safflower oils, canola oil, corn oil, soy oil, beef fat, and MCT. The fat content ranges from 37 to 50 g/L.

B. Chemically defined formulations

1. The chemically defined formulations are designed for 1- to 10-year-old children with severe protein allergies, malabsorption, and/or GI tract impairment. The nutrient content varies widely from product to product. Product selection should be determined by matching the disease condition with the appropriate nutrient composition. Peptide products with moderate MCT oil content are designed for children with malabsorption syndromes. Free amino acid products are indicated for children with severe protein allergies who demonstrate an allergic response to the extensively hydrolyzed protein found in the peptide products.

2. Formulation characteristics

a) Osmolality of the chemically defined formulas is typically higher than the that of general purpose pediatric formulations due to the predigested nature of the protein source. The most hypertonic formulas contain free amino acids as their protein source. The osmolalities of these products range from 260 to 820 mOsm per kg of water.

b) Caloric density ranges from 20 kcal/fluid ounce (0.8 kcal/mL) to 30 kcal/fluid ounce (1 kcal/mL).

c) Protein sources include whey hydrolysates, soy hydrolysates, pork hydrolysates, and free amino acids. The protein content ranges from 24 to 32 g/L (30–32 g/1000 kcal).

d) Carbohydrate sources include corn syrup solids, maltodextrin, modified cornstarch, and sucrose. All products are lactose-free. The carbohydrate content ranges from 107 to 138 g/L (107–162 g/1000 kcal).

e) Fat sources include high-oleic safflower oil, soy oil, canola oils, and MCT. The fat content ranges from 24 to 49 g/L (30–49 g/1000 kcal). MCTs range from 25% to 60% of the fat content.

C. High-MCT formulations

1. These formulations were initially designed for children with fat digestion, absorption, and transport disorders, as MCTs are easier to digest and absorb than LCTs. The use of a diet low in LCTs has also been recommended in the treatment of patients with chylous leak syndromes (chylothorax and chylous ascites) and in disorders of fatty acid transport (lymphangiectasia). As MCTs are transported via the portal system instead of the lymphatic system, they may minimize lymphatic flow.

2. Formulation characteristics

a) The high-MCT formulation is isotonic, with an osmolality of 350 mOsm per kg of water.

b) The caloric density is 30 kcal/ounce (1.01 kcal/mL).

c) The protein source is sodium caseinate. The protein content of the formulation is 35 g/L.

d) Carbohydrate sources include corn syrup solids and sucrose. The product is lactose-free and contains 114 g/L.

e) Fat sources include corn oil and MCTs. The MCT oil composes 87% of the fat. The product contains 48 g/L.

f) Because the LCT content is low, the content of essential fatty acids is also low (3.4 g linoleic acid/L). Long-term use of this product, particularly in patients with fat malabsorption, may induce essential fatty acid deficiency. When this product was labeled as an infant formulation, infants with hepatocellular disease fed the high-MCT formulation developed an increased triene:tetraene ratio consistent with essential fatty acid deficiency. When fed formulations containing only 50% of fat calories as MCT, the same infants were able to maintain essential fatty acid stores.[49] This high-MCT formulation should be avoided in infants with fat malabsorption. Infants requiring a high-MCT formulation for management of chylous leak syndromes may require a secondary source of essential fatty acids such as intravenous fat emulsions if the formulation is used for extended periods.

IV. Infant Enteral Formulations

A. Standard cow milk–based formulations for term infants

1. Cow milk formulations are indicated as routine feedings for infants.

2. Formulation characteristics

a) These formulations are isotonic, with osmolalities ranging from 280 to 300 mOsm per kg of water.

b) Standard energy density is 20 kcal/fluid ounce (0.67 kcal/mL). The formulations are also available in 24 kcal/fluid ounce ready-to-feed bottles (0.8 kcal/mL) for hospital use.

c) Protein sources include whey protein concentrate, sodium caseinate, nonfat milk, and hydrolyzed reduced-minerals whey protein concentrate. The protein content of these formulas, at standard dilution, is 1.4 g/100 mL (2.1 g/100 kcal).

d) Lactose is the carbohydrate source. The carbohydrate content at standard dilution ranges from 7.1 to 7.5 g/100 mL (10.6–11.2 g/100 kcal).

e) Fat sources include high oleic safflower and sunflower oils, soy oil, coconut oil, palm olein, and safflower oil. The fat content at standard dilution ranges from 3.4 to 3.6 g/100 mL (5.1–5.4 g/100 kcal).

f) The formulations are available with and without added ARA and DHA. Studies evaluating the effect of very long chain fatty acids on visual and neural development have had conflicting results, with some studies showing improved visual and mental development and others demonstrate no effect.[5,6] These differences in outcomes may reflect differing formula compositions, differing levels of very long chain fatty acid supplementation, and differing levels of essential fatty acids.

g) Some cow milk formulations contain added nucleotides. Studies have shown that the addition of a particular amount of nucleotides to infant feedings (72 mg/L) enhances antibody response to specific immunizations and lymphocyte maturation so that they are closer to those of breast-fed infants.[50]

h) Cow milk formulations are available with two levels of iron. Only the formulations with the higher iron content are indicated for routine use in infant feedings.[51]

i) Cow milk formulations are available in ready-to-feed, concentrated liquid (40 kcal/fluid ounce), and powder forms.

B. Cow milk–based lactose-free formulations

1. "Lactose-free formulations" are cow milk–based lactose-free products marketed as an alternative to soy formulations for infants

with symptoms thought to be related to lactose intake. The formulations are considered very low in lactose but are not indicated for use in infants with galactosemia.

2. Formulation characteristics
   a) These formulations are hypotonic, with osmolalities of approximately 200 mOsm per kg of water.
   b) Standard energy density is 20 kcal/fluid ounce (0.67 kcal/mL).
   c) The protein source is milk protein isolate. The protein content is 1.4 g/100 mL (2.1 g/100 kcal).
   d) Carbohydrate sources include maltodextrin, corn syrup solid, and sucrose. The carbohydrate content is approximately 7.2 g/100 mL (10.8 g/100 kcal).
   e) Fat sources include high oleic safflower and sunflower oils, soy oil, coconut oil, and palm olein. The fat content is approximately 3.6 g/100 mL (5.4 g/100 kcal). These formulations contain added ARA and DHA.
   f) These formulations contain added nucleotides.
   g) Cow milk–based lactose-free formulations are available in ready-to-feed, concentrated liquid (40 kcal/fluid ounce), and powder forms.

C. Soy-based lactose-free formulations
1. Soy-based formulations are cow milk protein–and lactose-free. They have been marketed for use with fussy babies and infants with allergies, lactose intolerance, or galactosemia. The American Academy of Pediatrics recommends the use of soy formulations for infants with galactosemia, infants with documented lactose intolerance, or infants with vegetarian parents who want a plant-based formulation for their children. Eighty six percent of patients with IgE-mediated cow milk protein allergy tolerated soy formula.[52] The academy states that soy formulations are not effective for treatment of colic and should not be used for infants with GI cow milk protein allergy or premature infants weighing less than 1800 g.[53]
2. Formulation characteristics
   a) These formulations are hypotonic, with osmolalities of approximately 200 mOsm per kg of water.
   b) Standard energy density of these formulations is 20 kcal/fluid ounce (0.67 kcal/mL).
   c) The protein source is soy protein isolate. L-methionine is added to improve the biological value of the soy protein. The protein content ranges from 1.6 to 1.9 g/100 mL (2.4–2.8 g/100 kcal).
   d) Carbohydrate sources include corn syrup, corn maltodextrin, and sucrose. The carbohydrate content ranges from 6.8 to 7.4 g/100 mL (10.1–11.1 g/100 kcal).
   e) Fat sources include high oleic safflower and sunflower oils, coconut oil, soy oil, and palm olein. The fat content ranges from 3.4 to 3.6 g/100 mL (5.1–5.5 g/100 kcal). These formulations are available with and without added ARA and DHA.
   f) One ready-to-feed soy formulation contains added soy fiber with a fiber content of 0.6 g/100 mL (0.9 g/100 kcal). Soy polysaccharide added to infant formulations has been found to improve stool consistency and reduce duration of diarrhea in infants and toddlers suffering from gastroenteritis or antibiotic-induced diarrhea.[54–56]
   g) Soy formulations are available in ready-to-feed, concentrated liquid (40 kcal/ounce), and powder forms.

D. Chemically defined formulations
1. Three different chemically defined formulations are available. Indications for each formulation vary. The first category contains extensively hydrolyzed protein and LCTs as the fat source. This formulation is designed for use in infants with cow milk or soy protein allergies. The second category contains extensively hydrolyzed protein and a blend of LCTs and MCTs. This formulation may be used for infants with cow milk or soy protein allergies but is also indicated for infants with malabsorption syndromes such as short-bowel syndrome and cystic fibrosis. The third category contains free amino acids and low amounts of MCTs. This formulation is indicated for infants who continue to demonstrate allergic symptoms on extensively hydrolyzed protein formulations. It is also often used for infants with serious malabsorption.
2. Formulation characteristics
   a) These formulations have osmolalities ranging from 320 to 500 mOsm per kg of water.
   b) Standard energy density is 20 kcal/fluid ounce (0.67 kcal/mL).
   c) Protein sources include extensively hydrolyzed casein and free amino acids. Casein hydrolysate formulations also contain added L-cystine, L-tyrosine, and L-tryptophan. The protein content ranges from 1.8 to 2.1 g/100 mL (2.7–3.1 g/100 kcal).
   d) Carbohydrate sources include corn syrup solids, modified cornstarch, modified tapioca starch, dextrose, and sucrose. All formulations are lactose-free. The carbohydrate content ranges from 6.8 to 9.1 g/100 mL (10.2–13.6 g/100 kcal).
   e) Fat sources include canola, coconut, corn, high oleic safflower, safflower, sunflower, and soy oils, as well as palm olein. Hydrolyzed casein formulations also contain ARA and DHA. Hydrolyzed casein formulations have an MCT content of 0% to 60% of fat calories. Free amino acid formulations have an MCT content of 5% to 33% of fat calories. The fat content ranges from 2.6 to 3.8 g/100 mL (4.2–5.7 g/100 kcal).
   f) Chemically defined formulations are available in a variety of forms. All products are available in a powder form, and the hydrolyzed formulations are also available in a ready-to-feed form. One hydrolyzed formulation is also available to hospitals as a concentrated liquid.
3. Approximately 2% to 3% of formula-fed infants will develop an allergy to cow milk protein. The incidence is increased in infants with a family history of allergy. Two forms of cow milk protein allergy/intolerance have been identified. The first form is immunoglobulin-E (IgE) mediated and presents as urticaria, respiratory difficulties, vomiting, and anaphylaxis. The second form, non-IgE mediated, presents as GI symptoms such as vomiting, diarrhea, bloody stools, and enterocolitis. Infants with IgE-mediated allergies will often tolerate soy formulations without development of a secondary allergy to soy. Infants with non-IgE-mediated GI protein intolerance are at high risk of developing a soy allergy. The American Academy of Pediatrics Committee on Nutrition recommends that breast milk, extensively hydrolyzed formulations, or free amino acid formulations be used for infants with "non-IgE-associated syndromes such as enterocolitis, proctocolitis, malabsorption syndrome, or esophagitis."[57]
4. Approximately 10% of infants with colic have a cow milk protein allergy that may respond to a chemically defined diet.[58]

E. Low electrolyte/mineral formulations for renal disease
1. Hypocalcemia and hyperphosphatemia are common complications in infants with renal disease. Diets low in phosphorus are indicated to minimize the development of bone disease.
2. Formulation characteristics
   a) Osmolality is isotonic, at 280 mOsm per kg of water.
   b) Standard energy density is 20 kcal/fluid ounce (0.67 kcal/mL).
   c) Protein sources include whey protein concentrate and sodium caseinate. The whey to casein ratio is 60:40. The protein content is 1.5 g/100 mL (2.2 g/100 kcal).

d) The carbohydrate source is lactose. The carbohydrate content is 6.8 g/100 mL (10.2 g/100 kcal).

e) Fat sources include corn, coconut, and soy oils. The fat content is 3.7 g/100 mL (5.6 g/100 kcal).

f) This product has a lower content of calcium, phosphorus, potassium, and chloride than standard cow milk formulations. It is also low in iron, containing 0.47 mg/100 mL (0.7 mg/100 kcal). An iron supplement is indicated for patients using this product.

g) This product is available in powder form only.

F. Thickened formulations

1. Gastroesophageal reflux and regurgitation are common symptoms in newborns, peaking at approximately 4 months of age and resolving by the end of the first year of life.[59] Although controversial, thickening of infant formulations is a common practice in the management of gastroesophageal reflux and has been recommended by the North American Society for Pediatric Gastroenterology and Nutrition as a treatment for this condition.[60] Thickening of infant formulas is often accomplished by adding rice cereal to a standard cow milk formula. This method of thickening formula increases the energy density and alters the nutrient composition of the product. An infant formulation product with added rice starch that thickens when exposed to gastric acid has been developed. Its nutrient composition is comparable to that of standard infant formulations.

2. Formulation characteristics

a) The osmolality is isotonic, at 240 mOsm per kg of water.

b) Energy density of the formula is 20 kcal/fluid ounce (0.67 kcal/mL).

c) Protein content is nonfat milk, with 1.7 g protein/100 mL (2.5 g/100 kcal).

d) Carbohydrate sources include lactose, rice starch, and maltodextrin. The carbohydrate content is 7.4 g/100 mL (11 g/100 kcal).

e) Fat sources include palm olein, soy oil, coconut oil, high oleic sunflower oil, and single-cell oils rich in DHA and ARA. The fat content is 3.4 g/100 mL (5.1 g/100 kcal).

f) The formulation is available in only a ready-to-feed form.

3. Several studies have shown that thickened infant formulations reduce overt signs of gastroesophageal reflux.[61,62] While thickening agents may reduce regurgitation, subclinical acid reflux may continue. Infant formulations thickened with carob bean gum have been found to reduce the frequency and reflux height of nonacid (pH > 4) regurgitations but not the frequency and duration of acid reflux (pH < 4).[62]

V. Preterm Infant Enteral Formulations

A. Human milk fortifiers

1. Preterm infants have increased needs for protein, minerals, and electrolytes to support the rapid growth and bone mineralization normally occurring during the final trimester of pregnancy. Human milk, ideal for term infants, requires supplementation to meet the needs of the growing preemie. Human milk fortifiers (HMFs) are powders or liquids that are mixed with human milk to increase the protein, mineral, electrolyte, and vitamin content.

2. Formulation characteristics

a) Osmolality of human milk fortified with HMF ranges from 285 mOsm per kg of water (liquid fortifier) to 320 to 385 mOsm per kg of water (powdered fortifier).

b) Energy density of preterm human milk mixed with a liquid fortifier at the standard dilution (1:1 ratio) is 22 kcal/fluid ounce (74 kcal/100 mL). The energy density of preterm human milk mixed with a powdered fortifier at standard dilution (4 packets HMF:100 mL breast milk) is 24 kcal/fluid ounce (80 kcal/100 mL).

c) Protein sources include nonfat milk, milk protein isolate, whey protein concentrate, and whey protein isolate hydrolysate. The protein content of the liquid fortifier is 2.2 g/100 mL, and fortified preterm milk made with the liquid fortifier at standard dilution contains 1.8 g/100 mL (2.4 g/100 kcal). The protein content of powdered fortifiers ranges from 1 to 1.1 g/4 packets, and fortified preterm milk made with the powdered fortifier at standard dilution contains 2.3 to 2.5 g/100 mL (2.9–3.1 g/100 kcal).

d) Carbohydrate sources include corn syrup solids and lactose. The carbohydrate content of the liquid fortifier is 8.5 g/100 mL, and fortified preterm milk made with the liquid fortifier at standard dilution contains 7.6 g/100 mL (9.5 g/100 kcal). The carbohydrate content of powdered fortifiers ranges from <0.4 to 1.8 g/4 packets, and fortified preterm milk made with the powdered fortifier at standard dilution contains 6.6 to 8.2 g/100 mL (8.2–10.2 g/100 kcal).

e) Fat sources include soy oil, coconut oil, and MCTs. The fat content of the liquid fortifier is 4.4 g/100 mL, and fortified preterm milk made with the liquid fortifier at standard dilution contains 4.1 g/100 mL (5.1 g/100 kcal). The fat content of powdered fortifiers ranges from 0.36 to 1 g/4 packets, and fortified preterm milk made with the powdered fortifier at standard dilution contains 4.1 to 4.9 g/100 mL (5.1–6.1 g/100 kcal).

f) Calcium and phosphorus content is increased in HMFs, and, when mixed at standard dilution, makes the calcium content 3 to 5 times greater than that found in preterm milk. The phosphorus content is increased to a greater degree, ranging by four- to six fold the content of preterm human milk. In general, the HMF provides a lower increase in mineral intake.

g) HMFs are available with and without added iron. Iron-containing HMFs have 1.4 mg iron/4 packets (1.8 mg iron/100 mL fortified human milk). Infants receiving HMFs without added iron require an oral iron supplement.

3. The addition of HMFs to human milk has been found to promote short-term increases in weight, length, and head circumference.[63]

B. Preterm formulations

1. Preterm infant formulations are designed to provide increased protein, mineral, electrolyte, and vitamin intakes in a form that is easy to digest and absorb.

2. Formulation characteristics

a) These formulations are isotonic, with osmolalities ranging from 280 to 310 mOsm per kg of water.

b) Standard energy density is 24 kcal/fluid ounce (0.8 kcal/mL). These products are also available in a 20 kcal/fluid ounce (0.67 kcal/mL) form.

c) Protein sources include nonfat milk and whey protein concentrate. The whey protein fraction is 50% to 60% of the total protein content. The protein content ranges from 2.2 to 2.4 g/100 mL (2.7–3 g/100 kcal).

d) Carbohydrate sources include corn syrup solids and lactose. The lactose content is approximately 50% of the total carbohydrate content. The carbohydrate content ranges from 8.5 to 9 g/100 mL (10.6–11.2 g/100 kcal).

e) Fat sources include soy oil, coconut oil, and MCTs. MCTs comprise approximately 40% to 50% of the total fat content.

The fat content ranges from 4.1 to 4.4 g/100 mL (5.1–5.5 g/100 kcal). Preterm infant formulations contain ARA and DHA.

f) Preterm infant formulations are available with or without iron. To meet the iron needs of the growing premature infant, the iron-containing form is recommended.

3. Clinical studies have shown improved early growth in infants fed preterm formulations versus standard formulations. Growth differences between the groups tend to disappear as the infants age into late childhood and early adolescence.[64] One study suggested that at the age of 7 to 8 years, neurodevelopmental outcome was improved in former preterm infants who received preterm formulations versus standard-term formulations in the first few weeks of life.[64]

C. Preterm discharge formulations

1. Preterm infants are frequently discharged to home before reaching term gestation. In addition, many preterm infants have delayed growth during hospitalization and will benefit from increased protein and mineral intakes after discharge to promote catch-up growth. The preterm discharge formulations are designed for preterm infants nearing hospital discharge and at home throughout the first year of life.

2. Formulation characteristics

a) These formulations are hypotonic, with osmolalities ranging from 230 to 250 mOsm per kg of water.

b) Standard energy density is 22 kcal/fluid ounce (0.74 kcal/mL).

c) Protein sources include nonfat milk and whey protein concentrate. The protein content is approximately 2 g/100 mL (2.7 g/100 kcal).

d) Carbohydrate sources include corn syrup solids and lactose. The lactose content is 40% to 60% of the total carbohydrate content. The carbohydrate content is approximately 7.7 g/100 mL (10.4 g/100 kcal).

e) Fat sources include high oleic sunflower oil, soy oil, coconut oil, and MCTs. MCTs comprise approximately 20% to 25% of the total fat content. The fat content is approximately 4 g/100 mL (5.4 g/100 kcal).

f) The calcium and phosphorus content of preterm discharge formulations is approximately 2.5 to 3 times the mineral content of term infant formulations.

g) All preterm discharge formulations have added iron (1.3 mg/100 mL).

3. Clinical studies suggest that the use of nutrient-enriched formulations in preterm infants after discharge improves growth in weight, length, and head circumference.[65,66] The benefit in weight was most pronounced in the first few months after discharge.[66] The difference in height has persisted as long as 18 months.[65]

D. Infant formulations with increased nutrient density

1. Infants with increased nutrient requirements or those requiring fluid restriction may require increased nutrient density formulations. Nutrient-dense formulations can be produced by concentrating formulas or by including modular nutrient additives of carbohydrate, protein, or fat. Before the nutrient density of formulations is altered, several consequences of the formulation change should be considered.

a) Maintaining nutrient balance. When increasing the nutrient density of formulations, it is important to keep in mind the actual nutrient requirements of the infant and the effect of changing formulation density on nutrient intakes. Fluid-restricted infants require formulations with an increased nutrient density of all nutrients. Energy, protein, minerals, electrolytes, and vitamins all need to be provided in smaller fluid volumes. These infants will benefit from concentrating formulations. When increased nutrient density formulations are produced by decreasing the amount of water added to formula powders or concentrates, the balance of nutrients is maintained. Infants with increased energy needs but little increase in other nutrient may tolerate the use of carbohydrate or fat modulars to increase the energy density of the formulation. Infants with increased protein needs, such as infants on peritoneal dialysis or small preterm infants, may benefit from concentrated formulations and/or the use of a protein modular.

b) Increasing nutrient density usually increases formulation osmolality. Concentrating formulations will cause a substantial increase in osmolality, particularly in formulations that are hypertonic at standard dilution. Carbohydrate modulars made from glucose polymers are also hypertonic and will generally increase osmolality to the same degree as an equicaloric increase in formulation concentration.[67] Fat modulars are isotonic and will therefore have no effect on formulation osmolality. As the protein used in protein modulars is a whole protein (whey protein concentrate or sodium, calcium caseinates), these products also have minimal effects on osmolality. Often, feeding osmolality is influenced more by the administration of hypertonic oral medication than by the increase in nutrient density. Best practice is to avoid mixing medications with enteral formulations. Medications should be given separately as boluses. In general, increases in formula osmolality are well tolerated if the concentration is advanced slowly and attention is paid to tolerance with each concentration change.

c) Infants, particularly newborns and preterm infants, have immature kidneys unable to concentrate urine when fluid intake is limited. Renal solute load refers to the amount of solute present in the diet (protein, sodium, potassium, chloride, and phosphorus) that must be excreted by the kidneys.[68] Formulations with a higher renal solute load will potentially require increased water content for excretion of the solutes. Increasing the concentration of the formulation and adding protein modulars will increase renal solute load, while adding carbohydrate or fat modulars will have minimal effect or may slightly decrease the renal solute load. Other factors must be considered when evaluating the risk of increasing renal solute load. As infants mature, their ability to concentrate urine increases and renal solute load becomes less of a problem. Rapidly growing infants will incorporate solutes into newly formed tissue and renal solute will decrease. Increased insensible fluid losses from fever or diarrhea and limited volume intake will increase the risk of dehydration, as less fluid is available for excretion of renal solutes. Generally, infants will tolerate moderate advances in renal solute load (ie, increasing formulation concentration to 24 or 27 kcal/fluid ounce). Infants will also tolerate increases in formulation concentration to 30 kcal/fluid ounce if fluid intake exceeds 100 mL/kg per day. It is important to carefully monitor hydration status in all infants receiving concentrated enteral formulations.

d) Products made from powders or concentrated liquids, particularly in a home environment with questionable sanitation, may put the infant at risk of receiving contaminated formulations. Sanitation issues are compounded as more and more additives are incorporated into the enteral formulation. Whenever possible, recipes for preparing formulations at home should be simple and have a limited number of additives, to minimize the risk of preparation errors and microbial contamination.

2. Methods
   a) Increasing nutrient density by concentrating formulation
      (1) Formulations are concentrated by using smaller volumes of water in formulation recipes. This method is easy to incorporate when formulations are available in a powder or concentrated liquid form.
      (2) In some instances (eg, preterm formulations), the products are available in only a ready-to-feed form. To increase the nutrient density of preterm formulations, term formulation concentrated liquids or powders or preterm infant discharge formulation powders must be added to the ready-to-feed preterm formulation. Concentrated liquids are preferred over powders in preterm infant formulations, as concentrated liquids are sterile. Addition of a term formulation to a preterm infant formulation will alter nutrient composition and reduce, in particular, the protein and mineral density.
      (3) Infants receiving breast milk who require formulations with increased nutrient density are a particular challenge. The nutrient density of term breast milk feedings may be increased by adding term infant formulation powders or concentrated liquids. In preterm infants, term infant concentrated liquids or preterm infant discharge formulation powders may be added to fortified human milk to increase nutrient density above 24 kcal/fluid ounce. Concentrated liquid are preferred over powders in preterm infant feedings because concentrated liquids are sterile. The addition of extra packets of HMF is generally discouraged because nutrient intakes of calcium and phosphorus increase substantially and may cause hypercalcemia and hyperphosphatemia.
   b) Increasing nutrient density by adding modular ingredients. Adding fat, carbohydrate, or protein modulars to infant formulations will alter the nutrient balance of the feeding regimen. When nutrient density is increased in this manner, careful attention must be paid to the effect of these additives on intakes of other nutrients.

VI. Reducing Contamination of Enteral Formulations

A. Complications related to contamination
1. Some degree of microbial contamination of formulations is almost inevitable during feedings. Contamination of enteral feedings may cause GI colonization, septicemia, nosocomial pneumonia, and diarrhea.[69–75] Sources of contamination include formulation ingredients, mixing equipment, delivery systems, handling during assembly of the administration system, unsanitary formula preparation areas and patient care units, health care providers, family members, and patients. Dangerous concentrations of organisms result from heavy initial contamination or inappropriately long hang times of the formulation or administration set.[69] Because infants are more susceptible to infection, guidelines for preparation, storage, and administration of infant feedings are more conservative than those for children and adults.[70]
2. Hazard Analysis Critical Control Point (HACCP) is a systematic approach to minimizing the potential for contamination. It is important to identify critical points where contamination of enteral formulations may occur to reduce the possibilities for microbial contamination and/or food-borne disease. HACCP also aids in providing safe and accurate nutrition products as mandated by the Joint Commission on Accreditation of Healthcare Organizations.
3. Reducing contamination during preparation.
   a) When possible, formulations should be mixed, reconstituted, and diluted in a centralized location (eg, enteral formulary room or pharmacy). Mixing equipment must be cleaned meticulously.
   b) In most instances, formulations can be reconstituted and diluted with tap water. However, in areas where the water supply is of questionable quality or in severely immunocompromised patients, it may be prudent to use distilled or sterile water.
   c) Infant feedings require additional formulation preparation safeguards. Whenever possible, sterile ready-to-feed formulations or concentrated liquid formulations should be used. Formulation powders should be weighed (not measured) and should be used only when no liquid forms are available.[70] Formulations should always be prepared with sterile water.[70]
4. Formulations should be stored according to manufacturers' recommendations.
   a) Expired or damaged formula containers should be discarded.[70]
   b) Unopened ready-to-feed formulations should be stored in a cool, dark place. They should not be stored in direct sunlight or near direct heat such as a radiator. Once opened, formulations may be stored in a refrigerator for up to 48 hours.[71]
   c) Reconstituted or diluted formulations be stored in a refrigerator for a maximum of 24 hours.[71]
   d) Additional guidelines for infant formulation storage include the following:
      (1) Prepared infant formulations should be chilled to 40°F within 1 hour of preparation.[70]
      (2) Opened ready-to-feed containers and prepared infant formulations should be stored in a refrigerator and used within 24 hours.[70]
      (3) Human milk may be stored frozen in a home-style freezer for 3 months. It may be stored in a deep freeze (−20°C or −4°F) for 12 months.[70]
      (4) Fresh human milk may be stored in a refrigerator for 48 hours. Thawed or fortified human milk should be stored and used within 24 hours.[70]
5. Reducing contamination during administration
   a) Formulation hang time
      (1) Canned, ready-to-use formulations generally can be hung for 8 to 12 hours at room temperature, but manufacturers' guidelines should be followed. In general, it is best to fill the reservoir using clean technique as infrequently as hang time restrictions allow.
      (2) Reconstituted powdered formulations generally can be hung for 4 to 6 hours at room temperature.
      (3) Prefilled administration sets (bag/container) can generally be hung for 24 to 48 hours, or according to the manufacturer's recommendations.[74]
   b) Administration set hang time
      (1) Refillable sets (bag/container and tubing) can be used in a short-term care setting for about 24 hours.[74]
      (2) It has been suggested that refillable administration sets (bags/containers and tubing) may be used for up to 72 hours in long-term care facilities; no differences in adverse effects (eg, fever, pneumonia, diarrhea, vomiting) were noted between delivery sets used for 24 versus 72 hours. However, no bacterial counts were performed. Thus, use of refillable delivery sets for longer than 24 hours in settings other than long-term care facilities requires further investigation.[75]
   c) Infant feeding delivery guidelines

(1) Hang times for human milk and infant formulas should not exceed 4 hours.[70]
(2) Syringe tubing should be changed every 4 hours in infants receiving continuous infusion feedings.[70]

(Enteral Formulations chapter from the 1st edition was contributed by Kelley Olree, Joseph Vitello, Jacqueline Sullivan, and Carol Kohn-Keeth)

REFERENCES

1. Storm HM, Lin P. Forms of carbohydrate in enteral nutrition formulas. *Support Line.* 1996;18:7–9.
2. Abrams SA, Griffin IJ, Davila PM. Calcium and zinc absorption from lactose-containing and lactose-free infant formulas. *Am J Clin Nutr.* 2002;76:442–446.
3. Bell SJ, Mascioli EA, Bistrian BR. Alternative lipid sources for enteral and parenteral nutrition: long- and medium-chain triglycerides, structured triglycerides, and fish oils. *J Am Diet Assoc.* 1991;91:74–78.
4. Innis S. Perinatal biochemistry and physiology of long-chain polyunsaturated fatty acids. *J Pediatr.* 2003;143:81–88.
5. Uauy R, Hoffman DR, Mena P, Llanos A, Birch EE. Term infant studies of DHA and ARA supplementation on neurodevelopment: results of randomized controlled trials. *J Pediatr.* 2003;143(suppl 4):S17–25.
6. Auestad N, Scott DT, Janowsky JS, et al. Visual, cognitive, and language assessments at 39 months: a follow-up study of children fed formulas containing long-chain polyunsaturated fatty acids to 1 year of age. *Pediatrics.* 2003;112(3 Pt 1):e177–183.
7. Mehta NR, Hamosh M, Bitman J, Wood DL. Adherence of medium-chain fatty acids to feeding tubes of premature infants fed formula fortified with medium-chain triglyceride. *J Pediatr Gastroenterol Nutr.* 1991;13:267–269.
8. Coster J, McCarty R, Hall J. Role of specific amino acids in nutritional support. *ANZ J Surg.* 2003;73:846–849.
9. Platell C, Kung S-E, McCauley R, Hall JC. Branched chain amino acids. *J Gastroenterol Hepatol.* 2000;15:706–717.
10. Lacey JM, Wilmore DW. Is glutamine a conditionally essential amino acid? *Nutr Rev.* 1990;48:297–309.
11. Neu J, DeMarco V, Li N. Glutamine: clinical applications and mechanisms of action. *Curr Opin Clin Nutr Metab Care.* 2002;5:69–75.
12. Spapen H, Diltoer M, Van Malderen C, Opdenacker G, Suys E, Huyghens L. Soluble fiber reduces the incidence of diarrhea in septic patients receiving total enteral nutrition: a prospective, double-blind, randomized, and controlled trial. *Clin Nutr.* 2001;20:301–305.
13. Spiegel JE, Rose R, Karabell P, et al. Safety and benefits of fructooligosaccharides as food ingredients. *Food Technol.* 1994;48:85–89.
14. Evans MA, Shronts EP. Intestinal fuels: glutamine, short-chain fatty acids, and dietary fiber. *J Am Diet Assoc.* 1992;92:1239–1246.
15. Daly JM, Lieberman MD, Goldfine J, et al. Enteral nutrition with supplemental arginine, RNA, and omega-3 fatty acids in patients after operation: immunologic, metabolic, and clinical outcome. *Surgery.* 1992;112:56–67.
16. Daly JM, Lieberman MD, Goldfine J, et al. Immune and metabolic effects of arginine in the surgical patient. *Ann Surg.* 1988;208:512–522.
17. Gianotti L, Braga M, Nespoli L, et al. A randomized controlled trial of preoperative oral supplementation with a specialized diet in patients with gastrointestinal cancer. *Gastroenterology.* 2002;122:1763–1770.
18. McCowen KC, Bistrian B. Immunonutrition: problematic or problem solving? *Am J Clin Nutr.* 2003;3:764–770.
19. Sax HC. Effect of immune enhancing formulas (IEF) in general surgery patients. *J Parenter Enteral Nutr.* 2001;25:S19–S23.
20. Fearon KCH, von Meyenfeldt MF, Moses AGW, et al. Effect of a protein and energy dense m-3 fatty acid enriched oral supplement on loss of weight and lean tissue in cancer cachexia. *Gut.* 2003;53:1479–1486.
21. Kudsk KA, Minard G, Croce MA, et al. A randomized trial of isonitrogenous enteral diets after severe trauma: an immune-enhancing diet reduces septic complications. *Ann Surg.* 1996;224:531–543.
22. Bower RH, Cerra FB, Bershadksy B, et al. Early enteral administration of a formula (Impact) supplemented with arginine, nucleotides and fish oil in intensive care unit patients: results of a multicenter, prospective, randomized, clinical trial. *Crit Care Med.* 1995;23:436–449.
23. Heys SD, Walker LG, Smith I, Eremin O. Enteral nutritional supplementation with key nutrients in patients with critical illness and cancer: a meta-analysis of randomized controlled clinical trials. *Ann Surg.* 1999;229:467–477.
24. Beale RJ, Bryg DJ, Bihari DJ. Immunonutrition in the critically ill: a systematic review of clinical outcome. *Crit Care Med.* 1999;27:2799–2805.
25. Kudsk KA, Moore F, Martindale RT, et al. Consensus recommendations from the U.S. Summit on Immune-Enhancing Enteral Therapy. *J Parenter Enteral Nutr.* 2001;25(suppl):S61–62.
26. Sacks GS, Kudsk KA. Maintaining mucosal immunity during parenteral feeding with surrogates to enteral nutrition. *Nutr Clin Pract.* 2003;18: 483–488.
27. Bower RH, Muggia-Sullam M, Vallgren S, et al. Branched chain amino acid-enriched solutions in the septic patient. A randomized, prospective trial. *Ann Surg.* 1986;203:13–20.
28. van den Berghe G, Wouters P, Weekers F, et al. Intensive insulin therapy in critically patients. *N Engl J Med.* 2001;345:1359–1367.
29. Franz MJ. 2002 diabetes nutrition recommendations: grading the evidence. *Diabetes Educ.* 2002;28:756–759, 762–764, 766.
30. American Diabetes Association. Nutrition principles and recommendations in diabetes. *Diabetes Care.* 2004;27(suppl):S36–46.
31. Munoz SJ. Nutritional therapies in liver disease. *Semin Liver Dis.* 1991;11: 278–291.
32. Silk DBA, O'Keefe SJD, Wick C. Nutritional support in liver disease. *Gut.* 1991;31(suppl):S29–33.
33. Sleisenger MH, Kim YS. Protein digestion and absorption. *N Engl J Med.* 1979;300:659–663.
34. Mowatt-Larson CA, Brown RO, Wojtysiak SL, et al. Comparison of tolerance and nutritional outcome between a peptide and a standard enteral formula in critically ill, hypoalbuminemic patients. *J Parenter Enteral Nutr.* 1992;16:20–24.
35. Heimburger DC, Geels WJ, Thiesse KT, Bartolucci AA. Randomized trial of tolerance and efficacy of a small-peptide enteral feeding formula versus a whole-protein formula. *Nutrition.* 1995;11:360–364.
36. Deitch EA, Xu D, Qi L, et al. Elemental diet-induced immune suppression is caused by both bacterial and dietary factors. *J Parenter Enteral Nutr.* 1993;7:332–336.
37. Serizawa H, Miura S, Tashiro H, et al. Alteration of mucosal immunity after long-term ingestion of an elemental diet in rats. *J Parenter Enteral Nutr.* 1994;18:141–147.
38. Windsor ACJ, Kanwar S, Li AGK, et al. Compared with parenteral nutrition, enteral feeding attenuates the acute phase response and improves disease severity in acute pancreatitis. *Gut.* 1998;42:431–435.
39. Kalfarentzos F, Kehagias J, Mead N, et al. Enteral nutrition is superior to parenteral nutrition in severe acute pancreatitis: results of a randomized prospective trial. *Br J Surg.* 1997;84:1665–1672.
40. Olah A, Pardavi G, Belagyi T, et al. Early nasojejunal feeding in acute pancreatitis is associated with a lower complication rate. *Nutrition.* 2002;18:259–262.
41. Al-Saady N, Blackmore C, Bennet ED. High fat, low carbohydrate enteral feeding reduces $PaCO_2$ and the period of ventilation in ventilated patients. *Intensive Care Med.* 1989;15:290–295.
42. Frankfurt JD, Fischer CE, Stansburg DW, et al. Effects of high- and low-carbohydrate meals on maximum exercise performance in chronic airflow obstruction. *Chest.* 1991;100:792–795.
43. Talpers SS, Romberger DJ, Bunce SB, et al. Nutritionally associated increased carbon dioxide production. Excess of total calories vs high proportion of carbohydrate calories. *Chest.* 1992;102:551–555.
44. Gadek J, DeMichele S, Karlstad M, et al. Effect of enteral with eicosapentanoic acid, γ-linolenic acid, and antioxidants in patients with acute respiratory distress syndrome. *Crit Care Med.* 1999;27:1409–1420.
45. Saffle JR, Wiebke G, Jennings K, et al. Randomized trial of immune-enhancing enteral nutrition in burn patients. *J Trauma.* 1997;42:793–802.
46. Shepherd AA. Nutrition for optimum wound healing. *Nurs Stand.* 2003; 18:55–58.

47. Gottschlich MM, Jenkins M, Warden GD, et al. Differential effects of three enteral dietary regimens on selected outcome variables in burn patients. *J Parenter Enteral Nutr.* 1990;14:225–236.
48. A.S.P.E.N. Board of Directors and the Clinical Guidelines Task Force. Guidelines for the use of parenteral and enteral nutrition in adult and pediatric patients. *J Parenter Enteral Nutr.* 2002;26:188SA–190SA.
49. Kaufman SS, Scrivner DJ, Murray ND, Vanderhoof JA, Hart MH, Antonson DL. Influence of portagen and pregestimil on essential fatty acid status in infantile liver disease. *Pediatrics.* 1992;89(1):151–154.
50. Pickering LK, Granoff DM, Erickson JR, et al. Modulation of the immune system by human milk and infant formula containing nucleotides. *Pediatrics.* 1998;101:242–249.
51. American Academy of Pediatrics. Committee on Nutrition. Iron fortification of infant formulas. *Pediatrics.* 1999;104:119–123.
52. Zeiger RS, Sampson HA, Bock SA, et al. Soy allergy in infants and children with IgE-associated cow's milk allergy. *J Pediatr.* 1999;134:614–622.
53. American Academy of Pediatrics. Committee on Nutrition. Soy protein-based formulas: recommendations for use in infant feeding. *Pediatrics.* 1998;101:148–153.
54. Vanderhoof JA, Murray ND, Paule CL, Ostrom KM. Use of soy fiber in acute diarrhea in infants and toddlers. *Clin Pediatr (Phila).* 1997;36: 135–139.
55. Burks AW, Vanderhoof JA, Mehra S, Ostrom KM, Baggs G. Randomized clinical trial of soy formula with and without added fiber in antibiotic-induced diarrhea. *J Pediatr.* 2001;139:578–582.
56. Brown KH, Perez F, Peerson JM, et al. Effect of dietary fiber (soy polysaccharide) on the severity, duration, and nutritional outcome of acute, watery diarrhea in children. *Pediatrics.* 1993;92:241–247.
57. American Academy of Pediatrics. Committee on Nutrition. Hypoallergenic infant formulas. *Pediatrics.* 2000;106:346–349.
58. Jakobsson I, Lothe L, Ley D, Borschel MW. Effectiveness of casein hydrolysate feedings in infants with colic. *Acta Paediatr.* 2000;89:18–21.
59. Nelson SP, Chen EH, Syniar GM, Christoffel KK. Prevalence of symptoms of gastroesophageal reflux during infancy. A pediatric practice-based survey. Pediatric Practice Research Group. *Arch Pediatr Adolesc Med.* 1997;6: 569–572.
60. Rudolph CD, Mazur LJ, Liptak GS, et al. Guidelines for evaluation and treatment of gastroesophageal reflux in infants and children: recommendations of the North American Society for Pediatric Gastroenterology and Nutrition. *J Pediatr Gastroenterol Nutr.* 2001;32(suppl 2):S1–31.
61. Vanderhoof JA, Moran JR, Harris CL, Merkel KL, Orenstein SR. Efficacy of a pre-thickened infant formula: a multicenter, double-blind, randomized, placebo-controlled parallel group trial in 104 infants with symptomatic gastroesophageal reflux. *Clin Pediatr (Phila).* 2003;42: 483–495.
62. Wenzl TG, Schneider S, Scheele F, Silny J, Heimann G, Skopnik H. Effects of thickened feeding on gastroesophageal reflux in infants: a placebo-controlled crossover study using intraluminal impedance. *Pediatrics.* 2003;111:e355–359.
63. Kuschel C, Harding J. Multicomponent fortified human milk for promoting growth in preterm infants. *Cochrane Database Syst Rev.* 2004;1:CD000343.
64. Morley R, Lucas A. Randomized diet in the neonatal period and growth performance until 7.5–8 y of age in preterm children. *Am J Clin Nutr.* 2000;71:822–888.
65. Lucas A, Fewtrell MS, Morley R, et al. Randomized trial of nutrient-enriched formula versus standard formula for postdischarge preterm infants. *Pediatrics.* 2001;108:703–711.
66. Carver JD, Wu PY, Hall RT, et al. Growth of preterm infants fed nutrient-enriched or term formula after hospital discharge. *Pediatrics.* 2001;107: 683–689.
67. Koo WW, Poh D, Leong M, Tam YK, Succop P, Checkland EG. Osmotic load from glucose polymers. *J Parenter Enteral Nutr.* 1991;15:144–147.
68. Fomon SJ, Ziegler EE. Renal solute load and potential renal solute load in infancy. *J Pediatr.* 1999;134:11–14.
69. Anderton A. Reducing bacterial contamination in enteral tube feeds. *Nutrition.* 1999;15:55–57.
70. Pediatric Nutrition Practice Group of the American Dietetic Association. *Infant Feedings: Guidelines for Preparation of Formula and Breast Milk in Health Care Facilities.* Chicago, IL: American Dietetic Association; 2003.
71. Campbell SM. *Preventing Microbial Contamination of Enteral Formulas and Delivery Systems.* Columbus, OH: Ross Products Division of Abbott Laboratories; 1995.
72. Kohn CL. The relationship between enteral formula contamination and length of enteral delivery set usage. *J Parenter Enteral Nutr.* 1991;15: 567–571.
73. Thurn J, Crossley K, Gerdts A, et al. Enteral hyperalimentation as a source of nosocomial infection. *J Hosp Infect.* 1990;15:203–217.
74. Donius MA. Contamination of a prefilled ready-to-use enteral feeding system compared with a refillable bag. *J Parenter Enteral Nutr.* 1993;17: 461–464.
75. Graham S, Chicone J, Gerard B, et al. Frequency of changing enteral alimentation bags and tubing, and adverse clinical outcomes in patients in a long term care facility. *Can J Infect Control.* 1993;8:41–43.

Linda Lord, NP, RN, MS, CNSN;
Michelle Harrington, MS, RD, CSP, CNSD, LDN

5

Enteral Nutrition Implementation and Management

Introduction

When the gastrointestinal (GI) tract is functional, enteral feeding is the preferred route for nutrition support. This type of feeding provides many physiologic, metabolic, safety, and cost benefits over parenteral feedings.[1] Tube feedings can range from providing adjunctive support to providing complete nutrition therapy. Enteral feedings can be administered and scheduled in a variety of ways. Practitioners who are familiar with these options can recommend regimens that accommodate each patient's needs and lifestyle. Selection of the optimal enteral regimen depends on a number of factors, such as the patient's nutritional and clinical status, GI function, age, and level of activity. Practitioners need to be aware of these factors so that enteral feedings can be administered successfully and safely. A well-tolerated enteral regimen that meets the patient's needs can reduce the length of time that support is necessary and improve the disease treatment outcome; it can also assist in the growth and development of the pediatric patient.[2]

I. Benefits, Indications, and Contraindications for Enteral Feedings

A. Benefits of enteral feeding
  1. Physiologic/metabolic benefits
    a) The gut can be used for the administration of complex nutrients (eg, intact protein, peptides, fiber) that cannot be given intravenously. Nutrients absorbed through the GI tract via the portal vein enter the liver and are processed before they enter the systemic circulation or are disposed of as waste products. Many nutrients enter the systemic circulation intact. This mechanism (first-pass metabolism) allows for more effective utilization of nutrients.
    b) In addition to the systemic benefits, enteral feedings have local, trophic beneficial effects on the GI mucosa, maintaining its absorptive structures by nourishing the enterocytes directly to support epithelial cell repair and replication. Enteral nutrients provide a complex systemic stimulus that leads to gut protection related to stress and corticosteroid use and reduces the risk of inflammation, ulceration, and bleeding. Luminal nutrients, such as glutamine and short-chain fatty acids, are used as fuel by the cells of the small bowel and colon, respectively. The presence of nutrients in the gut also helps maintain normal gut pH and flora and inhibits opportunistic bacterial overgrowth in the small bowel.
    c) The presence of nutrients in the gut, especially complex proteins and fats, supports the mucosa's critical immunologic barrier function by triggering feeding-dependent neuroendocrine activity. Subsequently, this activity appears to stimulate the manufacture of immunoglobulins in the gut, particularly secretory immunoglobulin A, which is important for preventing bacterial adherence and translocation.[3]
  2. Safety benefits. Enteral feeding is generally considered safer than parenteral feeding, when administered cautiously and with ongoing monitoring, and with the appropriate modifications made to the regimen as needed.
  3. Cost benefits. Enteral feeding generally costs less than parenteral feeding, including the costs for formula, equipment, administration, and monitoring in both the hospital and outpatient settings.

B. Indications for enteral feeding[4]
  1. Inability to consume or absorb adequate nutrients. Enteral support is considered in patients who have demonstrated inability to meet nutritional needs by mouth and are assessed as being at high risk for or as being malnourished. Enteral support is indicated when patients' volitional intake is inadequate to meet two thirds to three quarters of their daily energy needs. The duration of acceptable inadequate intake is based on several factors, such as a patient's age, nutritional status, expected illness and catabolic severity, length of illness, and expected duration of poor nutrient intake or absorption. Adult patients who do not eat or receive nutrition support for more than 10 to 14 days after hospital admission or after surgery have been reported to have worse clinical outcomes, longer hospitalizations, and higher costs of care.[5–7] However, it is often difficult to prospectively identify patients who will meet these criteria. Therefore, it may be prudent to initiate the appropriate modality of nutrition support in patients with inadequate oral intake for 7 to 14 days, or in those in whom inadequate oral intake is anticipated for more than 7 to 14 days.[5]
    a) Children. Children possess lower energy substrate stores relative to their rate of energy expenditure and therefore are at earlier risk for nutritional compromise than adults.[8] The nutrition goals for the pediatric patient are to provide adequate nutrition for growth, development, and the preservation of lean body mass.[9] Extended periods of malnutrition during childhood can manifest in growth failure, as well as have adverse effects on cognitive and behavioral development.[2,10]
    b) Additional criteria for consideration of enteral tube feeding in children who have a functioning GI tract include
      (1) no weight gain or weight loss for 3 consecutive months
      (2) weight for height less than the fifth percentile

(3) triceps skin fold measurement less than the fifth percentile for age

(4) total oral feeding time greater than 4 to 6 hours per day[11]

2. Functional or partially functional gut. Patients with a functional gut who are unable or not allowed to eat should receive enteral instead of parenteral feedings. Even patients with only a partially functional gut can often tolerate some enteral feeding, but may require a combined regimen (ie, both parenteral and enteral nutrition) to meet total nutritional needs.

C. Possible contraindications to enteral feeding. Contraindications to enteral feeding are usually relative or temporary rather than absolute. Potential contraindications include

1. Terminal illness. Before enteral nutrition support is initiated in patients who are terminally ill, the potential benefits should be weighed against the risk of potential problems. Potential problems include aspiration, diarrhea, overhydration, discomfort, and interference with personal dignity.
2. Short bowel. Patients with a short bowel often require parenteral nutrition (PN) for 1 to 3 months after surgery while the remaining bowel adapts to allow adequate nutrient absorption. Depending on the length of the remaining absorptive small bowel, some patients may require long-term PN or parenteral fluid, electrolyte, and mineral replacement.
3. Obstruction. Complete mechanical obstruction of the GI tract below the duodenum, or pseudo-obstruction that cannot be resolved, is a contraindication to enteral feeding. Partial obstruction of the GI tract often can be circumvented but requires ongoing monitoring of GI status as well as recurrent evaluation of the most appropriate feeding site, formula, and equipment.
4. GI bleeding. The etiology, severity, and location of acute GI bleeding, as well as the need for immediate GI evaluation and treatment, are determinants of the feasibility of enteral feedings. Chronic, slow upper GI bleeding is not necessarily a contraindication to enteral feedings but may be accompanied by anorexia and frequent nausea or vomiting. Small-bowel feedings may be better tolerated than gastric feedings in these patients.
5. Vomiting and diarrhea. Protracted vomiting and diarrhea are not absolute contraindications to enteral feedings; however, the cause(s) of either should be carefully assessed. Vomiting can make it difficult to keep a nasally placed tube in position. Patients with frequent episodes of nausea or vomiting may better tolerate small-bowel feedings with gastric decompression or may benefit from the use of prokinetic agents. Patients with diarrhea should be assessed for the type of diarrhea (osmotic or secretory) and for possible causes other than the enteral feedings, such as *Clostridium difficile* or oral medications (eg, sorbitol-containing medications; antibiotics; H2-receptor antagonists; antineoplastics; laxatives; antacids; prokinetic agents; potassium, magnesium, phosphorus supplements). In cases of mild to moderate vomiting or diarrhea, judicious waiting for symptomatic improvement is sometimes warranted. Depending on the patient's nutritional status and potential for depletion, PN may be indicated until symptoms abate.
6. Fistulas. When patients have fistulas, it is prudent to choose a feeding site away from the fistula to optimize nutrient absorption and minimize losses. Patients with fistulas in the more proximal or more distal gut are easier to feed enterally, and those with low to moderate fistula output are usually amenable to enteral feeding. High-output midgut (jejunal) fistulas are more problematic. Patients with fistulas require careful monitoring to ensure that nutrient, electrolyte, and fluid needs are met and that the feedings are not exacerbating the problem.
7. GI ischemia. Certain disease states or medical treatments can reduce blood flow to the gut and cause GI ischemia. Examples include critically ill patients with low cardiac output, sepsis, and multiorgan failure. Even a relatively brief reduction in mesenteric blood flow can cause rapid changes in the GI mucosa, reducing the absorptive and barrier functions of the gut. Therefore, the benefits of enteral feeding may be less clear-cut in patients with cardiopulmonary instability. However, enteral nutrition has been shown to improve blood flow in the gut and to maintain the barrier effect of the intestine.[12,13] The challenge with such patients is to determine when the physiologic balance has shifted and enteral feedings will clearly be beneficial rather than problematic. With chronic occlusive or compression syndromes that limit enteric blood supply, a potential risk for worsening ischemia and necrosis exists.
8. Ileus. Paralytic ileus occurs quite frequently in acutely ill patients. Common surgical causes include perforation, anastomotic leaks, intraperitoneal hemorrhage, peritonitis, and other intra-abdominal infections. Nonsurgical causes include ischemia, hypokalemia, head or spine injury, uremia, adverse drug effects, thyroid deficiency, and severe, uncontrolled diabetes. Ileus affects the small bowel to a lesser degree than the stomach and large bowel. Persistent gastric ileus usually can be circumvented with small-bowel feeding tube placement and gastric decompression.
9. GI inflammation. Inflammation or enteritis may have several etiologies, including inflammatory bowel disease, radiation, or chemotherapy. Bowel rest (with PN) has been prescribed in an effort to achieve remission during acute Crohn's disease flare-ups, but studies have failed to demonstrate any improvement in long-term outcomes.[14]
10. Pancreatitis. Bowel rest also is frequently prescribed for pancreatitis; however, several studies have reported successful use of enteral nutrition support without exacerbation of pancreatitis.[15,16] The degree of pancreatic stimulation is dependent on the location of the feeding tube in the GI tract, as well as the composition of the enteral formula. Less stimulation occurs when the feedings are delivered distally in the intestinal tract, and lower-fat formulations are tolerated best.[17,18]

II. Implementation of Enteral Feedings

The patient's type of access, tolerance of feedings, absorptive capacity, volume requirements, amount of oral intake, and lifestyle are determinants of the delivery method and duration of the daily tube feedings.[19]

A. Delivery methods

1. Gravity controlled. This manually controlled method of infusing formula is used almost exclusively for gastric feedings. A specific volume of formulation is hung in a plastic feeding bag or rigid plastic container with tubing on an intravenous (IV) pole above the insertion site of the feeding tube. The tubing is fitted with a roller clamp, to control the infusion rate of the formulation, and a connector, to permit attachment to the patient's feeding tube. Feedings may be provided over several minutes to hours depending on patient tolerance. A drawback to this method is that the formula infusion rate can fluctuate during the feeding as a result of positional changes or increases in gastric pressure.[20] Gravity-controlled feedings are indicated only for neurologically intact patients who can reliably protect their airways. Most often this method is used with ambulatory patients (ie, in-home care or long-term care facilities).

a) Continuous gravity feedings. These feedings are provided over 24 hours and can be accomplished with the use of high-quality gravity-feeding equipment and a roller clamp to control the infusion rate. This method may result in occasional incidents of unintentionally rapid infusion rates or interruptions. Poor-quality tubing or clamps make controlling the rate very difficult, and the patient may inadvertently receive a bolus feeding.

b) Intermittent gravity feedings. Intermittent feedings are generally well tolerated if a maximum of 200 to 300 mL is administered over 30 to 60 minutes every 4 to 6 hours.[21] A prescription for an intermittent gravity feeding might read as follows: provide 240 mL of formula every 4 hours; infuse over 1 hour; precede and follow with a 30-mL flush of tap water.

c) Bolus feedings. Bolus feedings are the infusion of a predetermined volume of formula at specified intervals by gravity or by syringe over a short period. The rate of infusion is controlled by either regulating the roller clamp or adjusting the syringe pressure. Feedings are generally accomplished over several minutes but may be best tolerated when provided at less than 60 mL/minute. In some settings, a large piston syringe (usually 50 mL or larger) is used to draw up and administer formula directly into the patient's feeding tube. When a syringe is used, the infusion rate can be gravity-controlled by either raising or lowering the syringe (plunger absent) or by slowly pushing the plunger inward. Rapid infusion of formula may cause discomfort, leading to the misconception that the formula instead of the administration method is not being tolerated. A feeding prescription might read as follows: provide 240 mL of formula every 3 hours over at least 4 minutes; precede and follow with a 30-mL flush of tap water. Bolus feedings are the easiest, least expensive delivery method and are more physiologic because they mimic normal feedings. The patient reaps the additional benefit of freedom of movement and breaks from feeding. Disadvantages include increased risk of aspiration, volume intolerance, vomiting, or delayed gastric emptying.[11]

2. Pump assisted. Continuous pump feedings are indicated when there is a high risk for aspiration, with volume sensitivity, with small-bowel feedings, sometimes with delayed gastric motility, and in sicker or hospitalized patients. Continuous feedings allow for maximal nutrient absorption and improved tolerance.[11] Pump-assisted feedings help to prevent GI complications associated with rapid infusion, such as nausea, cramping, and diarrhea. Pumps are also more appropriate in patients who have tenuous fluid balance; if programmed correctly, they can help to prevent fluid overload. Usual equipment includes a disposable pump set (container and tubing with drip chamber and connector) and the pump itself. Controlled infusion is accomplished by threading the tubing through the pump's electronic sensors and cassette or pumping mechanism. Portable "backpack"-style pumps are available for patients who require feedings while participating in their normal daily activities.

a) Continuous pump feedings are delivered via a stationary or ambulatory pump at a prescribed rate without interruption.[19]

b) Cyclic feedings are generally administered over 8 to 20 hours per day, depending on the patient's volume tolerance. This cycle allows for freedom from the feeding equipment for at least a few hours each day. Transitioning from continuous to cyclic feedings typically is attempted as the patient recovers mobility and independence. Feedings may be provided at night (nocturnal feedings) in an effort to allow patients to experience hunger and gradually increase their oral intake during the day.[22]

c) Intermittent pump feedings are used to deliver predetermined volumes more accurately over a specified period. This accuracy is helpful in managing patients that are at risk for aspiration resulting from a rapid infusion rate.

B. Initiation of enteral feedings. Currently, it is recommended that feedings in adults and children be initiated with full-strength formula at a slow rate and steadily advanced. This approach allows goal rates to be achieved earlier and reduces the risk of microbial contamination by minimizing the number of times the formula is manipulated. Experience has shown these regimens to be well tolerated, partially because of the widespread use of pumps for controlling infusion rates. Protocols for introducing tube feedings vary and should be individualized to fit the needs of the patient as well as the realities of the care environment.

During feeding advancement, only one change should be made at a time to allow for tolerance assessment. If poor tolerance of the enteral regimen is demonstrated, either the formula volume or the concentration should be decreased. It is important to allow adequate time for the patient to tolerate the modified regimen before further advances are attempted. Occasionally it becomes necessary to change the formula to achieve improved feeding tolerance. After the patient is receiving and tolerating the goal regimen, modifications to the feeding schedule may be attempted to accommodate the patient's and family's lifestyle.[22]

1. Bolus feedings and gravity-controlled feedings

a) Adults. Usually only gastric feedings are well tolerated when provided as a bolus or gravity feeding. The feedings are usually initiated with full-strength formula 3 to 8 times per day, with increases of 60 to 120 mL every 8 to 12 hours as tolerated up to the goal volume. Formula (ie, elemental, hypertonic, polymeric, or isotonic) does not require dilution unless additional water is necessary to meet fluid requirements. Careful monitoring of gastric residual volumes and GI tolerance may help to facilitate increases in formula intake to the goal volume. Some patients may require bolus feedings to be delivered by gravity over 15 to 20 minutes or in smaller volumes more frequently.

b) Children. Bolus feedings may be started with 25% of the goal volume divided into the desired number of daily feedings. Formula volume may be increased by 25% per day as tolerated, divided equally between feedings.[22]

2. Pump-assisted feedings. A pump is usually required for small-bowel feedings and is preferred for gastric feedings in critically ill patients, as the slower infusion rate of continuous feedings often enhances tolerance. Conservative initiation and advancement rates are recommended for patients who are critically ill, have not been fed enterally for some time, or require hydrolyzed or high-osmolality formula.

a) Adults. Formulas are initiated at full strength at 10 to 40 mL/hour and advanced to the goal rate in increments of 10 to 20 mL/hour every 8 to 12 hours as tolerated. This approach can usually be used with isotonic as well as high-osmolality or elemental products.

b) Children. A full-strength, isotonic formula can be started at 1 to 2 mL/kg/hour and advanced by 0.5 to 1 mL/kg/hour every 6 to 24 hours until the goal volume is achieved. Preterm, critically ill, or malnourished children who have not been fed enterally for an extended period may require a lower initial volume of 0.5 to 1 mL/kg/hour.[23]

III. Monitoring and Management of Enteral Feedings

A. Assessment of GI tolerance

1. Abdominal discomfort. Subjective signs of tube-feeding intolerance include feelings of abdominal fullness, cramping, and pain. Possible etiologies of GI discomfort that result from the provi-

sion of tube feedings include rapid administration of feeding, hyperosmolar solutions, medications, excess air in the stomach or intestines, tube migration from stomach to small intestine, infection, cold formula, bacterial contamination, and fat or lactose intolerance.[11]

a) If GI symptoms are attributable to hyperosmolar solutions, decrease the concentration of the formula and consider adding glucose polymers or fat to increase calories as needed.
b) If GI symptoms are thought to be caused by medications that are administered through the feeding tube, determine whether it is feasible to dilute the medication, change the form of the medication (ie, change to parenteral), or change to a different medication.
c) If GI symptoms are due to fat intolerance, consider using a formula that contains a higher proportion of fat from medium-chain triglycerides.
d) Intolerance can also be attributed to delayed gastric emptying, motility disorders of the small and large intestine, intestinal spasms or ischemia, and fiber-containing formulas.

2. Nausea and vomiting. Nausea and vomiting may be caused by gastric irritation or atony, rapid administration of the tube-feeding formula, medications, feeding tube migration from the intestine to the stomach, distal obstruction, anxiety, and other disease states. Nausea and vomiting may also indicate feeding tube migration, such as a balloon gastrostomy causing a gastric outlet obstruction.
3. Abdominal distension. Abdominal circumference can be measured daily at the level of the iliac crest to monitor changes in abdominal distension. Holding enteral feedings may be indicated if the circumference exceeds the baseline measurement by 8 to 10 centimeters.
4. Bowel sounds. The absence or presence of bowel sounds is not always a good indicator of bowel function. Fluid and air must be present in the GI tract for bowel sounds to be heard. For example, in patients with nasogastric tubes for decompression and suction, bowel sounds may not be heard despite good bowel function. Conversely, "bowel sounds" may be heard if the suction is not turned off prior to auscultation.
5. Stool pattern. Stool volume, frequency, consistency, and color should be noted for any patient receiving enteral tube feedings. The patient's baseline or normal bowel pattern should be noted and used as a basis for comparison.
   a) Diarrhea. Strategies to prevent and manage diarrhea include avoiding the provision of antibiotics or medications that cause diarrhea whenever medically feasible, decreasing the osmolality of hypertonic formulas, decreasing the tube-feeding infusion rate, altering the fat source and content when indicated, and increasing fluid replacement.
   b) Constipation. Possible dietary causes of constipation include inadequate fiber intake, inadequate fluid intake, or medications that slow peristalsis. Strategies to prevent or manage constipation include using fiber-containing formulas, monitoring that free water intake is adequate, supplementing with prune juice, and identifying medications that may be causing constipation (eg, narcotics) and finding appropriate substitutions when possible.[11]

B. Aspiration precautions

1. Tube-feeding residuals. Gastric residuals are frequently used to monitor the safety and gastric emptying of tube feedings. When gastric emptying is delayed or gastric secretion is excessive, fluid accumulates in the stomach and may result in vomiting, aspiration, abdominal distention, or cramping. To prevent these potential complications, the volume of fluid remaining in the stomach during feeding (the residual volume) is measured to monitor the safety of advancing or continuing enteral feeds.[24,25] Gastric motility is affected by disease, mechanical obstruction, and certain medications.[26]

One episode of high residual volume should not automatically prompt cessation of feedings in the absence of physical examination or radiographic abnormalities; rather, signs and symptoms of intolerance should be monitored carefully.[24–27] Patients with frequently elevated gastric residual volumes may benefit from feeding tube placement beyond the ligament of Treitz.[26]

a) Frequency of checking residuals. Gastric emptying of enteral feedings can be assessed by checking residuals prior to each intermittent feed or every 4 hours with continuous feeds.[11]
b) Method for obtaining residuals. Residuals are obtained by aspirating through the feeding tube with a syringe and measuring the formula and fluid withdrawn. The aspirating syringe needs to be fairly large, generally at least 50 mL for small-bore (12F or less) feeding tubes and at least 30 mL for gastrostomy tubes. Smaller syringes exert a higher pressure per square inch and may cause the tube to collapse. If unable to aspirate, inject 3 to 5 mL of air or water into the feeding tube and reattempt. Residuals contain formula, digestive juices, and electrolytes and therefore should be reinstilled through the feeding tube (unless there is a large amount).
c) Parameters for holding feedings. Isolated episodes of high gastric residuals are not always associated with abdominal symptoms. The amount of gastric residuals obtained depends on the amount and timing of the last feeding, medications, and the location of the feeding tube tip. The patient's activity and positioning may also affect the gastric emptying rate.[11] The residual may be clear, indicating the presence of gastric juices, or may contain partially digested formula.
   (1) Adults. When a residual reaches ≥200 mL with a nasogastric tube or ≥100 mL with a gastrostomy tube, associated signs or symptoms of intolerance should be assessed.[25]
   (2) Infants and children. Slowing or stopping feedings in infants and children has been recommended if residual volume exceeds twice the hourly infusion volume during continuous feedings or exceeds 50% of the infusion volume during bolus feedings.[28]
d) It is believed that aspiration from a gastrostomy tube is less likely to yield gastric residuals because of the tube's positioning in the anterior portion of the stomach, compared with a nasogastric tube. Therefore, high residuals from a gastrostomy tube are more worrisome. If abdominal discomfort or distension is present, feedings should be held. Further workup with roentgenograms may be indicated. If the abdominal exam is benign, feedings should be delayed for at least 1 hour and residuals rechecked. If high residuals persist without associated clinical signs and symptoms, a promotility agent (eg, erythromycin, metoclopramide) may be tried. Another option is to insert a transpyloric feeding tube and perform gastric decompression as necessary. Residuals cannot always be aspirated from jejunal or duodenal tubes.[11] Intolerance of small-bowel feedings can be identified when a patient experiences abdominal distention, discomfort, and/or diarrhea. If a patient develops feeding intolerance with small-bowel feedings, the previously tolerated formula strength or volume should be reinstituted and feeds gradually advanced as tolerated.[9]

2. Head-of-bed elevation. The effect of head elevation in patients fed through small-bore tubes or enterostomies has not been determined; however, the semirecumbent position (≥30° elevation) has been recommended for all tube-fed patients to minimize the potentially life-threatening consequences of aspiration.[29,30] Aspiration of pharyngeal and gastric secretions can still occur in some patients (even those not fed), and large-bore tubes may disrupt the function of the lower esophageal sphincter (LES), increasing the risk of aspiration.

C. Aspiration detection

1. Clinical signs and symptoms. When a significant amount of enteral formula is aspirated, sudden onset of dyspnea, tachypnea, wheezing, rales, tachycardia, cyanosis, decreased oxygenation, anxiety, and agitation can occur. Smaller amounts of formula may be aspirated over time with no apparent clinical symptoms. A subsequent fever can signal the development of aspiration pneumonia.
2. Roentgenogram findings are nonspecific and lack sensitivity for the detection of aspiration. There are many causes of pulmonary infiltrates, including pneumonia, contusion, atelectasis, and hemorrhage. The appearance of new infiltrates in dependent lung fields in a patient lacking other causes of infiltrates suggests aspiration.
3. Use of coloring agents. Blue dye has been used to tint tube-feeding formulas as a method for determining the presence of formula in tracheal aspirates. It was thought that this method would help detect pulmonary aspiration in tube-fed patients. The sensitivity, specificity, and safety of this method have not been adequately evaluated. The percentage of patients who will develop clinically significant aspiration whether or not coloring is detected has not been determined. Most important, a Food and Drug Administration Public Health Advisory issued September 29, 2003, reported blue discoloration and death in patients receiving tube feedings containing FD&C Blue No. 1 dye.[31] Blue discoloration of the skin, urine, feces, and serum has been reported in patients receiving this dye in their tube feedings, and in some the dye has been associated with refractory hypotension, metabolic acidosis, and death. Case reports reveal that critically ill patients, especially those who have increased intestinal permeability, are at risk for these complications. Based on these reports, patients with sepsis, severe burns, trauma, shock, surgical interventions, renal failure, celiac sprue, and inflammatory bowel disease may be at risk for systemic toxicity of blue dye absorption from enteral tube feedings. Other disadvantages of this method include the false elevation of gastric pH, positive Hemoccult stool tests, formula manipulation, and the potential to induce an allergic response. Blue food colorings or methylene blue may still be used when checking for fistulas (ie, tracheal-esophageal fistula) in hemodynamically stable patients, if provided in unit-of-use containers (ie, an ampule of methylene blue) to minimize contamination risk.
4. Tracheal glucose measurements. It has been reported that aspiration of tube-feeding formulas may be determined by a positive-glucose result in the tracheal aspirate,[32] but the sensitivity and specificity of this method have not been adequately tested. High tracheal concentrations of glucose have been found in intubated patients, both fed and not fed, and often are not associated with clinical evidence of aspiration. High tracheal concentrations of glucose also may be found in diabetic patients with high serum concentrations of glucose.[33]

D. Hydration status

1. Assessing hydration status
   a) Physical assessment. Possible clinical signs and symptoms of overhydration include edema, high urine output, dilute urine specific gravity, hypertension, respiratory insufficiency, congestive heart failure, and rapid weight gain. Possible signs of dehydration include decreased urine output or number of wet diapers in infants; concentrated, strong-smelling urine; elevated urine specific gravity; dry lips and mucous membranes; poor skin turgor; sunken eyes (and fontanelle in infants); flat neck veins; lethargy; hypotension; tachycardia; elevated blood urea nitrogen (BUN) level; constipation; and rapid weight loss.[34]
   b) Intake and output. In the euvolemic patient, fluid intake should approximately equal output. Fluid can be provided orally, with enteral feedings, or intravenously. Fluid output occurs primarily through the kidneys and, to a lesser extent, through the skin and lungs and in the feces. Insensible fluid loss in afebrile adult patients with intact skin approximates 10 mL/kg/day. Approximately 40 mL/100 kcal per 24 hours replaces insensible losses in pediatric patients.[35] Fluid needs increase with warmer weather, diarrhea, fever, vomiting, high nasogastric drainage, excessive diaphoresis, polyuria, open wounds, fistula/ostomy losses, and thermal injuries. These losses should be appropriately replaced with fluid and electrolytes. For each degree of body temperature above 38°C, insensible fluid loss is increased by 5 mL/kg per 24 hours. Diarrhea output should be monitored and replaced milliliter for milliliter.[35,36] In addition, liters of fluid can leak from the vascular compartment into the interstitial spaces in patients with vasodilatation or low serum oncotic pressure. In these conditions, fluid intake needs to be increased to compensate for the losses or fluid shifts and to maintain adequate intravascular volume. The clinician should also account for any factors or conditions that may result in fluid retention and could necessitate fluid restriction. Fluid restriction may be indicated in certain disease states, such as cardiac, liver, pulmonary, and renal dysfunction. Electrolyte disturbances and medications can also alter fluid needs.
   c) Weight changes. Fluid changes can be determined by daily changes in body weight. One kilogram of weight change is equivalent to 1 L of fluid.
2. Determining fluid requirements. Calculate water needs.
   a) Adults. There are several ways to calculate normal free water requirements for enterally fed, afebrile adults.[37] Either of the following methods is intended to replace urine and insensible fluid losses: provide 1 mL of water per calorie fed, or provide 30 to 35 mL of water per kilogram of body weight per day.
   b) Children. See Chapter 2 on nutrient requirements.
3. Providing extra fluids. Fluids can be given orally, intravenously, with medications, with the enteral tube feeding, and as tube-feeding flushes. Additional water requirements can be provided as tube flushes or intravenously. Calculate how much extra fluid a patient needs as follows:
   a) Determine how much fluid is being taken in orally and assess the patient's ability to consistently ingest that amount.
   b) Determine the volume of fluids being given intravenously.
   c) Determine the water content of the tube-feeding product being delivered. Most infant and pediatric enteral formulas contain approximately 85% to 90% free water (850 to 900 mL per L of formula), while most adult formulas contain 80% to 85% water (800 to 850 mL per L of formula). Calorically dense or concentrated formulas may contain as little as 60% water (600 mL per L of formula).[38]

d) Determine the amount of water being provided with flushes and medications that are being administered via the feeding tube.
e) Subtract the patient's fluid intake (total of steps a–d) from the daily amount required and provide the remainder throughout the day as water flushes via the enteral feeding tube. Note that if IV fluids are discontinued, water intake by the feeding tube may need to be increased.
f) Assess the patient's body weight, presence of edema, BUN, serum sodium, adequacy of intravascular volume, and urine output.

E. Assessment of nutrient intake
1. Assess actual nutrient intake. Calculate the macronutrients and energy being provided from the patient's oral intake, tube feedings, and dextrose-containing IV fluids. Often patients do not receive their full enteral nutrition prescriptions for various reasons, such as the scheduled administration of medications, tests or procedures, or daily therapies.
2. It is important for ongoing assessment of actual intake to determine whether changes in the nutrition support regimen are indicated to provide the daily prescribed volume of formulation more accurately and consistently.

F. Oral stimulation for children
1. Infants and young children who have received exclusive enteral tube feedings or PN for extended periods may experience difficulties when oral foods are introduced.[39] Early and frequent oral stimulation is necessary in such patients to minimize the potential for developing oral feeding difficulties and aversions.
2. Solid food feedings should be used particularly in infants in the first year of life at developmentally appropriate ages. Even though the nutrients may not be bioavailable, if these behaviors are not initiated and learned at this time, problems such as aversive behaviors toward eating are likely to manifest when the child is physiologically able to eat by mouth.[40]
3. If oral intake of fluids or solids is not medically feasible, non-nutritive sucking (sucking on a pacifier while being tube-fed) should be encouraged in infants.

G. Body weight
1. Ideal conditions. If possible, patients should be weighed in the morning—before eating, drinking, or the infusion of the tube-feeding formula but after voiding—using the same scale, and with minimal clothing.
2. Frequency. Patients should be weighed once or twice per week. More frequent measurements are useful in critically ill patients, in patients whose fluid status is unstable, or in infants and growing children.

H. Biochemical and hematological indices. The use of laboratory values as monitoring parameters during enteral nutrition support is individualized, and the frequency depends on the severity of the underlying medical condition, degree of malnutrition, level of metabolic stress, and presence of nutrient and electrolyte deficiencies.[41] Typically, laboratory monitoring is indicated less frequently in patients receiving enteral nutrition than PN because of the ability of the GI tract to regulate the absorption of electrolytes and minerals. However, baseline metabolic and nutrition assessment parameters should be obtained (see Chapter 1).[42] Follow-up laboratory work is then obtained based on the patient's clinical status.

I. Maintaining feeding tube patency
1. Method to irrigate the tube
a) Adults. To keep tubes patent, feeding ports should be flushed with warm water (at least 20–30 mL for adults) every 4 hours for continuous feedings as well as before and after each intermittent feeding or medication.[43] Medications should be administered separately, and 5 to 10 mL of water should be provided between each one. Gastric acids coagulate most intact protein formulations, so it is recommended that a feeding tube be flushed with 30 mL of warm tap water before and after checking for feeding residuals.[44] It is important to subtract the amount of water flushed from the obtained residual volume.
b) Children. Most pediatric tubes are not routinely flushed with water to prevent clogging unless recurrent problems occur. It is important to consider the size of the child when providing flushes. Infants' feeding tubes should be flushed with only 3 to 5 mL of water before and after medication administration, because they may not tolerate large amounts of calorie-free fluid. Older toddlers are also provided small volumes of flushes following medication administration in an effort to prevent fluid excess.[22]
2. Choice of irrigant. No irrigant has been shown to be more effective than water in preventing tube clogging. Water and carbonated beverages were shown to be equally effective in preventing tube clogging, and both were superior to cranberry juice. The lower pH of cranberry juice can cause clogging by precipitating certain proteins.[45]

J. The underlying medical condition(s) should be reassessed on an ongoing basis to evaluate the feasibility of transitional feeding and initiating or increasing oral intake.

IV. Complications and Management of Enteral Feedings[46–58]

A. Mechanical complications and management
1. Complications during placement of feeding tube (see Chapter 3).[57,59] Proper assessment of feeding-tube placement can prevent feedings from being delivered to the wrong site. Techniques for determining feeding-tube position include roentgenogram, tube-feeding aspiration (with assessment of pH, bile, volume of aspirate), use of special feeding tubes that measure pH or motility, auscultation, and laryngoscopy.
a) Upper airway injury during placement of feeding tubes may result in lacerations or bleeding of the nasal or oral cavity (especially in patients with coagulopathy or thrombocytopenia).
b) Lower airway injury during placement of feeding tubes may result in perforation of the trachea or pulmonary parenchyma (pneumothorax).[57,59] Pulmonary placement of feeding tubes is more likely in obtunded patients, in patients with impaired pharyngeal sensation (impaired cough or gag reflex), and with the use of small-bore feeding tubes.
c) GI tract injuries during feeding tube insertion include perforation (peritonitis) or laceration with GI bleeding. Other GI complications include intraperitoneal placement of the feeding tube and pneumoperitoneum.
d) Abdominal infection and abscess formation. Contamination of the peritoneum with resultant infection can occur from perforation of the GI tract or leakage following percutaneous or surgical tube placement.
e) Respiratory compromise may occur during feeding tube placement as a result of interference with oxygenation or aspiration of secretions.
f) Increased intracranial pressure and aggravation of brain ischemia may occur during tube placement in patients with intracranial lesions or bleeding.
2. Complications from the presence of a feeding tube[56]

a) Upper airway complications. Nasopharyngeal erosions and necrosis, sinusitis, otitis media, loosening and evulsion of teeth, bacteremia (especially in immunocompromised patients and patients with poor oral or dental hygiene), and interference with dental hygiene (oral tubes). Many of these complications are more common with the use of larger, stiffer tubes and can be minimized by the use of small-bore feeding tubes and meticulous nursing care.

b) Lower airway complications.[60] Feeding into the trachea or lung with resultant pneumonia, respiratory distress, acute respiratory failure, empyema, and adult respiratory distress syndrome. Proper assessment of tube location can prevent these complications.

c) GI injuries. Esophagus: erosions, aggravation of variceal bleeding (rarely occurs with soft, small-bore feeding tubes). Stomach: erosions, ulcer bleeding, and gastric outlet obstruction. Small intestine: erosions, ulcer bleeding, obstruction, and volvulus. Other: buried bumper syndrome (ie, percutaneous endoscopic gastrostomy placement), misplaced fasteners, necrotizing fascitis, wound infection, cellulitis, stomal leakage, hematoma, tube dislodgment, extrusion or migration of feeding tubes, subcutaneous emphysema, and enterocutaneous fistulas (eg, from percutaneous or surgical tube placement).

3. Tube clogging. Tube clogging is caused by viscous formulas, inappropriate medication administration, formula residue, and inadequate flushing.[26]

a) Tube clogging is more likely with intact protein products and viscous formulas (calorically dense and fiber-containing products).[44,61,62] Clogging may also be caused by product microbial contamination that leads to formula coagulation[63] or by the aspiration of residuals (gastric fluid coming in contact with formulation in the feeding tube).[64] To prevent tube clogging, the tubing should be flushed before and after each intermittent feeding and every 4 to 6 hours with continuous feeds.[65] Other strategies to prevent clogging include flushing the tube after aspirating for residuals, using an infusion pump to infuse viscous formulations, responding to an occlusion alarm on a pump as soon as possible, and using clean technique when administering enteral feedings to minimize contamination.

b) Clogging caused by medications. Inadequately crushed tablets, medications administered together (causing precipitation), interaction with formulation, or inadequate tube flushing can cause clogging. Clogging can be prevented by flushing feeding tubes with water (about 30 mL) before administering medication, as well as between each medication (at least 5 mL), and after the administration of all medications is complete (about 30 mL).[66] Avoid mixing a drug with any enteral formulation unless it has been shown to be compatible. Provide liquid forms of medications whenever possible and use elixirs or suspensions rather than syrups (which have a lower pH and can easily clump tube-feeding products).[67] Solid dosage forms, such as simple compressed tablets, should be crushed into a fine powder and diluted with enough water to dissolve the powder. Enteric-coated or sustained-release tablets should not be crushed. Bulk-forming agents should be avoided because they congeal rapidly when mixed with water and can clog the tube.[43,68,69] (See Chapter 9 for further discussion of medication administration via enteral feeding tubes.)

c) Clogging attributable to feeding-tube characteristics. Less clogging occurs with polyurethane tubes than with silicone tubes.[65,69,70]

4. Declogging methods. Feeding tubes are more successfully declogged when intervention is initiated immediately after the obstruction is noted and if the obstruction is close to the proximal tube opening.[71,72]

a) Irrigants. Warm water initially should be used as an irrigant. If ineffective, enzyme treatments can be initiated.[73] Papain (meat tenderizer) and carbonated beverages showed no significant advantage over distilled water in dissolving coagulated formula. However, a solution of digestive enzymes (pancrelipase) mixed with sodium bicarbonate (to activate the enzyme) has been shown to be fairly effective in dissolving formula occlusions.[73–75]

(1) With a 30- to 50-mL syringe, aspirate as much liquid as possible from the feeding tube so that the declogging solution can come in contact with the obstruction.

(2) Instill 5 mL of warm water with a 30- to 50-mL syringe under manual pressure for 1 minute and use a back-and-forth motion with the plunger to help dislodge the occlusion.

(3) Clamp the tube for 5 to 15 minutes.

(4) Try to aspirate or flush with warm water.

(5) If the tube remains clogged, prepare a pancrelipase solution buffered with a sodium bicarbonate tablet (eg, 1 crushed pancrelipase tablet or ¼ teaspoon of pancrelipase powder + 1 non-enteric-coated sodium bicarbonate [324 mg] tablet) or ⅛ tsp of baking soda dissolved in 5 mL of warm water. Follow steps 1 to 4 with the pancrelipase solution instead of water, and repeat once if necessary. When declogging feeding tubes, be certain the tube tip is not inadvertently positioned in the lung because enzymes or water can severely damage the pulmonary tissue.

b) Mechanical methods. Insertion of the following instruments into the feeding tube is generally used as a final attempt to declog the tube and should be performed by experienced practitioners only. In each case, the instrument used needs to be premeasured so it does not exceed feeding-tube length. Feeding-tube stylets should not be used to clear an obstruction, because they may cause tube perforation and trauma to the GI mucosa.[74]

(1) Small-diameter catheter. Introduce a small-diameter catheter into the clogged feeding tube. Instill declogging solution in close proximity to the obstruction.[71,73] After feeding-tube length is verified, mark the catheter appropriately and insert it into the feeding tube up to the point of obstruction. Initially, warm water is infused through the catheter and a back-and-forth motion is used to dislodge and dissolve the occlusion. If this method fails, the pancrelipase solution technique (see above) can be used.

(2) Endoscopy/cytology brushes.[61]—Insert an endoscopy/cytology brush through the tube lumen to break up an obstruction. The feeding tube is then flushed with water.

(3) Declogger devices. These devices are made of plastic and come in various lengths and diameters, which conform to various feeding-tube lengths and diameters. The threaded end of the device is inserted into the feeding tube with a twisting motion. After the clog is penetrated, the device is moved in a back-and-forth motion to dislodge the clog. This is followed by a water flush.

5. Aspiration is a potentially lethal complication of enteral feeding.[50,76,77] Clinically significant aspiration pneumonia is estimated to occur in 5% of gastric-fed patients. It can result in

cough, bronchospasm, pulmonary edema, pneumonia, empyema, and respiratory failure.

a) Risk factors include decreased level of consciousness, diminished cough or gag reflex, neurologic injury, incompetent LES, gastroesophageal reflux, supine position, use of large-bore feeding tubes, large gastric residuals, and gastroparesis. Most aspiration is of oral-pharyngeal secretions, not gastric contents.

b) Aspiration of gastric contents may be prevented by providing smaller, more frequent feedings in patients receiving intermittent tube feedings; using small-bowel feeding tubes (and gastric decompression); using promotility agents; periodically assessing gastric residuals; and keeping the head of the bed elevated (≥30°).

6. Miscellaneous. Other mechanical complications are tube knotting; perforation of the feeding tube with the guidewire (which also could perforate the bowel); inability to remove the guidewire because of knotting, kinking, or poor lubrication; tube deterioration; dislodgment; and migration.

B. GI complications

1. Gastroparesis is not a complication of feeding but may be present in patients who require enteral feeding. It predisposes the patient to gastroesophageal reflux and aspiration. Gastroparesis results from altered gut neurologic or muscular function (eg, neuropathy in patients with diabetes mellitus) and release of mediators that inhibit gastric emptying (eg, during critical illness). Consistently high gastric residuals may be an indicator of gastroparesis. For patients with impaired gastric motility, the use of promotility agents such as metoclopramide and erythromycin should be considered.

2. Gastroesophageal reflux occurs in most patients at some time.[78] Reflux can occur when gastric pressure exceeds LES pressure. Gastric pressure is increased by large gastric volumes and increased abdominal pressure due to fluid (eg, ascites). Reflux may be greater when the patient is in the supine position, especially if a large-bore feeding tube is in place.[30] Complications of reflux include esophagitis, vomiting, and aspiration. Gastroesophageal reflux and secondary aspiration can be minimized by maintaining low gastric volumes, keeping the head of the bed elevated, and using agents that increase LES pressure (eg, metoclopramide).

3. Duodenal-gastric (DG) reflux is common but does not usually present a clinical problem. The finding of bile or small-bowel feedings in the stomach is not a contraindication to enteral feedings. It is important to evaluate the clinical significance of the DG reflux. Large-volume DG reflux may indicate impaired small-bowel motility and can increase gastric residual volume. DG reflux is reduced by promotility agents and more distal placement of small-bowel feeding tubes. It is usually minimal when the feeding tube is beyond the ligament of Treitz.[79]

4. Diarrhea occurs in 2% to 63% of enterally fed patients, depending on how it is defined.[80–87] Diarrhea is generally defined as the passage of more than 200 grams of stool per day, but it is frequently defined clinically as three or more liquid stools per day.[86] It is important to note that the stool is usually pasty in patients fed non-fiber-containing liquid formulas. Many patients also develop rectal incontinence as a result of their illness. Thus, a patient with multiple small-volume bowel movements does not necessarily have diarrhea. Impaction should be ruled out in patients with oozing stools. Diarrhea rarely results from the enteral formula but rather indicates malfunction of the GI tract (eg, malabsorption, excess secretion), bacterial overgrowth, or the presence of toxins. Medications have been reported to cause 61% of the cases of diarrhea in tube-fed patients.[81–87] Antibiotics, H2-receptor antagonists, antineoplastics, laxatives, antacids, and potassium and phosphate supplements are medications that commonly contribute to the development of diarrhea. The cause of diarrhea is often multifactorial (Table 5-1). The best treatment for diarrhea remains unclear. It is rarely necessary to stop enteral feedings; diarrhea usually subsides as the cause is eliminated (eg, infection, drug, toxin, fecal impaction). However, in infants, increases in stool volumes of greater than 20 mL/kg per day are often an indication for less aggressive enteral feeding advancement.[40] Whenever possible, the offending medication(s) should be discontinued. It is important to rule out infection or the presence of enteric pathogens such as *C difficile* before using antimotility agents, because increased bowel motility is one mechanism for eliminating infecting organisms and toxins from the GI tract. Antimotility agents may enhance bacterial growth and toxin absorption. Agents used include adsorbents (eg, kaolin, pectin) and antimotility agents (eg, loperamide, diphenoxylate/atropine, paregoric, tincture of opium). Pancreatic enzymes may be useful in patients with pancreatic insufficiency. If diarrhea persists despite treatment of enteric pathogens or disease-related causes, antidiarrheal therapy, and medication adjustments, the enteral formulation should be evaluated. The addition of fiber to the enteral formulation may help bulk up the stool and promote more normal bowel function. Peptide-based and elemental enteral formulas have been associated with improved GI tolerance but should be used judiciously due to their higher cost.[87] Diluting the feeding formula or administering parenteral albumin rarely improves feeding tolerance and is not recommended. Hypoalbuminemia does not cause diarrhea but rather serves as a marker for patients with underlying inflammatory disease, increased gut permeability, and hypercatabolism.

TABLE 5-1. Possible Causes of Diarrhea in Tube-Fed Patients

Non-formula-related diarrhea

Medications (sorbitol-based elixirs, antibiotics, H2-receptor antagonists, laxatives, magnesium, and phosphorus)
Mediators released during inflammatory syndromes and sepsis
Pancreatic insufficiency
Delayed feedings causing bowel atrophy or long-term parenteral nutrition only
Increased bowel motility
Pathogenic bacteria (*Clostridium difficile,* enterotoxins)
Bacterial overgrowth
Cytomegalovirus
Inflammatory bowel disease
Impaction

Short-bowel syndrome

Formula-related diarrhea

Rapid infusion rate
Rapid initiation and progression of feedings in the small bowel
High fat intake
Lactose intolerance
Microbial contamination of formula

5. Constipation can result from inactivity, decreased bowel motility, decreased fluid intake, impaction, or lack of dietary fiber. Poor bowel motility and dehydration may lead to impaction and abdominal distension (from obstruction). Other common causes include the use of antimotility agents such as anticholinergics, opioids, calcium-channel antagonists, and certain chemotherapy agents such as vincristine. Neuromuscular blockers do not paralyze gut smooth muscle but may slow bowel motility via anticholinergic actions. Constipation is often improved by the provision of adequate hydration and the use of fiber-containing formulas, stool softeners, and bowel stimulants. Laxatives and enemas may improve symptoms in these patients. An abdominal roentgenogram may be needed as a diagnostic tool.
6. Malabsorption without diarrhea. The most common causes are medications (eg, antibiotics, sorbitol-containing medications, H2 antagonists), impaired digestion (pancreatic insufficiency, diminished gut mucosal enzymes, insufficient bile secretion), and impaired absorption (due to underlying injury or disease of the gut).

C. Metabolic complications. Metabolic complications are less prevalent with enteral than parenteral feedings due to the buffering effects of the gut and liver, which can help to prevent rapid metabolic changes.[34] However, it is still prudent to perform thorough ongoing assessments of patients receiving enteral nutrition support.

1. Hyperglycemia. Most enterally fed patients do not develop hyperglycemia. Hyperglycemia may occur in some patients because of underlying diabetes mellitus or insulin resistance (precipitated by the illness or by medications such as glucocorticoids). Carbohydrate feeding can increase blood glucose concentrations in these patients. Hyperglycemia should be treated because it impairs immune function, increases the risk of infection, increases post-ischemic neuronal damage, and results in fluid and electrolyte losses. In critically ill patients, hyperglycemia increases in-hospital mortality, bloodstream infections, incidence of acute renal failure requiring dialysis or hemofiltration, need for red cell transfusions, and critical illness polyneuropathy.[88] Blood glucose levels should be monitored at periodic intervals in all patients receiving enteral nutrition support. It is important to treat the underlying disease (eg, infection, inflammation), maintain intravascular volume, and prevent electrolyte disturbances. If blood glucose concentrations remain elevated (>110 mg/dL) in critically ill patients at the carbohydrate level needed by the patient, insulin should be administered and titrated to achieve blood glucose concentrations that are below this range. In nonacute hyperglycemic patients who have not been previously diagnosed with diabetes mellitus or are not being treated with corticosteroids, a workup for diabetes mellitus should be initiated.
2. Electrolyte and mineral deficiencies[89] (Table 5-2)
   a) Electrolytes are lost via stool, ostomies, fistulae, urine, and skin. Patients with excessive losses may need increased intake of various electrolytes. Potassium, magnesium, and phosphorus are required for optimal protein synthesis. The kidneys are primarily responsible for excretion of potassium, magnesium, and phosphorus; intake of these ions may need to be decreased in patients with renal insufficiency or failure. Serum concentrations should be monitored at intervals based on patient acuity, and electrolytes and minerals should be replaced as needed to keep serum levels within the normal range.
   b) Sodium is the primary extracellular cation in the body and the major controller of osmolality. Clinical features of hyponatremia and hypernatremia relate to the nervous system and include depressed mentation, confusion, irritability, obtundation, coma, seizures, nausea, vomiting, anorexia, and headache. Altered circulating levels of sodium primarily reflect the status of body water. An excess intake of water compared with sodium results in hyponatremia, while an excess intake of sodium compared with water results in hypernatremia. The most common cause of hyponatremia in hospitalized patients is the syndrome of inappropriate antidiuretic hormone (SIADH), which results in retention of water in excess of sodium. SIADH can result from a variety of causes, including intracranial hemorrhage, trauma, tumor, or encephalitis; carcinoma of the lung, duodenum, pancreas, thymus, or lymph nodes; and pneumonia, tuberculosis, lung abscess, cystic fibrosis, or certain medications. The most common cause of hypernatremia is dehydration due to water losses in excess of sodium (eg, excess sweating, excess urinary loss of water because of osmotic diuresis, limited water intake). Thus, hypernatremia is treated primarily by administration of fluid, and hyponatremia is treated by fluid restriction. Hypernatremia and hyponatremia also can be caused by high and low sodium intake, respectively, in relation to output. Most enteral formulas contain low amounts of sodium. Patients with increased sodium losses require replacement. Table salt may be judiciously added to the formula or the flush solution. The amount of salt used is based on the sodium deficit, the volume of fluid losses, and the organ from which the fluids came. Conversely, the sodium content of IV fluids needs to be calculated when hypernatremia is evaluated.
   c) Potassium is the primary intracellular cation in the body and is the major determinant of electrical membrane potential. Decreased concentrations of potassium result in cardiac arrhythmias, muscle weakness, and impaired protein synthesis. Potassium deficiency results from losses in the stool, GI secretions, and urine (especially with diuretics).
   d) Calcium is the primary divalent cation of the extracellular fluid and is essential for regulating processes that require movement in the body (eg, excitation-contraction coupling in cardiac, smooth, and skeletal muscle; neurotransmission; hormonal secretion; ciliary motion; or cell division).[89] Calcium circulates in the blood in three fractions: ionized, chelated, and protein bound. The ionized fraction is physiologically active and homeostatically regulated. Total calcium levels (measured by most laboratories) may not accurately reflect the ionized calcium status of sick patients. The best measure of circulating calcium status is the ionized calcium level. Ionized calcium levels are usually obtained with a parathyroid hormone level when serum total calcium values are persistently low despite attempts to normalize them. In the absence of an ionized calcium measurement, practitioners often use the following equation to determine a corrected value:

$$\begin{aligned}&[\text{normal serum albumin } (\text{mg/dL})\\ &- \text{observed serum albumin } (\text{mg/dL}) \times 0.8]\\ &+ \text{observed serum calcium } (\text{mg/dL})\\ &= \text{corrected serum calcium value } (\text{mg/dL})\end{aligned}$$

If adequate dietary calcium is not received over the short term, it will be mobilized from bone. However, long-term depletion of dietary calcium may lead to osteopenia or osteoporosis. Conversely, excess calcium administration during ischemic and septic states can cause cellular injury. Calcium should be administered to patients in only the amounts required to maintain normal concentrations. Some experts believe that calcium intake should be decreased or completely restricted for a short

TABLE 5-2. Electrolyte/Mineral Imbalances

Mineral	Physiologic Function	Clinical Features	Etiologies	Treatment
Sodium	1. Primary extracellular cation 2. Extracellular osmolality 3. Exchange of K^+, H^+, Ca^{++}, H_2O	Altered CNS function; disorientation, depressed mentation, confusion, irritability, coma, seizures, nausea, vomiting, weakness	1. Hyponatremia results from retention of water in excess of sodium (ie, from excess ADH or water intake); rarely does low sodium intake contribute. 2. Hypernatremia results from water loss in excess of sodium or excess intake of salt	1. Hyponatremia is treated by limiting the intake of free water and increasing water excretion. 2. Hypernatremia is treated with water administration or salt removal plus water repletion.
Potassium	1. Primary intracellular cation 2. Electrical membrane potential	1. Hypokalemia: cardiac arrhythmias, bradycardia, muscle weakness, paralysis, hyporeflexia, paresthesias, ileus, impaired protein synthesis 2. Hyperkalemia: bradycardia, heart block, dysrhythmias, diminished cardiac conduction, weakness, paralysis, paresthesias, hyporeflexia	1. Hypokalemia results from loss of potassium from the body in urine, stool, wounds, or through the skin (not matched by intake) or shift of K^+ into cells (refeeding) 2. Hyperkalemia results from excess excess entry of K^+ into the extracellular space from dietary intake or release from tissues (ie, cell necrosis) and/or decreased renal excretion.	1 Hypokalemia is treated by administering K^+. 2. Hyperkalemia is treated by antagonizing K^+ effect on the cell membrane with calcium (only emergencies), shifting K^+ into cells (insulin and glucose, bicarbonate), and removing K^+ from the body (diuretics, kayexalate).
Calcium	1. Primary extracellular divalent cation 2. Excitation-contraction coupling, secretion neurotransmission, cellular messenger, activator of enzymes 3. Major regulator of all processes that require movement	1. Hypocalcemia causes bone loss, weakening of bones, hypotension, poor cardiac contraction. 2. Hypercalcemia causes hypertension, impaired cardiac function, and altered mentation and can lead to renal stones and tissue calcification. 3 Calcium status is best determined using ionized calcium levels.	1. Hypocalcemia results from from decreased PTH or vitamin D action on bone; chelation may also cause hypocalcemia. 2. Hypercalcemia results from excess Ca^{++} intake or excess release of Ca^{++} from bone (ie, cancer, hyperparathyroidism, immobilization).	1. Hypocalcemia is treated with calcium administration; mild hypocalcemia is well tolerated over the short term (a few weeks) and may be protective against ischemic and inflammatory-mediated cellular injury.

(continued)

TABLE 5-2. Electrolyte/Mineral Imbalances

Mineral	Physiologic function	Clinical features	Etiologies	Treatment
				2. Hypercalcemia is treated by decreasing Ca^{++} intake, Ca^{++} excretion (with diuretics and sodium), and decreasing bone release of calcium.
Phosphorus	Cellular energy, second messengers, 2,3-DPG, DNA, RNA	1. Depletion results in diminished immune, muscle, hepatic, and other organ functions. 2. Excess usually causes symptoms by lowering Ca^{++} levels. 3. Ca-PO_4 precipitation is likely when Ca x PO_4 product >60 mg/dL.	1. Low levels result from decreased PO_4 intake, excess loss from the body, or shift of PO_4 into cells (ie, refeeding syndrome). 2. High levels result from excess intake, diminished renal excretion, or release of PO_4 from tissues (cell lysis).	1. Depletion is treated by administering enteral or IV PO_4. 2. Excess PO_4 states are y treated by decreasing PO_4 intake, increasing PO_4 loss from the body (diuretics, PO_4 binders such as aluminum-containing antacids), or shifting PO_4 intracellularly (glucose and insulin).
Magnesium	Regulates PTH and vitamin D secretion or action, Na^+-K^+ ATPase activity, cyclase activity, Ca^{++} channels; also a cofactor for many enzymes	1. Depletion results in cardiac arrhythmias, muscle weakness, hypokalemia, hypocalcemia. 2. Excess results in CNS depression, muscle weakness; very high levels can cause paralysis and cardiac arrest.	1. Depletion results from decreased intake and excess body losses (urine, stool, skin); levels may also decrease when Mg^{++} shifts into cells (ie, refeeding syndrome). 2. Excess states result from increased intake and decreased renal excretion.	1. Depletion is treated with enteral or IV Mg^{++}. 2. Excess states are treated by limiting intake and increasing losses from urine.

ADH, antidiuretic hormone; ATPase, adenosine triphosphatase; CNS, central nervous system; DPG, diphosphoglycerate ; IV, intravenous; PTH, parathyroid hormone.

period after the onset of critical illness, although this belief is controversial.

e) Phosphorus plays an important role in the body.[89] It is a source of cellular energy (eg, adenosine triphosphate, creatine phosphate), a component of cyclic adenosine monophosphate and cyclic guanosine monophosphate (important intracellular messengers), a component of 2,3-diphosphoglycerate (important for oxygen offloading from hemoglobin), and synthesis of nucleotides. Most circulating phosphorus is in the ionized form. Phosphorus depletion causes a sick-cell syndrome in which all cells of the body demonstrate diminished function (eg, immune system, muscle, liver). Respiratory arrest can occur with severe phosphorus depletion. Common causes of hypophosphatemia are administration of large amounts of carbohydrate (phosphorus shifts intracellularly when glucose enters the cell), administration of drugs (insulin, epinephrine, phosphate-binding antacids, sucralfate), and phosphate losses from the GI tract and kidneys. Serum phosphorus concentrations should be monitored based on patient acuity and replacement provided as necessary. If levels are severely low, IV phosphorus should be administered.

f) Magnesium is an important cofactor for many essential enzymes.[89] Magnesium depletion can result from losses in GI fluids or urine or from decreased intake in the diet. Magnesium depletion predisposes a patient to cardiac arrhythmias and cellular injury.

3. Refeeding syndrome
   a) Refeeding of severely malnourished patients may result in "refeeding syndrome," in which there are acute intracellular shifts of electrolytes as cell anabolism is stimulated.[90–92] Refeeding syndrome is a potentially life-threatening complication that may occur with the rapid reintroduction of carbohydrate-containing feedings in severely malnourished patients. Hematologic, neuromuscular, cardiac, and respiratory dysfunction has been observed in severe cases.[93] Refeeding syndrome can result in acute decreases in circulating levels of potassium, magnesium, and phosphorus. Serum levels should be monitored and replacement should be provided as needed to maintain normal circulating levels. Many of these patients also require thiamine supplementation.[92]
   b) Children. Malnourished children are at greater risk for metabolic problems. All moderately to severely malnourished children should have serum potassium, phosphorus, magnesium, and glucose levels checked at least daily during the first week of initiation of nutrition support, as well as periodically during the gradual advancement of feedings.[41]
4. Vitamin deficiencies may develop in patients who receive nutrition support. Deficiencies commonly result from inadequate vitamin intake (which fails to match requirements or losses) or poor absorption. Malnourished patients are at higher risk of developing vitamin deficiencies due to their depleted state when nutrition support is initiated. (See Chapter 1 for clinical manifestations of vitamin deficiencies.)
   a) Fat-soluble vitamins (vitamins A, D, E, and K) require pancreatic enzymes and bile for absorption. Concentrations may be low in patients with pancreatic insufficiency, cirrhosis, or malabsorption syndromes. Vitamin K is synthesized by gut bacteria, and concentrations may be decreased in patients who receive antibiotics. Vitamin K is required for synthesis of coagulation proteins, while vitamin D is necessary for the maintenance of circulating calcium.
   b) Water-soluble vitamins. The most common deficiencies are of folate, ascorbic acid, and thiamine. Humans are almost entirely dependent on dietary sources for these vitamins and require constant intake to maintain normal stores. Thiamine is an essential vitamin for carbohydrate metabolism (including glucose). In the United States, chronic alcoholism, advanced age, long-term malnutrition, malabsorption syndromes, prolonged antacid therapy (thiamine is destroyed in alkaline pH), and dialysis are the most common causes of thiamine deficiency. Thus, many of these patients are provided thiamine upon hospital admission.
5. Dehydration is a risk for patients receiving enteral nutrition support, and the etiology is multifactorial. Water needs average 1 mL per calorie consumed in adults. Dehydration may result from the use of concentrated formulations, which contain less water. In addition, high-protein feeds may cause an osmotic (urea) diuresis and loss of body water. Dehydration also may result when body fluid losses are not met by fluid intake (eg, water loss from skin during fever, from urine, from stool, or from fistula/ostomy output). An increasing serum sodium concentration, BUN, or BUN/creatinine ratio suggests dehydration. Treatment is aimed at restoring intravascular volume and fluid balance.

V. Transitioning from Enteral Nutrition Support

Before beginning the process of weaning from tube feedings, the patient should have an adequate nutrition status or the ability to return to normal status by eating. In addition, it is important to ensure that the patient's fluid needs are being met either by tube or orally during the transitional phase.

A. Transitioning from continuous tube feedings. When a patient is transitioning from full enteral nutrition support, physiologic preparation should be initiated by providing the patient bolus feedings throughout the day to simulate meals and snacks. This strategy is implemented in an effort to stimulate hunger and to achieve the association of satiety with feedings.[11] Initially, oral intake can be minimal and coupled with supplemental feedings via tube after each meal to provide the majority of nutrition needs. As oral intake increases, tube-feeding formula volume is decreased, keeping the combined regimen isocaloric.[94] Another option is to provide a portion of the tube feedings by continuous drip at night, ending at least 1 hour before the first meal. This allows freedom from tube feeding during the day and helps promote an appetite. This also is useful in patients who have short-bowel syndrome and require small, frequent feedings to optimize intestinal absorption. If the patient is receiving elemental tube feedings due to intestinal malabsorption or if weight gain is deemed inadequate, additional calories may need to be provided via the feeding tube, but efforts to continue to increase the intake of oral foods should still be encouraged.

B. Discontinuing tube feedings. When the patient is able to consume 75% of nutrition needs by mouth, the tube feeding can be discontinued but the feeding tube left in place. Before the feeding tube is removed, factors that should be considered include the type of tube placement (ie, nasogastric vs. a more permanent gastrostomy), the underlying medical condition(s) that necessitated the tube, whether fluid needs can be met, and whether medications can be administered without the tube. It is especially helpful to observe patients who have received long-term enteral nutrition support during an acute illness to determine the future necessity of the tube.[11]

(Enteral Nutrition Management chapters from the 1st edition were contributed by Linda Lord, Linda Trumbore, Gary Zaloga, Kristy Gibbons, Nancy Cyr, Michael L. Christensen, and Richard A. Helms)

REFERENCES

1. Braunschweig CL, Levy P, Sheean PM, et al. Enteral compared with parenteral nutrition: a meta-analysis. *Am J Clin Nutr.* 2001;74:534–542.
2. Kang A, Zamora SA, Scott RB, Parsons HG. Catch-up growth in children treated with home enteral nutrition. *Pediatrics.* 1998;102:951–955.
3. Alverdy J. Effect of nutrition on gastrointestinal barrier function. *Sem Respir Infections.* 1994;9:248–255.
4. A.S.P.E.N. Board of Directors. Guidelines for the use of parenteral and enteral nutrition in adult and pediatric patients. *J Parenter Enteral Nutr.* 1993;17:8SA.
5. A.S.P.E.N. Board of Directors. Guidelines for the use of parenteral and enteral nutrition in adult and pediatric patients. *J Parenter Enteral Nutr.* 2002;26:18SA–19SA.
6. Hernandez G, Velasco N, Wainstein C, et al. Gut mucosal atrophy after a short enteral fasting period in critically ill patients. *J Crit Care.* 1999;14:73–77.
7. Holter AR, Fisher JE. The effects of perioperative hyperalimentation on complications in patients with carcinoma and weight loss. *J Surg Res.* 1977; 23:31–34.
8. Cunningham J. Body composition and nutrition support in pediatrics: what to defend and how soon to begin. *Nutr Clin Pract.* 1995;10:177–182.
9. Marian M. Pediatric nutrition support. *Nutr Clin Pract.* 1993;8:199–209.
10. A.S.P.E.N. Board of Directors. Guidelines for the use of parenteral and enteral nutrition in adult and pediatric patients. *J Parenter Enteral Nutr.* 2002;26:13SA–14SA.
11. Smith B, Pederson A. Nutrition focus tube feeding update. *Nutr Focus.* 1990;5:1–6.
12. Lord LM, Sax H. The role of the gut in critical illness. *AACN Clin Issues Crit Care Nurs.* 1994;5:450–458.
13. Martindale RG. Enteral feeding during states of marginal visceral blood flow. In: *Current Issues in Enteral Nutrition Support: Report of the First Ross Conference on Enteral Devices.* Columbus, OH: Ross Products; 1996:59–61.
14. Greenberg GR, Fleming CR, Jeejeebhoy KN, et al. Controlled trial of bowel rest and nutritional support in the management of Crohn's disease. *Gut.* 1988;29:1309–1315.
15. Fleming CR. Nutrition in patients with Crohn's disease: another piece of the puzzle [editorial]. *J Parenter Enteral Nutr.* 1995;19:93–94.
16. Simpson WG, Marsano L, Gates L. Enteral nutritional support in acute alcoholic pancreatitis. *J Am Coll Nutr.* 1995;14:662–665.
17. A.S.P.E.N. Board of Directors. Guidelines for the use of parenteral and enteral nutrition in adult and pediatric patients. *J Parenter Enteral Nutr.* 2002;26:68SA–70SA.
18. Ragins H, Levenson SM, Singer R, et al. Intrajejunal administration of an elemental diet at neutral pH avoids pancreatic stimulation. *Am J Surg.* 1973; 126:606–614.
19. Weckwerth J, Nelson J, O'Shea R. Home nutrition support. In: Gottschlich M, Matarese L, Shronts E, eds. *Nutrition Support Dietetics Core Curriculum.* Silver Spring, MD: A.S.P.E.N; 1993:467–473.
20. Nevin-Folino N, Miller M. Enteral nutrition. In: Queen Samour P, King Helm K, Lang CE, eds. *Pediatric Nutrition.* Gaithersburg, MD: Aspen Publishers; 1999:513–549.
21. Heitkemper M, Martin D, Hansen B, et al. Rate and volume of intermittent enteral feeding. *J Parenter Enteral Nutr.* 1981;5:312–316.
22. Harrington M, Lyman B. Special considerations for the pediatric patient. In: Guenter P, Silkroski M, eds. *Tube Feeding: Practical Guidelines and Nursing Protocols.* Gaithersburg, MD: Aspen Publishers; 2001:139–188.
23. Akers SM, Groh-Wargo SL. Normal nutrition during infancy. In: Queen Samour P, King Helm K, Lang CE, eds. *Pediatric Nutrition.* Gaithersburg, MD: Aspen Publishers; 1999:65–97.
24. Burd RS, Lentz C. The limitations of using gastric residual volumes to monitor enteral feedings: a mathematical model. *Nutr Clin Pract.* 2001;16: 349–354.
25. McClave SA, Snider HI, Lowen CC, et al. Use of residual volume as a marker for enteral feeding intolerance: prospective blinded comparison with physical examination and radiographic findings. *J Parenter Enteral Nutr.* 1992;16:99–105.
26. A.S.P.E.N. Board of Directors. Guidelines for the use of parenteral and enteral nutrition in adult and pediatric patients. *J Parenter Enteral Nutr.* 2002;26:33SA–35SA.
27. Murphy LM, Bickford V. Gastric residuals in tube feeding: how much is too much? *Nutr Clin Pract.* 1999;14:304–306.
28. Schanler RJ. The low birth weight infant: perinatal nutrition. In: Walker WA, Watkins JB, eds. *Nutrition in Pediatrics: Basic Science and Clinical Applications.* Hamilton, Ontario; B.C. Decker; 1996:387–407.
29. Torres A, Serra-Batlles J, Ros E, et al. Pulmonary aspiration of gastric contents in patients receiving mechanical ventilation: the effect of body position. *Ann Intern Med.* 1992;116:540–543.
30. Ibanez J, Penafiel A, Raurich JM, et al. Gastroesophageal reflux in intubated patients receiving enteral nutrition: effect of supine and semirecumbent positions. *J Parenter Enteral Nutr.* 1992;16:419–422.
31. FDA Public Health Advisory. *Reports of Blue Discoloration and Death in Patients Receiving Enteral Feedings Tinted with the Dye, FD&C Blue no. 1.* Rockville, MD. US Food and Drug Administration; 2003.
32. Winterbauer RH, Durning RB Jr, Barron E, et al. Aspirated nasogastric feeding solution detected by glucose strips. *Ann Intern Med.* 1981;95:67–68.
33. Kinsey GC, Murray MJ, Swensen SJ, et al. Glucose content of tracheal aspirates: implications for the detection of tube feeding aspiration. *Crit Care Med.* 1994;22:1557–1562.
34. Nardella M. Practical tips on tube feedings for children. *Nutr Focus.* 1995;10:1–8.
35. A.S.P.E.N. Board of Directors. Guidelines for the use of parenteral and enteral nutrition in adult and pediatric patients. *J Parenter Enteral Nutr.* 2002;26:26SA–27SA.
36. Ellis KJ, Shypailo RJ, Wong WW. Measurement of body water by multifrequency bioelectrical impedance spectroscopy in a multiethnic pediatric population. *Am J Clin Nutr.* 1999;70:847–853.
37. Lipp J, Lord LM, Scholer LH. Fluid management in enteral nutrition. *Nutr Clin Pract.* 1999;14:232–237.
38. Mahan L, Arlin M, eds. *Krause's Food, Nutrition & Diet Therapy.* 8th ed. Philadelphia, PA: WB Saunders; 1992.
39. Huggins PS, Tuomi SK, Young C. Effects of nasogastric feeding tubes on the young normal swallowing mechanism. *Dysphagia.* 1999;14: 157–161.
40. Vanderhoof JA, Young RF. Overview of considerations for the pediatric patient receiving home parenteral and enteral nutrition. *Nutr Clin Pract.* 2003;18:221–226.
41. A.S.P.E.N. Board of Directors. Guidelines for the use of parenteral and enteral nutrition in adult and pediatric patients. *J Parenter Enteral Nutr.* 2002;26:16SA–17SA.
42. A.S.P.E.N. Board of Directors. The 1995 standards for nutrition support of hospitalized patients. *Nutr Clin Pract.* 1995;10:206–207.
43. Scanlan M, Frisch S. Nasoduodenal feeding tubes: prevention of occlusion. *J Neurosci Nurs.* 1992;24:256–259.
44. Marcuard S, Perkins A. Clogging of feeding tubes. *J Parenter Enteral Nutr.* 1988;12:403–405.
45. Methany N, Eisenberg P, McSweeney M. Effect of feeding tube properties and three irrigants on clogging rates. *Nurs Res.* 1988;37:165–169.
46. Kudsk KA, Minard G. Enteral nutrition. In: Zaloga GP, ed. *Nutrition in Critical Care.* St Louis, MO: Mosby; 1994:331–360.
47. Silk DBA, Payne-James JJ. Complications of enteral nutrition. In: Romeau JL, Caldwell MD, eds. *Clinical Nutrition: Enteral and Tube Feeding.* 2nd ed. Philadelphia, PA: WB Saunders; 1990:510–531.
48. Bastow MD. Complications of enteral nutrition. *Gut.* 1986;27(suppl 1): 51–55.
49. Kirby DF, DeLegge MH. Enteral nutrition: the challenge of access. In: Kirby DF, Dudrick SJ, eds. *Handbook of Nutrition in Clinical Practice.* Boca Raton, FL: CRC Press; 1994:87–104.
50. Zaloga GP. Enteral nutrition in the critically ill. In: Chernow B, ed. *The Pharmacologic Approach to the Critically Ill Patient.* 3rd ed. Baltimore, MD: Williams & Wilkins; 1994:1034–1050.
51. Cabre E, Gassull MA. Complications of enteral feeding. *Nutrition.* 1993; 9:1–9.

52. Eddy VA, Snell JE, Morris JA Jr. Analysis of complications and long-term outcome of trauma patients with needle catheter jejunostomy. *Am Surg.* 1996;62:40–44.
53. Fleming CR. Hepatobiliary complications in adults receiving nutrition support. *Dig Dis.* 1994;12:191–198.
54. O'Keefe KP. Complications of percutaneous feeding tubes. *Emerg Med Clin North Am.* 1994;12:815–826.
55. Bowling TE, Silk DB. Enteral feeding: problems and solutions. *Eur J Clin Nutr.* 1994;48:379–385.
56. Bohnker BK, Artman LE, Hoskins WJ. Narrow bore nasogastric feeding tube complications. A literature review. *Nutr Clin Pract.* 1987;2:203–209.
57. Miller KS, Tomlinson JR, Sahn SA. Pleuropulmonary complications of enteral tube feedings. *Chest.* 1985;88:230–233.
58. Metheny N. Minimizing respiratory complications of nasoenteric tube feeding: state of the science. *Heart Lung.* 1993;22:213–223.
59. Roubenoff R, Ravich WJ. Pneumothorax due to nasogastric feeding tubes. Report of four cases. *Arch Intern Med.* 1989;149:184–188.
60. Montecalvo MA, Steger KA, Farber HW, et al. Nutritional outcome and pneumonia in critical care patients randomized to gastric versus jejunal tube feedings. The Critical Care Research Team. *Crit Care Med.* 1992;10: 1377–1387.
61. Caos A, Gogel HK. A simple method for clearing obstructed enteral feeding tubes [letter]. *Gastrointest Endosc.* 1986;32:55.
62. Hofstetter J, Allen LV Jr. Causes of nonmedication-induced nasogastric tube occlusion. *Am J Hosp Pharm.* 1992;49:603–607.
63. Kohn CL. The relationship between enteral formula contamination and length of enteral delivery set usage. *J Parenter Enteral Nutr.* 1991;5:567–571.
64. Powell KS, Marcuard SP, Farrior ES, et al. Aspirating gastric residuals causes occlusion of small-bore feeding tubes. *J Parenter Enteral Nutr.* 1993;17: 243–246.
65. Sensibile J, Agrecy J, Griggs M, Lovoy K, Smart J. Breakout session. Group II: salvage of the clogged feeding tube: tricks of the trade. *Nutr Clin Pract.* 2000;15:S74–S75.
66. Williams PJ. How do you keep medicines from clogging feeding tubes? *Am J Nurs.* 1989;89:181–182.
67. Altman E, Cutie AJ. Compatibility of enteral products with commonly employed drug additives. *Nutr Supp Serv.* 1984;4:8, 10, 11, 14.
68. Holtz L, Milton J, Sturek JK. Compatibility of medications with enteral feedings. *J Parenter Enteral Nutr.* 1987;11:183–186.
69. Hearne BE, Besser PM, Groshen S, et al. In vitro flow rates of enteral solutions through nasoenteric tubes. *J Parenter Enteral Nutr.* 1984;8:456–459.
70. Petrosino BM, Meraviglia M, Becker H. Mechanical problems with small-diameter enteral feeding tubes. *J Neurosci Nurs.* 1987;19:276–280.
71. Bommarito AA, Heinzelmann MJ, Boysen DA. A new approach to the management of obstructed enteral feeding tubes. *Nutr Clin Pract.* 1989:4: 111–114.
72. Mateo MA. Maintaining the patency of enteral feeding tubes. *Online J Knowledge Synth Nurs.* 1994;1(Doc 9):1–13.
73. Marcuard SP, Stegall K, Trogdon S. Clearing obstructed feeding tubes. *J Parenter Enteral Nutr.* 1989;3:81–83.
74. Webber-Jones J, Sweeney K, Winterbottom A, et al. How to declog a feeding tube. *Nursing.* 1992;22:62–64.
75. Marcuard SP, Stegall KS. Unclogging feeding tubes with pancreatic enzyme. *J Parenter Enteral Nutr.* 1990;14:198–200.
76. Hamaoui E. Gastroesophageal reflux during gastrostomy feeding. *J Parenter Enteral Nutr.* 1995;19:172–173.
77. Gustke RF, Varma RR, Soergel KH. Gastric reflux during perfusion of the proximal small bowel. *Gastroenterology.* 1970;59:890–895.
78. Mullan H, Roubenoff RA, Roubenoff R. Risk of pulmonary aspiration among patients receiving enteral nutrition support. *J Parenter Enteral Nutr.* 1992;16:160–164.
79. Pratt JC, Tolbert CG. Tube feeding aspiration. *Am J Nurs.* 1996;96:37.
80. Koruda MJ. Diarrhea-diagnosis and treatment. In: Zaloga G, ed. *Nutrition in Critical Care.* St. Louis, MO: Mosby; 1994:815–829.
81. Edes TF, Walk BE, Austin JL. Diarrhea in tube-fed patients: feeding formula not necessarily the cause. *Am J Med.* 1990;88:91–93.
82. Mobarhan S, DeMeo M. Diarrhea induced by enteral feeding. *Nutr Rev.* 1995;53:67–70.
83. Eisenberg PG. Causes of diarrhea in tube-fed patients: a comprehensive approach to diagnosis and management. *Nutr Clin Pract.* 1993;8:119–123.
84. Bowling TE. The Sir David Cuthbertson Medal Lecture. Enteral-feeding-related diarrhoea: proposed causes and possible solutions. *Proc Nutr Soc.* 1995;54:579–590.
85. Heimburger DC, Sockwell DG, Geels WJ. Diarrhea with enteral feeding: prospective reappraisal of putative causes. *Nutrition.* 1994;10:392–396.
86. Bliss DZ, Guenter PA, Settle RG. Defining and reporting diarrhea in tube-fed patients—what a mess! *Am J Clin Nutr.* 1992;55:753–759.
87. Fuhrman MP. Diarrhea and tube feeding. *Nutr Clin Pract.* 1999;4:83–84.
88. Van den Berghe G, Wouters P, Weekers, F, et al. Intensive insulin therapy in critically ill patients. *New Engl J Med.* 2001;345:1359–1367.
89. Zaloga GP, Chernow B. Divalent ions: calcium, magnesium, and phosphorus. In: Chernow B, ed. *The Pharmacologic Approach to the Critically Ill Patient.* 3rd ed. Baltimore, MD: Williams & Wilkins; 1994:777–804.
90. Jolly AF, Blank R. Refeeding syndrome. In: Zaloga G, ed. *Nutrition in Critical Care.* St. Louis, MO: Mosby; 1994:765–782.
91. Bowling TE, Silk DB. Refeeding remembered. *Nutrition.* 1995;11:32–34.
92. Solomon SM, Kirby DF. The refeeding syndrome: a review. *J Parenter Enteral Nutr.* 1990;14:90–97.
93. A.S.P.E.N. Board of Directors. Guidelines for the use of parenteral and enteral nutrition in adult and pediatric patients. *J Parenter Enteral Nutr.* 2002;26:39SA–41SA.
94. Reimers K, Carlson S, Lombard K. Nutritional management of infants with bronchopulmonary dysplasia. *Nutr Clin Pract.* 1992;7:127–132.

SUGGESTED READINGS

Clevenger F, Rodriguez D. Decision-making for enteral feeding administration: the why behind where and how. Nutr Clin Pract. 1995;10:104–113.

Ideno K. Enteral nutrition. In: Gottschlich M, Matarese L, Shronts E, eds. Nutrition Support Dietetics: Core Curriculum. 2nd ed. Silver Spring, MD: A.S.P.E.N.; 1993:71–104.

Kudsk K. Clinical applications of enteral nutrition. *Nutr Clin Pract.* 1994;9: 165–171.

Rolandelli R, DePaula J, Guenter P, et al. Critical illness and sepsis. In: Rombeau J, Caldwell M, eds. *Clinical Nutrition: Enteral and Tube Feeding.* 2nd ed. Philadelphia, PA: WB Saunders; 1990:288–305.

Elizabeth A. Krzywda, RN, APN, MSN;
Charles E. Edmiston, Jr., PhD

6

Parenteral Nutrition Access and Infusion Equipment

Introduction

The development of central venous access devices is closely linked to the development of total parenteral nutrition. Today, the use of central venous access has become a standard for a multitude of intravenous (IV) therapies. Vascular access is both an art and a science. Decisions and practices related to device selection, placement, and maintenance as well as appropriate use of infusion systems affect the success of parenteral nutrition administration. This chapter addresses the following:

I. Central Venous Access: General Principles
II. Central Venous Catheter Placement
III. Central Venous Catheter Features
IV. Central Venous Catheter Types
V. Central Venous Catheter Selection
VI. Central Venous Catheter Care and Maintenance
VII. Peripheral Access
VIII. Infusion Delivery Devices
IX. Infusion Delivery Device Selection Criteria
References

I. Central Venous Access: General Principles

A. Central venous access provides for infusion and blood withdrawal from the central circulation.
B. Access is facilitated through the use of specialized catheters with distal tip placement into the vena cava adjacent to the right atrium.
C. The most common venipuncture sites are the subclavian, jugular, femoral, cephalic, and basilic veins.
D. Primary indications for central venous infusions include chemotherapy, antibiotic administration, and parenteral nutrition (PN). Central access allows for use of therapy toxic to the endothelium of small veins due to medication pH, osmolarity, and volume; vesicant properties of some medications; and length of therapy.
E. The risk of infectious complications decreases with standardization of aseptic care, staff experience with device placement, and adequate nursing staff. Specialized IV teams have been effective in decreasing catheter-related infections.[1]

II. Central Venous Catheter Placement

A. Methods
   1. Percutaneous approach: Commonly used to access subclavian, internal and external jugular, or antecubital vessels. The subclavian vein is often easiest to cannulate in emergent situations such as profound volume depletion or shock. Ultrasound guidance during internal jugular venous catheterization reduces the number of catheterization failures, the mechanical complications, and the time required for insertion.[2]
      a) Modified Seldinger technique: Venipuncture and passage of a guidewire through the needle are followed by removal of the needle and catheter placement over the guidewire.
      b) Peel-away introducer sheath and tissue dilator: The catheter passes through the introducer into the vein and the introducer tears longitudinally, leaving the catheter in place.
      c) Introducers should be 0.2F to 0.5F sizes larger than the catheter to prevent bleeding or air embolism.
   2. Cut down: Surgical dissection is followed by isolation of the vessel and catheter placement. This technique is most often used to access the cephalic, external, or internal jugular vessels.
   3. Tunneled: A catheter segment of approximately 6 cm is tunneled from the selected skin exit site through the subcutaneous tissues to the venipuncture site.

B. Complications
   1. Pneumothorax is the most common immediate complication of percutaneously placed subclavian catheters. The incidence is 1% to 4%.[3]
   2. Arterial puncture is the most common complication associated with the percutaneous internal jugular approach.[3]
   3. A wide variety of technical and mechanical complications during catheter placement have been reported, including pneumothorax, catheter malposition, arrhythmias, air and catheter embolization, vascular injury, cardiac injury, pleural injury, mediastinal injury, neurologic injury, and thoracic duct injury.[3]
   4. Pericardial tamponade is the most lethal complication, with a mortality rate between 65% and 90%. The relationship of this complication to catheter placement is addressed by the Food and Drug Administration with the recommendation that the catheter tip not be placed in or allowed to migrate into the heart. This recommendation is controversial and is not universally supported by clinical practice or research.[3]

C. Setting
   1. Catheter placement can take place in the operating room or a variety of other settings, such as bedsides, minor procedure rooms, physicians' offices, and interventional radiology suites.
   2. Currently, implanted and tunneled catheters are most commonly placed in the operating room or interventional radiology suite. Fluoroscopy is often used to verify catheter placement, and the patient receives local anesthesia and at times supplemental IV sedation.
   3. Regardless of the setting in which central venous catheters (CVCs) are placed, it is imperative that catheter tip location be confirmed by chest x-ray or fluoroscopy before the start of therapy. In the pediatric population, proper catheter tip placement should be confirmed and/or revalidated as the patient grows and matures.

D. Patient preparation
   1. Placement of CVCs for PN should always be done on an elective basis, allowing for adequate patient preparation (Section II.F).

2. Appropriate explanation to the patient is essential.
3. Patient or parent/guardian consent is required.

E. Strategies for preventing infection
1. The best results are achieved when strict infection control protocols are followed, regardless of the type of catheter and dressing.[1]
   a) Hand washing
   b) Aseptic site and hub care
   c) Port sterilization before access
   d) Monitoring of the catheter site appearance
2. Maximal sterile barrier precautions consist of mask, cap, sterile gloves, sterile gown, and large sterile drape. The use of maximal barrier precautions during CVC placement minimizes catheter contamination and subsequent catheter infections.[4]
3. Site choice may influence infection risk. Subclavian veins have a lower risk than jugular or femoral veins. Internal jugular catheters that are close to oropharyngeal secretions and difficult to immobilize may have the highest risk of infection.[1,2]
4. Techniques used to decrease infections include placing catheters with a minimal number of lumens, using silver-chelated cuffs, tunneling catheters, and using antibiotic-impregnated catheters.
5. Blood sampling through catheters, especially in acutely ill patients, should be minimized.
6. CVCs that are no longer needed should be removed.
7. Routine CVC exchange over a guidewire is no longer recommended in view of increased mechanical and infectious complications.[1,2]

F. Patient evaluation: before catheter placement
1. Vascular access history: previous lines, infection, thrombosis, or difficult placement
2. Physical findings at or near access site: lesions, tumors, previous surgical procedures, venous abnormalities, or burns
3. Specific disease states: lung and breast cancers, pneumonia, coagulopathies, cervical masses, and adenopathy
4. Medication history: attention to anticoagulants, including aspirin, nonsteroidal anti-inflammatory drugs, warfarin, and unfractionated as well as low–molecular weight heparins. Warfarin should be withheld the day before CVC placement, and prothrombin time should be checked the day of catheter placement. Unfractionated heparin infusions should be withheld 4 hours before the procedure.[3] Low–molecular weight heparin therapy should be discontinued 12 hours prior to the procedure.
5. Laboratory evaluation: A complete blood cell count, including platelet count and the differential, is necessary. The need for additional laboratory evaluations is based on the clinician's assessment.[3] Neutropenia has been identified as a significant risk factor in the placement of tunneled CVCs.[5]

III. Central Venous Catheter Features

A. Materials
1. Polyvinyl chloride[6]
   a) Relatively stiff
   b) Common complications: thrombosis and phlebitis
   c) Infrequently used
2. Polyethylene[7]
   a) High tensile strength
   b) Minimal intimal irritation when used for short-term access
   c) Associated with platelet adherence and fibrous capsule formation in long-term access
3. Polyurethane[8]
   a) Great range of flexibility, excellent physical strength, and resistance to hydrolytic enzymes
   b) When used for short-term access, results in more infrequent inflammatory changes and thrombophlebitis than with polytetrafluoroethylene, polyvinyl chloride, or polyethylene
   c) When used for long-term access, requires anticoagulation to prevent thrombus formation
4. Polytetrafluoroethylene (Teflon, DuPont)[8]
   a) Extremely stable; demonstrates nonadhesive, antifriction properties; resistant to degradative enzymes
   b) catheter surface
   c) Generally unsuitable for long-term use because of rigidity, which causes irritation of the intima, leading to thrombus formation
5. Silicone elastomer (Silastic, Dow Corning)[9]
   a) High degree of elasticity and flexibility, causing minimal damage to the intima
   b) Biomaterial most often used for long-term indwelling devices
   c) Resistant to hydrolytic enzymes; hydrophobic surface resists bacterial adherence
   d) Considered to be chemically inert in blood because of the ability of the surface to adsorb host protein without triggering the complement cascade.
   e) Guidewire or peel-away introducer required for insertion because of soft texture
6. Coated/bonded catheters[10]
   a) Antimicrobial-impregnated catheters, either chlorhexidine and silver sulfadiazine or minocycline and rifampin, are the most frequently used.
   b) The use of these catheters may reduce the risk of catheter-related bloodstream infections and associated costs in high-risk patient populations.
   c) Long-term studies will be required to determine whether microbial resistance is an issue with these catheters.

B. Lumens
1. Many catheters are available in multilumen versions.
2. Multilumen catheters provide for simultaneous infusion of multiple or incompatible drugs.
3. The design varies across manufacturers in terms of both lumen size and intravascular or lumen openings. Lumens may exit at the catheter tip or along the distal side of the catheter.
4. While studies have not consistently demonstrated an increased risk of infectious complications, selection of the catheter with the minimal number of lumens required to administer therapy is recommended.[11]

C. Cuffs: a subcutaneous anchor and a mechanical barrier to infection[12]
1. Polyethylene eterphthalate (Dacron, DuPont) cuffs are attached to tunneled catheters. These cuffs, positioned in the subcutaneous tissue, anchor the catheter by facilitating fibrous ingrowth.[1]
2. Collagen cuffs impregnated with silver ions can be attached to the catheter at insertion or are available preattached. The gradual release of the silver ion exerts a short-term antimicrobial activity, but studies have not demonstrated efficacy. The use of silver-impregnated cuffs with tunneled devices has not been shown to offer an added benefit.[1]

D. Specialized valve: A pressure-sensitive three-way slit valve (Groshong, Bard) prevents retrograde blood flow, possible catheter occlusion, and air embolism. This valve is positioned distally along the side of the catheter; the distal end is closed. The design to prevent retrograde blood flow eliminates the need for daily heparinized saline flushes and catheter clamping.

E. Catheter diameter/circumference
   1. Diameter: expressed in millimeters defining both the internal and external diameters
   2. French size: circumference of the outer diameter in millimeters
   3. Gauge: inversely related to the catheter's outer diameter
   4. Catheters with similar external diameters can have a 30% difference in internal lumen size depending on the catheter material. A ratio of the inner to the outer diameter represents this feature. For example, polytetrafluoroethylene, polyurethane, and polyethylene have a ratio of 0.75, compared with 0.38 for silicone catheters.
   5. Catheter length
      a) Catheter length is dependent on the site of insertion.
      b) Silicone catheters can be trimmed at the time of insertion.
      c) Tapered-tipped catheters are inserted without alteration.

IV. Central Venous Catheter Types[1,12,13]

A. Nontunneled central venous access catheters
   1. Description: single- and multilumen catheters, placed using a percutaneous approach into the jugular, subclavian, or femoral vessels. The preferred site is the subclavian vein. Length, 6 to 30 cm; gauge, 14 to 27.
   2. Indication: usually used in the acute-care setting for short-duration therapy, such as inpatient PN. An exception is the Hohn (Bard) catheter, which is made of silicone and may be placed for home infusions.
   3. Advantages: economical, easily removed, and easily exchanged over a guidewire.
   4. Disadvantages: requires heparin flushing and sterile dressing changes. Patient self-care is difficult, and catheter breakage is possible. There are sutures at the exit site, which may become detached and result in catheter dislodgment.

B. Tunneled cuffed catheters (Hickman/Broviac/Groshong [Bard])
   1. Description: single and multilumen catheters placed percutaneously, most often into the jugular or subclavian veins or via cut down into the cephalic vein. These catheters use a Dacron cuff and are tunneled in the subcutaneous tissue. Length, 55 to 90 cm; gauge, 2.7 to 19.7 (dual lumen).
   2. Indication: extended IV therapy often administered on an outpatient basis, including home PN, chemotherapy, and pain management.
   3. Advantages: can be used for extended periods of time, require minimal dressing care, can be repaired externally, can be cared for by patients, and are secured with a subcutaneous cuff.
   4. Disadvantages: require an operating room or a special room for placement and routine heparin flushes (exception: Groshong); may be difficult to remove.

C. Peripherally inserted central catheter (PICC)[11]
   1. Description: single- or double-lumen catheters, placed percutaneously into the antecubital vessels. Length, 33.5 to 60 cm; gauge, 14 to 60.
   2. Indications: used for patients requiring access for several weeks to several months. PICCs have been used in the acute-care setting as well as for outpatient therapies including PN.
   3. Advantages: eliminate the risks associated with thoracic catheter placement. For adults, placement can occur at the patient's bedside or home. In most states, placement can be performed by specially trained registered nurses, thereby decreasing the cost associated with placement.
   4. Disadvantages: require routine heparin flushing and site care. There is a higher rate of catheter malposition, self-care is difficult and therefore greater costs may be incurred for long-term home care, external catheter breakage is possible, and repairs may be difficult because no standard repair kit is available. Infection prevention protocols should be followed as for centrally placed catheters.

D. Ports
   1. Description: a subcutaneous injection port with a self-sealing silicone septum and a catheter. Septum diameters are 6.4 to 19.1 mm; septum depth, 5.1 to 13 mm. A septum can withstand approximately 1000 to 2000 punctures using a special noncoring needle. The anterior chest wall is the most common placement site, although a smaller peripheral port can be placed in the abdomen, groin, or antecubital vessels. Ports are available in a dual-lumen version, with preattached or separate catheters for attachment to the port chamber at the time of placement.
   2. Alternative port designs include reservoirs without corners and possible areas of residual or "sludge" collection; ports with access parallel to the skin rather than perpendicular to the skin, which is the more common design; and a "needleless" port that is accessed with a needlelike device.
   3. Indications: used for long-term intermittent IV access; at times, this has included daily PN.
   4. Advantages: Site care is needed only when the port is accessed, heparinization is needed only monthly if the port is not in use, the patient's body image remains intact, and there are no external components for breakage.
   5. Disadvantages: Needle access is required, needle displacement from the reservoir is possible, placement must occur in an operating room or a special room, and removal requires a minor surgical procedure.

V. Central Venous Catheter Selection

A. Clinicians experienced in the many facets of vascular access are key to appropriate device selection. Interdisciplinary collaboration as well as input from the patient and caregivers will enhance device selection.

B. CVC device selection is a process that appropriately matches the patient, the disease, the therapy, and the catheter.

C. Patient assessment
   1. Preoperative evaluation (Section II.F)
   2. Activity level
   3. Body image concerns
   4. Physical ability to care for catheter
   5. Cognitive abilities
   6. Caregiver involvement
   7. Patient's diagnosis and future activity level
   8. Financial considerations
      a) Cost of the device
      b) Cost of the insertion
      c) Costs associated with care and maintenance
      d) Potential costs of complications

D. Duration and type of therapy
   1. Length (see Table 6-1): Estimated length of therapy is one of the most significant variables in catheter choice.
      a) Patients requiring long-term outpatient therapy are best served by a tunneled cuffed catheter, an implanted port, or a PICC. If therapy is daily, implanted ports may not be the optimal choice, as frequent needle access can lead to skin irritation and may make patient self-care difficult.
      b) Either peripheral access or nontunneled central venous access and PICCs can serve patients requiring acute short-

TABLE 6-1. Length of Therapy for Various Types of Venous Access

Type of Access	Length of Therapy
Nontunneled CVC	Weeks
Tunneled CVC	Months to years
PICC	Months
Port	Months to years

CVC, central venous catheter; PICC, peripherally inserted central catheter.

term infusion therapy, depending on whether the prescribed therapy mandates central access.

2. Type: Single infusion or multiple infusions differentiate the need for single- versus multiple-lumen catheters. Most patients requiring home PN can be managed with a single-lumen catheter, infusing PN nightly and other IV medications around the scheduled PN infusion.
3. Need for frequent blood sampling
4. Drug volume and rate of administration

VI. Central Venous Catheter Care and Maintenance

A. Site care: considered one of the most important measures for decreasing catheter-related infections; aimed at reducing microbial colonization through skin antisepsis and dressings at the insertion site
   1. Common antiseptics include chlorhexidine 2%, povidone-iodine 10%, alcohol 70%, and tincture of iodine. The use of acetone to defat the skin has been shown to have no efficacy in reducing catheter infections. A 2% chlorhexidine–based preparation is the agent of choice for cleaning the skin prior to access.[1,12]
   2. Antimicrobial ointments should not be used.[1] Studies addressing the application of antimicrobial ointments to the skin site have contradictory findings. There is concern that fungal infections may be associated with the use of antibacterial ointments.
   3. Protocols vary with the type of catheter dressing, the interval for dressing changes, and the frequency of site observation for signs of local infection. The two types of dressings most often used are transparent dressings and gauze dressings. Either sterile gauze or sterile transparent semipermeable dressing can be used to cover the catheter site. Tunneled CVC sites that are well healed may not require a dressing.[1,14]
      a) Gauze dressings should be replaced every 2 days; transparent dressings should be changed every 7 days.[1]
      b) The simplicity of gauze dressings makes patient self-care easier.
      c) Transparent dressings allow for continuous inspection of the site and aid in securing the catheter.
   4. A sustained-release chlorhexidine gluconate patch is available for placement around the catheter insertion or exit site. A gauze or transparent dressing is then applied over the patch. Limited studies have shown a reduction in the rate of catheter-related bloodstream infections.
   5. Collodion, a solution of pyroxylin in ether and alcohol that provides an occlusive transparent film after application, has been used as a dressing. This dressing is both bacteriostatic and inexpensive, but very limited studies are available to date.[15]

B. Flushing: maintains catheter patency and reduces fibrin or thrombus formation. In addition, very low doses (1 mg/day) of warfarin can protect against thrombosis in patients with long-term central venous access.[16]
   1. Frequency and dosage are dependent on catheter type, usage, and institutional protocols.
   2. Although saline and heparin have been shown to be equally efficacious for flushing peripheral catheters, most protocols endorse a heparin solution for routine flushing of CVCs (except Groshong).
   3. There is a lack of consensus regarding the volume, frequency, and concentration of heparinized solutions for flushing.
      a) Flushing volumes range from 1 to 5 mL.
      b) Heparin concentrations range from 1 to 1000 units/mL; the concentration most frequently used is 10 units/mL.
      c) Flushing is most often done daily, except for with ports, which are flushed every 4 weeks.
   4. Groshong catheters are flushed weekly with sodium chloride 0.9% (normal saline).

C. Hub care: reduces intraluminal contamination at the catheter hub. Disinfection, often with 70% alcohol, is done during manipulations (eg, tubing changes) at the catheter hub.[1]

D. In the hospital setting, IV tubing is changed no more frequently than every 72 hours, with the exception of tubing used for blood infusions and intravenous fat emulsions, which should be changed within 24 hours.[1] In the home setting, PN tubing should be changed daily.

E. Port access mandates skin antisepsis before needle insertion. Protocols vary from aseptic technique to sterile technique with a mask and sterile gloves when ports are accessed.

F. Specific CVC care and maintenance (see Table 6-2)

G. Long-term complications[17]
   1. Infection (see Chapter 8)
   2. Occlusion and thrombosis (see Chapter 8)
   3. Catheter breakage
      a) External catheter segment. Tunneled, cuffed long-term catheters can be repaired with proprietary repair kits. If these kits are not immediately available, a temporary repair can be done with a 16-gauge blunt-end needle inserted into the catheter and secured. Catheters that cannot be repaired must be removed and replaced.
      b) Fracture of the internal catheter segment is related to catheter "pinch-off syndrome." Access devices are inserted via the subclavian vein course between the clavicle and the first rib. In certain patients, this anatomical angle is narrow and causes catheter compression that presents as occlusion. This syndrome is confirmed when the occlusion is relieved with postural changes, such as raising the arm, and by radiologic findings of catheter luminal narrowing in this area. Although this complication is rare, it can result in catheter embolus. Catheter removal is appropriate with pinch-off syndrome. Replacement should be on the opposite side if possible; use of a more lateral approach may prevent this complication.[18]
   4. Catheter malposition can present as a catheter malfunction with symptoms of thrombosis, occlusion, or perforation. Catheters with tip malposition can be replaced or repositioned under fluoroscopic guidance.

VII. Peripheral Access[19]

A. Parenteral nutrition may be administered by peripheral venous access when the therapy is expected to be short term (10–14 days),

TABLE 6-2. CVC Maintenance

Catheter Type	Site Care	Flushing
Nontunneled CVC	Dressing: transparent or gauze Transparent enhances catheter stability Performed as a sterile dressing Skin antisepsis protocols include one or a combination of the following: (1) 70% alcohol(3 swabs); (2) 10% povidone-iodine (3 swabs).	Internal volume: 0.1±0.53 mL 1±2 mL flush is adequate Frequency: usually daily
Tunneled cuffed CVC	Dressing: transparent or gauze until incision heals Dressings often discontinued once incision heals and suture is removed. Performed as sterile dressing antisepsis (see above) Hydrogen peroxide may be used to remove crusting at the site	Internal volume: 0.15–1.8 mL Frequency: usually daily Groshong catheters: 5 mL 0.9% saline weekly
PICC	Dressing: transparent preferred to enhance catheter stability Performed as sterile dressing antisepsis (see above) Dressings required as long as catheter is in place	Internal volume: 0.04–1.2 mL 2–3 mL flush adequate Frequency: daily
Ports	Dressing until incision healed (several days postop) Transparent dressing when port is accessed to stabilize needle Huber needle change at least every 7 days Skin antisepsis as above prior to needle placement Sterile approach is recommended during needle insertion and dressing change	Internal volume: 0.5–1.5 mL At least 3 mL adequate Frequency: every 4 weeks

CVC, central venous catheter; PICC, peripherally inserted central catheter.
Reprinted with permission from Krzywda EA, Andris DA, Edmiston CE, Wallace JR. Parenteral access devices. In: Gottschlich MM, ed. *The Science and Practice of Nutrition Support: A Case-Based Core Curriculum.* Dubuque, IO: Kendall Hunt/American Society for Parenteral and Enteral Nutrition; 2001:225–250.

fluid restriction is not necessary, and formulation osmolarity is <600 to 900 mOsm/L.

B. Adequate peripheral veins are necessary for successful peripheral venous access administration.
C. General principles of catheter care and maintenance, as noted above, apply to peripheral catheters.
D. Peripheral catheters include standard peripheral cannulas, midline catheters, and midclavicular catheters. Often referred to as extended-dwell peripheral catheters, midline catheters are advanced approximately 5 to 7 inches into the vein, and midclavicular catheters involve distal tip placement at the axillary and subclavian junction. Neither of these placements provides central venous access. Midline catheters are not recommended for administration of PN due to the risk of upper extremity thrombosis.
E. Peripheral catheters remain at risk for complications associated with infection and occlusion; however, the principal complication is peripheral vein thrombophlebitis.
F. Catheter recommendations for peripheral venous access
   1. Use fine-bore cannulas.
   2. Polyurethane is the preferred catheter material.
   3. Use large veins and avoid placement across joints.
   4. Inspect cannula site daily.
   5. Standard peripheral cannulas require site rotation every 72 to 96 hours in adult patients but are not routinely changed in the pediatric population. Midline catheters may be used for up to 4 weeks, and midclavicular catheters may be used for 2 to 3 months.[19]
   6. The cannula should be removed as soon as thrombophlebitis develops. The replacement cannula should be inserted at some distance from the site of thrombophlebitis, preferably on the contralateral side.
G. Prophylaxis against peripheral vein thrombophlebitis during peripheral venous access[19]
   1. Combine heparin (1 unit/mL) and hydrocortisone (10 mg/L). This approach has not been evaluated in the pediatric population, however.
   2. Use topical nonsteroidal anti-inflammatory creams and gels.
   3. Minimize solution osmolarity to <600 mOsm/L. There are some reports of infusions of 800 to 1000 mOsm/L with the use of measures such as the addition of heparin and hydrocortisone.
   4. Buffer infusion formulations with sodium bicarbonate within the pH range 7.2 to 7.4.
   5. Include iso-osmolar lipid emulsions to provide additional calories and lower osmolarity.

VIII. Infusion Delivery Devices

A. Infusion delivery devices provide for accurate and safe administration of IV therapies, including PN.
B. Significant technological advancements in these devices are related to the expansion of home IV therapies over the past 2 decades.
C. Device classification[1]
   1. Gravity infusion devices: manual regulation of drop chamber, associated with a high degree of inaccuracy, not used for PN infusions
   2. Controllers: maintain a regular drop rate with no mechanical parts, incapable of high volumes, not used for PN
   3. Syringe devices: control fluid delivery from a syringe and a

TABLE 6-3. Summary of Ambulatory and Stationary Infusion Devices[20–22]

	Ambulatory infusion devices	Stationary infusion devices
Availability	>25 devices marketed	Approximately 10 devices marketed
Size	Small and lightweight (approximately 8 ounces)	Heavier (approximately 12 pounds)
Patient mobility	Designed for patient to remain ambulatory	Mounted on pole—requires patient to remain homebound
Flow rate/volumes	Wide range	Wide range
Alarms/safety measures	Wide range	Wide range
Automatic programming	Yes	Yes
Administration set	Many require proprietary set	May use generic set
Cost acquisition	Usually 20% to 25% more expensive	Lower up-front cost
Patient indications	Allows for mobility	Use for nighttime infusions

CVC, central venous catheter; PICC, peripherally inserted central catheter.
Reprinted with permission from Krzywda EA, Andris DA, Edmiston CE, Wallace JR. Parenteral access devices. In: Gottschlich MM, ed. *The Science and Practice of Nutrition Support: A Case-Based Core Curriculum.* Dubuque, IO: Kendall Hunt/American Society for Parenteral and Enteral Nutrition; 2001:225–250.

motor-driven piston, appropriate for low-volume infusions, used for neonatal PN

4. Infusion pumps
   a) Electronic devices that provide accurate volume (rate) control and free-flow protection; visual and auditory safety alarms indicate increased pressure or air within the system and signal infusion completion. Additional features may include programmable automatic cycling and rate tapering
   b) The basic types commonly used for PN administration are ambulatory infusion devices and stationary infusion devices.

D. Comparative features of ambulatory infusion devices and stationary infusion pumps (see Table 6-3)

IX. Infusion Delivery Device Selection Criteria[20–22]

A. Appropriate device selection, especially in the outpatient setting or alternative site, is dependent on the patient, the therapy (length and type), and cost-effectiveness/reimbursement.

B. Key patient characteristics
   1. Age, diagnosis, and overall condition
   2. Ambulation status
   3. Lifestyle and mobility
   4. Manual dexterity
   5. Cognitive ability
   6. Caregiver involvement

C. Therapy
   1. Single infusion or multiple drugs
   2. Continuous or intermittent infusion
   3. Length of infusion cycle
   4. Volume of infusion

D. Cost-effectiveness of the infusion device[21,22]
   1. Ease of staff training
   2. Ease of patient training
   3. Complications associated with device
   4. Pharmacy time
   5. Amount of waste and ease of disposal
   6. Storage space at both patient's home and provider's location
   7. Product availability and manufacturer's support
   8. Downtime and repair costs
   9. Inventory costs
   10. Overall product reliability

E. Reimbursement: Increasingly, providers are choosing stationary infusion devices because of the lower acquisition prices and the ability to use less costly administration sets.

(Parenteral Nutrition Access and Infusion Equipment chapters from the first edition were contributed by Elizabeth A. Krzywda, Charles E. Edmiston, Jr, Kristy Gibbons, Nancy Cyr, Michael L. Christensen, and Richard A. Helms)

REFERENCES

1. O'Grady NP, Alexander M, Dellinger EP, et al. Guidelines for the prevention of intravascular catheter-related infections. Centers for Disease Control and Prevention; Aug 9, 2002. *MMWR Recomm Rep.* 51(RR-10):1–29.
2. McGee DC, Gould MK. Preventing complications of central venous catheterization. *N Engl J Med.* 2003;348:1123–1133.
3. Whitman ED. Complications associated with the use of central venous access devices. *Curr Probl Surg.* 1996;33:311–378.
4. Raad II, Hohn DC, Gilbreath BJ, et al. Prevention of central venous catheter-related infections by using maximal sterile barrier precautions during insertion. *Infect Control Hosp Epidemiol.* 1994;15:231–238.
5. Howell PB, Walters PE, Donowitz GR, Farr PM. Risk factors of infection of adult patients with cancer who have central venous catheters. *Cancer.* 1995;15:1367–1374.
6. Kim SW, Petersen RV, Lee ES. Effect of phthalate plasticizers on blood compatibility of polyvinyl chloride. *J Pharm Sci.* 1976;65:670–673.
7. Williams D. Implantable prostheses. *Phys Med Biol.* 1980;25:611–636.
8. Larsson N, Stemberg K, Linder L, Curelaru I. Cannula thrombophlebitis: a study in volunteers comparing polytetrafluoroethylene, polyurethane, and polyamide-ether-elastomer cannula. *Acta Anaesthesiol Scand.* 1989;33:223–231.
9. Trooskin SZ, Mikulaschek AW. Biomaterials used for catheters. In: Greco RS, ed. *Implantation Biology.* Boca Raton, FL: CRC Press; 1994:270–271.
10. Shorr AF, Humphreys CW, Helman DL. New choices for central venous catheters. *Chest.* 2003;124:275–284.
11. Orr M. Issues on the management of percutaneous central venous catheters: single and multiple lumens. *Nurs Clin North Am.* 1993:28:911–919.
12. Crnich CJ, Maki DG. The promise of novel technology for the prevention of intravascular device-related bloodstream infection, I: pathogenesis and short-term devices. *Clin Infect Dis.* 2002;34:1232–1242.
13. Crnich CJ, Maki DG. The promise of novel technology for the prevention of intravascular device-related bloodstream infection, II: long-term devices. *Clin Infect Dis.* 2002;34:1362–1368.
14. Zitella L. Central venous catheter site care for blood and marrow transplant recipients. *Clin J Oncol Nurs.* 2003;3:289–298.

15. Babycos CR, Barracos A, Mancuso J, Turner-Marse T. Collodion as a safe, cost-effective dressing for central venous catheters. *South Med J.* 1990;83:1286–1288.
16. Bern MM, Lokich JJ, Wallach SR, et al. Very low doses of warfarin can prevent thrombosis in central venous catheters. *Ann Intern Med.* 1990;112:423–428.
17. Moureau N, Poole S, Murdock MA, Gray SM, Semba CP. Central venous catheters in home infusion care: outcomes analysis in 50,471 patients. *J Vasc Interv Radiol.* 2002;13:1009–1016.
18. Andris D, Krzywda EA, Schulte W, Ausman R, Quebbeman EJ. Pinch-off syndrome: a rare etiology for central venous catheter occlusion. *J Parenter Enteral Nutr.* 1994;18:531–533.
19. Payne-James J, Khawala HT. First choice for total parenteral nutrition: the peripheral route. *J Parenter Enteral Nutr.* 1993;17:468–478.
20. Saladow J. Ambulatory systems for I.V. antibiotic therapy: making sense of the options. *Infusion.* April 1995:17–29.
21. Saladow J. Ambulatory electronic infusion systems: making sense of the options. *Infusion.* July 1995:9–21.
22. Saladow J. Stationary infusion pumps used in home care: making sense of the options. *Infusion.* September 1995:11–17.

SUGGESTED READINGS

Holcombe BJ. Adult parenteral nutrition. In: Young LY, Koda-Kimble MA, eds. *Applied Therapeutics: The Clinical Use of Drugs.* 8th ed. Philadelphia, PA: Lippincott Williams and Wilkins; 2004:35.

Task Force for the Revision of Safe Practices for Parenteral Nutrition. Safe practices for parenteral nutrition. *J Parenter Enteral Nutr.* 2004;28:S29-S70.

Vanek VW. The ins and outs of venous access: part I. *Nutr Clin Pract.* 2002;17:85–98

Vanek VW. The ins and outs of venous access: part II. *Nutr Clin Pract.* 2002;17:142–155.

Vanessa J. Kumpf, PharmD, BCNSP;
Jay M. Mirtallo, MS, RPh, BCNSP;
Craig Petersen, RD, CNSD

7

Parenteral Nutrition Formulations: Preparation and Ordering

Introduction

Parenteral nutrition (PN) is defined as nutrients provided intravenously. From a pharmaceutical perspective, a PN formulation is a complex admixture of individual chemicals, all having physicochemical properties that influence their behavior when combined in a single container. A thorough understanding of the available nutrient products used in the PN admixture is necessary to formulate a safe and clinically appropriate end product. The many factors that influence the end product include concentration, composition, and pH of base solutions; stability of base solutions; microbial growth potential; and compatibility of nutrient components. This chapter provides an overview of these issues in both the adult and pediatric populations. Guidelines regarding appropriate ordering and labeling of PN formulations are also provided with the intent to promote safe practice.

I. Formula Design

A. Components of a PN admixture

1. Protein source: Amino acids are included in the PN admixture as the source for new protein synthesis.
   a) Crystalline amino acid solutions are classified as either standard or specialized. The standard amino acid solutions contain a balanced or physiologic mixture of essential and nonessential amino acids.[1] The base solutions are available in a range of concentrations from 3% to 20%. The specialized amino acid solutions contain mixtures of amino acids designed to meet disease- or age-specific amino acid requirements.
   b) Amino acid compositions of commercially available formulations intended for infant use have an amino acid profile that has been demonstrated to result in plasma amino acid levels in the same range as those seen 2 hours postprandial in the breast-fed infant. These specialized amino acid formulations also contain taurine, which is involved in the conjugation of bile acids. Cysteine can be added separately at the time of preparation. Infant amino acid formulations are more acidic than standard amino acid products.[2] This acidity enhances calcium and phosphorus solubility and allows higher concentrations of these two nutrients without causing precipitation.
2. Carbohydrate source: Carbohydrate serves as the primary energy substrate in a PN formulation. The patient's energy requirements and glucose oxidation rate, and the desired balance of carbohydrate and fat calories, determine the amount of carbohydrate in a given PN admixture.
   a) Dextrose monohydrate is used almost exclusively in PN solutions as the source of carbohydrate calories. Dextrose monohydrate provides 3.4 kcal/g, and base solutions are available in a range of concentrations, from 5% to 70%.
   b) Glycerol is a naturally occurring sugar alcohol that is used as an alternative source of energy in some PN formulations. It yields 4.3 kcal/g and has been shown to be protein sparing when used concomitantly with amino acids.[3]
3. Fat source: Fat is delivered in the form of stabilized emulsions. These emulsions provide essential fatty acids and are a concentrated source of calories.
   a) Long-chain fatty acid (LCFA) emulsions currently are the only commercially available source of intravenous fat emulsions (IVFE) in the United States. These fat emulsions are made from either soybean oil or a mixture of safflower and soybean oils.[4,5] They are available as concentrations of 10%, 20%, and 30% fat emulsions. IVFE also contain egg phosphatides as an emulsifier and glycerol to adjust the osmolarity.
   b) Medium-chain fatty acid (MCFA)/LCFA physical mixtures are available in Europe. Two separate triglyceride sources, MCFA and LCFA, are combined to create these mixtures. MCFA/LCFA mixtures take advantage of the fact that MCFAs are more rapidly oxidized for energy than LCFAs. The LCFA provides a source of essential fatty acids.[6]
   c) MCFA/LCFA structured lipids are similar to the MCFA/LCFA physical mixture in that they combine the properties of the two types of fatty acids. However, the structured lipid is created through hydrolysis of triglycerides and transesterification of fatty acids to form a composite triglyceride molecule that has various proportions of both MCFA and LCFA. The structured lipids are thought to have an advantage over the physical mixture of MCFA and LCFA because of a slower rate of release and utilization of the MCFA.[6] These products are currently investigational only.
4. Water: Sterile water is added to most PN admixtures to adjust the total volume of fluid needed to meet the prescribed 24-hour fluid intake via PN. This is a convenient and economical way to create a PN admixture when concentrated dextrose, amino acids, and IVFE are used as the base products.
5. Electrolytes: Electrolytes are included in the PN admixture to maintain electrolyte homeostasis. Electrolyte balance is dependent on many factors, such as renal function, acid-base balance, gastrointestinal losses, and medications. Therefore, electrolyte

intake needs to be individualized in many patients. In stable, uncomplicated patients, a multiple-electrolyte formulation containing standard doses of several electrolytes or several single-entity electrolyte solutions may be used in a PN admixture. The electrolyte composition of PN admixtures is also dependent on the compatibility of each electrolyte with the other components of the PN admixture (see Section II.B).

a) Sodium is available as the chloride, acetate, bicarbonate, phosphorus, or lactate salt. The bicarbonate form should not be used in PN admixtures, as it may cause precipitation of other additives, particularly calcium and magnesium. Lactate is considered an inferior choice relative to acetate, as acetate is more readily metabolized to bicarbonate intravenous (IV) sodium and is dosed in milliequivalent units.

b) Potassium is available as the chloride, acetate, or phosphorus salt. IV potassium is dosed in milliequivalent units.

c) Phosphorus is available as the sodium or potassium salt. IV phosphorus is dosed in millimoles.

d) Magnesium is available as the sulfate or chloride salt. IV magnesium is dosed in milliequivalent units.

e) Calcium is available as the chloride or gluconate salt. Calcium gluconate is the preferred form of calcium for PN admixtures because it is more stable in solution and, therefore, is less likely to dissociate and form a precipitate with phosphorus. IV calcium is dosed in milliequivalent units.

f) The choice of the chloride versus acetate salt of sodium and potassium depends on the patient's acid-base status. Generally, acid-base balance can be maintained by using approximately equal amounts of chloride and acetate (ie, a 1:1 ratio). Acetate and chloride are also present in the base amino acid solutions in various amounts. If a patient has altered acid-base status, the chloride-acetate ratio may need to be adjusted. For example, if metabolic acidosis is present, maximum acetate and minimum chloride should be used in the PN admixture. Conversely, if metabolic alkalosis is present, maximum chloride and minimum acetate should be used.

6. Vitamins are added to the PN admixture daily, usually as a fixed dose using a multivitamin preparation. Parenteral vitamins have limited stability once they are added to the PN admixture. In general, they are stable for 24 hours.[7]

a) Adult: Available parenteral multivitamin products for adults contain 12 or 13 known vitamins (with or without vitamin K). In 2000, the US Food and Drug Administration (FDA) amended requirements for marketing an "effective" adult parenteral vitamin formulation and recommended changes to the 12-vitamin formulation that had been available for over 20 years.[8] The new requirements call for increased dosages of vitamins B_1 (thiamine), B_6 (pyridoxine), C (ascorbic acid), and folic acid as well as addition of vitamin K. An adult parenteral vitamin formulation meeting the 2000 reformulation requirements but without vitamin K has also received FDA approval and is commercially available.

b) Pediatric: Parenteral multivitamin products are available for pediatric patients who are up to age 11 years or who weigh up to 40 kg. They are formulated to comply with the Subcommittee on Pediatric Parenteral Nutrient Requirements of the Committee on Clinical Practice Issues of the American Society for Clinical Nutrition.[9]

c) Individual vitamin products are used to supplement multivitamin doses when a deficiency state exists or when there are increased needs because of a disease or clinical condition. Single-entity parenteral vitamin products include vitamin B_1 (thiamine), vitamin B_2 (riboflavin), vitamin B_6 (pyridoxine), vitamin B_{12} (cyanocobalamin), folic acid, vitamin C, vitamin A, and vitamin K. Vitamin D can also be given by intramuscular administration.

7. Trace minerals are essential to normal metabolism and growth. Although relatively minute amounts of trace minerals are required, deficiency states may develop fairly rapidly when increased metabolic requirements (eg, burn injury), increased losses (eg, large-volume fistula output), or rapid growth are present. The recommended daily requirement (plus supplemental replacement doses as needed for increased requirements or losses) should be included in all PN admixtures. There are, however, clinical conditions necessitating trace mineral restriction (eg, decreased copper and manganese excretion with biliary disease), and therefore the recommended daily requirement may need adjustment. Trace minerals available for parenteral admixture include chromium, copper, iodine, iron, manganese, molybdenum, selenium, and zinc.

a) Standard multiple–trace element solutions are available in several combinations with as few as four (chromium, copper, manganese, zinc) and as many as seven (chromium, copper, iodine, manganese, molybdenum, selenium, zinc) trace elements. The doses of each trace element in the recommended daily volume for admixture usually are based on the American Medical Association National Advisory Group recommendations for daily parenteral trace element intake.[10] Separate products exist for adult and pediatric patients.

b) Single-entity trace element solutions are available to use when individual trace element requirements cannot be met with the multiple–trace element products. Single-entity products exist for chromium, copper, iodine, iron, manganese, molybdenum, selenium, and zinc. Iron dextran may be added to non-IVFE-containing PN formulations but requires caution due to compatibility limitations.[11] It should not be added to a total nutrient admixture (TNA) because it can destabilize the IVFE (see Section II.C.2). Iron sucrose and sodium ferric gluconate provide therapeutic options for the parenteral supplementation of iron, but compatibility data with PN formulations are not available.[11]

B. Contaminants of PN formulation components: Many components of the PN formulation have been shown to be contaminated with trace elements such as zinc, copper, manganese, chromium, selenium, and aluminum.[12] Manganese and aluminum appear to be the most clinically relevant trace element contaminants.

1. Aluminum: Toxicity due to aluminum contamination in PN formulations can cause significant clinical problems.[13] As a result, the FDA developed regulations that require manufacturers to disclose on the label the aluminum content of small- and large-volume parenteral products used in the preparation of PN (as of July 2004).[14]

a) The safe limit of aluminum in PN has been set at 5 mcg/kg/day.[14]

b) The intent of the regulation is to educate health care practitioners about aluminum exposure and facilitate the preparation of low-aluminum parenteral solutions to patients in high-risk groups.

c) High-risk groups include infants and neonates receiving PN for a period longer than 10 days and any patient receiving long-term PN who has renal compromise.

d) Renal compromise is associated with central nervous system manifestations of aluminum toxicity.

e) Infants and neonates are extremely vulnerable to aluminum toxicity, which is manifested by alterations in bone formation and mineralization, encephalopathy, and impaired neurologic development.[13,14] These patients are at higher risk because of the excess aluminum burden per kg body weight infused with PN, the infant's inability to regulate the body's aluminum content due to immature renal function, and the impact of aluminum on growth and development.

f) Aluminum contamination of products used in PN preparation comes primarily from raw materials during the manufacturing process and can therefore vary by manufacturer and lot. The aluminum sources of most concern are calcium and phosphate salts.

g) Adults receiving long-term home PN have had problems with osteopenia and bone mineralization, in part caused by aluminum.[13] This problem has been partially improved by the replacement of casein hydrolysates with crystalline amino acid products as the source of protein and reduction in the aluminum in PN formulations.

2. Manganese: Manganese toxicity associated with PN has been reported, most notably in long-term home PN patients.[15] Hypermanganesemia may lead to manganese deposition in the basal ganglia and neurological symptoms. Manganese contamination of PN additives has been identified as a factor contributing to hypermanganesemia. The level of contamination appears to vary by manufacturer and lot number. Manganese concentrations ranging from 8 to 22 mcg per total daily volume have been reported in PN formulations with no added manganese.[16] It may, therefore, be necessary to eliminate the use of multiple–trace element products that contain added manganese in long-term home PN patients with hypermanganesemia and instead use single-entity trace element solutions.

C. Types of PN formulations

1. Dextrose/amino acids (2-in-1): Dextrose and amino acids are mixed with electrolytes, vitamins, and trace elements. These formulations are typically mixed in single-liter volumes. However, in some circumstances the components may be in a container that provides a 24-hour supply of nutrients. IVFE are infused separately.

2. TNAs: Under specific circumstances, IVFE can be admixed with the other components of PN to create a TNA.[17] All the parenteral nutrient components are mixed in one container that supplies the 24-hour nutrient intake. There are both advantages and disadvantages associated with a TNA when compared to a 2-in-1 formulation with a separate IVFE infusion.[18]

a) Advantages

(1) Decreased nursing time: Since a TNA system uses only one container per day, nursing time involved in IV setup and administration is decreased.

(2) Decreased risk of touch contamination: Fewer manipulations of the catheter and administration set are required, decreasing the risk of touch contamination. This may decrease the risk of catheter-related infection.

(3) Decreased pharmacy preparation time: Compared with admixing multiple single-liter containers of the PN admixture for each patient each day, it takes less time to admix a single 24-hour supply of the PN admixture, especially if an automated compounder is available.

(4) Cost savings: Less nursing and pharmacy time plus fewer materials used in admixing and administering the PN formulation result in lower cost. For example, the infusion pump and administration set for a separate IVFE infusion are not required.

(5) Ease of administration for home PN patients: Using a single container per day rather than piggybacking a separate container of lipid into the PN admixture is simpler for most patients. It eliminates the need for two separate infusion pumps and administration sets. As a result, it can significantly improve quality of life.

(6) Better fat utilization: A slow, continuous infusion of IVFE has been shown to be better tolerated than a shorter IVFE infusion period, as demonstrated by reticuloendothelial system impairment.[18,19]

b) Disadvantages

(1) Diminished stability and compatibility: Addition of IVFE to the PN admixture decreases the overall stability of the fat emulsion. If the fat emulsion separates from the other components after it is prepared and then is infused, there could be potentially life-threatening consequences (see Section III.B). There are limitations to the amounts of nutrients that can be combined when IVFE is present in the PN admixture. This is due to the properties of the fat emulsion and the ease with which it can be disrupted by substances such as divalent and trivalent electrolytes (see Section II.B.).

(2) Impaired visual inspection of the TNA: Addition of IVFE renders the PN admixture opaque. Therefore, visual inspection, one of the most frequently used methods of checking for solution impurities or precipitates, is obscured. This increases the risk of infusing an admixture that may harm the patient.[20-21]

D. Order of admixing: The order in which the components of a PN admixture are combined can affect the overall stability of the final product. The additive sequence in compounding must be optimized and validated as a safe and efficacious method.[22] The order of admixing is determined by the method used (eg, automated vs gravity).

1. Automated compounding: The procedure depends on the specific automated compounding device being used. Assistance in optimizing the compounding order for automated devices should be obtained through consultation with the manufacturer of macronutrients being used as well as the manufacturer of the compounding device because brand-specific issues might influence the compatibility of the final formulation.[22]

2. Gravity transfer: The steps below should be followed in the order presented (step *a* first and step *j* last) to optimize the stability of the PN admixture.[23]

a) Combine dextrose, amino acids, and water.

b) Add phosphorus.

c) Add sodium, potassium, and magnesium (in any order).

d) Add trace minerals.

e) Agitate the solution well.

f) Add calcium (or a calcium-containing multielectrolyte solution) and agitate the solution well again.

g) Observe the solution for precipitates or contaminants (eg, rubber cores). If either is present, discard the solution. If a precipitate is present, review the quantities of additives for incompatibilities (especially calcium and phosphorus; see Section II.B.1) and adjust nutrient doses as needed to achieve compatibility (see Section II.B.1.e). Review the order of mixing and remix the solution.

h) If a TNA is being admixed, add the IVFE next, gently agitate, and observe for signs of the emulsion cracking (see Section III.B.2).

i) Add vitamins last, as close to the time of administration of the PN admixture as possible. For home PN patients, the patient or caregiver should add vitamins just prior to infusion.

j) Note that when a TNA is admixed, dextrose and IVFE should never be added directly to one another. The low pH of dextrose solutions will disrupt the IVFE.

E. Admixture osmolarity refers to the osmoles of solute per liter of solution. Osmolarity is measured in milliosmoles per liter (mOsm/L). PN admixture osmolarity is important because the IV access site used for a given infusion is dictated by admixture osmolarity. The higher the osmolarity, the larger the vein needed to accommodate the formulation. A formulation with high osmolarity infused into a small peripheral vein will cause irritation and pain, with damage to the vessel (phlebitis), which will necessitate frequent changes of the IV site.

1. Central vein infusion guidelines: Due to the high osmolarity of most PN formulations, they are limited to administration through a central venous access catheter with tip placement in the superior vena cava adjacent to the right atrium.[22,24] Because of the high rate of blood flow through the central vein, the formulation is rapidly diluted and is not harmful to the vessel. There are no known upper limits to solution osmolarity via the central vein; however, the maximum is usually limited by the concentration of available base solutions used in compounding the PN formulation.
2. Peripheral vein infusion guidelines: Typically, a peripheral vein can tolerate a formulation of up to 600 mOsm/L without any irritation or damage. As the osmolarity of the formulation increases above 600 mOsm/L, the likelihood of vein irritation and damage increases. Data indicate that an appropriate standard maximum osmolar concentration for a peripheral PN admixture is 900 mOsm/L.[25]
3. Estimating osmolarity: Formulation osmolarity can be estimated by adding the osmolar contribution from each component of the PN formulation and dividing by the total volume (in liters) of the formulation. The approximate osmolar contribution of commonly used components of a PN admixture is as follows[22]:
   a) Amino acids: 1 g = 10 mOsm
   b) Dextrose: 1 g = 5 mOsm
   c) 20% IVFE: 1 g = 0.71 mOsm (product dependent)
   d) Calcium gluconate: 1 mEq = 1.4 mOsm
   e) Magnesium sulfate: 1 mEq = 1 mOsm
   f) Potassium (chloride, acetate, or phosphate salt): 1 mEq = 2 mOsm
   g) Sodium (chloride, acetate, or phosphate salt): 1 mEq = 2 mOsm

II. Compatibility Issues

A. General considerations: Ensuring compatibility among all the components of a PN admixture is a prerequisite to using PN safely. Every effort must be made to ensure compatibility to avoid complications.[20–22] Although data do not exist to predetermine the compatibility of every possible nutrient combination in a PN admixture, general guidelines do exist and are key to minimizing the risk of incompatibility. An appropriate caution, however, is "When in doubt, don't." The factors known to affect the compatibility of any given additive include concentration, temperature, pH, length of time of exposure of the additive and the PN admixture, and order of mixing.[26] The most common compatibility issues will be discussed here.

B. Nutrient additives

1. Calcium and phosphorus: Solid precipitates can develop when an incompatible combination of salts is added to a PN formulation; this results in the formation of insoluble product. Calcium salts are one of the most reactive compounds and readily form insoluble products with a number of additives. Dibasic calcium phosphate is one of the most dangerous combinations and has resulted in embolic deaths when infused.[20] Although the potential for precipitation of calcium phosphate is well documented, this precipitation remains difficult to predict because of the many contributing factors.[21] Some of the known factors include the following:
   a) Increased temperature increases the likelihood of a precipitate forming because of increased dissociation of calcium from gluconate and of potassium and sodium from phosphate. This increases the chance for collision between the calcium and phosphate ions.
   b) Calcium gluconate is the preferred salt form of calcium, as it is more stable than an equivalent amount of calcium chloride.[22]
   c) Increased solution pH increases the likelihood of precipitation because the amount of dibasic phosphate is increased. An acidic pH is more favorable to calcium phosphate solubility. Acidity is especially influenced by the type and amount of amino acid solution used, as pH varies with the many available amino acid products. The pH of the amino acid solution helps maintain the pH of the PN admixture because of its buffering capacity. Neonatal/infant amino acid solutions are specifically designed with a lower pH to enhance calcium and phosphorus solubility. Addition of L-cysteine hydrochloride to the PN formulation containing neonatal/infant amino acid solutions will further reduce pH and improve solubility.[27]
   d) Order of mixing is extremely important to avoid the formation of an insoluble precipitate (see Section I.D). In general, phosphate should be added first, and calcium should be added near the end of the compounding sequence to take advantage of the maximum volume of the PN formulation.[22]
   e) Increased quantities of calcium and phosphorus in the PN admixture favor precipitation. Clinicians should refer to documented solubility curves provided by the manufacturers of amino acid products and published sources to guide calcium and phosphorus limitations.[2] When a PN order is written for potentially incompatible amounts of calcium and phosphorus, verification of the patient's requirements should be obtained and adjustments in the doses should be made as appropriate.[28] In some cases, if high calcium or phosphorus requirements exist, the requirement for one of the electrolytes may need to be met by some route and vehicle other than the PN admixture.
   f) Increased time of exposure of calcium and phosphorus in the PN admixture may result in formation of an insoluble precipitate. The likelihood increases as the PN admixture warms. Therefore, frequent agitation and observation for precipitates in the product are important.
   g) It should be emphasized that precipitation of calcium phosphate (or any other substance) is obscured by the presence of IVFE in a TNA. Therefore, additional caution is warranted when a TNA is prepared, and calcium and phosphorus limitations must be known and followed.
2. Bicarbonate salts are incompatible with PN admixtures and should not be used. Bicarbonate reacts with calcium to form the insoluble product calcium carbonate.[22] The addition of bicarbonate to the acidic PN admixture can also result in formation of carbon dioxide and loss of the bicarbonate ion.

C. TNA

1. General considerations: Adding IVFE to a PN admixture changes the overall physiochemical properties of the product. Most notable

is the fact that when dextrose and IVFE alone are combined, they are incompatible with each other because the low pH of IV dextrose solutions disrupts the IVFE. The presence of the amino acids serves as a buffer and facilitates a stable admixture. The presence of IVFE also further limits the compatibility of other additives. Strict adherence to published compatibility guidelines[5] is critical to avoid disrupting the TNA (see Section III.B) or developing a potentially lethal precipitate.[20,21]

2. Iron dextran: Iron is a trivalent cation (Fe^{+3}) that can destabilize the TNA when iron dextran is added to the formulation. The higher the cation valence, the greater the destabilizing power; thus, iron is more disruptive than calcium and magnesium (divalent cations), which are more disruptive than sodium and potassium (monovalent cations). There is no safe concentration of iron dextran in any TNA.[22,29] However, iron dextran can be added to non-IVFE-containing PN formulations, within limits.[11]

D. Medication additives

1. In general, the PN admixture should not be used as a drug delivery vehicle. Data on medication compatibility with PN formulations are limited, identifying physical compatibility, which is only one of several variables that influence complete bioavailability of both the drug and the nutrient provided by PN.[21]
2. In some cases there is no reasonable alternative to medication administration with PN. When medications are being admixed with the PN formulation, the following issues need to be addressed[30]:
   a) Medication stability and compatibility with 2-in-1 or TNA is assured.
   b) Evidence supports the efficacy of the medication administered in this manner.
3. Studies of medication compatibility in PN found compatibility to differ for TNA or 2-in-1 formulas.[31,32] Therefore, compatibility with one PN admixture does not predict compatibility with another.
   a) The physical compatibility of 102 drugs with 2-in-1 PN formulations simulating y-site administration has been determined.[32] Twenty drugs, including amphotericin B, acyclovir, sodium bicarbonate, and ciprofloxacin, were found to be incompatible.
   b) The physical compatibility of 106 drugs with TNA formulations simulating y-site administration has been determined.[32] Twenty-three drugs were found to be incompatible.
   c) Many of these interactions and incompatibilities could be identified by careful inspection of the PN formulas for precipitates, discoloration, haziness, or breaking of the emulsion.
   d) Compatibility information should be derived for the PN formulation that most closely matches the one prescribed for the patient in question.
4. Coadministration or admixture of medications known to be incompatible with PN should be prevented.[33] In the absence of reliable information concerning compatibility of a specific drug with PN, the medication should be administered separate from the PN.[33]

III. Stability Issues

A. General considerations: As with compatibility, many factors influence the stability of PN admixtures. Stability and compatibility are often overlapping issues, as the conditional incompatibility of individual nutrients renders the admixture less stable. Each nutrient additive in a PN admixture has its own inherent stability profile, which once combined with the other PN admixture components may be dramatically altered. The general factors affecting PN admixture stability are discussed below.

1. Temperature: Whereas it typically is assumed that increasing temperature helps substances dissolve or stay in solution better, the converse is true for PN admixtures. With increased temperature, there is increased dissociation of electrolytes, resulting in an increased likelihood of the formation of salts that will precipitate, for example, calcium phosphate (see Section II.B.1.a). Furthermore, the degradation of several amino acids (eg, tryptophan, arginine, methionine) is hastened by room temperature, compared to refrigerator temperature.[22]
2. pH: pH has variable effects, depending on the nutrient in question. For example, IVFE are more stable at higher pH values, whereas a lower pH value is favorable to calcium phosphate solubility. Therefore, the specific composition of an individual PN admixture must be taken into consideration when stability is evaluated relative to pH.
3. Light and oxygen exposure: Light and oxygen exposure enhances the degradation of some nutrients, including selected vitamins and amino acids. During storage, PN admixtures should be protected from light. Light protection is generally not considered necessary while a PN admixture is being infused into the patient because of the relatively short time of exposure (eg, ≤24 hours). However, it may be prudent to consider using light-protective coverings for PN formulations exposed to high levels of ultraviolet light (phototherapy lights) or fluorescent light, due to the susceptibility of vitamins, particularly vitamin A, to photodegradation.
4. Composition: The specific doses and combinations of nutrients can greatly affect the stability of a PN admixture. As discussed in Section II, some nutrients have a destabilizing effect when in the presence of other nutrients. For example, dextrose and IVFE cannot be directly admixed because of the effect of the low pH of the dextrose solution on the integrity of the IVFE. Divalent and trivalent cations are known to be potentially disruptive of a TNA admixture because of the effect of these ions on IVFE integrity.
5. Order of admixing (see Section I.D)

B. TNAs

1. General considerations: The issues of TNA stability are frequently related to compatibility. The presence of IVFE in the TNA alters the physicochemical character of the PN admixture. The TNA is an oil-in-water emulsion that is inherently less stable than a 2-in-1 formulation, which is completely water-based. All the factors that affect stability in a PN formulation tend to do so to a greater extent with a TNA. Therefore, a more conservative approach to interpreting admixture guidelines for compatibility is needed followed to avoid disruption of the TNA or formation of a visually undetectable precipitate.[20,21]
2. Stages of TNA deterioration: The integrity of a TNA is dependent on the oil droplets remaining dispersed throughout the aqueous phase. If the oil droplets are allowed to aggregate, they can eventually cause complete separation into oil and water phases, and the TNA that is no longer safe for infusion. The stages of deterioration or cracking of the TNA are as follows[17]:
   a) Aggregation (flocculation): Fat droplets aggregate to form larger droplets but can be redispersed with gentle agitation.
   b) Creaming: The larger fat droplets that have aggregated rise to the surface and form a cream layer; this stage can be reversed with gentle agitation.
   c) Coalescence: The fat droplets aggregate into significantly larger droplets, creating an irreversible separation of the oil and water phases and an unusable TNA.

d) Oiling out: There is continued coalescence, with total, irreversible separation of the oil and water phases and an unusable TNA.

C. Vitamins

1. General considerations: Light exposure and time are the primary factors affecting vitamin stability in PN admixtures. Vitamins should be added as the last component when a PN admixture is prepared (see Section I.D). Once the vitamins have been added, the PN admixture should be infused within 24 hours to limit loss of potency.
2. Specific vitamin considerations
   a) Ascorbic acid (vitamin C) breakdown is hastened by the presence of copper. The addition of ascorbic acid in a batch fashion has caused degradation, resulting over time in the formation of oxalic acid. Oxalic acid readily reacts with free calcium to form calcium oxalate precipitates.[22]
   b) Thiamine may be destroyed by sodium bisulfite but appears to be stable in the presence of sodium hydrosulfite. Sodium bisulfite or sodium hydrosulfite is used in some commercially prepared crystalline amino acid solutions as an antioxidant.
   c) Riboflavin degradation is increased by light exposure.
   d) Vitamin A may adsorb to plastic bags and tubing. Vitamin A in the form of retinol is less susceptible to adsorption than retinol palmitate. Substantial amounts of vitamin A can also be lost over time due to degradation.[34]

D. 2-in-1 base solutions are stable for various lengths of time depending on the storage conditions; 2-in-1 solutions cannot be commercially premixed because the temperatures required for autoclave sterilization caramelize the dextrose (a process known as the Maillard reaction). Caramelization is detected by the presence of a brown coloration in the 2-in-1 formulation.

IV. Microbial Growth Potential

A. General considerations: Safe administration of a PN admixture is dependent on the product being free of microbial contamination. Strict adherence to infection control admixing guidelines and validation of an aseptic compounding technique are imperative. Professional organizations have published guidelines for compounding and dispensing sterile products. The American Society of Health-System Pharmacists has published guidelines[35] on quality assurance for pharmacy-prepared sterile products, while the United States Pharmacopeia publishes the official compendium *The United States Pharmacopeia and The National Formulary,* which includes a chapter on pharmaceutical compounding of sterile preparations.[36] The following factors influence the sterility of the PN admixture:

1. Sterile compounding procedure: Sterile products are divided into three levels of risk on the basis of the probability of exposing multiple patients to microbial and physical contaminants.[35,36] Drawing a sterile product into a sterile syringe or transferring a sterile product from a vial into a commercially produced intravenous bag is an example of a low-risk process. Medium risk is the level assigned for automated compounding of PN formulations.
   a) PN admixtures should be prepared in a class 100 environment (ie, fewer than 100 particles of a size 0.5 μm/cu ft of air). This is best achieved by using a laminar flow hood.
   b) Personnel are required to wear clean gowns or coveralls, as scrub attire by itself is not acceptable. Gloves and masks are recommended during the compounding process.
   c) Process validation of aseptic procedures is recommended for PN formulations.[35] Individuals involved in PN compounding should successfully complete a process validation of aseptic technique before being allowed to admix PN. Process simulation of the PN formulation may also be used but is more difficult since the PN formulation itself may limit or inhibit microbial growth if inadvertently contaminated during the compounding process.
2. Nutrient composition
   a) PN admixtures can serve as an ideal growth environment for some microorganisms. These organisms may be introduced into the admixture when it is compounded or when the it is manipulated during administration.
   b) The ability of the PN admixture to support the growth of contaminants depends on nutrient composition. When the individual base components are compared, IVFE are better than amino acids, which are better than dextrose, in supporting microbial proliferation. When nutrient components are admixed, TNAs are more likely to support microbial proliferation than 2-in-1 formulations.
3. Temperature: Room temperature facilitates and refrigerator temperature retards microbial growth.
4. pH: An acidic environment inhibits bacterial growth, which is partly why a 2-in-1 formulation is less likely than a TNA to support proliferation of bacteria. However, fungi can rapidly proliferate in a 2-in-1 formulation despite the lower pH.
5. Time frame
   a) Lipid emulsions support the growth of bacteria and fungi that can reach clinically significant numbers within 24 hours. The Centers for Disease Control and Prevention (CDC) recommends that IVFE infused separately from PN formulations be completed within 12 hours of hanging the container.[37]
   b) TNAs support the growth of bacteria and fungi but at a slower rate than IVFE alone. The CDC recommends that a TNA be completed with 24 hours of hanging the solution.[37]
   c) 2-in-1 formulations support fungi but do not support bacteria. Like TNAs, they should be infused within 24 hours of initiating the infusion to avoid clinically significant fungal proliferation.[22]

B. Microbes of greatest clinical significance: There have been reports of infectious complications associated with a contaminated PN admixture. The following organisms related to PN contamination have been reported:

1. *Candida albicans* in 2-in-1 formulations[7]
2. *Malassezia furfur* in IVFE[38]
3. Coagulase-negative staphylococci in neonates receiving IVFE in the intensive care unit[39]
4. *Staphylococcus saprophyticus* in TNAs[40]

V. Automated Compounding

A. General characteristics

1. An automated compounding device (ACD) is a mechanical system usually made up of numerous stations, each designated for a component of the PN admixture. Some ACDs are limited to preparation of the base components (dextrose, amino acids, sterile water, and IVFE), whereas other systems include up to 23 channels to accommodate micronutrients as well.
2. ACDs admix PN formulations under computer-assisted commands connected to special hardware housed with sterile, disposable compounding sets. Based on prescribed dose, information regarding the specified volume of each ingredient is fed to the appropriate channels for the compounding process.

B. Guidelines on safe use: Due to the risk level of the compounding procedure, it is recommended that automated PN compounding include the following[22,41]:
   1. Pharmacist validation of data entered into the compounding device prior to PN preparation
   2. Performance of end-product checks to verify compounding accuracy
   3. Periodic observation by the operator of the device to ensure that it is working properly
C. Advantages (compared with manual compounding)
   1. Potential reduction in labor
   2. More efficient use of materials: Bulk volumes of additives can be used for compounding multiple patients' PN admixtures. Fewer needles and syringes are needed for manually adding components.
   3. Less likelihood of contamination during compounding because of less manual manipulation
   4. Availability of safety and quality assurance checks
D. Disadvantages (compared with manual compounding)
   1. Potential user error
   2. Potential equipment malfunction
   3. Susceptibility to power outages

VI. Off-Site Compounding Centers

A. Definition: an off-site IV admixture center providing IV compounding services that are shared by multiple institutions, eliminating the need for each institution to have its own dedicated IV admixture facility[42]
B. Potential advantages
   1. Greater efficiency in staffing, materials use, and inventory control, especially in institutions with a small volume of PN patients
   2. Standardization of procedures with improved quality control
   3. More efficient use of space
C. Potential disadvantages
   1. Logistics of communicating orders and order changes
   2. Logistics of transporting products from the off-site admixture center to the institution
   3. Less ability to assess quality control measures at the outside facility

VII. Ordering PN Formulations

A. General considerations: Many of the errors associated with the use of PN formulations are related to the complex nature of the ordering process. Clinical errors have been associated with the manner in which orders were created and communicated and lack of uniformity in the ordering process from institution to institution.[22] Standardizing the order-writing process has been shown to reduce prescribing errors.[43–45] A set of minimum standards for creating a PN order form have been recommended to reduce errors and improve patient safety.[22]
B. Clarity of the order form: A PN order form should be designed so that all health care professionals who use it understand it. The following principles have been recommended to promote order form clarity[22]:
   1. Organization: The form should be organized simply and be easy to scan for completeness.
   2. All nutrients should be clearly identified.
   3. Adequate space should be provided to allow clear handwriting. However, the use of a standardized PN order form should dramatically reduce the need for the prescriber to hand write items, thus reducing the likelihood of misinterpretation.
   4. Trailing zeroes should never be used, and the use of decimals should be avoided whenever possible. Leading zeroes should be used for doses less than one measurement unit.[46]
   5. Units of measure on the PN order form should be consistent with the recommended PN label format (see Section VIII).
   6. Ingredients should be listed in the same order on the PN order form and the PN label to facilitate verification of the PN contents against the PN order.
C. Mandatory components of the order form: The design of PN order forms may differ from institution to institution to account for specific needs and concerns. However, the following recommendations are deemed to be necessary for all PN order forms[22]:
   1. Type of access (central or peripheral vein)
   2. Height, weight, diagnosis, PN indication
   3. Contact number for reference person and prescriber
   4. Hang time guidelines
   5. Safeguards to avoid incompatibilities
   6. Warning mechanism for excessive rate of nutrient administration
D. Recommended components of the order form: Although not considered mandatory, these items are strongly recommended for inclusion on the PN order form (or back of the form)[22]:
   1. Nutrient dosing guidelines based on weight and age
   2. Recommended nutrient ranges, including maximum and minimum amounts, when applicable
   3. Guidelines to assist in nutrient and volume calculations
   4. Monitoring guidelines
   5. Guidelines for stopping or interrupting the PN infusion
   6. Specific content of multivitamin and trace element preparations available
   7. Specific amino acid and IVFE brands available
   8. Insulin guidelines
E. Sample order form (Figure 7-1): A sample adult PN order form is provided as a guide to meeting criteria for mandatory and strongly recommended items for inclusion. Its content must be adapted to meet the needs of the individual institution based on patient population, prescribing patterns, and judgment by the health care professional.

VIII. Labeling PN Formulations

A. General considerations: The way PN ingredients are labeled varies considerably.[22] PN base components (dextrose, amino acids, and IVFE) have been labeled as the volume of the percent of original concentration added, the percent of final concentration after admixture, and either the grams per liter or the grams per total volume of PN admixed. Additives, especially electrolytes, have been labeled as mEq or mmol and as quantity per day, per kg, per liter, or per 100 mL.
   1. Misinterpretation of the dextrose content of a PN label led to an error in PN preparation that caused a patient's death.[47] Hepatic toxicity resulted from an iron overdose caused by the misinterpretation of a PN label for iron dextran (1 mL) where the original solution containing 50 mg/mL was used rather than a pre diluted product having a concentration of 1 mg/mL.[48]
   2. Quantity per total volume: With use of a 24-hour nutrient infusion system, quantity per total volume is most consistent with that of a nutrient label, requiring the least number of calculations to determine the nutrient dose per day.
B. PN label template (see Figures 7-2 through 7-4): Due to the complex nature of the label, there are several points that should be clarified.
   1. Amount/day is the only column required on the adult label (Figure 7-2). A second, optional column may be added reflecting amount/L.

FIGURE 7-1. Parenteral Nutrition Order Form Template

Physician Orders
PARENTERAL NUTRITION (PN) - ADULT

Primary Diagnosis: ______________________ **Ht:** ________cm **Dosing Wt:**_____kg

PN Indication:______________________ **Allergies:** ______________________

Instructions: This form must be completed for a new order or continuation of PN and faxed to the Pharmacy by **[Insert Time]** to receive same day preparation. PN administration begins at **[Insert Time]**. Contact the Nutrition Support Service at (XXX) XXX-XXXX for additional information.

Administration Route: ☐ CVC or PICC *Note: Proper tip placement of the CVC or PICC must be confirmed prior to PN infusion*

☐ Peripheral IV (PIV) (*Final PN Osmolarity ≤ ________ mOsm/L*)

Monitoring: Daily weights, Strict input & output, Bedside glucose monitoring every _____ hours

☐ Na, K, Cl, CO_2, Glucose, BUN, SCr, Mg, PO_4 every ________________

☐ T. Bili, Alk Phos, AST, ALT, Albumin, Trigl ycerides, Calcium every ____________

Base Solution: *Select one* — *Parenteral nutrition **MUST** be administered through a dedicated infusion port and filtered with a 1.2-micron in-line filter at all times. Discard any unused volume after 24 hours.*

☐ PERIPHERAL 2-in-1

Dextrose _____ g

Amino Acids (*Brand* _________) _____ g

For patients with PIV and established glucose tolerance; Provides ______ kcal; Maximum Rate not to exceed ______ mL/hour

☐ CENTRAL 2-in-1

Dextrose _____ g

Amino Acids (*Brand* _________) _____ g

For patients with CVC or PICC and established glucose tolerance; Provides ______ kcal; Maximum Rate not to exceed ______ mL/hour

☐ CENTRAL 3-in-1

Dextrose _____ g

Amino Acids (*Brand* ___________) _____ g

Fat Emulsion (*Brand* ___________) _____ g

For patients with CVC or PICC and established glucose / fat emulsion tolerance; Provides ______ kcal; Maximum Rate not to exceed ______ mL/hour

Use of additional fat emulsion not required with 3-in-1 base solution

RATE & VOLUME: ______ mL/hour for _____ hours = ______ mL/day
Must specify

or **CYCLIC INFUSION:** ______ mL/hour for _____ hours, then ______ mL/hour for _____ hours = ______ mL/day

Fat Emulsion (*Brand* ___________) ***– via PIV or CVC with 2-in-1 base solutions*** *(Select caloric density & volume)*

☐ 10% ☐ 250 mL Infuse at ______ mL/hour over _____ hours Frequency _____________

☐ 20% ☐ 500 mL *(Note: Infusions < 4 or > 12 hours not recommended)* *Discard any unused volume after 12 hours.*

Additives: *(per day)*		***Normal Dosages***
Sodium Chloride	_______ mEq	*1-2 mEq Sodium/kg/day*
as Acetate	_______ mEq	*pH or CO_2 dependent*
as Phosphate	_______ mmol of PO_4	*Consider if hyperkalemic*
Potassium Chloride	_______ mEq	*1-2 mEq Potassium/kg/day*
as Acetate	_______ mEq	*pH or CO_2 dependent*
as Phosphate	_______ mmol of PO_4	*20-40 mmol/day (1 mmol Phos = 1.5 mEq K)*
Calcium **Gluconate**	_______ mEq	*5-15 mEq/day*
Magnesium **Sulfate**	_______ mEq	*8-24 mEq/day*
Adult **Multivitamins**	______ mL/day	*Contains Vitamin K 150 mcg*
Adult **Trace Elements**	______ mL/day	*Zn __ mg, Cu __ mg, Mn __ mg, Cr __ mcg, Se __ mcg (with normal hepatic function)*
H_2 Antagonist _________	_______ mg	*____ mg/day with normal renal function*
Other:		

Additives: *(per day)*

Regular Insulin ________ units

Recommend if hyperglycemic, start with 1 unit for every 10 g of dextrose

***Pharmacy Use Only: Ca/PO_4* Limit Checked ____**

(Note: Some brands of amino acids contain phosphate)

Physician's Signature: ______________________**PagerNumber:**_________**Date/time:**_________

Orders transcribed by: __________ **Date/time:** ___________ **Orders verified by:** ___________**Date/time:**________

SEND COMPLETED ORDERS TO PHARMACY File under: Physician Orders

Reprinted from Task Force for the Revision of Safe Practices for Parenteral Nutrition. Safe practices for parenteral nutrition. *J Parenter Enteral Nutr.* 2004;28:S39–S70 with permission.

FIGURE 7-2. Standard PN Label Template: Adult Patient

Institution/Pharmacy Name, Address, and Pharmacy Phone Number

Name ________________ Dosing Weight __________

Location ______________

Administration Date/Time _________ Expiration Date/Time _________

Base formula	Amount/day	(Amount/L)
Dextrose	g	(g/L)
Amino acids[a]	g	(g/L)
IVFE[a]	g	(g/L)
Electrolytes		
Sodium chloride	mEq	(mEq/L)
Sodium acetate	mEq	(mEq/L)
Sodium phosphate	mmol of P	(mmol/L)
	(mEq of Na)	(mEq/L)
Potassium chloride	mEq	(mEq/L)
Potassium acetatem	Eq	(mEq/L)
Potassium phosphate	mmol of P	(mmol/L)
	(mEq of K)	(mEq/L)
Calcium gluconate	mEq	(mEq/L)
Magnesium sulfate	mEq	(mEq/L)
Vitamins, trace elements, and medications		
Multiple vitamins[a]	mL	
Multiple trace elements[a]	mL	
Insulin	units	(units/L)
H_2 antagonists[a]	mg	

Rate ___ mL/hour Volume ___ mL Infuse over ___ hours

Formulation contains _____ mL plus _____ mL overfill

Discard any unused volume after 24 hours

Central Line Use Only

[a] Specify product name.

Reprinted from Task Force for the Revision of Safe Practices for Parenteral Nutrition. Safe practices for parenteral nutrition. *J Parenter Enteral Nutr.* 2004;28:S39–S70 with permission.

FIGURE 7-3. Standard Parenteral Nutrition Label Template: Neonate or Pediatric Patient

Institution/Pharmacy Name, Address, and Pharmacy Phone Number

Name ________________ Dosing Weight __________

Location ______________

Administration Date/Time _______ Do Not Use After: Date/Time ______

Base formula	Amount/day	(Amount/L)
Dextrose	g/kg	g
Amino acids[a]	g/kg	g
Electrolytes		
Sodium chloride[b]	mEq/kg	mEq
Sodium acetate[b]	mEq/kg	mEq
Potassium chloride	mEq/kg	mEq
Potassium acetate[b]	mEq/kg	mEq
Potassium phosphate	mmol of P/kg	mmol of P
	(mEq of K)/kg	(mEq of K)
Sodium phosphate[b]	mmol of P/kg	mmol of P
	(mEq of Na)/kg	(mEq of Na)
Calcium gluconate	mEq/kg	mEq
Magnesium sulfate	mEq/kg	mEq
Vitamins, trace elements, and medications		
Multiple vitamins[a]	mL/kg	mL
Multiple trace elements[a]	mL/kg	mL
L-cysteine	mg/kg	mg
H_2 antagonists[a]	mg/kg	mg
L-carnitine	mg/kg	mg

Rate ___ mL/hour Volume ___ mL Infuse over 24 hours

Admixture contains _____ mL plus _____ mL overfill

Central Line Use Only

[a] Specify product name.

[b] Since the admixture usually contains multiple sources of sodium, potassium, chloride, acetate, and phosphorus, the amount of each electrolyte/kg provided by the PN admixture is determined by adding the amount of electrolyte provided by each salt.

Reprinted from Task Force for the Revision of Safe Practices for Parenteral Nutrition. Safe practices for parenteral nutrition. *J Parenter Enteral Nutr.* 2004;28:S39–S70 with permission.

2. For neonatal or pediatric patients, nutrient doses should be labeled as amount/kg/day. PN labels for these patients should include a column for amount/day and amount/kg/day (Figure 7-3). Optional columns may be added to reflect amount/L or amount/100 mL.
3. If IVFE are not included in the PN formulation, this line may be omitted from the label. Figure 7-4 provides a label template for IVFE administered separate from the PN formulation.
4. The dosing weight (the weight used to calculate nutrient doses) is required on the label.
5. The PN label should specify the route of administration.
6. If the PN contains overfill, it should be clearly stated on the label.
7. The administration date and time and expiration date and time should be expressed clearly on the label.
8. The phosphorus content should be expressed as both the mmol quantity of phosphorus and the mEq quantity of the salt's cation, potassium, or sodium.
9. Rate should be expressed in mL/hour over 24 hours. If the PN is cycled, the infusion duration and rates are to be expressed on the label.
10. For use in the home setting, ingredients to be added at home should be labeled as patient additives.
11. An auxiliary label may be used to provide supplemental information thought to be useful but not required on the PN label.

C. Practice guidelines[22]

1. Labels for PN formulations shall be standardized.
   a) The amount per day of nutrients and medications is required on the label.
   b) Using the quantity per liter option supports programs that continue to admix PN in 1-liter volumes.
   c) The dosing weight is required on the label.

FIGURE 7-4. Standard IVFE Label Template: Adult, Neonate, or Pediatric Patient

Institution/Pharmacy Name, Address, and Pharmacy Phone Number

Name ____________________ Dosing Weight __________

Location ______________

Administration Date/Time _______ Expiration Date/Time ______

	Volume	Amount/kg/day	Amount/day
Intravenous fat emulsion[a](%)	___ mL	________ g/kg	_______ g

Infusion rate ___ mL/hour Infuse over ___ hours

May contain overfill—Discard any unused volume after 12 hours

For peripheral or central line administration

[a] Specify product name.

Reprinted from Task Force for the Revision of Safe Practices for Parenteral Nutrition. Safe practices for parenteral nutrition. *J Parenter Enteral Nutr.* 2004;28:S39–S70 with permission.

2. Auxiliary labels may be used to provide information not already included on the label.
3. Pharmacist-to-pharmacist communication is required when a patient transfers between health care environments, to ensure the accurate transfer of the PN prescription.
4. The PN label must be compared to the PN order for accuracy and to verify expiration date prior to administration.

(Parenteral Nutrition Formulation chapters from the 1st edition were contributed by Kathleen M. Strausburg, Kristy Gibbons, Nancy Cyr, Michael L. Christensen, and Richard A. Helms)

REFERENCES

1. Kearns LR, Phillips ML, Ness-Abramof R, Apovian CM. Update on parenteral amino acids. *Nutr Clin Pract.* 2001;16:219–225.
2. Amino acid injection. In: Trissel LA, ed. *Handbook on Injectable Drugs.* 12th ed. Bethesda, MD: American Society of Health-System Pharmacists; 2003:45–90.
3. Singer P, Bursztein S, Kirvela O, et al. Hypercaloric glycerol in injured patients. *Surgery.* 1992;112:509–514.
4. Driscoll DF. Intravenous lipid emulsion: 2001. *Nutr Clin Pract.* 2001;16: 215–218.
5. Fat emulsion, intravenous. In: Trissel LA, ed. *Handbook on Injectable Drugs.* 12th ed. Bethesda, MD: American Society of Health-System Pharmacists; 2003:562–582.
6. Driscoll DF, Adolph M, Bistrian BR. Lipid emulsions in parenteral nutrition. In: Rombeau JL, Rolandelli RH, eds. *Clinical Nutrition: Parenteral Nutrition.* 3rd ed. Philadelphia, PA: WB Saunders; 2001:35–39.
7. Mirtallo JM. Parenteral formulas. In: Rombeau JL, Rolandelli RH, eds. *Clinical Nutrition: Parenteral Nutrition.* 3rd ed. Philadelphia, PA: WB Saunders; 2001:118–137.
8. Food and Drug Administration. Parenteral multivitamin products: drugs for human use: drug efficacy study implementation: amendment. *Federal Register.* April 20, 2000;65(77):21200–21201
9. Greene HL, Hambidge KM, Schanler R, Tsang RC. Guidelines for the use of vitamins, trace elements, calcium, magnesium, and phosphorus in infants and children receiving total parenteral nutrition: report of the Subcommittee on Pediatric Parenteral Nutrient Requirements from the Committee on Clinical Practice Issues of the American Society for Clinical Nutrition. *Am J Clin Nutr.* 1988;48:1324–1342.
10. American Medical Association Department of Foods and Nutrition. Guidelines for essential trace element preparations for parenteral use. A statement by an expert panel. *JAMA.* 1979;241:2051–2054.
11. Kumpf V. Update on parenteral iron therapy. *Nutr Clin Pract.* 2003;18: 318–326.
12. Pluhator-Murton MM, Fedorak RN, Audette RJ, et al. Trace element contamination of total parenteral nutrition, I: contribution of component solutions. *J Parenter Enteral Nutr.* 1999;23:222–227.
13. ASCN/ASPEN Working Group on Standards for Aluminum Content of Parenteral Nutrition Solutions. Parenteral drug products containing aluminum as an ingredient or a contaminant: response to food and drug administration notice of intent and request for information. *Am J Clin Nutr.* 1991;53:399–402.
14. Aluminum in large and small volume parenterals used in total parenteral nutrition. Food and Drug Administration, Docket No. 90N-0056. *Federal Register.* January 26, 2000;65(17):4103–4111.
15. Dickerson RN. Manganese intoxication and parenteral nutrition. *Nutrition.* 2001;17:689–693.
16. Kurkus J, Alcock NW, Shils ME. Manganese content of large-volume parenteral nutrition solutions and of nutrient additives. *J Parenter Enteral Nutr.* 1984;8:254–257.
17. Brown R, Quercia RA, Sigman R. Total nutrient admixture: a review. *J Parenter Enteral Nutr.* 1986;10:650–658.
18. Driscoll DF. Total nutrient admixtures: theory and practice. *Nutr Clin Pract.* 1995;10:114–119.
19. Jensen GL, Mascioli EA, Seidner DL, et al. Parenteral infusion of long- and medium-chain triglycerides and reticuloendothelial system function in man. *J Parenter Enteral Nutr.* 1990;14:467–471.
20. Hill SE, Heldman LS, Goo EDH, et al. Fatal microvascular pulmonary emboli from precipitation of a total nutrient admixture solution. *J Parenter Enteral Nutr.* 1996;20:81–87.
21. McKinnon BT. FDA safety alert: hazards of precipitation associated with parenteral nutrition. *Nutr Clin Pract.* 1996;11:59–65.
22. Task Force for the Revision of Safe Practices for Parenteral Nutrition. Safe practices for parenteral nutrition. *J Parenter Enteral Nutr.* 2004;28:S39–S70.
23. Bertch KE, McKinnon BT. Pharmaceutical issues for parenteral nutrition solutions. In: Christensen ML, McKinnon BT, eds. *Nutrition Support Pharmacy: Selected Cases for Self-Study.* Silver Spring, MD: A.S.P.E.N.; 1995:7-1 to 7-17.
24. A.S.P.E.N. Board of Directors and the Clinical Task Force. Guidelines for the use of parenteral and enteral nutrition in adult and pediatric patients. *J Parenter Enteral Nutr.* 2002;26(suppl):1SA–138SA.
25. Isaacs JW, Millikan WJ, Stackhouse J, et al. Parenteral nutrition of adults with 900-milliosmolar solution via peripheral vein. *Am J Clin Nutr.* 1977;30:552–559.
26. Johnson GC, Anderson JD. Compounding considerations. In: Teasley-Strausbury KM, ed. *Nutrition Support Handbook: A Compendium of Products with Guidelines for Usage.* Cincinnati, OH: Harvey Whitney Books; 1992:133–146.
27. Eggert LD, Risho WJ, MacKay MW, et al. Calcium and phosphorus compatibility in parenteral nutrition solutions for neonates. *Am J Hosp Pharm.* 1982;39:49–53.
28. Mirtallo JM. The complexity of mixing calcium and phosphate. *Am J Hosp Pharm.* 1994;51:1535–1536.
29. Driscoll DF, Bhargava HN, Li L, et al. Physicochemical stability of total nutrient admixtures. *Am J Hosp Pharm.* 1995;52:623–634.
30. Driscoll DF, Baptista RJ, Mitrano FP, et al. Parenteral nutrient admixtures as drug vehicles. Theory and practice in the critical care setting. *Ann Pharmacother.* 1991;25:276–283.
31. Trissel LA, Gilbert DL, Martinez JF, et al. Compatibility of parenteral nutrient solutions with selected drugs during simulated Y-site administration. *Am J Health-Syst Pharm.* 1997;54:1295–1300.
32. Trissel LA, Gilbert DL, Martinez JF, et al. Compatibility of medications with 3-in-1 parenteral nutrient admixtures. *J Parenter Enteral Nutr.* 1999;23:67–74.
33. A.S.P.E.N. Board of Directors and the Clinical Guidelines Task Force. Drug-nutrient interactions, IX: guidelines for the use of parenteral and enteral nutrition in adult and pediatric patients. *J Parenter Enteral Nutr.* 2002;26(suppl):42SA–44SA.

34. Howard L, Chu R, Feman S, et al. Vitamin A deficiency from long-term parenteral nutrition. *Ann Intern Med.* 1980;93:576–577.
35. American Society for Health-System Pharmacists. ASHP guidelines on quality assurance for pharmacy-prepared sterile products. *Am J Health-Syst Pharm.* 2000;57:1150–1169.
36. USP General Chapter <797> pharmaceutical compounding–sterile preparations. United States Pharmacopeial Convention. *Pharmacopeial Forum.* 2003;29(4):940–965.
37. Centers for Disease Control and Prevention. Guidelines for the prevention of intravascular catheter-related infections. *MMWR.* 2002;51(No RR-10):1–29.
38. Shek YH, Tucker MC, Viciana AL, et al. *Malassezia furfur*-disseminated infection in premature infants. *Am J Clin Pathol.* 1989;92:595–603.
39. Freeman J, Goldmann DA, Smith NE, et al. Association of intravenous lipid emulsion and coagulase-negative staphylococcal bacteremia in neonatal intensive care units. *N Engl J Med.* 1990;323:301–308.
40. Llop JM, Mangues I, Perez JL, et al. *Staphylococcus saprophyticus* sepsis related to total parenteral nutrition admixture contamination. *J Parenter Enteral Nutr.* 1993;17:575–577.
41. American Society for Health-System Pharmacists. ASHP Guidelines on Safe Use of Automated Compounding Devices for the Preparation of Parenteral Nutrition Admixtures. *Am J Health-Syst Pharm.* 2000;57:1343–1348.
42. Fauber WS, Cosnotti SJ, Mady RL. Offsite intravenous admixture center shared by health-system facilities. *Am J Hosp Pharm.* 1995;52:2550–2555.
43. Petros WP, Shank WA. A standardized parenteral nutrition solution: prescribing, use, processing, and material cost implications. *Hosp Pharm.* 1986;21:648–656.
44. Mitchell KA, Jones EA, Mequid MM, et al. Standardized TPN order form reduces staff time and potential for error. *Nutrition.* 1990;6:457–460.
45. Cerra FB. A standardized TPN order form reduces staff time and potential error [editorial]. *Nutrition.* 1990;6:498–499.
46. ISMP list of error-prone abbreviations, symbols, and dose designations. *ISMP Medication Safety Alert.* 2003;8(24):3–4.
47. Carey LC, Haffey M. Incident: home TPN formula order misinterpreted after hospital admission. *Home Care Highlights.* spring 1995:7.
48. Iron overdose due to miscommunication of TPN order. Error alert. *Pharm Today.* September 1995:52.

Gordon S. Sacks, PharmD, BCNSP, FCCP;
Susan Mayhew, PharmD, BCNSP;
Debbie Johnson, RN, MSN

8

Parenteral Nutrition Implementation and Management

Introduction

Parenteral nutrition (PN) is the provision of intravenous nutrients to patients whose gastrointestinal (GI) tract is not functioning or cannot be accessed and to patients whose nutritional needs cannot be met with oral diets or enteral tube feeding. Recognized as a major medical advance in the past 50 years, PN has provided lifesaving therapy for patients who could not otherwise be nourished. Because of its complexity, PN therapy requires careful monitoring by trained clinicians to avoid serious complications. New knowledge and technological advances have resulted in appropriate patient selection and therapies that have steadily improved patient safety.

I. Background

PN refers to a combination of nutrients—crystalline amino acids, dextrose, fat emulsions, electrolytes, vitamins, and minerals—administered intravenously.

A. PN was developed in the late 1960s to provide nutrition for those without a functioning GI tract.
B. PN was initially called intravenous (IV) hyperalimentation, but now the terms PN and central PN are more often used.
C. PN administered via a peripheral vein is called peripheral PN (PPN).
D. PN admixtures are of two types.
   1. Mixtures of dextrose, amino acids, vitamins, and minerals are referred to as 2-in-1. IV fat emulsions (IVFE) are infused separately.
   2. Total nutrient admixtures (TNAs), 3-in-1, or all-in-one formulations are terms for PN that contains IVFE in the same container with crystalline amino acids, dextrose, vitamins, and minerals.

II. Situations in Which PN Is Commonly Used

A. The indication for PN is a nonfunctioning or inaccessible GI tract.
B. The anticipated duration of PN is at least 7 days.
C. The American Society for Parenteral and Enteral Nutrition (A.S.P.E.N.) has developed specific guidelines for implementation of PN in adult patients.[1]
D. A.S.P.E.N. has also developed specific guidelines for implementation of PN in pediatric patients[1]

III. Initiation of PN

A. PN may be initiated in adult patients who are hemodynamically stable, who are able to tolerate the fluid volume necessary to provide significant macronutrient intake, and who have central vascular access. If access to a central vein cannot be obtained, PPN should be considered. PPN is more commonly used in neonatal and pediatric populations than in adults.
B. For preterm neonates, PN is a cornerstone of postnatal care and initiation is advocated as soon as clinically possible after birth, often on day 1 of life. Goals for initiation and advancement of protein, carbohydrate, fat, and fluid intake in term and preterm neonates are listed in Chapter 26. Goals for fluid intake, energy, and protein in infants, children, and adolescents are listed in Chapter 2.
C. The usual goals for protein, carbohydrate, fat, and fluid intake for adult patients on PN are presented in Table 8-1.
D. Guidelines for mineral and electrolyte intake are presented in Table 8-2 for pediatric patients and in Table 8-3 for adult patients.[2–4]
E. Electrolytes may be manipulated to avoid electrolyte and acid-base imbalance. Although it is inappropriate to use PN to manage short-term fluid and electrolyte shifts, the fluid, mineral, and electrolyte content of PN is frequently individualized. Consideration is given to the patient's existing deficits, dry weight, ongoing losses, and changes in organ function or drug therapy.
F. Recommendations for vitamin and trace element intake are given in Tables 8-4 and 8-5 for adult PN formulations and in Tables 8-6 and 8-7 for pediatric PN formulations.[5,6]
G. Generally, the patient should have satisfactory hydration, electrolyte, and acid-base status prior to the initiation of PN. Individualized PN may help balance hydration, electrolytes, and acid-base status. However, to best achieve nutritional goals with PN, the hydration, electrolyte, and acid-base status of the patient should be corrected as much as possible before PN is started.
H. The initial PN for adults is based on ability to tolerate volume and macronutrients.
   1. As protein intake in an adult is associated with minimal metabolic side effects, the maximum amount of protein (up to 60–70 g/L) can be given on day 1. The initial maximum carbohydrate given in an adult is usually 150 to 200 g per day or a 15% to 20% final dextrose concentration. For adult patients with diabetes mellitus or hyperglycemia of stress, 100 to 150 g per day of dextrose or a 10% to 15% final dextrose concentration can be administered initially.[7]
   2. For most adult patients, PN may be increased so that energy and protein goals are achieved by day 2 or 3. Many institutions, how-

TABLE 8-1. Suggested Nutrient Intake for Adult Patients on Parenteral Nutrition*

	Critically ill patients	Stable patients
Protein	1.2–1.5 g/kg/d	0.8–1.0 g/kg/d
Carbohydrate	Not >4 mg/kg/min	Not >7 mg/kg/min
Lipid	1 g/kg/d	1 g/kg/d
Total calories	25–30 kcal/kg/d	30–35 kcal/kg/d**
Fluid	Minimum needed to deliver adequate macronutrients	30–40 mL/kg/d***

*Estimated dry weight is used as the basis of calculations. For obese patients, 120% of ideal weight is used as the basis for calculations.
**Varies according to activity levels.
***May vary if the patient has ongoing fluid losses.

TABLE 8-3. Daily Electrolyte Guidelines for Adult Parenteral Nutrition Formulations[2–4]

Nutrient	Standard daily requirement	Factors Tthat increase needs	Dosage form
Calcium	10–15 mEq	High protein intake	Ca gluconate
Magnesium	8–20 mEq	GI losses, drugs, refeeding	Mg sulfate
Phosphorus	20–40 mmol	High dextrose loads, refeeding	Na phosphate K phosphate
Sodium	1–2 mEq/kg		Na phosphate Na chloride Na acetate Na lactate
Potassium	1–2 mEq/kg	Diarrhea, vomiting, NG suction	K phosphate K acetate K chloride

GI, gastrointestinal; NG, nasogasric.

ever, can provide patient-specific PN formulations with increased nutrient density, so volume is not a limiting factor.

a) The dextrose content of the PN can be increased if the patient has capillary blood glucose values consistently ≤180 mg/dL.

b) The IVFE in the PN can be increased if the patient has serum triglycerides ≤400 mg/dL.

I. The initiation rate of PN for neonatal and pediatric patients will often replace maintenance IV fluids, thereby meeting maintenance fluid requirements. Generally, the time to reach energy and protein goals with PN is inversely related to age. For example, 3 to 5 days of PN therapy (advanced incrementally each day) are generally required for neonatal patients before nutritional goals are reached, whereas for children and adolescents, PN goals can often be met in 48 to 72 hours.

1. Daily protein requirements are inversely related to developmental age and weight. Initial protein doses for preterm neonates range from 1 to 2 g/kg/day and are increased daily by 0.5 to 1 g/kg/day to a goal of 3 g/kg/day for most neonates and infants. Protein requirements in healthy individuals decline to about 1.5 to 2 g/kg/day around 1 year of age and by adolescence approach adult values, with requirements generally ranging from 0.8 to 1.5 g/kg/day.
2. Dextrose infusions are generally initiated at doses that approximate endogenous glucose production rates (about 6–8 mg/kg/minute for neonates and infants) and are increased gradually in daily increments until energy goals are achieved or the maximum of 12 to 14 mg/kg/minute is reached (about 19 g/kg/day).[1] The upper limit of carbohydrate intake appears to peak between the ages of 1 to 3 years and gradually decreases with age, approaching adult values (5–6 mg/kg/minute or 9 g/kg/day) during adolescence (8–10 mg/kg/minute or 12–14 g/kg/day).[8] When IVFE are administered to supplement nonprotein calories, dextrose intake at or below the upper limit is generally sufficient for adequate weight gain.
3. IVFE provide a concentrated source of energy and prevent essential fatty acid deficiency (EFAD). Preterm neonates are especially prone to developing EFAD because of low body fat stores. For neonates receiving PN, IVFE should be initiated within 3 days of birth and are usually started at doses of 0.5 to 1 g/kg/day and advanced daily (in increments of 0.5–1 g/kg/day) to a goal dose of 3 g/kg/day. For term neonates, infants, and children, IVFE are commonly initiated at 1 g/kg/day and advanced daily to a goal of 2 to 3 g/kg/day for children and generally 2 g/kg/day for adolescents.

TABLE 8-2. Daily Electrolyte and Mineral Requirements for Pediatric Patients*[2–4]

Electrolyte	Preterm neonates	Infants/children	Adolescents and children >50kg
Sodium	2–5 mEq/kg	2–5 mEq/kg	1–2 mEq/kg
Potassium	2–4 mEq/kg	2–4 mEq/kg	1–2 mEq/kg
Calcium	2–4 mEq/kg	0.5–4 mEq/kg	10–20 mEq/d
Phosphorus	1–2 mmol/kg	0.5–2 mmol/kg	10–40 mmol/d
Magnesium	0.3–0.5 mEq/kg	0.3–0.5 mEq/kg	10–30 mEq/d
Acetate	As needed to maintain acid-base balance	As needed to maintain acid-base balance	As needed to maintain acid-base balance
Chloride	As needed to maintain acid-base balance	As needed to maintain acid-base balance	As needed to maintain acid-base balance

*Assumes normal age-related organ function.

TABLE 8-4. Recommendations for Vitamin Intake in Adults[5–6]

Vitamin	Daily dose
Vitamin A	3300 IU
Vitamin D	200 IU
Vitamin E	10 IU
Vitamin K	150 mcg
Thiamine (B_1)	6 mg
Pyridoxine (B_6)	6 mg
Cyanocobalamin (B_{12})	5 mcg
Pantothenic acid	15 mg
Biotin	60 mcg
Ascorbic acid	200 mg
Folic acid	600 mcg
Niacin	40 mg
Riboflavin	3.6 mg

J. After a review of organ function, medication profile, and serum concentrations, electrolytes are manipulated according to the following general guidelines:
   1. Because magnesium, phosphorus, and potassium needs increase with anabolism and are carbohydrate dependent, repletion levels of these minerals may be needed for the first few days of PN.
   2. Potassium, magnesium, and phosphorus administration is adjusted according to changes in the serum concentrations and renal function.

K. Elevated serum or capillary glucose concentrations or fluid volume intolerance may preclude an increase in glucose concentration or PN volume, respectively. If fluid restriction is necessary, the required amounts of protein and energy substrate are concentrated within the volume tolerated.

L. Because of reduced dextrose concentration and osmolarity, PPN can be initiated at greater volumes than central PN formulations.
   1. If PPN is 5% dextrose, it may be initiated at the same rate as peripheral IV fluids.
   2. Osmolarity restrictions usually preclude adding large amounts of electrolytes to PPN. The maximum osmolarity for PPN is 900 mOsm/L. A formula to estimate the osmolarity of formulations is in Chapter 7. Additional electrolyte supplements may be delivered via the GI tract or a peripheral vein.

TABLE 8-5. Recommended Trace Element Intake in Adult Patients on Parenteral Nutrition[5–6]

Trace element	Standard daily intake
Chromium	10–15 mcg
Copper	0.3–0.5 mg
Manganese	60–100 mcg
Selenium	20–60 mcg
Zinc	2.5–5 mg

TABLE 8-6. Daily Dose Recommendations for Pediatric Multivitamins*[5–6]

Manufacture		AMA-NAG	
Weight (kg)	Dose	Weight (kg)	Dose
<1	1.5 mL	<2.5	2 mL/kg
1–3	3.25 mL	>2.5	5 mL
>3	5 mL		

*Assumes normal age-related organ function. Pediatric multivitamin formulation (5 mL): A 2300 IU, D 400 IU, E 7 IU, K 200 mcg, ascorbic acid 80 mg, thiamine 1.2 mg, riboflavin 1.4 mg, niacin 17 mg, pantothenic acid 5 mg, pyridoxine 1 mg, cyanocobalamin 1 mcg, biotin 20 mcg, and folic acid 140 mcg.

IV. Administration of PN

A. Proper central venous catheter (CVC) tip placement must be confirmed prior to initial PN administration as well as any time signs and symptoms indicate a compromised catheter position.

B. Because it is hypertonic, central PN is administered via a CVC with the distal tip placed in the superior vena cava adjacent to the right atrium.[1,9,10]

C. Infusion of PN via a peripheral vein requires careful consideration of the formulation's osmolarity along with judicious monitoring of the venous access site for signs of phlebitis and/or infiltration.

D. The use of femoral catheters for adult PN administration should be avoided unless no other access can be obtained. These catheters are associated with a higher risk of venous thrombosis and catheter-related sepsis.[11,12] However, in pediatric patients, femoral catheters have a lower incidence of mechanical complications and may have an infection rate similar to catheters not placed in the femoral vein.[12]

E. The use of in-line filters is recommended during the administration of PN because the filters can eliminate or reduce the infusion of particulates, microprecipitates, microorganisms, pyrogens, and air.[13–15]
   1. A 0.22-micron filter should be used for 2-in-1 formulations.

TABLE 8-7. Trace Element Daily Requirements for Pediatric Patients*[5–6]

Trace	Preterm neonates <3 kg	Term neonates, infants 3–10 kg	Children 10–40 kg	Adolescents >40 kg
Zinc	400	50–250	50–125	2–5 mg
Copper	20	20	5–20	200–500 mcg
Manganese	1	1	1	40–100 mcg
Chromium	0.05–0.2	0.2	0.14–0.2	5–15 mcg
Selenium	1.5–2	2	1–2	40–60 mcg

*Assumes normal age-related organ function. Recommended intakes of trace elements cannot be achieved through the use of a single pediatric multiple–trace element product. Only through the use of individualized trace element products can recommended intakes of trace elements be achieved.

2. A 1.2-micron filter should be used for TNA formulations.
3. Alternatively, a 1.2-micron filter may be used for all PN formulations.
4. Occlusion of a filter during PN infusion could be indicative of a problem; the filter may be replaced but should never be removed altogether.

F. PN final containers and administration sets free of the plasticizer di(2-ethylhexyl)phthalate (DEHP) should be used to prevent DEHP contamination of TNAs or separate IVFE infusions.[16] DEHP is highly lipophilic, and IVFE are capable of extracting DEHP from the polyvinyl chloride (PVC) containers/administration sets. DEHP is a known neurotoxic, hepatoxic, and carcinogenic agent in animal models. The use of DEHP-free bags and tubing is especially important in chronic long-term patients, pregnant patients, and pediatric patients receiving PN.

G. Administration sets[9,12]
1. PN administration sets are changed using aseptic technique and universal precautions.
2. TNA administration sets are changed every 24 hours and immediately upon suspected contamination, or if the product integrity has been compromised.
3. 2-in-1 administration sets are changed every 72 hours.
4. Administration sets for a separate IVFE infusion are discarded after use, or at least every 12 hours if the IVFE is infused continuously.

H. PN is to administered via an infusion pump having adequate protection from "free flow" and reliable audible alarms.[9,17,18]
1. Infusion pumps ensure accurate volume (rate) control and contain safety alarms (visual and auditory) for sensing air and pressure changes in the IV tubing; some pumps also have a programmable rate-cycling feature to minimize infusion errors. These infusion pump features are key to ensuring safe PN administration because of the hypertonic nature, fluid volume, dextrose content, and potassium content of the PN formulation.
2. Regular infusion pump preventative maintenance and testing should be performed, as health care practitioners administering the PN rely on the pump and its alarms to optimize safe infusion of the PN formulation.

I. Medical devices for PN administration should minimize the risk of needle-stick injuries and patient/caregiver exposure to blood-borne pathogens.[19–21]
1. Federal agencies have published standards to prevent needle-stick injuries in health care settings and enforcement procedures regarding occupational exposure to blood-borne pathogens. These standards are laws and are enforced in the same manner as other Occupational Safety and Health Administration laws.
2. Health care providers administering PN should take an active role in identifying, evaluating, and selecting available effective medical devices to reduce exposure to blood-borne pathogens, for instance, needle-less systems to draw blood or the application of a needle-free catheter patency device to the CVC that eliminates the backflow of blood into the catheter lumen.

J. The PN infusion should be completed within 24 hours of initiation.[12]

K. IVFE infused separately from the PN formulation should be completed within 12 hours of entry into the original container.[12]

L. Each PN formulation should be inspected prior to administration, and the PN formulation should not be infused if visual changes or precipitates are apparent.[14] The pharmacist evaluates the PN formulation before dispensing, and the nurse, patient, or caregiver is responsible for ongoing evaluation of the PN prior to and during the infusion.

M. Patients may tolerate the PN infusion better if the refrigerated PN is removed from the refrigerator 30 to 60 minutes prior to the infusion time; patients occasionally complain of discomfort when the chilled formulation is infused into the central circulation.[9]

N. Patients receiving PN formulation for the first time should be monitored closely for any adverse reactions.

V. Monitoring and Management of PN

A. Serious complications can be associated with PN administration. The potential for serious complications with PN is unacceptably high unless careful monitoring is conducted by experienced clinicians.

B. Monitoring by experienced clinicians can control costs and minimize complications. Suggested protocols for monitoring PN in neonates/pediatric patients and adults are shown in Tables 8-8 and 8-9, respectively.

C. Once it is determined that an individual requires PN, the goals for specialized nutrition support should be set with specific markers and outcomes.[1,22] These goals may include the following:
1. Stabilization of weight or moving toward goal weight
2. Improvement or replenishment of protein stores
3. Normalization of clinical laboratory values
4. Reduction in morbidity/mortality
5. Improvement in quality of life
6. Optimization of clinical outcomes

D. Nutrition monitoring should be conducted and monitored parameters compared to the goals of the nutrition care plan.
1. All individuals receiving PN should be monitored for fluid, electrolyte, and acid/base imbalances.

TABLE 8-8. Monitoring—Neonates/Pediatric Patients on PN

Parameter	Initial	Daily	Weekly
Anthropometric			
Weight	•	•	
Length	•		•*
Head circumference	•		•*
Physical examination	•	•	
Fluid balance	•	•	
Metabolic assessment			
Na, K, Cl, CO_2	•	•	•**
Ca, Phos, Mg	•		•
Glucose	•	•	•**
BUN/Cr	•		•
Liver profile	•		•
Triglycerides	•***		•
Urine glucose	•	•	
Complete blood count	•		•
Prealbumin	•****		•

BUN, blood urea nitrogen.
*Weekly until 3 months of age.
**Daily until stable, then once or twice weekly.
***Initially and before each advancement of intravenous fat emulsions, then once weekly. If septic, more frequent monitoring is prudent.
****Prealbumin approaches adult values at approximately 3 months of age.

TABLE 8-9. Monitoring for Adult Patients on Parenteral Nutrition

Parameter	Baseline	Critically ill patients	Stable patients
Chemistry screen (Ca, Mg, LFTs, P)	Yes	2–3x/week	Weekly
Electrolytes, BUN, creatinine	Yes	Daily	1–2x/week
Serum triglycerides	Yes	Weekly	Weekly
CBC with differential	Yes	Weekly	Weekly
PT, PTT	Yes	Weekly	Weekly
Capillary glucose	3x/day	3x/day (until consistently <200 mg/dL)	3x/day (until consistently <200 mg/dL)
Weight	If possible	Daily	2–3x weekly
Intake and output	Daily	Daily	Daily unless fluid status is assessed by physical exam
Nitrogen balance	As needed	As needed	As needed
Indirect calorimetry	As needed	As needed	As needed

BUN, blood urea nitrogen; CBC, complete blood count; LFT = liver function test; PT, prothrombin time; PTT, partial thromboplastin time.

a) In general, it is inappropriate to manage short-term fluid, electrolyte, and acid-base imbalances by PN alone. However, adjustments in fluid, electrolyte, and acid-base content of PN may avoid the risk and expense inherent in providing supplemental fluids and electrolytes.
b) PN volume may be concentrated for patients at risk for volume overload or expanded to meet the needs of patients with increased fluid requirements.
c) The electrolyte composition of PN may be varied based on the electrolyte profile, changes in clinical status, organ function, and medications.
d) Acid-base disorders of metabolic origin may respond to adjustments in the amount of chloride or acetate in PN.
e) Acid-base disorders of respiratory origin will usually respond to correction of the underlying problem or adjustments of the ventilator.[23]

2. All patients receiving PN should be monitored for proper glucose control.
3. One or more visceral protein concentrations (eg, albumin, prealbumin, transferrin) should be evaluated with consideration given to their half-life and changes in patient fluid status, organ function, and presence of infection. If an unsatisfactory response is observed, a nitrogen-balance study may be used to guide nutrient intake. Serum albumin concentration is a poor marker of nutritional repletion or depletion because of its long half-life and large body pool. However, serum albumin has been shown to be an excellent prognostic marker for patient outcome.
4. Typically, laboratory monitoring of serum chemistries and visceral proteins is more frequent when PN is initiated and decreases in frequency once a degree of metabolic stability is demonstrated. The health care provider needs to be alert to potential changes in fluid status and should closely monitor intake and output, presence of edema, vital signs, and weight with attention to changes, patterns, or trends that could indicate problems or progress toward achieving nutrition goals.

E. It is important that the health care provider periodically compare the actual PN infused into the patient with the recommended, measured, or estimated nutrition needs to ensure optimal treatment.
F. The nutrient content of the administered PN should be regularly compared with predicted energy and protein needs. Changes in clinical condition and activity level may require periodic reassessment of energy requirements.
G. GI function and readiness for oral/enteral feeding should be assessed whenever the patient's clinical condition changes.
H. Adjustments of the PN formula may be necessary as oral intake begins or improves.
I. Regular assessments and meticulous care of the parenteral access device ensure a reliable delivery system for the PN and minimize infection.
J. Extensive attention is directed toward monitoring the patient's physiological response to PN therapy, but it is equally important to assess, monitor, and manage the patient's developmental, emotional, and psychological response to PN.

VI. Complications of PN

Although widely reported, complications of PN can be minimized when a multidisciplinary team of trained professionals monitors PN therapy and venous access devices.

A. Peripheral venous access catheters for PN
   1. The indication for PPN infusion is a short-term need for PN.
   2. The patient receiving PPN should have no fluid restrictions.
   3. Infusion of PN via a peripheral vein requires careful consideration of the formulation's osmolarity (<900 mOsm/L) along with judicious monitoring of the venous access site for phlebitis and/or infiltration.
   4. The peripheral venous access catheter should be removed as soon as thrombophlebitis develops or an infiltration is noted.
   5. The Centers for Disease Control and Prevention (CDC) recommends the following[12]:
      a) Replace peripheral venous catheters at least every 72 to 96 hours in adults to prevent phlebitis and bacterial catheter colonization. However, in pediatric patients, the risk for phlebitis is not increased with the duration of catheter days, so the peripheral venous catheter should be left in place until the IV therapy is completed unless complications (phlebitis, infiltration) occur.
      b) Use a transparent, semipermeable polyurethane dressing or a gauze dressing to cover the peripheral access site.
      c) Replace the dressing when the catheter is removed or replaced, or when the dressing becomes damp, loosened, or soiled.
   6. Hydrocortisone and heparin may be added to 2-in-1 PN formulations to decrease phlebitis.

B. CVCs for PN
   1. General information
      a) Central PN is administered via a CVC with the distal tip placed in the superior vena cava adjacent to the right atrium.[14]
      b) Proper CVC tip placement must be confirmed before initiating PN, as well as any time signs or symptoms indicate an improper catheter position.

c) Venous access catheters should be promptly removed when no longer needed.

2. Catheter occlusion: the inability to infuse a solution and/or aspirate a blood sample
   a) Thrombotic occlusion[9,17]
      (1) Intraluminal clotting as a result of inadequate flushing or blood reflux. Treat by instilling a thrombolytic agent directly into the catheter, not to exceed the volume capacity of the catheter. Protocols for the organizational use of thrombolytic agents to restore catheter patency must be developed.
      (2) Fibrin sheath/fibrin sleeve at the distal catheter tip: parenteral admixtures can be infused without trouble, but blood samples cannot be aspirated. Thrombolytic agents directly instilled into the catheter exceeding the volume capacity of the catheter may correct this problem, or an endovascular procedure to remove the fibrin sheath may be needed to salvage the catheter.
      (3) Subclavian vein thrombosis. Subclavian vein thrombosis can occlude a catheter and manifest clinical symptoms of vascular obstruction. Symptoms include neck vein distention, edema, pain or tingling over the ipsilateral arm and neck, throat tightness, and prominent anterior chest wall vein distention. This situation is serious and requires immediate physician intervention. Catheter-related subclavian thrombosis is the most common cause of upper arm extremity deep vein thrombosis, and there is a 12% incidence of pulmonary embolus with a subclavian thrombosis.[24,25] Treatment of the subclavian thrombosis may include catheter removal, elevation of the affected arm, catheter-directed thrombolytic agent infusion, systemic infusion of a thrombolytic agent, and/or endovascular stenting.
   b) Nonthrombotic occlusion
      (1) Intraluminal drug precipitates can result in catheter occlusions.
      (2) Catheter irrigations with 0.1N hydrochloric acid may dissolve occlusions caused by calcium phosphate or other mineral precipitates by decreasing the pH and improving solubility.[26]
      (3) Catheter irrigations with a 70% ethanol-in-water solution or 0.1N sodium hydroxide may be used to clear an occlusion caused by fat emulsion.[27,28]
      (4) Protocols for the organizational use of precipitant clearance agents to restore catheter patency must be developed.
   c) Mechanical occlusion
      (1) Catheter malposition, external catheter or infusion clamps, kinking of the catheter, and/or constricting sutures should be assessed for and corrected.
      (2) "Pinch-off syndrome": Intermittent mechanical obstruction/occlusion is related to postural changes caused by catheter compression between the clavicle and first rib.[29] In certain patients, an anatomic narrow triangle exists at the junction of the axillary and subclavian vein. This junction is in the lateral aspect of the clavicle, and "pinch-off" may occur with medial placement of the CVC. Changing the patient's position by raising the ipsilateral arm (opening the angle) relieves the occlusion. Chest x-rays will demonstrate a luminal narrowing of the catheter at this site. Catheter removal is recommended, as the pinch-off syndrome can lead to catheter transection and embolus.

3. Infectious complications
   a) It has been estimated that over 200,000 nosocomial bloodstream infections occur yearly in the United States and that the majority of these infections are associated with venous access devices.[30]
   b) Catheter-related infection accounts for nearly 75% of all complications seen in pediatric patients receiving PN therapy.[31]
   c) The multidisciplinary health care team providing and monitoring the efficacy of the PN therapy has a responsibility to minimize catheter infections.
      (1) Reductions in catheter-associated sepsis occur when specially trained registered nurses care for the CVC.[1]
      (2) Proper hand hygiene procedures—involving hand washing with conventional antiseptic-containing soap and water or with waterless alcohol-based gels or foams—must be observed.
      (3) Care and maintenance of the CVC must be performed according to published standards.[9,12]
      (4) Aseptic technique must be observed for the insertion and care of the intravascular catheter.
      (5) The CDC also makes the following recommendations[12]:
         (a) To prevent catheter-related infections, adult CVCs or percutaneously inserted central catheters (PICCs) should not be routinely replaced. The CDC makes no recommendations in this area for pediatric patients.
         (b) CVCs or PICCs should not be removed on the basis of fever alone. Use clinical judgment regarding removal of the catheter if infection is detected elsewhere or if a noninfectious cause of fever is suspected.
         (c) If no evidence of infection is present, guidewire exchange to replace a nontunneled catheter should be performed only to replace a malfunctioning catheter.
         (d) If a multilumen catheter is used for fluids, one port should be designated exclusively for PN administration. A CVC should have the minimum number of ports/lumens necessary for clinical management of the patient.
         (e) Antibiotic lock solutions should not be routinely used in an attempt to prevent catheter-related bloodstream infection.
         (f) Clean skin should be disinfected with an appropriate antiseptic before catheter insertion and during dressing changes. A 2% chlorhexidine-based prep is preferred (no recommendations for chlorhexidine in infants <2 months can be made), though tincture of iodine, an iodophor, or 70% alcohol can be used. No topical antibiotic ointment or creams should be placed on catheter insertion sites (except dialysis catheters) because of the potential for antimicrobial resistance and fungal infections. Organic solvents (eg, acetone, ether) should never be applied to the skin. The catheter insertion site should then be covered with either a sterile gauze or a sterile, transparent, semipermeable dressing. Gauze dressings should be changed every 2 days, and sterile, transparent dressings should be changed at least weekly, depending on the patient's clinical circumstances.
         (g) All catheter injection ports should be cleansed with 70% alcohol or an iodophor before the system is accessed.
         (h) The CDC has published specific guidelines for the care of umbilical catheters.[12]

C. GI tract
1. Disuse of the GI tract can lead to some degree of villous atrophy and possibly bacterial translocation.
2. Bacterial translocation may be avoided with enteral feeding, but the amount and type of enteral feeding required to prevent bacterial translocation is unknown.
3. Hepatobiliary complications[32]
   a) Mildly elevated transaminase and alkaline phosphatase concentrations usually occur 2 weeks after PN is initiated.
   b) Elevated serum bilirubin is seen less often, and jaundice does not occur in most adults.
   c) Elevated enzyme concentrations may return to normal while the patient is still on PN but almost always normalize when PN is stopped.
   d) Causes of hepatic abnormalities related to PN include steatosis, especially with infusion of carbohydrate at rates greater than 5 mg/kg/minute, and sepsis.
   e) A metabolic complication seen more frequently in the pediatric population than in adults is the development of PN-associated cholestasis (PNAC), the most life-threatening long-term complication of PN therapy in children.
   f) The incidence of PNAC in children receiving long-term PN is estimated at 30% to 60%.[33]
   g) The etiology of PNAC is believed to be multifactorial. It has been associated with recurrent sepsis, delays in enteral feeding, bacterial overgrowth, excessive dextrose administration, altered amino acid profiles, prematurity, low birth weight, long duration of PN, short-bowel syndrome, and elevated levels of lithocholic acid.
   h) While no definitive preventive measure is known, efforts to minimize the incidence of PNAC should be directed toward early initiation of EN, prevention and aggressive treatment of sepsis, avoidance of overfeeding, and use of cyclic PN for prolonged therapy.[1]
   i) A sustained upward trend of conjugated bilirubin and alkaline phosphatase serve as a warning that the patient may be at risk of developing PNAC and should prompt reevaluation of the PN regimen and transition to EN when medically possible.
4. Management of PN-induced hepatobiliary abnormalities usually includes giving about one third of calories as IVFE, cycling the PN so that the patient is off PN 8 to 10 hours per day, and using enteral nutrition to stimulate bile flow.

D. Metabolic
1. Osteopenia of prematurity, also commonly termed metabolic bone disease (MBD), is a complication of long-term PN therapy. While the incidence of MBD is unknown, the patient population at highest risk of developing MBD is premature infants (<34 weeks gestation at birth or <1.5 kg birth weight). Major factors compromising bone mineralization are deficiencies in phosphorus, calcium, and vitamin D. Aluminum, found as a contaminant in PN formulations, may also decrease the rate of bone formation and mineralization. Amounts of aluminum exceeding 5 mcg/kg/day may be associated with bone toxicity. The severity of MBD can vary from mild subclinical bone undermineralization to nontraumatic fractures. Maximizing calcium and phosphorus intake soon after birth to match intrauterine accretion rates can help prevent the development of MBD. Calcium and phosphorus intake at a ratio of 1.7:1 (Ca:P) by weight has produced mineral retention of approximately 90% in very low birth weight infants receiving PN.[34]
2. MBD can also occur in adults on long-term PN therapy. See Table 8-10 for monitoring and management guidelines for MBD.

TABLE 8-10. Suggested Guidelines for Monitoring and Managing PN-Associated MBD

1. Evaluate all patients receiving long-term PN >1 year for MBD.
2. Monitor for physical signs of MBD: loss of height, bone or back pain.
3. Provide adequate amounts of minerals in the PN solution for bone remodeling, including calcium 15 mEq, phosphorus 15 mM, magnesium (adjust amount for serum and urine levels).
4. Reduce higher protein doses to 1 g/kg/day once nutritional status is stable.
5. Treat metabolic acidosis with adequate amounts of acetate in PN solutions.
6. Monitor serum (at least monthly) calcium, phosphorus, magnesium, and acetate concentrations. Maintain normal concentrations by adjusting amounts in the PN solutions. Specific markers of bone metabolism may be of further help.
7. Obtain 24-hour urine collection for calcium and magnesium every 6 to 12 months. Adjust PN to maintain positive balances.
8. Obtain DEXA measurement and refer patient to endocrinologist for evaluation and pharmacologic therapy if low bone mineral density (T-score below −1). Repeat DEXA every 1 to 2 years.
9. Minimize steroid use and all medications known to cause bone resorption.
10. Promote exercise or refer to physical therapist.
11. Encourage cessation of smoking.

Reprinted with permission from Hamilton C. Parenteral nutrition-associated metabolic bone disease. *Support Line*. 2003;25(5):7–13.

3. Refeeding syndrome is defined as a constellation of fluid, micronutrient, electrolyte, and vitamin imbalances that occurs within the first few days after refeeding of starved adult patients.[35] It is potentially life-threatening if not recognized and treated promptly.
   a) This syndrome may involve hemolytic anemia, respiratory distress, paresthesias, tetany, and cardiac arrhythmias.
   b) Biochemical findings include hypophosphatemia, hypomagnesemia, and hypokalemia.
   c) Proposed risk factors for refeeding syndrome include alcoholism, anorexia nervosa, marasmus, rapid refeeding, and excessive dextrose infusion.
   d) Suggested prevention of refeeding syndrome in the adult includes addressing repletion of serum potassium, magnesium, and phosphorus concentrations before initiating PN; limiting initial carbohydrate to 150 g/day and fluid to 800 mL/day in at-risk patients; providing adequate amounts of potassium, magnesium, phosphorus, and vitamins in initial PN; and increasing carbohydrate-dependent minerals in proportion to increases in carbohydrate when PN is advanced.
4. Hyperglycemia
   a) The incidence of hyperglycemia appears to be inversely related to developmental age and weight in the pediatric population. In neonates, hyperglycemia is defined as a plasma glucose concentration >150 mg/dL or a whole-blood glucose concentration >125 mg/dL. Prematurity, excessive dextrose infusions via PN, sepsis, surgery, or respiratory distress may

contribute to hyperglycemia. To minimize the risk of hyperglycemia in pediatric patients, as well as to avoid elevations in CO_2 in the systemic circulation, dextrose infusion rates in PN should not exceed 10 to 14 mg/kg/min.[1] To control PN-associated hyperglycemia in infants, continuous insulin infusion can be administered in a safe and effective manner.[36]

b) Risk factors for hyperglycemia (nonfasting blood glucose >180 mg/dL) in adults include metabolic stress, medications, obesity, and diabetes mellitus.

c) Techniques to minimize hyperglycemia in an adult receiving PN include glucose monitoring every 6 hours with initiation of PN; administration of dextrose in amounts less than the maximum glucose oxidation rate (<4 mg/kg/minute); and administration of decreased amounts of dextrose initially in at-risk patients (100–150 g/day or 2–3 mg/kg/minute).

d) For patients previously treated with insulin or oral hypoglycemic agents, a basal amount of human regular insulin should be added to the PN formulation to keep blood glucose concentrations below 180 mg/dL.

e) Only regular human insulin is compatible with PN formulations. Other insulin products such as NPH, ultralente, lente, lispro, aspart, and glargine are not compatible with PN.

f) A regimen of 0.1 units of insulin per gram of dextrose in the PN infusion can be used as a starting dose.[37,38] If the blood glucose is >300 mg/dL, PN should not be initiated until glycemic control is improved (<180 mg/dL).

g) In general, the dextrose content of the PN should not be increased until glucose concentrations during the previous 24-hour period are consistently <180 mg/dL.

h) If hyperglycemia persists when 0.3 units of insulin per gram of PN dextrose is exceeded, initiation of a separate IV insulin infusion should be considered to achieve more appropriate glycemic control.

i) The amount of insulin that adheres to the PN bag and tubing made from ethyl vinyl acetate or PVC is approximately 5% to 15%[39]; therefore, insulin requirements may appear slightly higher than they actually are.

5. Hypoglycemia can develop rapidly in neonates, young infants, and some adults upon interruption of PN.

a) Preterm neonates are at increased risk for developing hypoglycemia because of immature homeostatic mechanisms, limited glycogen stores, and increased glucose requirements.[40]

b) Hypoglycemia can be seen within 15 to 30 minutes after stopping PN, suggesting that glucose concentrations should be checked within 15 to 60 minutes.[41] PN can be tapered over 1 to 2 hours prior to discontinuation to prevent hypoglycemia episodes.[1] This tapering process is usually accomplished during the transition period between PN and enteral feeding.

6. Hyperlipidemia

a) Triglyceride (TG) levels provide a reasonable estimate of lipid clearance and should be maintained below 200 mg/dL in pediatric patients. Hypertriglyceridemia in pediatric populations is usually due to excessive fat administration, uncontrolled hyperglycemia, excessive carbohydrate administration without hyperglycemia, prematurity, low birth weight, or sepsis.

b) If baseline TG concentrations are <200 mg/dL, IVFE can be administered and TG concentrations monitored. A rise of ≥50 mg/dL warrants a temporary discontinuation or reduction in the infusion rate. Clinical consequences of hypertriglyceridemia include reduced oxygenation, impaired leukocyte function, deposition of lipids in the reticuloendothelial cells, and displacement of albumin-bound bilirubin by free fatty acids.[1]

c) In adult patients, IVFE should be limited to the provision of essential fatty acids (eg, 250 mL of 20% IVFE, once or twice weekly) when triglyceride concentrations rise above 400 mg/dL.[42]

d) Withholding IVFE must be considered when triglyceride concentrations are greater than 500 mg/dL or in the presence of lipemic serum. Topical administration of soybean or safflower oil may be a useful alternative under these conditions since topical linoleic acid is transcutaneously absorbed directly into plasma without exacerbating hypertriglyceridemia.[42]

E. Fluid and electrolytes[43]

1. Hyponatremia is frequently noted in patients receiving PN. The most common cause of hyponatremia is administration of excessive hypotonic fluid. Other causes include nephritis, adrenal insufficiency, congestive heart failure, the syndrome of inappropriate antidiuretic hormone, and cirrhosis with ascites. Symptoms of hyponatremia include confusion, hypotension, irritability, lethargy, and seizures. Depending on the etiology, hyponatremia is usually treated with fluid restriction or diuretics. If sodium intake is inadequate and the clinical condition warrants additional sodium intake, sodium may be increased in the PN formulation.

2. Hypernatremia occurs infrequently. Possible causes of hypernatremia include inadequate free water administration, excessive water loss (as with fever, burns, osmotic diuresis hyperventilation), or excessive sodium intake. Symptoms of hypernatremia include thirst, decreased skin turgor, and mild irritability. Increasing fluid intake usually treats hypernatremia; less often, reducing sodium content in the PN formulation treats it.

3. Hypokalemia may be caused by inadequate potassium intake, refeeding syndrome, or excessive losses with diarrhea or intestinal fluids. Drugs such as loop and thiazide diuretics, cathartics, and some antibiotics or antifungals (eg, amphotericin B) may increase urinary potassium losses. Hypomagnesemia may also give rise to hypokalemia. Symptoms of hypokalemia include nausea, vomiting, confusion, arrhythmias, respiratory depression, and cardiac arrest. Increasing the potassium content of the PN by providing it through a peripheral vein or by the GI route may treat hypokalemia. If potassium is to be administered via a peripheral vein or via the GI tract, it is necessary to collaborate with the pharmacist, as potassium supplements are very hypertonic and can cause significant irritation to the peripheral vein or the GI mucosa. If hypomagnesemia is present, it should be corrected first to facilitate correction of hypokalemia.

4. Hyperkalemia may be caused by renal dysfunction, administration of excessive potassium, metabolic acidosis, or potassium-sparing medications (eg, angiotensin-converting enzyme [ACE] inhibitors). Symptoms of hyperkalemia include diarrhea, paresthesia, tachycardia, oliguria, and cardiac arrest. Hyperkalemia may be managed by reducing potassium intake or, if severe, by using potassium exchange resins, insulin and dextrose, inhaled beta agonists, or dialysis.

5. Hypocalcemia may caused by decreased vitamin D intake, hypoparathyroidism, citrate binding of calcium with blood product administration, or hypoalbuminemia. Hypomagnesemia may also contribute to hypocalcemia. Symptoms of hypocalcemia include tetany, irritability, seizures, and ventricular arrhythmias. Hypocalcemia that is independent of hypoalbuminemia may be treated with calcium supplementation.

6. Hypercalcemia may be caused by renal failure, tumor lysis syndrome, bone cancer, administration of excess vitamin D, prolonged immobilization and stress, or hyperparathyroidism. Symptoms of hypercalcemia include confusion, dehydration, muscle weakness, nausea, vomiting, and coma. Hypercalcemia may be treated by administering isotonic saline, inorganic phosphate, corticosteroids, bisphosphonates, or mithramycin.
7. Hypomagnesemia may be caused by refeeding syndrome, alcoholism, diuretic use, prolonged nasogastric suction, increased stool output, diabetic ketoacidosis, or magnesium-wasting medications. Symptoms of hypomagnesemia include cardiac arrhythmias, tetany, convulsions, and muscular weakness. Parenteral magnesium supplementation should be used to treat moderate and severe hypomagnesemia since orally administered magnesium products are poorly absorbed.
8. Hypermagnesemia may be seen with excessive magnesium intake in renal insufficiency. Symptoms of hypermagnesemia include respiratory paralysis, hypotension, premature ventricular contractions, lethargy, coma, liver dysfunction, and cardiac arrest. Hypermagnesemia is usually treated by decreasing magnesium intake. Severe hypermagnesemia may necessitate dialysis.
9. Hypophosphatemia may be seen with refeeding syndrome, long-term alcoholism, and inadequate phosphorus intake. Symptoms of hypophosphatemia include congestive heart failure, arrhythmias, nausea and emesis, altered red blood cell morphology, hemolytic anemia, leukocyte dysfunction, ataxia, short-term paralysis, lethargy, confusion, coma, acute respiratory failure, acute tubular necrosis, and bicarbonate and glucose wasting. Moderate and severe hypophosphatemia should be treated with IV phosphate supplementation since oral phosphate products are poorly absorbed.
10. Hyperphosphatemia may be seen with administration of excess phosphate or with renal insufficiency. Symptoms of hyperphosphatemia include paresthesias, flaccid paralysis, mental confusion, hypertension, and cardiac arrhythmias. Tissue calcification may occur with prolonged elevated levels. Decreasing phosphorus intake and/or using enteral phosphate binders may treat hyperphosphatemia.

VII. Transitional Feeding and Discontinuing PN[44,45]

A. The ultimate goal for patients receiving PN is to return to as nearly normal food intake as tolerated. The period during which oral or enteral feeding is initiated and PN is discontinued may be termed the transitional period. The transition from PN to oral intake or enteral tube feeding should be accomplished in an orderly fashion to avoid the potential for deterioration in nutritional status when PN is discontinued.
   1. In pediatric patients, discontinuation of PN is generally a more gradual process than in adult patients.
      a) PN is tapered as enteral feeds are advanced. Ideally, the combination of PN and enteral feedings will meet all estimated nutritional goals during the transitional period.
      b) In practice, PN is generally continued until about 75% to 80% of energy needs (90–100 kcal/kg) are met enterally.
   2. For many adult patients, PN may be discontinued as soon as they are able to tolerate solid foods. These patients are usually younger, well nourished before PN, not debilitated, free of malignancy, and without oral intake for less than 1 to 2 weeks.
   3. For other adult patients, a detailed transitional feeding plan may be needed. Candidates for transitional feeding include those who are elderly or debilitated, those with malignancy, and those who eat ethnic foods not available in the hospital setting.
   4. Adult patients with known diabetes mellitus or clinically induced insulin resistance require special monitoring to set up a safe transitional feeding plan.

B. To guide the transition from PN to full oral intake, a bedside calorie count may be performed when the patient is eating a substantial amount of food with a consistent appetite or effort but unsure of how much may have been tolerated or consumed. This count may be used to guide the reduction or discontinuation of PN.

C. Although it has been documented that nondiabetic adult patients suffer minimal ill effects, abrupt discontinuance of PN may potentiate rebound hypoglycemia in patients who are not being fed orally or enterally.
   1. PN may be rapidly discontinued in an adult patient who is tolerating tube feeding in amounts adequate to maintain serum glucose levels.
   2. Decreasing the PN infusion rate by one-half for 1 to 2 hours before discontinuation may minimize the risk of rebound hypoglycemia.
   3. If PN is abruptly discontinued, a 10% dextrose solution may be administered for a few hours. This practice is unnecessary when discontinuing PPN.
   4. Capillary glucose concentrations may be measured 30 to 60 minutes after cessation of a central PN formulation, and oral or IV carbohydrate can be given as appropriate if hypoglycemia is suspected.

D. Oral or enteral tube feeding may be initiated when the patient has demonstrated return of GI function.

E. Initiation of oral intake requires GI function, minimal risk for aspiration, and patient motivation.

F. In some circumstances, a swallowing evaluation may be useful in determining readiness for oral feeding and can dictate the type and texture of foods introduced.

G. PN may have a negative effect on appetite. If more than 25% of caloric needs are provided as PN, reduced oral intake can be expected.[46]
   1. When oral intake equals 500 kcal/day in an adult patient, the carbohydrate and protein in the PN should be reduced by an amount equal to the amount consumed orally.
   2. Subsequent decreases in the PN should continue as oral intake increases.
   3. Once an adult patient is taking 60% of goal energy and protein via the oral route, PN may be stopped.

H. For adults who do not achieve acceptable oral intake within a few days, enteral tube feeding should be considered.

I. For adults who have been receiving substantial amounts of electrolytes in the PN, oral or IV electrolyte supplements may be needed.

(Parenteral Nutrition Management chapters from the 1st edition were contributed by Annalynn Skipper, Keith Millikan, Kristy Gibbons, Nancy Cyr, Michael L. Christensen, and Richard A. Helms)

REFERENCES

1. A.S.P.E.N. Board of Directors and the Clinical Guidelines Task Force. Guidelines for the use of parenteral and enteral nutrition in adult and pediatric patients. *J Parenter Enteral Nutr.* 2002;26(suppl):1SA–138SA.
2. Institute of Medicine. Minerals. *Recommended Dietary Allowances.* 10th ed. Washington, DC: National Academy Press; 1989:174–194.

3. Baumgartner TG. *Clinical Guide to Parenteral Micronutrition.* 3rd ed. Fujisawa USA; Deerfield, IL 1997.
4. Rudman D, Millikan WJ, Richardson TJ, et al. Elemental balances during intravenous hyperalimentation of underweight adult subjects. *J Clin Invest.* 1975:55:94–104.
5. American Medical Association Department of Foods and Nutrition. Multivitamin preparations for parenteral use: a statement by the Nutrition Advisory Group. *J Parenter Enteral Nutr.* 1979:3:258–262.
6. American Medical Association Department of Foods and Nutrition. Guidelines for essential trace element preparations for parenteral use: a statement by an expert panel. *J Am Med Assoc.* 1979;241:2051–2054.
7. McMahon M, Manji N, Driscoll DF, Bistrian BR. Parenteral nutrition in patients with diabetes mellitus: theoretical and practical considerations. *J Parenter Enteral Nutr.* 1989;13:545–553.
8. Kalhan SC, Kilic I. Carbohydrate as nutrient in the infant and child: range of acceptable intake. *Euro J Clin Nutr.* 1999;53(suppl 1):S94–S100.
9. Intravenous Nurses Society. Infusion nursing: standards of practice. *J Intravenous Nurs.* 2000;23(suppl):S1–S88.
10. A.S.P.E.N. Board of Directors and the Task Force on Standards for Specialized Nutrition Support for Hospitalized Adult Patients. Standards for specialized nutrition support: adult hospitalized patients. *Nutr Clin Pract.* 2002;17:384–391.
11. Harden JL, Kemp C, Mirtallo J. Femoral catheters increase risk of infection in total parenteral nutrition patients. *Nutr Clin Pract.* 1995;10:60–66.
12. Centers for Disease Control and Prevention. Guidelines for the prevention of intravascular catheter-related infections. *MMWR.* 2002;51(No. RR-10).
13. Bethune K, Allwood M, Grainger C, Wormleighton C. British Pharmaceutical Nutrition Group Working Party. Use of filters during the preparation and administration of parenteral nutrition: position paper and guidelines prepared by a British pharmaceutical nutrition group working party. *Nutrition.* 2001;17:403–408.
14. Task Force for Safe Practices for Parenteral Nutrition. Safe practices for parenteral nutrition. *J Parenter Enteral Nutr.* 2004;28:S39–S70.
15. Food and Drug Administration. Safety alert: hazards of precipitation associated with parenteral nutrition. *Am J Hosp Pharm.* 1994;51:1427–1428.
16. Dickerson RN. Di(2-ethylhexyl)phthalate as a plasticizer for intravenous bags and tubing: a toxicological quandary. *Nutrition.* 1997;13:1010–1012.
17. Krzywda EA, Andris DA, Edmiston CE, Wallace JR. Parenteral access devices. In: Gottschlich MM, ed. *The Science and Practice of Nutrition Support: A Case-Based Core Curriculum.* Dubuque, IA: Kendall/Hunt; 2001:225–250.
18. JCAHO. 2005 National Patient Safety Goals FAQs. www.jcaho.org/accredited+organizations/patient+safety/05+npsg/05_npsg.html Accessed December 8, 2004
19. US Department of Health and Human Services, Public Health Service, Centers for Disease Control and Prevention, National Institute for Occupational Safety and Health Settings (NIOSH). *Preventing Needlestick Injuries in Health Settings.* NIOSH Publication No 2000-108. Cincinnati, OH:NIOSH;November; 1999.
20. US Department of Labor, Occupational Safety and Health Administration. *Enforcement Procedures for the Occupational Exposure to Bloodborne Pathogens. Directives No CPL 2-2.44D.* Effective date: November 5, 1999. US Department of Labor, Washington DC, 1999.
21. US Department of Labor, Occupational Safety and Health Administration. *Occupational Exposure to Bloodborne Pathogens; Needlesticks and Other Sharp Injuries; Final Rule Federal Legislation, Public Law 106-430.* Effective date: April 18, 2001. US Department of Labor, Washington DC, 2001.
22. A.S.P.E.N. Board of Directors. *Clinical Pathways and Algorithms for Delivery of Parenteral and Enteral Nutrition in Adults.* Silver Spring, MD: American Society for Parenteral and Enteral Nutrition; 1998.
23. Nehme AE. Nutritional support of the hospitalized patient: the team concept. *JAMA.* 1980;243:1906–1908.
24. Kerr TM, Lutter KS, Moeller DM, et al. Upper extremity venous thrombosis diagnosed by duplex scanning. *Am J Surg.* 1990;160:202–206.
25. Horattas MC, Wright DJ, Fenton AH, et al. Changing concepts of deep venous thrombosis of the upper extremity: report of a series and review of the literature. *Surgery.* 1988;104:561–567.
26. Shulman RJ, Reed T, Pitre D, et al. The use of hydrochloric acid to clear obstructed central venous catheters. *J Parenter Enteral Nutr.* 1988;12:509–510.
27. Pennington CR, Pithie AD. Ethanol lock in the management of catheter occlusion. *J Parenter Enteral Nutr.* 1987;11:507–508.
28. Borg FT, Timmer J, de Kam SS, Sauerwein HP. Use of sodium hydroxide solution to clear partially occluded vascular access ports. *J Parenter Enteral Nutr.* 1993;17:289–291.
29. Andris DA, Krzywda EA. Catheter pinch-off syndrome: recognition and management. *J Intravenous Nurs.* 1997;20:233–237.
30. Maki DG, Stolz SM, Wheeler S, et al. Prevention of central venous catheter–related bloodstream infection by use of an antiseptic-impregnated catheter: a randomized, controlled trial. *Ann Intern Med.* 1997;127:257–266.
31. Adal KA, Farr BM. Central venous catheter-related infections: a review. *Nutrition.* 1996;12:208–213.
32. Fleming CR. Hepatobiliary complications in adults receiving nutrition support. *Dig Dis.* 1994;12:191–198.
33. Suita S, Ikeda K, Nagasaki A, et al. Follow-up studies of children treated with a long-term intravenous nutrition during the neonatal period. *J Pediatr Surg.* 1982;17:37–42.
34. Pelegano JF, Rowe JC, Carey DE, et al. Simultaneous infusion of calcium and phosphorus in parenteral nutrition for premature infants: use of physiologic calcium/phosphorus ratio. *J Pediatr.* 1989;114:115–119.
35. Brooks MJ, Melnik G. The refeeding syndrome: an approach to understanding its complications and preventing its occurrence. *Pharmacotherapy.* 1995;15:713–726.
36. Collins JW Jr, Hoppe M, Brown K, et al. A controlled trial of insulin infusion and parenteral nutrition in extremely low birth weight infants with glucose intolerance. *J Pediatr.* 1991;118:921–927.
37. McCowen KC, Malhotra A, Bistrian BR. Stress-induced hyperglycemia. *Crit Care Clin.* 2001;17:107–124.
38. McCowen KC, Bistrian BR. Hyperglycemia and nutrition support: theory and practice. *Nutr Clin Pract.* 204;19:235–244.
39. Marcuard SP, Dunham B, Hobbs A, Caro JF. Availability of insulin from total parenteral nutrition solutions. *J Parenter Enteral Nutr.* 1990;14:262–264.
40. Farrag HM, Cowett RM. Glucose homeostasis in the micropremie. *Clin Perinatol.* 2000;27:1–22.
41. Werlin SL, Wyatt D, Camitta B. Effect of abrupt discontinuation of high glucose infusion rates during parenteral nutrition. *J Pediatr.* 1994;124:441–444.
42. Sacks GS, Mouser JF. Is IV lipid emulsion safe in adult patients with hypertriglyceridemia? *Nutr Clin Pract.* 1997;3:120–123.
43. Brown RO, Dickerson RN. Drug-nutrient interactions. *Am J Managed Care.* 1999;5:345–352.
44. Wagman LP, Miller KB, Thomas RB, Newsome HH, Weir GC. The effect of acute discontinuation of total parenteral nutrition. *Ann Surg.* 1986;204:524–529.
45. Winkler MF, Pomp A, Caldwell MD, Albina JE. Transitional feeding: the relationship between nutritional intake and plasma protein concentrations. *J Am Diet Assoc.* 1989;89:969–970.
46. Gil KM, Skeie B, Kvetan V, Askanazi J, Freidman MI. Parenteral nutrition and oral intake: effect of glucose and fat infusions. *J Parenter Enteral Nutr.* 1991;15:426–432.

SUGGESTED READINGS

Klein S, Kinney J, Jeejeebhoy K, et al. Nutrition support in clinical practice: review of published data and recommendations for future research directions. *J Parenter Enteral Nutr.* 1997;21:133–156.

Rombeau JL, Rolandelli RR, eds. *Clinical Nutrition: Parenteral Nutrition.* 3rd ed. Philadelphia, PA: WB Saunders; 2001.

Michael S. Nyffeler, PharmD, BCNSP;
Eric Frankel, PharmD, BCNSP; Edmund Hayes, PharmD;
Stephanie Mighdoll, PharmD

9

Drug-Nutrient Interactions

Introduction

The goal of a multidisciplinary approach to monitoring enterally and parenterally fed patients for drug-nutrient interactions is to maximize the therapeutic response to the medication administered without adversely affecting enteral nutrition tolerance. This chapter addresses principles of drug absorption, distribution, and metabolism along with potential drug-nutrient interactions in these patients.

I. Background

A. Absorption

1. Enteral

a) Absorption requires movement of medication from the gastrointestinal (GI) tract into the general circulation. Not all of a drug dose is necessarily absorbed, and not all absorbed drug reaches the systemic circulation as active drug. Some of the absorbed drug is eliminated or metabolized in the GI tract or liver before it reaches its site of action. Absorption of medication is generally what is affected when drug-nutrient interactions occur in enterally fed patients.

b) Bioavailability is the percentage of the original dose that reaches the systemic circulation as active drug[1]; the process of bioavailability is distinctly different from absorption.

c) Disintegration and dissolution of a drug in the aqueous digestive fluid must occur prior to absorption, if the medication is not already in solution. Medications that are formulated as suspensions must also undergo dissolution. Once a medication has dissolved, it can then diffuse across the intestinal mucosa.[2]

(1) For most solid-dose forms (tablets, capsules), the rate-limiting step of absorption is dissolution.[2] Disintegration is the process of a solid-dose form breaking down into smaller particles, which improves the rate at which a drug then dissolves so that absorption may occur. Stomach churning in the presence of aqueous fluids aids in disintegration and dissolution. Once the components of the tablet have been adequately reduced in size, they leave the stomach and enter the small bowel, where the majority of absorption occurs. The small bowel provides a large surface area and is well perfused to enhance the absorption process.[2]

(2) For liquid medications in solution, the rate-limiting step to absorption is blood perfusion of the intestines, where absorption takes place.[2] Adequate perfusion of the small bowel is necessary for proper absorption. Disease states, edema, surgery, and sepsis may decrease perfusion.

(3) Absorption of medication may be altered by factors such as the presence of other drugs, the gastric emptying rate, the route of administration, the location of the distal tip of the enteral tube, or the presence of food.

d) Factors that alter medication absorption

(1) Approaches to enhance absorption

(a) Use liquid medications to bypass the dissolution step; if tablets are used, they should be pulverized to enhance dissolution and subsequent absorption.[3]

(b) Administer liquid medications or pulverized tablets with adequate fluid. Fluid helps expand the stomach, thereby enhancing the rate of gastric emptying.

(c) Many enterally fed patients do not meet their daily fluid requirements with enteral feeding alone, and they require additional free water throughout the day. Whenever possible, administer additional free water flushes in conjunction with scheduled medications. These flushes provide an excellent medium for delivery of medication, enhance its absorption, and maintain enteral tube patency.

(2) Factors that may inhibit optimal absorption

(a) Enteral tubes are placed with the distal tip in the stomach, duodenum, or jejunum. Absorption may become an issue for medications when the distal end of the enteral feeding tube is placed beyond the main site of absorption.

i) Itraconazole is a medication that requires an acidic environment to ensure proper dissolution when administered as a solid dosage form. Absorption will be poor if delivered in the jejunum because dissolution is inadequate. The liquid form, on the other hand, is already dissolved and does not require the acidic environment of the stomach for dissolution to occur; therefore, it is amenable to postpyloric administration. Extemporaneous preparations of itraconazole are not reliably absorbed.[4–5] No studies to date have evaluated itraconazole absorption with concurrent enteral feedings.

ii) The main site of absorption of ciprofloxacin is the upper part of the intestinal tract.[6] Studies have indicated mixed results with respect to ciprofloxacin absorption via feeding tubes. When ciprofloxacin is administered via a jejunostomy tube, reduction in absorption may result in treatment failure; therefore, this type of administration is not advised.[7]

(b) Medications delivered directly into the jejunum rather than the stomach can be expected to have a decreased transit time, reducing the amount of time during which the medication can be absorbed. Tablets delivered directly into the jejunum lose the positive churning and dissolution activity of the stomach, yet the jejunum is still a viable option for administration of most medications.[3]

(c) Some medications (eg, penicillin, tetracycline, rifampin), are better absorbed when taken "on an empty stomach." Patients who receive continuous feeding by gastric tube never have an empty stomach. To optimize absorption of such medications, tube feeding should be held approximately 30 to 60 minutes before and 30 minutes after the medication is administered; the tube-feeding schedule should then be readjusted to meet the patient's total 24-hour nutritional needs.

(d) If patients develop GI intolerances during tube feedings (eg, nausea, vomiting, diarrhea, increased gastric residuals, cramping), the medication profile should be reviewed for potential causative agents. Whenever possible, change to medications with therapeutic equivalents or change the route of administration before considering discontinuation of tube feeding.

(e) Use of prokinetic agents (eg, metoclopramide) may decrease transit time, alter absorption of some medications, and contribute to diarrhea.[8]

(f) Medications that delay gastric emptying or decrease GI motility

i) Anticholinergics (eg, antihistamines, tricyclic antidepressants, phenothiazines, medications for Parkinson's disease) cause smooth muscle relaxation and inhibit gastric motility.[9]

ii) Aluminum-containing antacids delay gastric emptying.

iii) Narcotics interfere with normal peristalsis and delay gastric emptying.[9]

2. Parenteral

a) Parenteral routes of drug delivery. Technically, the term parenteral refers to all drug administration other than by the GI tract. Commonly, the term is used to refer to the intravenous (IV) route, where the drug is injected into the body. Parenteral delivery of medication avoids the issue of absorption, as the entire dose will enter the body. Once the drug is in the bloodstream, the action of the drug is the same without regard for administration route. With few exceptions, oral administration of drugs is favored, as is oral administration of nutrients.

b) Effect of route on kinetics. A large variety of drug delivery routes fall under the umbrella of parenteral administration. Rapid IV infusion (IV push), controlled IV infusion over a short period of time (IV piggyback or secondary administration), and continuous IV infusion (IV drip) are all common parenteral drug administration methods. Intra-arterial delivery is also done for certain drugs to deliver a concentrated dose to a specific organ.

c) Effect of entry point into bloodstream (first-pass effect or lack of same affecting systemic dose). The point at which a drug enters the bloodstream can affect its bioavailability. Most parenterally administered drugs enter the bloodstream via the capillary or venous circulation. In contrast, enterally administered drugs (with a few exceptions for gastric, sublingual, and buccal administration) will enter the portal circulation and be transported to the liver before entering the general circulation. Since this occurs only after initial absorption, it is referred to as the first-pass effect. The liver is the major site of biotransformation of organic substances and exerts a profound effect on many enterally absorbed substances. Dosage differences for drugs given orally versus parenterally can be large; in the case of propranolol, for instance, the oral dose is approximately 10 times the IV dose. First-pass effect can also change the action of a drug. The composition of early pediatric parenteral amino acids was based on the amino acids in human breast milk. However, because human breast milk undergoes biotransformation by the liver before entering the general circulation and parenteral amino acids bypass the liver entirely, parenteral amino acids for neonates are now designed to match the serum aminograms of breast-fed infants, not the amino acid composition of human breast milk.

B. Distribution

1. Volume of distribution defined. When a substance enters the body, it is distributed via the bloodstream to many tissues. It achieves varying concentrations in these tissues based on the solubility of the drug and its affinity for each tissue. If a drug has a high affinity for muscle or fat, serum levels of the drug will be lowered. An artificial construct called apparent volume of distribution or simply volume of distribution (V_d) is used to predict the kinetics of a substance. Volume of distribution is defined as the volume in which the substance entering the body would need to be diluted to achieve the observed serum levels. The volume of distribution is expressed in liters per kilogram of body weight to correct for differing body weights. If the drug is highly water soluble and primarily found in body water, it will have a volume of distribution of 0.6 L/kg. The same dose of a drug that is lipid soluble will achieve lower serum levels, and its volume of distribution will be greater than 0.6 L/kg. For example, digoxin is widely distributed in body tissue and has a V_d of 7 L/kg. A drug that is concentrated intravascularly will have a V_d less than 0.6 L/kg. Sulfisoxazole has a V_d of 0.16 L/kg.[10]

2. Protein binding. Many substances bind to protein. Protein binding may increase the length of time a drug remains in the body while also attenuating its serum levels. The metabolism of the substance by the liver may be decreased, as only the unbound substance is available for biotransformation.

3. Solubility and tissue distribution. The solubility of a substance has a profound effect on its distribution within the body. Water-soluble or hydrophilic substances are principally distributed within the fluid compartments of the body.

C. Metabolism.

1. Liver enzyme systems. Many drugs are metabolized via the cytochrome P-450 (CYP450) enzyme system. Although numerous enzyme families within CYP450 have been identified, CYP3A4 is involved with the metabolism of most drugs currently on the market.[11] Other isoenzymes commonly associated with drug metabolism include CYP1A2, CYP2C19, and CYP2D6.[12] Nutrients, like drugs, can inhibit or induce the effects of these metabolic enzymes. When the enzyme that is responsible for the metabolism of a particular drug is induced, the serum level of the drug is decreased. The opposite effect on the drug would occur if the

enzyme were being inhibited. Following are examples of some nutrients that affect the various CYP450 enzymes:

a) Broccoli, brussels sprouts, and charcoal-broiled meats can induce CYP1A2. Therefore, any drug that is metabolized by CYP1A2 could become toxic when taken with either broccoli or brussels sprouts. Some of the drugs that are metabolized by CYP1A2 are acetaminophen, amitriptyline, caffeine, clozapine, cyclobenzaprine, desipramine, diazepam, ethinyl estradiol, fluvoxamine, haloperidol, imipramine, methadone, naproxen, nortriptyline, olanzapine, ondansetron, propranolol, ritonavir, tamoxifen, theophylline, verapamil, and warfarin.

b) Grapefruit (juice) inhibits CYP1A2 and CYP3A4, and therefore any drug metabolized by either of these two CYP isoenzymes could become toxic when routinely taken with grapefruit juice. Some drugs metabolized by CYP1A2 are listed above. Examples of drugs that are metabolized by CYP3A4 are acetaminophen, alprazolam, amiodarone, amitriptyline, atorvastatin, buspirone, caffeine, carbamazepine, cerivastatin, chlorpheniramine, chlorpromazine, cimetidine, cisapride, clarithromycin, clindamycin, clomipramine, clonazepam, cocaine, codeine, cyclophosphamide, cyclosporine, delavirdine, dexamethasone, dextromethorphan, diazepam, diltiazem, disopyramide, dolasetron, donepezil, doxorubicin, enalapril, erythromycin, estrogens (oral), felodipine, fentanyl, flutamide, glyburide, haloperidol, hydrocodone, imipramine, indinavir, itraconazole, ketoconazole, lansoprazole, lidocaine, losartan, lovastatin, methadone, miconazole, midazolam, mirtazapine, nelfinavir, nifedipine, nimodipine, ondansetron, oral contraceptives, paclitaxel, pravastatin, prednisone, quinidine, quinine, rifampin, ritonavir, saquinavir, sertraline, sildenafil, simvastatin, tacrolimus (oral), tamoxifen, temazepam, teniposide, terfenadine, testosterone, theophylline, trazodone, triazolam, verapamil, vinblastine, and vincristine.

2. Cranberry juice has been recently reported in the literature to inhibit CYP2C9 and thus warfarin metabolism, resulting in an increased International Normalized Ratio (INR) and bleeding.[13]

D. Excretion. Excretion is the process by which a drug or a metabolite is eliminated from the body without further chemical change.[14]

1. Urinary. Renal excretion is the major pathway for the elimination of most water-soluble drugs and their metabolites. Alteration in renal function will have a profound effect on the clearance of drugs and may result in increased serum levels or prolonged half-life. Dosage adjustments may be necessary according to a patient's renal function. Antibiotics such as penicillins, cephalosporins, aminoglycosides, vancomycin, and fluoroquinolones are cleared renally.[15] Ranitidine is primarily eliminated via the urine; approximately 70% of an IV dose is excreted unchanged.[16] Analgesics that are excreted in the urine unchanged or as metabolites include nonsteroidal anti-inflammatory drugs, COX-2 inhibitors (eg, celecoxib), opioids, and tramadol.[17]

2. GI. Drugs and their metabolites are also excreted into the bile. Protein transporters usually mediate this process. Drugs and their metabolites enter the duodenum via the common bile duct, move through the small intestine, and are excreted in the stool. The drugs may be reabsorbed from the intestine. Some drugs will be reabsorbed back into the bloodstream and return to the liver by the enterohepatic circulation. The drug then undergoes further metabolism or is secreted back into bile. This process, referred to as enterohepatic cycling, may extend the duration of action of a drug. Drugs that undergo enterohepatic cycling include ethinyl estradiol[18] and antibiotics such as macrolides, ceftriaxone, nafcillin, and doxycycline.[19]

II. Enteral Incompatibilities.

Every available dosage form has the potential to cause undesirable effects or incompatibilities when combined with enteral feeding formulations or administered to the enterally fed patient.

A. Physical incompatibility is a chemical instability that occurs when two susceptible substances are mixed together. This incompatibility results in an actual physical change between two substances. A typical example is the formation of a precipitate.

1. A common reaction that may occur with enteral formulations is formation of a precipitate (eg, curdling, flocculation, altered enteral formulation consistency, viscosity [coagulation, thickening, gelling, or thinning]).
2. Physical incompatibilities may cause feeding tubes to occlude.
3. See Table 9-1 for physical compatibilities with selected enteral feeding formulations.

B. Pharmaceutical incompatibility is an alteration in the drug form itself that interferes with drug efficacy, potency, or tolerance. Medications in specialized dosage forms (ie, enteric coated, sustained release, or sublingual) typically are not amenable to administration via a feeding tube. A pharmacist should evaluate all dosage forms prior to administration via a feeding tube to determine appropriateness.

C. Physiologic incompatibility is the result of a nonpharmacologic action incurred by the medication itself or by the medium in which it is suspended. This type of incompatibility occurs when liquid medications have a high osmolality or contain a significant amount of sorbitol. Patients typically experience nausea, increased gastric residuals, bloating, cramping, and diarrhea.

D. Pharmacologic incompatibility results when a medication alters tolerance of the enteral nutrition or PN regimen because of the medication's mechanism of action. This incompatibility frequently leads to either a greater pharmacologic effect of the medication than initially intended (eg, abdominal cramping or diarrhea related to use of prokinetic agents) or an unintended side effect of the medication (eg, increased gastric residuals caused by narcotic analgesics).

E. Pharmacokinetic incompatibilities occur when the enteral or parenteral feeding regimen alters the bioavailability, absorption, distribution, metabolism, and/or elimination of the medication, or when the medication alters nutrient function. Common medications that cause pharmacokinetic interactions involving enteral nutrition include phenytoin, warfarin, ciprofloxacin, and any medication that should be taken on an empty stomach in order to maximize absorption.

III. Medication Administration via Enteral Feeding Tubes

A. Medication dosage forms that can be administered via enteral tubes. Medications that can be given via enteral tubes include immediate-release oral tablets, hard gelatin capsules, soft gelatin capsules, and liquid formulations. All medications should be mixed with appropriate diluents and administered separately; the feeding tube should be flushed with water before and after each medication is administered to minimize incompatibilities and prevent occlusion.

1. Immediate-release oral medications. Most simple, compressed tablets, including film- and sugar-coated and hard gelatin cap-

TABLE 9-1. Physical Compatibilities With Enteral Feeding Products

Drug	TwoCal HN	Ensure Plus	Ensure HN	Osmolite 1 cal	Osmolite HN	Vivonex	Comments
Acetaminophen/Codeine Elixir				C	C	C	
Acetaminophen Elixir	C	C	C	C	C	C	
Actifed Syrup		C	C	C	C	C	
Amoxicillin Suspension	C		C		C	C	
Amphogel				I	C	C	Thickens on contact
Bactrim Suspension	C	C	C	C	C	C	
Benadryl Elixir	C	C	C	C	C	C	
Bentyl Liquid					I	C	Thickens on contact
Benylin DM		C	C	C	C	C	
Cephalexin Suspension	C	C	C	C	C	C	
Cephulac		C	C	C	C	C	
Cibalith-S		I	I	I	I	C	Clumping
Compazine Elixir	C				C		
Dexamethasone Elixir	C	C	C	C	C	C	
Dimetane Elixir	I	I	I	I	I	C	Gelatinous formation
Dimetapp Elixir	I	I	I	I	I	C	Enteral product breaks down
Docusate Liquid	C	C	C	C	C	C	
Donnatal Elixir	C	C	C	C	C	C	
Doxepin Concentrate	C	C	C	C	C	C	
EES Granules		C	C	C	C	C	
Feosol Elixir	I	I	I	I	I	C	Complete gel formation
Fleet Phospho-Soda	I			I	I	C	Instant clumping
Gantrisin Suspension	C	C	C	C	C	C	
Gevrabon Liquid	I					C	
Griseofulvin Suspension		C		C			
Guaifenesin Liquid	I	I	I	I	I	C	Flocculate precipitate
Haldol Drops	C	C	C	C	C	C	
Imodium Liquid				C	C	C	
KCl Oral Liquid		I	I	I	I	I	Interphase incompatibility
Klorvess Granules		C	C		C	C	
Lanoxin Elixir	C	C	C	C	C	C	
Lasix Liquid	C	C		C	C	C	
Mandelamine Granules		C	C	C	C	C	
Mandelamine Suspension			I	I	I	I	Gelatinous tacky formation
MCT Oil		I		I			Adhesive gelatinous mass formation
Mellaril Concentrate	C					C	
Mellaril Solution		I	I	I	I	C	Granular formation
Mestinon Suspension		C	C	C	C	C	
Milk of Magnesia	C						
Morphine Liquid				C	C	C	
Mylanta				C	C	C	
Mylanta II				I	I		Thickening on contact
Navane Concentrate	C	C	C	C	C	C	
Neo-Calglucon Syrup	I	I	I	I	I	C	Adhesive gelatinous mass
Nitrofurantoin Suspension	C	C	C	C	C	C	
Organidin Elixir		C	C	C	C	C	
Paregoric Elixir	I			I	I	C	Instant clumping
Periactin				C	C	C	
Phenergan Syrup		C	C	C	C	C	

(Continued)

TABLE 9-1. Physical Compatibilities With Enteral Feeding Products (*Continued*)

Drug	TwoCal HN	Ensure Plus	Ensure HN	Osmolite 1 cal	Osmolite HN	Vivonex	Comments
Phenobarbital Elixir	C	C	C	C	C	C	
Reglan Syrup	C					C	
Riopan				I	C		Thickening on contact
Simethicone Drops	C	C	C	C	C	C	
Slo-Phyllin Syrup		C	C	C	C	C	
SSKI Liquid		C	C	C	C	C	
Sudafed Syrup	C	I	I	I	I	C	Viscous gelatinous formation
Sumycin Syrup	C	C		C		C	
Tagamet Elixir	C			I	I	C	Thickening on contact
Terpin Hydrate Elixir		C	C	C	C	C	
Theolair Liquid	C	C		C		C	
Theragran Liquid	C		C		C	C	
Thorazine Concentrate		I	I	I	I	C	Granulation and particle formation
Triaminic Syrup	I	C	C	C	C	C	
Zinc Sulfate	I						

C, compatible; I, incompatible

References

Lutomski DM, Gora ML, Wright SM, Martin JE. Sorbitol content of selected oral liquids. *Ann Pharmacother.* 1993;27:269–274.

Miller SJ, Oliver AD. Sorbitol content of selected sugar-free liquid medications. *Hosp Pharm.* 1993;28:741–744, 755.

Niemiec PW, Vanderveen TW, Morrison JI, Hohenwarter MW. Gastrointestinal disorders caused by medications and electrolyte solution osmolality during enteral nutrition. *J Parenter Enteral Nutr.* 1983;7:387–389.

sules filled with a fine powder, are amenable to administration via a feeding tube.

a) Tablets must be crushed to a fine powder (eg, with a mortar and pestle) and mixed with water before administration. The finer the powder the better, both to enhance absorption and reduce the risk of tube occlusion.

b) Hard gelatin capsules filled with a fine powder should be opened and mixed thoroughly with water before administration. Soft gelatin capsules can be emptied by creating a pinhole in one end of the capsule and squeezing out the contents. The contents can then be mixed with water. Precise dosing may not be possible, as it is difficult to remove all the capsule's contents.

2. Liquid medications[20–22] are the preferred alternative for administration via an enteral feeding tube because of better absorption and decreased potential for enteral tube occlusions. However, liquid medications are not without potential for producing adverse effects.

   a) Liquid medications may cause physiologic incompatibilities (eg, diarrhea, elevated gastric residuals, distended abdomen, cramping).

   b) These responses may not be attributed initially to the enteral feeding formulation and may be misdiagnosed as a tube-feeding intolerance.

   c) The "intolerance" may in fact be attributable to the liquid medication preparation, as these medications often have a high osmolality or contain large amounts of sorbitol.[23–26]

   d) Hyperosmolar liquid medications may cause diarrhea, cramping, and increased gastric residuals. The osmolality of GI tract secretions is approximately 300 mOsm/kg. Liquid medications exceeding 300 mOsm/kg require GI dilution to approach the isotonic state to aid absorption; if the amount of fluid that moves into the GI tract exceeds the absorptive capacity of the intestinal tract, diarrhea will result.

   e) The stomach may be more tolerant of hyperosmolar medications than the small intestine because of the stomach's inherent ability to dilute hypertonic solutions with gastric juice before emptying the gastric contents into the duodenum.

   f) Administration of undiluted hyperosmolar liquid medications directly into the duodenum or jejunum should be approached cautiously, as it causes a significant influx of water and electrolytes into the GI tract, which could contribute to bloating, nausea, cramping, diarrhea, and electrolyte imbalances.

   g) Complications can be avoided by diluting hypertonic liquid medications with an appropriate amount of water. The site of medication delivery and the tonicity of the medication influence the amount of water required. More diluent may be needed to dilute medications administered into the small intestine than into the stomach.

   h) Coordinate the patient's need for additional water with amounts of water needed to dilute hypertonic medications.

   i) Osmolalities of liquid medications can reach as high as 9000 mOsm/kg of water. Check with the manufacturer or read the package insert for more information.[23,24]

   j) Medications that contain sorbitol often cause a physiologic incompatibility (eg, diarrhea, bloating, cramping). Doses as low as 10 g have been known to cause mild GI distress, with 20 g or more causing more severe symptoms.[26] Children may be more susceptible to the effects of sorbitol than adults.

(1) Sorbitol is considered an inert ingredient that is added to enhance palatability and improve stability. Sorbitol may be present in all liquid medications except tinctures and emulsions. None of the reconstituted antibiotic preparations are known to contain sorbitol.[27]

(2) The sorbitol content of a liquid medication may vary among manufacturers. Manufacturers do not list the sorbitol content on the label. The best source for determining whether sorbitol is present is the package insert, but the manufacturer must be contacted to obtain the actual sorbitol content.

(3) The total daily dose of sorbitol provided by all liquid medication preparations administered must be considered.

(4) Common offending agents are acetaminophen elixir, theophylline solutions, valproate, and guaifenesin syrup. These medications contain large quantities of sorbitol, and numerous doses may be given in a 24-hour period. Any product may have a high concentration of sorbitol, but if the product dose in milliliters is small, the actual dose of sorbitol may also be quite small.

(5) Options for avoiding problems with sorbitol include changing to another manufacturer's product, using therapeutically equivalent products that have less or no sorbitol, changing the route of administration, and using tablets or capsules that do not exhibit pharmaceutical incompatibility.

3. Suspensions
   a) Suspensions present few incompatibility concerns
   b) Suspensions do not contain sorbitol.
   c) Suspensions may be hyperosmolar; adding water to the dose will reduce tonicity.
   d) Antibiotics are often available as suspensions. The diarrhea that may occur is a direct side effect of the antibiotic and is not related to the suspension form. Recolonization of the GI tract may be useful in these cases.
4. Granular-type medications
   a) Psyllium hydrophilic mucilloid and cholestyramine resin may be added to a patient's regimen to control diarrhea. Cholestyramine resin may also be added as a hypercholesterolemia agent.
   b) These medications require dilution with water before administration. The granules rapidly absorb water and expand to form a gelatinous mixture that may occlude the enteral tube; small-bore feeding tubes are more problematic than larger gastric tubes.
   c) Metamucil may be administered by mixing 4 g with 80 mL of water and completing the dose administration within 5 minutes or less.[28] The quick administration minimizes expansion of the granules and decreases the risk of tube occlusion.
   d) A therapeutically equivalent medication should be considered if the patient has a small-bore feeding tube.

B. Medication dosage forms *not* recommended for administration via tube

1. Enteric coated medications[20,21]
   a) Crushing these medications may induce a pharmaceutical incompatibility. A therapeutic equivalent or alternative administration route should be considered.
   b) It is important to understand the purpose of the enteric coating and the location of the tip of the feeding tube.

(1) Enteric coating may protect the stomach lining. Certain formulations of aspirin are coated to decrease the gastric irritation often associated with its use. Administering a crushed enteric-coated aspirin may produce some GI upset or irritation associated with aspirin, but the overall efficacy of the medication will most likely be unaltered.

(2) Enteric coating protects a number of medications (eg, erythromycin base, erythromycin stearate, pancrelipase) from destruction in the acidic environment of the stomach prior to absorption in the small intestine. Upon entering the alkaline environment of the duodenum, the enteric coating will dissolve and release the medication for absorption. These medications require an intact enteric coating to preserve the integrity of the active drug during its passage through the stomach to ensure bioavailability.[29]

(3) If a medication has an enteric coating solely for the purpose of preventing destruction from acidic acid, administration via a feeding tube beyond the pylorus is acceptable. Check with a pharmacist to verify the purpose of the enteric coating.

2. Sublingual or buccal medications[20]
   a) These medications are placed under the tongue or in the cheek pouch and absorbed into the systemic circulation.
   b) Administration via feeding tube is not recommended.
3. Sustained-release (SR) tablets or SR capsules.[20,21] Crushing these medications is not recommended, as significant pharmaceutical incompatibilities or toxicities could occur.
   a) Administering crushed SR tablets or capsules delivers a bolus of drug that was intended to be delivered over 6 to 24 hours. The bolus causes high peaks with a potential for toxicity followed by low troughs and inadequate coverage.
   b) Emptying capsules with extended-release beads into feeding tubes is not recommended because it increases the potential for tube occlusions.
   c) Dissolving the beads in water or NaCl 0.9% solution is not recommended because it will adversely affect the integrity of the beads' outer coating. This can affect the integrity of the medication and compromise the time-release properties.
   d) Alternative therapeutic equivalents must be considered.

(1) Use a liquid therapeutic equivalent or a crushable immediate-release medication, or choose an alternative delivery route (eg, parenteral, rectal).

(2) If a therapeutically equivalent immediate-release medication is available as a tablet or liquid, it will require more frequent administration, usually at the same total daily dose as the SR form.

(3) Monitor for appropriate clinical response and, whenever warranted, adequate blood concentrations.

4. A comprehensive list of oral solid dosage products that should not be crushed is available.[20]
5. Syrups[29–31]
   a) A physical incompatibility may occur when syrups are mixed with enteral formulations. Syrups with a pH of ≤4 can denature the protein in the enteral formulation, leading to an increase in viscosity that may contribute to feeding tube occlusions.
   b) It is important to be aware of the protein source of the enteral formula. Syrup preparations administered with whole-protein formulations have been shown to cause physical incompatibilities; those with free amino acids or hydrolyzed formulations are not as affected by concurrent administration of syrup.
   c) Physical incompatibilities (clumping, etc) cannot be avoided by diluting the syrup or the enteral formulation. Not all syrup products have an acidic pH ≤4. If there is suspicion that the product has a low pH, the pH may be tested with pH paper or

a small amount of the syrup may be mixed with a sample amount of the enteral formulation to observe any affect on the formulation stability.

d) Alternatively, a compatible therapeutically equivalent medication (ie, a tablet or capsule form that could be sufficiently pulverized and diluted in water) can be selected or an alternative route of administration can be used. If the incompatible syrup must be administered via the feeding tube, the steps below should be followed:
   (1) Stop the tube feeding.
   (2) Flush the feeding tube with 30 mL of water to clear the tube of all formulation.
   (3) Administer the syrup via the tube.
   (4) Flush the tube with 30 to 60 mL of water to clear the tube of residual syrup and ensure tube patency.
   (5) Resume the tube feeding.

C. Drug-nutrient interactions. Drug-nutrient interactions are situations in which the ultimate effect of a drug is altered by a nutrient or the ultimate effect of a nutrient is altered by a drug. Interactions could involve any of the previously mentioned types of incompatibilities.

1. Proton pump inhibitors available as capsules or tablets[32]
   a) Capsules containing enteric-coated beads
      (1) Enteric coating preserves the integrity of the medication until it reaches the alkaline pH of the duodenum, where the coating dissolves and absorption begins.
      (2) Dissolving the beads in water removes the protective enteric coating, exposing the medication inside to a basic environment. In this basic environment, the active medication begins to degrade, thereby decreasing its overall effectiveness. Mixing with water also causes the beads to clump as the enteric coating dissolves. Clumping contributes to occlusion of enteral feeding tubes.
      (3) Two alternative methods of delivery have published support.
         (a) The contents of the capsule (omeprazole, lansoprazole, esomeprazole) may be mixed in an acidic fruit juice such as orange juice or apple juice. The enteric coating will remain intact until the beads reach the basic environment of the duodenum. One concern with this approach is that the intact beads may occlude small-bore feeding tubes. Not all of the dose is administered to the patient, as the beads can collect and remain lodged in the syringe hub.[32,33]
         (b) The beads can be dissolved in sodium bicarbonate 8.4% solution, creating a simplified suspension. Stability is maintained at this high pH.[34]
         (c) Extemporaneous simplified suspensions of omeprazole and lansoprazole can be prepared. These formulations have proven to be effective in maintaining adequate buffering of stomach contents in the critically ill population.[35,36] One study involving healthy individuals administered esomeprazole via a feeding tube immediately after the drug was mixed with water demonstrated good results.[37]
         (d) The commercially available lansoprazole packets should not be administered via a feeding tube. The product contains particles or gums that will occlude a feeding tube.[38]
         (e) Simplified suspensions of proton pump inhibitor should be administered via feeding tubes to avoid tube occlusion.
         (f) An orally disintegrating form of lansoprazole is available. This dosage form circumvents the feeding tube route, as the pellets dissolve in the patient's mouth and do not require swallowing.
         (g) A powder formulation of omeprazole is commercially available and can be reconstituted for administration via enteral feeding tubes.
   b) Enteric-coated tablets
      (1) Crushing enteric-coated tablets has the same effect as crushing the enteric-coated beads in capsules.
      (2) A pantoprazole extemporaneous solution can be prepared using sodium bicarbonate 4.2% solution.[39,40]
   c) Alternative options. Use an H_2 antagonist when possible.
      (1) H_2 antagonists are available in liquid form and in easily dissolved tablets and capsules.
      (2) Use parenteral proton pump inhibitor or H_2 antagonists only when the GI tract cannot be used.

2. Phenytoin. Impaired absorption of phenytoin is a pharmacokinetic incompatibility[41–44] that is well documented in the literature.
   a) There appears to be impairment in absorption, but there is debate about where and how the interaction occurs. Possible reasons for impaired absorption include the following:
      (1) The protein source of the enteral formulation may contribute to the interaction. Calcium caseinate protein sources may impair absorption more than sodium caseinates.
      (2) The phenytoin suspension may bind to the enteral feeding tube.
      (3) The phenytoin suspension has poor solubility and may contribute to poor absorption.
      (4) There may be decreased gastric emptying, with subsequent destruction of phenytoin by gastric acid.
      (5) Drug administration via a tube placed in the distal jejunum reduces transit time and time for drug absorption.
      (6) Patients have decreased GI transit time (ie, the drug spends less time in the GI tract).
   b) Patients receiving enteral formulations may need much higher phenytoin doses than usual to maintain therapeutic blood levels.
   c) Seizures are a potential consequence of inadequate phenytoin blood levels.
   d) Strategies to maintain therapeutic phenytoin levels and provide adequate protection from seizures include the following:
      (1) Hold the tube feeding 2 hours before and 2 hours after administering the phenytoin dose. Adjust the tube-feeding schedule to accommodate the total 24-hour requirement.
      (2) Dilute the phenytoin with water (30–60 mL) before administration. The water may enhance dissolution and improve absorption.
      (3) Monitor blood levels more frequently when changing from an established therapeutic parenteral dose via vein to the suspension form administered via the feeding tube.
      (4) Consider administering the parenteral form of phenytoin via enteral tube if problems persist in maintaining therapeutic levels. Supporting evidence at this time is limited to a single-dose trial in healthy subjects, which is not adequate to establish this route as a reliable alternative. The parenteral form is hyperosmolar and must be diluted before administration.[45]
      (5) Phenytoin toxicity can occur as the patient transitions from tube feeding to oral feedings, because of the removal of the

offending interaction. Monitor the phenytoin levels closely until stable.

(6) Consider the use of IV phenytoin or fosphenytoin in difficult situations.

3. Warfarin. A decreased therapeutic response to warfarin has been noted in patients receiving enteral tube feeding.[46–48]
   a) The altered response was initially thought to be related to the high vitamin K content of enteral formulations.
      (1) The vitamin K content could antagonize warfarin activity.
      (2) Subsequently, the vitamin K content was reduced in most enteral products.
      (3) Warfarin resistance continues to be reported in the literature.
   b) Warfarin is a highly protein-bound drug.
      (1) It has a protein-binding level in serum of 97.4% to 99.9%.
      (2) It may bind to the protein in the enteral formulation.
   c) One letter to the editor indicated success in one patient when the warfarin was administered during the 6-hour break in the patient's daily 18-hour cycle.[49]
   d) Warfarin drug-nutrient interactions are less consistent than phenytoin drug-nutrient interactions.
   e) Monitor anticoagulant activity closely while the patient is on enteral tube feeding.
   f) Evaluate warfarin dose, anticoagulant goals, and monitoring parameters closely as the patient transitions to an oral diet or begins a bolus, intermittent gravity tube-feeding regimen.
4. Quinolones
   a) Significant controversy surrounds the use of quinolones administered simultaneously with enteral feedings. Efficacy is best measured by evaluating the area under the curve (AUC) data and comparing these data to the minimum inhibitory concentration (MIC) of the bacterial strain being treated.
   b) The AUC measures the total amount of quinolone that is absorbed over time. The AUC/MIC ratio is the most important predictor of efficacy.[50]
   c) Concurrent administration of quinolones with medications that are high in aluminum, magnesium, iron, and calcium can impair absorption, resulting in a clinically significant decrease in absorption.[51]
   d) High concentrations of the following cations in enteral feeding formulations may also impair quinolone absorption.
      (1) Ofloxacin
         (a) A single-dose trial with a crushed tablet administered with a bolus of Ensure (Ross Products) produced a 10% reduction in the AUC.[52]
         (b) This was not a significant reduction compared to taking on an empty stomach with water.
      (2) Ciprofloxacin
         (a) There have been mixed results depending on what patient groups were studied and how the medication was administered.
            i) Single-dose trials in which the tablet was crushed and administered simultaneously with a bolus of enteral feedings demonstrated reduced absorption.[53–55]
            ii) Nonsurgical, critically ill patients receiving continuous enteral tube feeding and receiving multiple doses of ciprofloxacin have demonstrated adequate absorption.[56,57]
         (b) Adequate GI tract function must be established prior to changing ciprofloxacin from the parenteral route to the enteral route.[58]
            i) It may not be advisable to change ciprofloxacin to the feeding tube route if pseudomonal respiratory tract infection is being treated. The feeding tube route should be acceptable for patients with urinary tract infections.
            ii) For a more detailed discussion on this topic, refer to a review article by Nyffeler.[59]
      (3) Levofloxacin. No information is presently available.
      (4) Gatifloxacin. A single-dose prospective two-way crossover trial in critically ill patients comparing AUC for the parenteral product to a single dose administered via a feeding tube with concurrent enteral feeding did not demonstrate a difference in overall bioavailability.[60]
5. Atovaquone. A single-dose trial of atovaquone suspension administered to healthy patients within 1 hour of an enteral supplement produced levels of absorption similar to those taking it with a normal breakfast.[61]
6. Carbamazepine
   a) Administration with concurrent tube feedings should not be a problem if an appropriate dilution-and-flush routine is used.
   b) One trial demonstrated that administration of undiluted carbamazepine suspension via a polyvinyl feeding tube resulted in decreased absorption. Diluting the suspension prior to administration produced more normal delivery.[62]
   c) An insignificant reduction in overall absorption was demonstrated in a small trial of healthy patients. This was a crossover trial that demonstrated 90% bioavailability of carbamazepine suspension when taken after fasting or with continuous enteral feedings.[63]
   d) Serum concentrations should be monitored closely after patients are started on carbamazepine and enteral feedings. A consistent method of administration should be used.
   e) A report describes the use of an extended-release version of carbamazepine (Carbatrol) via feeding tubes in pediatric patients.[64] This trial administered the contents of the capsule via feeding tubes. No mention was made of carbamazepine levels or side effects, but the patient's family noted frequent occlusion of the feeding tube. Administering capsule contents via feeding tubes always presents the potential for occluding the feeding tube and is probably best avoided.
7. Carbidopa/levodopa
   a) No trials have evaluated absorption of carbidopa/levodopa with concurrent enteral feedings.
   b) Extrapolations have been made from the data showing a decreased effect when the medication was taken with a high-protein meal. The amino acids in the high-protein meal inhibited transport across the blood-brain barrier via a competitive uptake mechanism.
   c) If patients are receiving intermittent feedings, doses should be administered during off-time. Another option is to explore alternative medications for Parkinson's that do not exhibit this interaction.
8. Clarithromycin. Administration of suspension, which contains granules, may result in occluded feeding tubes.
9. Hydralazine. Absorption in continuous enteral feedings is comparable to that of fasted patients.[65]
10. Fluconazole
   a) A number of trials in patients in intensive care unit support the administration of fluconazole via a feeding tube in conjunction with continuous enteral feedings.[66,67]

b) Postpyloric administration in trauma patients has also demonstrated adequate absorption.[68]

11. Tacrolimus. One study demonstrated that absorption of tacrolimus was no different whether the enteral feedings (Osmolite, Ross Products) were held 1 hour before and 8 hours after tacrolimus administration or administered in conjunction with continuous enteral feedings.[69]
12. Theophylline
    a) Theophylline and/or aminophylline absorption is probably not impaired when the medication is administered with enteral feedings, but serum levels may be affected by the presence of enteral feedings.
    b) The initiation of enteral feeding stimulates liver enzymes that contribute to the metabolism of theophylline, subsequently reducing theophylline levels.[70]
    c) Two single-dose trials in healthy patients did not demonstrate a reduction in absorption when a long-acting theophylline preparation was taken and an hourly enteral supplement drunk. Neither trial used feeding tubes.[71,72]
13. Sucralfate
    a) Sucralfate is a medication that may be used for stress ulcer prophylaxis, esophageal ulcerations, or gastric reflux disease. Sucralfate must be administered into the acidic environment of the stomach in order to be converted to the active moiety. This is difficult to accomplish when patients are on continuous enteral feedings.
    b) An additional problem with mixing enteral feedings and sucralfate is the risk of developing a bezoar. This occurs when a complex forms between the sucralfate and the protein component of the enteral feeding supplement.[73,74]
14. Levothyroxine
    a) There is concern that interaction with the soy content in an enteral feeding formulation could impair the absorption of levothyroxine.
    b) Only data to support this direct interaction was done a at a time when it was more common for adult enteral formulations to be soy based.[75] Although some adult formulas may contain some soy protein, this interaction has not been studied using currently available enteral formulations. Without supporting evidence, it is not necessary to hold enteral feedings for administration of levothyroxine.

D. Summary

1. Develop multidisciplinary standards and practice protocols to ensure the safe, consistent care and monitoring of the enterally fed patient who needs to receive medication via an enteral tube. Doing so will have the following results:
    a) Ensures optimal therapeutic response to medication and enteral nutrition
    b) Minimizes side effects and complications of administration of the medication
    c) Optimizes effectiveness of therapies and interventions
    d) Optimizes cost-effectiveness of therapies and interventions
2. Consult a pharmacist to review the patient's medication profile before administering a medication via an enteral feeding tube.
3. Confirm proper placement of the enteral tube before administration of medication.
4. Do not mix any medications directly with enteral formulations.
5. Administer each medication separately.
6. Flush the enteral feeding tube with water before and after each medication is administered.
7. Differentiate medication-induced GI intolerance from enteral delivery system- or formula-induced GI intolerance.
8. Continually and consistently monitor the patient's therapeutic drug response to all medications.

IV. Parenteral Considerations.

Patients receiving parenteral nutrition (PN) are often treated concomitantly with medications, both orally and parenterally. The clinician should be aware of the physical compatibility of parenteral medications as well as the effects of medications on laboratory measurements and the overall nutrition status of the patient. The compatibility of PN formulations infused with other additives is often influenced by the exposure time between the nutrients and additives present. A useful reference for the compatibility of medications and PN formulations is by Trissel (see Suggested Readings).

A. Secondary medications (Y site). Usually, secondary or IV piggyback medications are coinfused simultaneously with a primary infusion. In most cases, the primary IV infusion contains relatively low concentrations of electrolytes and poses few compatibility problems. Also, the of time for contact with the secondary IV infusion is relatively short. Most significant interactions are time and concentration dependent. The situation becomes more complicated if a PN formulation is used as the primary IV infusion. Numerous additives may be, either individually or in combination, incompatible with concentrated secondary medications. In the presence of limited venous access, medications with borderline stabilities should be diluted or administered at a Y site proximal to the patient. Otherwise, a separate infusion port or injection site should be used for secondary medications where stability after exposure to PN is questionable.

B. Stability of added ingredients. Numerous additives are combined in a PN formulation. PN is frequently considered as a vehicle for medication administration. However, because of the complexity of the formulations and the potential for incompatibilities and interactions, admixing PN with medications is not advised. See Chapters 7 and 8 for discussions on PN formulations and physicochemical interactions.

C. Administration sets. Regular insulin is often either coadministered or added to the PN formulation for glucose management. Insulin binds to the surface of the delivery container and the administration set. Binding is particularly problematic with polyvinyl chloride containers. The extent of binding to a particular container is also influenced by the formulation within the container. The effect of the formulation on the extent of insulin binding to container surface is as follows (from greatest binding to least)[76]: NaCl 0.9% (normal saline) > dextrose > amino acids > albumin. Therefore, the same dose of insulin will have a different amount of activity depending on the vehicle in which it is administered. The higher the concentration of insulin, the lower the extent of binding, because there are a limited number of binding sites per container. The route of administration and the insulin product (insulin lispro, insulin aspart, insulin regular, insulin NPH, insulin glargine) will also have a major effect on the action of this drug.[77]

D. Predicting interactions

1. Reviewing the package insert for the pH of a medication may provide information for predicting compatibility with a PN formulation. Medications that are weak acids or bases are formulated at a pH that optimizes their solubility. IV medications that produce extreme changes in the final pH of the reconstituted product, such as phenytoin, tend to be most reactive and therefore capable of significant incompatibilities.

2. Injectable medications that contain cosolvents, such as propylene glycol or ethanol, have the greatest potential for interaction if coadministered with a PN formulation or other large-volume parenteral infusion. Examples include furosemide, diazepam, digoxin, phenytoin, and etoposide.

V. Effects of Medications on Clinical Laboratory Values

A. Interference of drugs with laboratory tests. Drugs may interfere with substrates within the body and alter clinical laboratory values. In some cases, organ dysfunction can produce aberrant values, which may be misinterpreted as related to nutrition therapy. It is important for the clinician to differentiate between the adverse effects of medications and other causes of changes in nutrition indices. Table 9-2 lists some of the more prevalent and clinically significant alterations in laboratory values.

B. Analytical interference of medications. Medication interactions with laboratory tests can occur through several mechanisms of interference.[78] Medications can both increase and decrease laboratory values through different mechanisms.

VI. Effects of Drugs on Nutrition and Metabolism

A. Drug-nutrient interactions. The following is not intended to be an all-inclusive list. Individual agents are mentioned only to provide a concrete illustration of the root cause of interactions.
   1. Antibiotics inhibit or kill susceptible bacteria. These may include gut bacteria responsible for vitamin K production. Since vitamin K is essential for the production of clotting factors II (prothrombin), VII, IX, and X, reduced vitamin K can result in decreased coagulation and bleeding. Antibiotics differ in the extent of this effect.[79]
   2. Some medications may affect hepatic protein synthesis. Chloramphenicol is one of these. It also decreases the amount of iron incorporated into heme, resulting in decreased hemoglobin synthesis.[80]
   3. Certain diuretics may increase urinary excretion of potassium, magnesium, and zinc.[79] Other diuretics may spare potassium while increasing the urinary excretion of sodium.
   4. Medications used to treat or prevent ulcer disease, such as histamine$_2$ receptor antagonists and proton pump inhibitors, raise the gastric pH. This can result in decreased iron absorption. There may also be a decrease in the secretion of intrinsic factor.[79] Histamine$_2$ receptor antagonists can prevent metabolic alkalosis, which occurs when patients have losses of gastric secretions such as through nasogastric tubes connected to external suction. This is an example of a medication affecting nutrient absorption.
   5. Drugs may also affect the pharmacodynamics of a nutrient at its site of action. There is a report of hydralazine interfering with the activity of pyridoxine, resulting in peripheral neuropathy.[79] Phenytoin can increase inactivation of 25-hydroxy vitamin D, potentially leading to osteomalacia or rickets.[79]

B. Medication-metabolic interactions. Drugs can alter metabolism. Alterations are seen in appetite, digestion, and absorption; organ integrity and nutrient-processing capabilities; nutrient incorporation; and nutrient metabolism and excretion. The following are examples of drugs that affect general nutritional status:
   1. Growth hormone is a potent anabolic agent that affects protein, carbohydrate, and fat metabolism. It increases protein synthesis and nitrogen retention.[81]
   2. Drugs that affect metabolic rate include thyroid hormones and steroids (anabolic, corticosteroid).[82,83]
   3. Chemotherapeutic agents. Emetogenic agents stimulate the chemotherapeutic trigger zone in the central nervous system. Examples include cisplatin, high-dose methotrexate, and doxorubicin.[84,85]
   4. Drugs that affect appetite or taste[86,87]
      a) Drugs that cause anorexia: diuretics, estrogens, sympathomimetics (including decongestants), and serotonin uptake antagonists such as fluoxetine and sertraline
      b) Drugs that stimulate appetite: methylprogesterone, dronabinol, cyproheptadine, and tricyclic antidepressants such as amitriptyline and imipramine
      c) Drugs that cause dry mouth: anticholinergics, diuretics, methyldopa, and antihistamines
      d) Drugs that cause a bad taste[87]: gold products, metronidazole, penicillins, and some other antibiotics
      e) Drugs that decrease taste[87]: azathioprine and phenytoin
      f) Drugs that affect taste acuity[87]: captopril and other angiotensin-converting enzyme inhibitors, chlorpromazine
   5. Drugs with GI effects[86]
      a) Drugs that cause nausea or vomiting: anticholinergics, autonomic agents, beta blockers such as propranolol or labetalol, and emetogenic cancer chemotherapeutic agents
      b) Drugs that cause gastritis or ulcers: corticosteroids such as dexamethasone, methylprednisolone, hydrocortisone, nonsteroidal anti-inflammatory agents (indomethacin, ketorolac), and serotonin reuptake antagonists
      c) Drugs that alter intestinal motility[86]: decrease in motility—opiates, anticholinergics, and phenothiazines such as chlorpromazine; increase in motility—metoclopramide, erythromycin, and cisapride
      d) Drugs that can damage GI tract mucosa: colchicine and cytotoxic agents
      e) Drugs that can cause diarrhea: Many drugs can induce diarrhea as a result of an adverse reaction or toxicity. Additionally, drugs can significantly alter GI flora, which can precipitate diarrhea. Antibiotics, quinidine, digoxin, and theophylline are examples of medications that induce diarrhea.[84]
      f) Drugs that can cause abdominal pain and cramping: estrogens[79,86]
   6. Drugs that can affect the pancreas[79,84,86]
      a) Drugs that can cause or exacerbate pancreatitis: diuretics, estrogens, anticonvulsants, corticosteroids, azathioprine, cyclosporine, carbamazepine, alcohol, antibiotics, and asparaginase
      b) Drugs that can alter pancreatic secretions: octreotide
      c) Drugs that can alter pancreatic hormone release: insulin, asparaginase, beta blockers, glucocorticosteroid, octreotide, growth hormone
   7. Drugs that can affect liver function
      a) Thiazides: increase glycogen synthesis and increase glycogenolysis
      b) Drugs that can induce drug-metabolizing enzymes: barbiturates, alcohol, theophylline, diazepam, cimetidine, and erythromycin[88]
      c) Drugs that inhibit drug-metabolizing enzymes: cyclosporine, isoniazid, chloramphenicol, amphotericin B, cytotoxic agents, tricyclic antidepressants, steroids, long-acting antihistamines such as terfenadine and astemizole, thiazides, allopurinol, anesthetics, antibiotics, and anti-inflammatory agents[81,89]

TABLE 9-2. Drug Interference With Clinical Laboratory Values (*Continued*)

Drug	Laboratory test	Increase/ decrease	Mechanism of action
Acetaminophen	Alkaline phosphatase	Increase	Hepatic necrosis associated with high drug concentration
	Bilirubin	Increase	Hepatic damage with overdose
	Glucose	Decrease	GOD-PERID method, measured by MediSense Precision QID
Acyclovir	Alkaline phosphatase	Increase	Increased liver function tests
		Decrease	Leukopenia
	Bilirubin	Increase	Increased liver function tests
	Creatinine	Increase	Reversible renal failure
Aluminum antacids	Phosphorus	Decrease	Binds to phosphorus in gastrointestinal tract
Amiodarone	Alkaline phosphatase	Increase	Hepatitis, asymptomatic change in liver function enzyme
	Bilirubin	Increase	Cholestasis, hepatitis
	Prealbumin	Decrease	Probable direct effect on clearance or synthesis
Amitriptyline	Alkaline phosphatase	Increase	May rarely cause hepatitis, hypersensitivity
Amphotericin B	Bilirubin	Increase	May cause hepatocellular dysfunction
	BUN	Increase	Nephrotoxic effect
	Creatinine	Increase	Nephrotoxic effect
	Magnesium	Decrease	Nephrotoxic effect
	Potassium	Decrease	Altered distal tubule permeability
Ampicillin	Sodium	Increase	Measured by ISE without predilution
Ascorbic acid	Bilirubin	Increase	SMA 12/60 method
	Urine sugar	(False +)	Clinitest
Atenolol	Glucose	Increase or decrease	Altered glucose regulation mediated by beta-2 receptors
Barium	Potassium	Decrease	Impaired cellular discharge
Beta-2 agonists	Potassium	Decrease	Facilitates intracellular uptake
Beta-adrenergic blockers	Potassium	Increase	Aldosterone effect
Bicarbonates	Chloride	Decrease	Induced metabolic alkalosis
	Potassium	Decrease	Induced metabolic alkalosis
Calcium	Potassium	Increase	Emission spectrum interferes with that of potassium in direct flame photometric method
	Sodium	Increase	Emission spectrum interferes with that of sodium in direct flame photometric method
Captopril	Potassium	Increase	Hypoaldosterone, impaired excretion
Carbamazepine	Alkaline phosphatase	Increase	Hepatotoxicity
	Bilirubin	Increase	Hepatotoxicity
Cephalexin	Alkaline phosphatase	Increase	Transient hepatitis and cholestatic jaundice reported
	Creatinine	Increase	Jaffe methods, Technicon SMAC, Serno Centrifichem
Chlorambucil	Bilirubin	Increase	Hepatotoxicity

TABLE 9-2. Drug Interference With Clinical Laboratory Values (*Continued*)

Drug	Laboratory test	Increase/ decrease	Mechanism of action
Chloramphenicol	Bilirubin	Increase	Hepatotoxicity
	BUN	Decrease	Berthelot method
		Increase	Nesslerization method
Chlordiazepoxide	Bilirubin	Increase	Infrequent cholestatic effect
Chlorfibrate	Sodium	Decrease	Increased ADH
Chloroquine	Bilirubin	Increase	Hemolytic anemia due to G6PD deficiency
Chlorpromazine	Alkaline phosphatase	Increase	Hepatic sensitivity to drug (up to 2% of patients)
	Glucose	Increase	Abnormally high after repeated doses
Chlorpropamide	Sodium	Decrease	Increased inappropriate ADH secretion
Cholestyramine	Cholesterol	Decrease	Increases fecal excretion of bile acids
Cisplatin	Magnesium	Decrease	Renal wasting
	Potassium	Decrease	Renal wasting
Citrates	Calcium	Decrease	EDTA titration method
	Magnesium	Decrease	Complexes with calcium in fluorometric test
Clonidine	Sodium	Increase	By effect on renal tubules
Corticosteroids	Calcium	Decrease	Metabolic effect
	Chloride	Decrease	Decreased reabsorption
		Increase	By salt/water retention
	Glucose	Increase	Gluconeogenesis
	Phosphorus	Decrease	Glucose utilization
	Potassium	Decrease	Renal potassium wasting
	Sodium	Increase	By salt/water retention
Cyclophosphamide	Bilirubin	Increase	Hepatotoxicity
	Sodium	Decrease	Increased ADH/water retention
Cyclosporine	Potassium	Increase	Impaired excretion
Diethylstilbestrol	Bilirubin	Increase	Hepatotoxicity
	Calcium	Increase	Elevations over baseline level
Digoxin	Potassium	Decrease	Impaired K/Na pump
Diltiazem	Alkaline phosphatase	Increase	Mild increases in enzyme activity
	Bilirubin	Increase	Mild transient increase
	Uric acid	Increase	May cause gout as a side effect
Enalapril	Potassium	Increase	Hypoaldosterone, impaired excretion
Erythromycin	Alkaline phosphatase	Increase	May cause intrahepatic cholestasis (reversible)
	Bilirubin	Increase	Cholestatic effect in 15% of patients
Estrogens	Dexamethasone suppression test	(False +)	Due to increased corticosteroid binding globulin

(*Continued*)

TABLE 9-2. Drug Interference With Clinical Laboratory Values (*Continued*)

Drug	Laboratory test	Increase/ decrease	Mechanism of action
Ethacrynic acid	Bicarbonate	Increase	By alkalosis
	Calcium	Decrease	Renal wasting
	Chloride	Decrease	By diuretic effect
	Magnesium	Decrease	Impaired reabsorption
	Potassium	Decrease	By diuretic action
	Sodium	Decrease	By diuretic effect
Fat emulsion	Bilirubin	Decrease	May affect accuracy
Furosemide	BUN	Increase	Nephrotoxic effect: usually dehydration
	Calcium	Decrease	Diuretic action
	Chloride	Decrease	Diuretic effect
	Glucose	Increase	Diabetogenic action of drug
	Magnesium	Decrease	Diuretic action
	Potassium	Decrease	Diuretic action
	Sodium	Decrease	Diuretic effect
Gentamicin	Magnesium	Decrease	Associated with massive urinary loss of magnesium and potassium and renal tubular toxicity
	Potassium	Decrease	Associated with massive urinary loss of magnesium and potassium and renal tubular toxicity
Glutamine	Phenytoin	Increase	Significant increase in children
Growth hormone	Phosphate	Increase	Metabolic effect
	Total protein	Increase	Increased protein synthesis
Heparin	Calcium	Decrease	EDTA titration method
		Decrease	Fluorometric titration method
	Potassium	Increase	Impaired aldosterone synthesis
	Sodium	Decrease	Increases sodium excretion
Hydrochlorothiazide	Bicarbonate	Increase	By alkalosis
	Bilirubin	Increase	Cholestatic jaundice
	Calcium	Increase	Impaired excretion
	Glucose	Increase	Glucose intolerance associated with potassium depletion
	Potassium	Decrease	By diuretic action
Indomethacin	Alkaline phosphatase	Increase	Hepatotoxicity
	Bilirubin	Increase	Cholestatic jaundice
	Glucose	Increase	No mechanism known
	Potassium	Increase	ISE method
	Urea nitrogen	Increase	Occasionally to upper normal
Insulin	Potassium	Decrease	Intracellular shift
	Total protein	Increase	Increased protein synthesis

TABLE 9-2. Drug Interference With Clinical Laboratory Values (*Continued*)

Drug	Laboratory test	Increase/ decrease	Mechanism of action
Isoniazid	Alkalinc phosphatase	Increase	Hepatotoxicity
	Bilirubin	Increase	Cholestatic jaundice
Laxatives	Magnesium	Decrease	From malabsorption and diarrhea
	Potassium	Decrease	From malabsorption and diarrhea
	Sodium	Decrease	From malabsorption and diarrhea
Lithium	Magnesium	Increase	Affect membrane transport
Magnesium hydroxide	Phosphorus	Decrease	Binding effect
Magnesium salts	Calcium	Increase	EDTA titration method
Mannitol	Sodium	Decrease	By diuretic effect
Meperidine	Glucose	Increase	Mechanism unknown
Metformin	Bicarbonate	Decrease	Acidosis
	Iron	Decrease	Impaired B_{12} absorption
Methotrexate	Alkaline phosphatase	Increase	Hepatotoxicity
	Bilirubin	Increase	Hepatotoxicity
Methyldopa	Bilirubin	Increase	Hepatotoxicity
	Chloride	Increase	By salt/water retention
	Sodium	Increase	By salt/water retention
	Urine ketone	Increase	Affect alkaline nitroprusside procedure
Metoclopramide	Potassium	Decrease	About 0.3 mmol/L
Metoprolol	Alkaline phosphatase	Increase	Increased enzyme activity
Metronidazole	Glucose	Decrease	Hexokinase/G6PD method
			Du Pont academic method
Morphine	Urine volume	Decrease	Increased ADH
Niacin	Alkaline phosphatase	Increase	Hepatic impairment
	Bilirubin	Increase	Hepatic impairment
	Glucose	Increase	Glucose intolerance may occur
	Uric acid	Increase	Hyperuricemia may occur
Nitrofurantoin	Bicarbonate	Decrease	By nephrotoxicity
	Creatinine	Increase	Jaffe-Fading-Fraction method
Nonsteroidal anti-inflammatory drugs	Potassium	Increase	Impaired potassium secretion, hypoaldosteronism
Oral contraceptives	Glucose	Increase	Alters glucose tolerance test
	Sodium	Increase	By salt/water retention
	Total protein	Decrease	Decreased protein synthesis; increases 3 years after administration
Oxazepam	Bilirubin	Increase	Possible hepatotoxicity
	Glucose	Increase	Affects *o*-toluidine/neocuprion method
Oxytocin	Sodium	Decrease	At induction of labor, also observed in infant

(*Continued*)

TABLE 9-2. Drug Interference With Clinical Laboratory Values (*Continued*)

Drug	Laboratory test	Increase/ decrease	Mechanism of action
Penicillin	Albumin	Decrease	BCG method
	Potassium	Decrease	If intravenous sodium penicillin infused
		Decrease	Large doses given intravenously (especially carbenicillin and ticarcillin) may cause hypokalemia due to the large amount of non-reabsorbable anion in the distal renal tubules
	Urine glucose	Increase	Ames Clinitest tablets
Phenobarbital	Calcium	Decrease	Metabolic effect with long-term therapy
	Folate	Decrease	Low levels in 27% to 91% of treated epileptics
Phenothiazines	Bilirubin	Increase	Intrahepatic cholestatic syndrome
	Phosphate	Decrease	Affects methods using phosphomolybdate
Phenytoin	Alkaline phosphatase	Increase	Hepatotoxicity (in 42% of 60 patients treated for >10 yrs)
	Folate	Decrease	Low level after extended therapy
	Glucose	Increase	Inhibitory effect on insulin secretion
Phosphates	Calcium	Decrease	Emission flame method
Probenecid	Bilirubin	Increase	Hepatotoxicity
	Urine protein	Increase	Nephrotoxic effects
Procainamide	Potassium	Increase	ISE method
Propranolol	Glucose	Decrease	May precipitate overt diabetes
		Increase	In long-term dialysis, due to beta blockade
	Triglycerides	Increase	After therapy for >10 wks
Quinidine	Bilirubin	Increase	Hemolysis effect
Rifampin	Bilirubin	Increase	Yellow coloration interferes with several analytical methods
	Glucose	Increase	Du Pont academic method
Risperidone	Glucose	Increase	Infrequent diabetes mellitus observed
	Potassium	Decrease	Hypokalemia observed
	Sodium	Decrease	Hyponatremia observed
Saline infusions	Chloride	Increase	Without addition of other anions, normal saline is hyperchloric with respect to physiologic extracellular fluid
Sildenafil	Alkaline phosphatase	Increase	Abnormal liver function tests
	Glucose	Increase	Unstable diabetes or hyperglycemia observed
		Decrease	Hypoglycemic reactions observed
Spironolactone	Potassium	Increase	Blunted normal response to aldosterone
	Sodium	Decrease	By diuretic effect
Succinylcholine	Potassium	Increase	Transient effect: general anesthesia
Sulcrafate	Phosphate	Decrease	Comparable to aluminum hydroxide
Sulfonylureas	Alkaline phosphatase	Increase	Elevation with cholangiolitis
	BUN	Increase	Diacetyl method

TABLE 9-2. Drug Interference With Clinical Laboratory Values (*Continued*)

Drug	Laboratory test	Increase/ decrease	Mechanism of action
Sulfonylureas (*Continued*)	Sodium	Decrease	Potentiates vasopressin, causes water retention
Tetracycline	Glucose	Decrease	Ascorbic acid in preparation may affect glucose oxidase procedure, by GOD/POD-PAP method.
		Increase	MBTH procedure of Neeley, slight effect on hexokinase, *o*-toluidine methods
	Phosphate	Decrease	May occur with Fanconi syndrome
		Increase	May occur with nephrotoxicity
	Sodium	Increase	May cause hypernatremia with renal impairment
Theophylline	Bilirubin	Decrease	Diazo reaction (general)
	Glucose	Decrease	Hypoglycemia observed with acute and chronic overdoses
	Potassium	Decrease	Renal/gastrointestinal cellular shift
Thiazide diuretics	Bilirubin	Increase	Cholestatic hepatitis
	Calcium	Increase	Renal retention: up to 0.25 mEq/L
	Chloride	Decrease	Impaired tubular reabsorption
	Glucose	Increase	Decreased glucose tolerance
	Magnesium	Decrease	Diuretic effect
	Sodium	Decrease	Diuretic effect
Thyroid preparations	Glucose	Increase	Promotes mobilization of glycogen stores
Tolbutamide	Alkaline phosphatase	Increase	Hepatotoxicity
	Cholesterol	Decrease	Inhibits hepatic synthesis
Triamterene	Bicarbonate	Decrease	By nephrotoxicity
Tube feedings	Magnesium	Increase	Especially in high rate and renal failure
Valproic acid	Alkaline phosphatase	Increase	Acute hepatic centrilobular necrosis
	Bilirubin	Increase	Abnormal liver function tests
	Sodium	Decrease	Hyponatremia and inappropriate ADH secretion
	Sodium	Increase	Technicon SRA-2000
Valsartan	Potassium	Increase	Serum potassium may increase 20%
Vancomycin	BUN	Increase	Nephrotoxicity
Vasopressin	Sodium	Decrease	Water retention
Verapamil	Urine sodium	Increase	Marked increase in hypertensives
Vincristine	Sodium	Decrease	Increased inappropriate secretion of ADH
Vitamin K	Bilirubin	Increase	Increases bilirubin by hemolyzing G6PD-deficient red blood

ADH, antidiuretic hormone; BUN, blood urea nitrogen; EDTA = ethylenediaminetetraacetic acid; G6PD = glucose-6-phosphate dehydrogenase; ISE, ion-sensitive electrode (laboratory method)

References

Abernethy DR, Greenblatt DJ, Divol M, et al. Alterations in drug distribution and clearance due to obesity. *J Pharmacol Exp Ther.* 1981;217:681–685.

Anderson KE, Conney AH, Dappas A. Nutrition and oxidative drug metabolism in man: relative influence of dietary fat, carbohydrate, and protein. *Clin Pharmacol Ther.* 1979;26:493–501.

Buchanan N, Eyberg C. Intramuscular tobramycin administration in kwashiorkor [letter]. *South Afr J Med.* 1978;25(Feb):273–274.

Buchanan N, Eyberg C, Davis MD. Isoniazid pharmacokinetics in kwashiorkor. *South Afr J Med.* 1979;25(Aug):299–300.

Buchanan N, Robinson R, Koornfoh HF, et al. Penicillin pharmacokinetics in kwashiorkor. *Am J Clin Nutr.* 1979;32:2233–2236.

(*Continued*)

TABLE 9-2. Drug Interference With Clinical Laboratory Values (*Continued*)

Buchanan N, Van Der Walt LA. The binding of antitubercular drugs in normal and kwashiorkor serum. *South Afr Med J.* 1977;17(Sept):522.
Buchanan N, Van Der Walt LA, Strickland B. Pharmacology of malnutrition, III: binding of digoxin to normal and kwashiorkor serum. *J Pharm Sci.* 1972;236:914–916.
Christian D. Drug interference with laboratory blood chemistry determinations. *Am J Clin Pathol.* 1970;54:118–142.
Henderson RP, Covinsky JO. Effect of protein on renal function and drug disposition. *Drug Intell Clin Pharm.* 1986;20:842–844.
Jagadeesan V, Krishnaswamy K. Drug binding in the undernourished: a study of the binding of propranolol to alpha-acid glucoprotein. *Eur J Clin Pharmacol.* 1985;27:657–659.
Ladenson JH, Bowers GN. Free calcium in serum. Determination with the ionspecific electrode, and factors affecting the results. *Clin Chem.* 1973;19:565–574.
Letellier G, Desjarlais F. Analytical interference of drugs in clinical chemistry: interference of 3-cephalosporin with the determination of serum creatinine concentration by the Jaffe reaction. *Clin Biochem.* 1985;18:352–356.
Lewis DP, VanDyke DC, Willhite LA, et al. Phenytoin-folic acid interaction. *Ann Pharmacother.* 1995;29:726–735.
Maslakowski CJ. Drug-nutrient interactions/interrelationships. *Nutr Supp Serv.* 1981:1:14–17.
McEvoy G, ed. *American Hospital Formulary Service, Drug Information 1997.* Bethesda, MD: American Society of Health System Pharmacists; 1997.
Mehta S, Kalsi HK, Mather VS. Chloramphenicol metabolism in children with protein calorie malnutrition. *Am J Clin Nutr.* 1975;26:977–981.
Muther RS. Drug interferences with renal function tests. *Am J Kidney Dis.* 1983;3(2):118–120.
Nozue T, Kobayashi A, Kodama T, et al. Clinical and laboratory observations: pathogenesis of cyclosporineinduced hypomagnesemia. *J Pediatr.* 1992;120:638–640.
Obama M, Cangir A, Van Eys J. Nutrition status and anthracycline cardiotoxicity in children. *South Med J.* 1983;76:577–578.
Pantuck EJ, Pantuck CB, Weisman C, et al. Stimulation of oxidative parenteral feeding. *Gastroenterology.* 1984;89:241–245.
Powers DE, Moore AO. *Food Medication Interactions.* 5th ed. Phoenix, AZ: F-MI Publishing; 1986.
Raghurham TC, Krishnaswamy K. Pharmacokinetics of tetracycline in nutritional oedema. *Chemotherapy.* 1982;28:428–433.
Reidenberg MM. Obesity and fasting: effects on drug metabolism and drug activity in man. *Clin Pharmacol Ther.* 1976;22:729–734.
Ryan MP. Diuretics and potassium/magnesium depletion: directions for treatment. *Am J Med.* 1987;82(suppl):3A.
Sher PP. Drug interferences with clinical laboratory tests. *Drugs.* 1982;24:24–63.
Smith CH, Bidlack WR. Dietary concerns associated with the use of medications. *J Am Diet Assoc.* 1984;84:901–914.
Smith SR, Bledsoe T, Chetri MK. Cortisol metabolism and the pituitary adrenal axis in adults with protein calorie malnutrition. *J Clin Endocrinol Metab.* 1975;40:43–52.
Wirth WA, Thompson BS. The effect of various conditions and substances on the results of laboratory procedures. *Am J Clin Pathol.* 1965;43:579–589.
Young DS. *Effects of Drugs on Clinical Laboratory Tests.* 3rd ed. Washington, DC: AACC Press; 1995.
Young DS, Pestaner LC, Gibberman V. Effects of drugs on clinical laboratory tests. *Clin Chem.* 1975;21(5):1D–3D.

C. Effects of nutrition on drug disposition
1. Protein and calorie malnutrition. Body weight is often considered in dosing medications, particularly those with a high potential for toxicity (narrow therapeutic index). Body composition may also affect drug distribution, depending on the affinity of the drug for muscle, fat, and water.
2. Hypoalbuminemia and hypoproteinemia. Decreased hepatic transport protein levels may affect drug disposition. Physiologically active calcium is the ionized calcium in the blood. Much of the calcium in the blood is bound to albumin. Since most clinical laboratories measure total serum calcium, which includes both the ionized and the bound calcium, in the presence of a low serum albumin concentration a decreased serum total calcium concentration may not be indicative of a low ionized calcium level. This may lead to unnecessary treatment of hypocalcemia.
3. Obesity/body composition. Different drugs may behave differently in relation to a patient's body composition. Dosages of some drugs, such as aminoglycosides and ceftazidime, are best based on lean body mass.[90] Chemotherapy drugs are best dosed on body surface area.[91] Since greater than 90% of the metabolism is thought to occur in lean tissue and adipose tissue is not considered metabolically active, many drug effects correlate best with lean body mass. Exceptions to this generality are extremely lipophilic substances such as barbiturates and benzodiazepines.[92] Lower serum concentrations may be seen for such drugs, with a longer elimination half-life in obese patients than nonobese patients. Dosing based on actual drug levels or titration to patient response are preferred schemes for dosing medications in obese patients.

(Drug-Nutrient Consideration chapters from the 1st edition were contributed by Deborah R. Johnson, Michael S. Nyffeler, Mark G. Klang, Edmund M. Hayes, and Cynthia S. Bloss)

REFERENCES

1. Notari RE. *Biopharmaceutics and Clinical Pharmacokinetics: An Introduction.* 3rd ed. New York, NY: Marcel Dekker; 1980.
2. Gubbins PO, Bertch KE. Drug absorption in gastrointestinal disease and surgery. *Clin Pharmacol Dis Process.* 1991;21:431–447.
3. Melnik G. Pharmacologic aspects of enteral nutrition. In: Rombeau JL, Caldwell MD, eds. *Clinical Nutrition: Enteral and Tube Feeding.* 2nd ed. Philadelphia, PA: WB Saunders; 1990, 472–509.
4. Christensen KJ, Gubbins PO, Gurley BJ, et al. Relative bioavailability of itraconazole from an extemporaneously prepared suspension and from the marketed capsules. *Am J Health Syst Pharm.* 1998;55:261–265.
5. Villarreal JD, Erush SC. Bioavailability of itraconazole from oral liquids in question. *Am J Health Syst Pharm.* 1995;52:1707–1708.
6. Staib AH, Beermann D, Harder S, et al. Absorption differences of ciprofloxacin along the human gastrointestinal tract determined using a remote-control drug delivery device (HF-capsule). *Am J Med.* 1989; 5A(suppl 87):66s–69s.
7. Healy DP, Brodbeck MC, Clendening CE. Ciprofloxacin absorption is impaired in patients given enteral feedings orally and via gastrostomy and jejunostomy tubes. *Antimicrob Agents Chem.* 1996;40:6–10.
8. Ramirez B, Richter JE. Review article: promotility drugs in the treatment of gastro-oesophageal reflux disease. *Aliment Pharmacol Ther.* 1993;7:5–20.
9. Chaudhuri TK, Fink S. Update: pharmaceuticals and gastric emptying. *Am J Gastroenterol.* 1990;3:223–230.
10. Gibaldi M. *Biopharmaceutics and Clinical Pharmacokinetics.* 3rd ed. Philadelphia, PA: Lea & Febiger, 1984:214.
11. Hansten PD. Drug interactions. In: Koda-Kimble MA, Young LY, eds. *Applied Therapeutics: The Clinical Use of Drugs.* Vancouver, BC: Applied Therapeutics; 1995.
12. Hayes E. Cytochrome P450 tables. Available at: http://www.edhayes.com/startp450.html Accessed November 21, 2004.
13. Suvarna R, Pirmohamed M, Henderson L. Possible interaction between warfarin and cranberry juice. *BMJ.* 2003;327(7429):1454.
14. Woolf T. *The Handbook of Drug Metabolism.* New York, NY: Marcel Dekker; 1999:175–183.

15. Rajagopalan S. Antimicrobial treatment in the elderly. *Med Clin North Am.* 2001;85:133–147.
16. Micromedex. Ranitidine. *Drugdex* [online database]. Available at: www. Micromedex.com/products/drugdex/ Accessed March 22, 2004.
17. Raffa RB. Mechanism of action of analgesics used to treat osteoarthritis pain. *Rheum Dis Clin North Am.* 2003;294:733–745.
18. Archer JS. Oral contraceptive efficacy and antibiotic interaction: a myth debunked. *J Am Acad Dermatol.* 2002;46:917–923.
19. Cunha BA. Antibiotic side effects. *Med Clin North Am.* 2001;85:149–185.
20. Mitchell JF, Leady MA. Oral solid dosage forms that should not be crushed—1996. *Hosp Pharm.* 1996;31:27–37.
21. Estoup ME. Approaches and limitations of medication delivery in patients with enteral feeding tubes. *Crit Care Nurse.* 1994;14:68–72, 77–79.
22. Eisenberg PG. Causes of diarrhea in tube-fed patients: a comprehensive approach to diagnosis and management. *Nutr Clin Pract.* 1993;8:119–123.
23. Miyagawa CI. Drug-nutrient interactions in critically ill patients. *Crit Care Nurse.* October 1993:69–90.
24. Dickerson RN, Melnik G. Osmolality of oral drug solutions and suspensions. *Am J Hosp Pharm.* 1988;45:832–834.
25. Niemiec PW, Vanderveen TW, Morrison JI, Hohenwarter MW. Gastrointestinal disorders caused by medications and electrolyte solution osmolality during enteral nutrition. *J Parenter Enteral Nutr.* 1983;7:387–389.
26. Lutomski DM, Gora ML, Wright SM, Martin JE. Sorbitol content of selected oral liquids. *Ann Pharmacother.* 1993;27:269–274.
27. Miller SJ, Oliver AD. Sorbitol content of selected sugar-free liquid medications. *Hosp Pharm.* 1993;28:741–744, 755.
28. Heather DJ, Howell L, Montana M, et al. Effect of a bulk-forming cathartic on diarrhea in tube-fed patients. *Heart Lung.* 1991;20:409–413.
29. Cutie AJ, Altmen E, Lenkel L. Compatibility of enteral products with commonly employed drug additives. *J Parenter Enteral Nutr.* 1983;7:186–191.
30. Burns PE, McCall L, Wirsching R. Physical compatibility of enteral formulas with various common medications. *J Am Diet Assoc.* 1988;9:1094–1096.
31. Fagerman KE, Ballou AE. Drug compatibilities with enteral feeding solutions coadministered by tube. *Nutr Supp Serv.* 1988;8:31–32.
32. Dunn A, White CM, Reddy P, Quercia RA, Chow MS. Delivery of omeprazole and lansoprazole granules through a nasogastric tube in vitro. *Am J Health Syst Pharm.* 1999;56:2327–2330.
33. Sharma VK. Comparison of 24-hour intragastric pH using four liquid formulations of lansoprazole and omeprazole. *Am J Health Syst Pharm.* 1999;56(suppl 4):S18–S21. Erratum in *Am J Health Syst Pharm.* 2000; 57(7):699.
34. DiGiacinto JL, Olsen KM, Bergman KL, Hoie EB. Stability of suspension formulations of lansoprazole and omeprazole stored in amber-colored plastic oral syringes. *Ann Pharmacother.* 2000;34:600–605.
35. Phillips JO, Metzler MH, Palmieri TL, et al. A prospective study of simplified omeprazole suspension for the prophylaxis of stress-related mucosal damage. *Crit Care Med.* 1996;24:1793–1800.
36. Tsai WL, Poon SK, Yu HK, et al. Nasogastric lansoprazole is effective in suppressing gastric acid secretion in critically ill patients. *Aliment Pharmacol Ther.* 2000;1:123–127.
37. Sostek MB, Chen Y, Skammer W, et al. Esomeprazole administered through a nasogastric tube provides bioavailability similar to oral dosing. *Aliment Pharmacol Ther.* 2003;18:581–586.
38. Prevacid [package insert]. Lake Forest, IL: TAP Pharmaceuticals; 2003. 03-5316-R22-Rev.
39. Ferron GM, Ku S, Abell M, et al. Oral bioavailability of pantoprazole suspended in sodium bicarbonate solution. *Am J Health Syst Pharm.* 2003;60(13):1324–1329.
40. Dentinger PJ, Swenson CF, Anaizi NH. Stability of pantoprazole in an extemporaneously compounded oral liquid. *Am J Health Syst Pharm.* 2002;59:953–956.
41. Bauer LA. Interference of oral phenytoin absorption by continuous nasogastric feedings. *Neurology.* 1982;32:570–572.
42. Hooks MA, Lange RL, Taylor AT, et al. Recovery of phenytoin from an enteral formula. *Am J Hosp Pharm.* 1986;43:685–688.
43. Fleischer D, Sheth N, Kou JH. Phenytoin interaction with enteral feedings administered through nasogastric tubes. *J Parenter Enteral Nutr.* 1990;14:513–516.
44. Rodman DP, Stevenson TL, Ray TR. Phenytoin malabsorption after jejunostomy tube delivery. *Pharmacotherapy.* 1995;15:801–805.
45. Doak KK, Haas CE, Dunnigan KJ, et al. Bioavailability of phenytoin acid and phenytoin sodium with enteral feedings. *Pharmacotherapy.* 1998;18: 637–645.
46. Martin JE, Lutomski DM. Warfarin resistance and enteral feedings. *J Parenter Enteral Nutr.* 1989;2:206–208.
47. Kuhn TA, Garnett WR, Wells BK, Karnes HT. Recovery of warfarin from an enteral nutrient formula. *Am J Hosp Pharm.* 1989;46:1395–1399.
48. Penrod LE, Allen JB, Cabacungan LR. Warfarin resistance and enteral feedings: 2 case reports and a supporting in vitro study. *Arch Phys Med Rehabil.* 2001;82:1270–1273.
49. Petretich DA. Reversal of osmolite-warfarin interaction by changing warfarin administration time [letter]. *Clin Pharm.* 1990;9:93.
50. Forrest A, Nix DE, Ballow CH, Goss TF, Birmingham MC, Schentag JJ. Pharmacodynamics of intravenous ciprofloxacin in seriously ill patients. *Antimicrob Agents Chemother.* 1993;37:1073–1081.
51. Hoffken G, Boner K, Glatzel PD, et al. Reduced enteral absorption of ciprofloxacin in the presence of antacids [letter]. *Eur J Clin Microbiol.* 1985;3:345.
52. Mueller BA, Brierton DG, Abel SR, Bowman L. Effect of enteral feeding with Ensure on oral bioavailabilities of ofloxacin and ciprofloxacin. *Antimicrob Agents Chemother.* 1994;38:2101–2105.
53. Piccolo ML, Toossi Z, Goldman M. Effect of coadministration of a nutritional supplement on ciprofloxacin absorption. *Am J Hosp Pharm.* 1994;51:2697–2699.
54. Noer BL, Angaran DM. The effect of enteral feedings on ciprofloxacin pharmacokinetics [abstract]. *Pharmacotherapy.* 1990;10:254.
55. Yuk JH, Nightingale CH, Quintiliani R, et al. Absorption of ciprofloxacin administered through a nasogastric or a nasoduodenal tube in volunteers and patients receiving enteral nutrition. *Diagn Microbiol Infect Dis.* 1990;13:99–102.
56. de Marie S, VandenBergh MFQ, Buijik SLCE, et al. Bioavailability of ciprofloxacin after multiple enteral and intravenous doses in ICU patients with severe gram-negative intra-abdominal infections. *Intensive Care Med.* 1998;24:343–346.
57. Mimoz O, Binter V, Jacolot A, et al. Pharmacokinetics and absolute bioavailability of ciprofloxacin administered through a nasogastric tube with continuous enteral feeding to critically ill patients. *Intensive Care Med.* 1998;24:1047–1051.
58. Cohn SM, Cohn KA, Rafferty MJ, et al. Enteric absorption of ciprofloxacin in early postsurgical patients. *Arch Surg.* 1995;133:1221–1225.
59. Nyffeler MS. Ciprofloxacin use in the enterally fed patient. *Nutr Clin Pract.* 1999;14:73–77.
60. Kanji S, McKinnon PS, Barletta JF, et al. Bioavailability of gatifloxacin by gastric tube administration with and without concomitant enteral feeding in critically ill patients. *Crit Care Med.* 2003;31:1347–1352.
61. Freeman CD, Klutman NE, Lamp KC, Dall LH, Strayer AH. Relative bioavailability of atovaquone suspension when administered with an enteral nutrition supplement. *Ann Pharmacother.* 1998;32:1004–1007.
62. Clark-Schmidt AL, Garnett WR, Lowe DR, Karnes HT. Loss of carbamazepine suspension through nasogastric feeding tubes. *Am J Hosp Pharm.* 1990;47:2034–2037.
63. Bass J, Miles MV, Tennison MB, Holcombe BJ, Thorn MD. Effects of enteral tube feeding on the absorption and pharmacokinetic profile of carbamazepine suspension. *J Clin Pharmacol.* 2001;41:183–186.
64. Riss JR, Kriel RL, Kammer NM, Judge MK, Montgomery MJ. Administration of Carbatrol to children with feeding tubes. *Pediatr Neurol.* 2002;27:193–195.
65. Semple HA, Koo W, Tam YK, Ngo LY, Coutts RT. Interactions between hydralazine and oral nutrients in humans. *Ther Drug Monit.* 1991;13: 304–308.
66. Nicolau DP, Crowe H, Nightingale CH, Quintiliani R. Bioavailability of fluconazole administered via a feeding tube in intensive care unit patients. *J Antimicrob Chemother.* 1995;36:395–401.
67. Buijk SL, Gyssens IC, Mouton JW, Verbrugh HA, Touw DJ, Bruining HA. Pharmacokinetics of sequential intravenous and enteral fluconazole in crit-

ically ill surgical patients with invasive mycoses and compromised gastrointestinal function. *Intensive Care Med.* 2001;27:115–121.
68. Davis GA, Rapp RP, Kearney PA, Ensom MH. Pharmacokinetics of fluconazole in trauma patients with postpyloric feeding tubes. *Ann Pharmacother.* 2001;35:1492–1494.
69. Murray M, Grogan TA, Lever J, Warty VS, Fung J, Venkataramanan R. Comparison of tacrolimus absorption in transplant patients receiving continuous versus interrupted enteral nutritional feeding. *Ann Pharmacother.* 1998;32:633–636.
70. Fagan TC, Walle T, Oexmann MJ, et al. Increased clearance of propranolol and theophylline by high-protein compared with high-carbohydrate diet. *Clin Pharmacol Ther.* 1987;41:402–406.
71. Plezia PM, Thornley SM, Kramer TH, Armstrong EP. The influence of enteral feedings on sustained-release theophylline absorption. *Pharmacotherapy.* 1990;10:356–361.
72. Bhargava VO, Schaaf LJ, Berlinger WG, Jungnickel PW. Effect of an enteral nutrient formula on sustained-release theophylline absorption. *Ther Drug Monit.* 1989;11:515–519.
73. Carraugher SG, Barrilleaux CN. Esophageal bezoars: the sucralith. *Crit Care Med.* 1991;19:837–839.
74. Lentsch EJ, Bumpous JM. Early postoperative esophageal obstruction caused by enteral feeding concretions in patients who have undergone laryngectomy. *Otolaryngol Head Neck Surg.* 1999;120(4):617–618.
75. Pinchera A, MacGillivray MH, Crawford JD, et al. Thyroid refractoriness in an athyreotic cretin fed soybean formula. *N Engl J Med.* 1965;273:83–87.
76. Seres DS. Insulin adsorption to parenteral infusion systems: case report and review of the literature. *Nutr Clin Pract.* 1990;5:111–117.
77. *AHFS Drug Information 2003.* Bethesda, MD: American Society of Health System Pharmacists; 2003.
78. Christian D. Drug interference with laboratory blood chemistry determinations. *Am J Clin Pathol.* 1970;54:118–142.
79. Powers DE, Moore AO. *Food Medication Interactions.* 5th ed. Phoenix, AZ: F-MI Publishing; 1986.
80. Mehta S, Kalsi HK, Mather VS. Chloramphenicol metabolism in children with protein calorie malnutrition. *Am J Clin Nutr.* 1975;26:977–981.
81. Anderson KE, Conney AH, Dappas A. Nutrition and oxidative drug metabolism in man: relative influence of dietary fat, carbohydrate, and protein. *Clin Pharmacol Ther.* 1979;26:493–501.
82. Smith SR, Bledsoe T, Chetri MK. Cortisol metabolism and the pituitary adrenal axis in adults with protein calorie malnutrition. *J Clin Endocrinol Metab.* 1975;40:43–52.
83. Buchanan N, Van Der Walt LA. The binding of antitubercular drugs in normal and kwashiorkor serum. *South Afr Med J.* 1977;52:522–525.
84. McEvoy G, ed. *American Hospital Formulary Service, Drug Information 2004.* Bethesda, MD: American Society of Health-System Pharmacists; 2004.
85. Obama M, Cangir A, Van Eys J. Nutrition status and anthracycline cardiotoxicity in children. *South Med J.* 1983;76:577–578.
86. Smith CH, Bidlack WR. Dietary concerns associated with the use of medications. *J Am Diet Assoc.* 1984;84:901–914.
87. Maslakowski CJ. Drug-nutrient interactions/interrelationships. *Nutr Supp Serv.* 1981;1:14–17.
88. Henderson RP, Covinsky JO. Effect of protein on renal function and drug disposition. *Drug Intell Clin Pharm.* 1986;20:842–844.
89. Pantuck EJ, Pantuck CB, Weisman C, et al. Stimulation of oxidative parenteral feeding. *Gastroenterology.* 1984;89:241–245.
90. Morgan DJ, Bray KM. Lean body mass as a predictor of drug dosage: implications for drug therapy. *Clin Pharmacokinet.* 1994;26(4):292–307.
91. Traynor AM, Nafziger AN, Bertino JS. Aminoglycoside dosing weight correction factors for patients of various body sizes. *Antimicrob Agents Chemother.* 1995;39:545–548.
92. Ogunnaike BO, Jones S, Jones D, Provost D, Whitten C. Anesthetic considerations for bariatric surgery. *Anesth Analg.* 2002;95:1793–1805.

SUGGESTED READINGS

Abernethy DR, Greenblatt DJ, Divol M, et al. Alterations in drug distribution and clearance due to obesity. *J Pharmacol Exp Ther.* 1981;217:681–685.

Dager WE, Inciardi JG, Howe TL. Estimating phenytoin concentrations by the Sheiner-Tozer method in adults with pronounced hypoalbuminemia. *Ann Pharmacother.* 1995;29:667–670.

Pantuck EJ, Pantuck BA, Garland WA, et al. Stimulatory effect of brussels sprouts and cabbage on human drug metabolism. *Clin Pharmacol Ther.* 1979;25:88–95.

Roe DA. *Handbook on Drug and Nutrient Interactions.* Chicago, IL: American Dietetic Association; 1989.

Trissel LA. *Handbook on Injectable Drugs.* 13th ed. Bethesda, MD: American Society of Health-System Pharmacists; 2004.

Young DS. *Effects of Drugs on Clinical Laboratory Tests.* Vol 2, 5th ed. Washington, DC: AACC Press; 2000.

SECTION EDITOR
Karen Ringwald-Smith, MS, RD

II

Immune Driven Conditions

Cade Fields-Gardner, MS, RD, LD, CD

10

HIV Infection/Acquired Immunodeficiency Syndrome

Introduction

Infection with the human immunodeficiency virus (HIV) has become a global pandemic, with prevalence ranging from 0.5% in the United States and many Western countries to nearly 40% in some transitional and developing nations.[1] While death rates have declined dramatically in the United States, there are an estimated 40,000 new infections yearly, with a trend toward increasing numbers of HIV diagnoses.[2,3] A dramatic (>80%) decline in perinatal transmission has been seen with the use of antiretroviral (ARV) therapies, which are nearly 100% effective in preventing transmission from mothers to children.[4,5] The majority of new infections in the United States are seen in the population categories of women and ethnic minorities.[6] The natural history of HIV infection and its symptomatic manifestation of acquired immunodeficiency syndrome (AIDS) vary widely among individuals.[7–9] HIV infects many cells and proliferates in activated CD4+ T cells. A background on the life cycle of HIV is helpful, and several online sources are available.[10]

I. Overview of HIV Infection and AIDS

A. Several aspects of primary (initial) and chronic infection with HIV can affect health and nutritional well-being.
   1. The acute viral syndrome that develops 2 to 4 weeks after exposure to HIV may include weight loss, fatigue, and fever. Gastrointestinal manifestations during this time include abdominal pain, vomiting, and diarrhea.[11]
   2. Immune deficiency resulting from the dysfunction and destruction of immune cells can lead, predictably, to opportunistic infection and neoplasm.[12]
   3. HIV is found in many tissues and may continue to be harbored regardless of viral load measures and ARV therapy.[13]
   4. Various manifestations of chronic HIV infection and treatments can directly affect the maintenance and restoration of nutritional status.[11]
      a) Chronic HIV infection can result in various metabolic alterations, including hypertriglyceridemia, hyperglycemia, lactic acidosis, insulin resistance, and altered body shape.
      b) Oral manifestations are more common in immunosuppressed patients and may include candidiasis (oral and esophageal), aphthous ulcers, gingival erythema, *Herpes spp.* lesions, oral hairy leukoplakia, and Kaposi's sarcoma.
      c) Gastrointestinal manifestations include esophageal ulcers, abdominal pain, biliary tract dysfunction, pancreatitis, and diarrhea (often associated with opportunistic infection).
      d) Weight loss episodes are commonly associated with opportunistic infections.
      e) Hematologic, neurologic, and neoplastic problems are associated with chronic or untreated HIV disease and immune dysfunction.

B. Treatments include ARV drugs targeted to various segments of the HIV life cycle, prevention and treatment for opportunistic infections, and prevention and treatment for a variety of symptoms that complicate disease treatment.
   1. The introduction and routine use of combination ARV therapies has resulted in a 50% decline in death rates in the United States. It is speculated that use of ARV therapies may also reduce the incidence of HIV infection for the future, assisting in efforts to eradicate the pandemic.[14–17]
   2. ARV treatment is not universally used or available. General recommendations suggest the initiation of ARV therapy if there is severe immune compromise as evidenced by CD4 cell counts of <200/uL in adults, adolescents, and children older than 6 years; or <500/uL in children aged 1 to 5 years; or <750/uL in children under 1 year old.[18,19] In addition, patient medical and nutritional history should play a role in choosing the most appropriate regimens. For instance, for a patient with a history of cardiovascular disease, regimens less likely to elevate blood lipids may be preferred.
   3. Prophylaxis for opportunistic infections may include antibiotic medications.[12] Interactions with ARVs and additive risk for side effects should be considered in choices for prevention and treatment for opportunistic infections.[20]
   4. Additional treatment may be required for diseases affecting nutritional status, such as diabetes, cancer, and cardiovascular disease. Please refer to chapters on individual disease states for treatment recommendations. Prior to treatment, special attention should be paid to potential interactions of diet and therapies with ARV medications
   5. Variations in quality of care have been documented and may be related to several factors, including CD4 count and medical insurance.[21]

II. Nutritional Aspects of HIV Infection

A. Nutritional alterations occur in primary infection and throughout the disease process.

1. Individuals experience primary infection differently. As with other infections, primary infection with HIV can lead to catabolism of lean tissues and alterations in nutrient metabolism. Symptoms associated with primary infection that specifically affect nutritional status may include anorexia, nausea, vomiting, diarrhea, and fever.
2. Malnutrition, wasting, and altered metabolism are relatively common and in some cases clinically significant, particularly in symptomatic phases of the disease.
   a) Malnutrition may start early in chronic HIV infection, with altered body composition and mild to moderate gastrointestinal dysfunction.[22–24]
   b) Weight loss and wasting, while common, are not necessarily a component of the natural history of HIV disease.[25,26] Weight loss episodes continue to be common regardless of the use of ARV medications.[27]
   c) Weight loss is related to the following:
      (1) Reduced intake or loss of nutrients that may be due to oral manifestations, diarrhea, vomiting, fever, and sweating[28,29]
      (2) Malabsorption of nutrients related to HIV or other infection in the gastrointestinal tract, hepatobiliary dysfunction, and pancreatic dysfunction[30,31]
      (3) Increased catabolism of body tissues in response to HIV or opportunistic infection and neoplasm[32]
      (4) Viral load with each log increase in levels associated with a 1.68 kg weight loss and a 1.58 increased likelihood of weight loss[33]
   d) Altered metabolism of nutrients may include changes in absorption, utilization, and losses.[34,35]
      (1) Altered organ function related to inflammatory response, HIV or opportunistic infection, and cancers can lead to changes in nutrient needs and tolerances.
      (2) Nutrients associated with inflammatory response may indicate more about infection severity than nutritional status but are still important indicators of disease and nutritional status changes.[36,37]
         (a) HIV is a chronic inflammatory disease, and long-term alterations in nutrient status may be related to disease process as well as nutritional status changes.
         (b) Albumin levels that quickly drop are more likely to be indicative of infection than of a change in nutritional status.[38,39]
         (c) Nutrients bound to albumin are also likely to be altered during an inflammatory response, with or without a significant change in nutritional status.[40] For instance, changes in zinc status may be related to inflammation, hydration, or hemolysis.[41] Whether albumin can be used as an adequate indicator of nutritional status may depend on the severity of an inflammatory response. Additional information, such as C-reactive protein levels, may help to establish the severity of inflammation.
         (d) Nutrients such as iron may be shunted to storage forms during inflammatory responses. Care should be taken in both diagnosing iron deficiency and treating potential deficiency with supplements (which may be contraindicated in chronic inflammatory conditions, such as HIV infection).[42,43]

B. Alterations in organ and other tissue function can be related to HIV infection.

1. HIV can infect and affect organ function. Gastrointestinal, liver, kidney, pancreas, adrenal, and sex organ functions may be adversely affected.
   a) If HIV infection is introduced through the gastrointestinal tract, gastrointestinal compromise may occur early.[44,45]
      (1) Symptoms and risk factors for compromise may include malabsorption of macronutrients and micronutrients, diarrhea, and lactose intolerance.
      (2) Reduced food and nutrient intake may result in weight loss.
   b) Liver manifestations are common in persons who are infected with HIV and are being treated for it.[46,47]
      (1) Alterations may be due to inflammatory response to infection.
      (2) Additional alterations may result from medication, nutrients, and other treatments.
      (3) Coinfection with hepatitis A, B, or C or other hepatitis viruses may lead to additional nutritional risk. Patients with hepatitis C coinfection on ARV therapies may be at higher risk for developing disease- and nutrition-related complications, such as diabetes.[48] ARV therapies may interact with treatments for hepatitis C coinfection and should be closely monitored to maintain the efficacy of both therapies.[49,50]
   c) Pancreatic function affects both absorption and metabolism of nutrients.
      (1) Exocrine pancreatic function can be compromised by infection and by medication interactions. Altered exocrine pancreatic function can lead to fat malabsorption and steatorrhea in some cases.[51,52]
      (2) Endocrine pancreatic function can be compromised by infection and altered hormonal milieu.[53]
   d) Adrenal gland function may be altered, leading to changes in inflammatory responses and other hormones.[54–56]
   e) Sex hormone alterations may be related to other hormonal alterations and to weight and subcutaneous fat losses.[57]
   f) Changes in growth hormone levels and circadian rhythms have been reported and may lead to weight loss, alterations in body composition, and anabolic blocks.[58]
   g) Alterations in thyroid hormone levels have been documented. Hypothyroidism may be more prevalent in HIV-infected men than in women and more commonly associated with low CD4 counts. The potential of ARVs to alter thyroid levels remains equivocal.[59,60]

C. Nutritional compromise can be related to chronic HIV infection and opportunistic conditions.

1. Chronic HIV infection and intermittent opportunistic infections or cancers related to immune compromise can also alter nutritional status according to the site affected and the severity of the infection or cancer.
2. Nutritional compromise can further impair immune function and the ability to withstand opportunistic events.[61]

D. Nutritional alterations occur with ARV and other treatments.

1. The introduction of combination therapy with ARVs has resulted in a 50% decline in the death rate due to HIV infection.[6]
2. Medication interactions with food and nutrient metabolism can compromise nutritional status and lead to additional acute and/or chronic disease characterized by gastrointestinal, liver, kidney, pancreatic, and other organ dysfunction. See Table 10-1 for potential interactions and other effects of ARVs.[20]
   a) Once initiated, it is likely that medication therapies will be long-term and possibly lifelong. Adherence is an important part of an integrated health care plan. Adherence is supported

TABLE 10-1. Potential Nutrition Interactions With Antiretroviral Therapies

Generic name (brand name) Class of drug (manufacturer)	Diet and nutrition interactions
Abacavir (Ziagen) Protease inhibitor (GlaxoSmithKline)	Diet interactions: Take with or without food; caution with alcohol Potential side effects: nausea/vomiting, anorexia, abdominal pain, diarrhea, anemia, pancreatitis, lactic acidosis (rare); may increase triglycerides, slight glucose intolerance
Amprenavir (Agenerase) Protease inhibitor (GlaxoSmithKline)	Diet interactions: Take with or without food but not with high-fat meal (>50 g); avoid vitamin E supplements; take 1 hour apart from antacids Potential side effects: diarrhea, nausea/vomiting, taste changes, stomach upset, diabetes, fatigue, increased cholesterol, increased triglycerides, anemia
Atazanavir (Reyataz) Protease inhibitor (Bristol-Myers Squibb)	Diet interactions: Take with food Potential side effects: abdominal pain, anorexia, aphthous stomatitis, colitis, constipation, gastroenteritis, taste changes, increased high-density lipoprotein cholesterol, increased bilirubin, lactic acidosis, potential for altered fat deposition
Delavirdine (Rescriptor) NNRTI (Agouron)	Diet interactions: Take with or without food; do not take with antacids or magnesium-containing supplements; can take with acidic beverage (eg, cranberry juice); avoid alcohol Potential side effects: increased thirst, anorexia, dry mouth, nausea/vomiting, gastritis, diarrhea, constipation, flatulence
Didanosine (Videx) NRTI (Bristol-Myers Squibb)	Diet interactions: Take without food on an empty stomach; do not take with acidic beverage or food, aluminum-containing antacids, or magnesium-containing supplements; avoid alcohol Potential side effects: anorexia, diarrhea, weight loss, anemia, nausea/vomiting, constipation, dry mouth, taste changes, pancreatitis (increased risk with alcohol; decreased risk in pediatric patients), lactic acidosis (rare), increased triglycerides
Efavirenz (Sustiva) NNRTI (Bristol-Myers Squibb)	Diet interactions: Do not take with high-fat meal (>40–60 g); avoid alcohol Potential side effects: anorexia, nausea/vomiting, diarrhea, increased cholesterol, increased triglycerides
Emtricitabine (Emtriva) NRTI (Gilead)	Diet interactions: Take with or without food Potential side effects: nausea/vomiting, diarrhea
Enfurvitide (Fuzeon) Fusion inhibitor (Roche)	Diet interactions: Subcutaneous injection with no food interactions Potential side effects: diarrhea, nausea, fatigue, taste change, decreased appetite, potential for pancreatitis
Fosamprenavir (Lexiva) Protease inhibitor (GlaxoSmithKline)	Diet interactions: Take with or without food Potential side effects: nausea/vomiting, diarrhea, increased triglycerides
Indinavir (Crixivan) Protease inhibitor (Merck)	Diet interactions: Take without food on an empty stomach or with very low calorie/low protein snack (note: no food restriction when taken with ritonavir); take with plenty of fluids Potential side effects: nausea/vomiting, abdominal pain, taste changes, diarrhea, kidney stones, diabetes (rare), insulin resistance, increased triglycerides, increased cholesterol; increased indirect bilirubin in pediatric patients should be closely monitored

TABLE 10-1. Potential Nutrition Interactions With Antiretroviral Therapies (*Continued*)

Generic name (brand name) Class of drug (manufacturer)	Diet and nutrition interactions
Lamivudine (Epivir) **NRTI (GlaxoSmithKline)**	Diet interactions: Take with or without food Potential side effects: nausea/vomiting, abdominal cramps, diarrhea, anorexia, pancreatitis, lactic acidosis (rare)
Lopinavir (Kaletra) **Protease inhibitor (Abbott)**	Diet interactions: Take with or without food; meals with >15 g fat increase absorption Potential side effects: abdominal pain, diarrhea, nausea, increased triglycerides, increased cholesterol
Nelfinavir (Viracept) **Protease inhibitor (Agouron)**	Diet interactions: Take with food; mixing powder with acidic food or beverage results in bitter taste Potential side effects: diarrhea, flatulence, nausea, abdominal pain, diabetes (rare), increased or decreased glucose
Nevirapine (Viramune) **NNRTI (Roxane)**	Diet interactions: Take with or without food Potential side effects: nausea/vomiting, abdominal pain, fatigue, hepatotoxicity
Ritonavir (Norvir) **Protease inhibitor (Abbott)**	Diet interactions: Take with food; meals with >15 g fat increase absorption Potential side effects: nausea/vomiting, diarrhea, taste changes, anorexia, upset stomach, abdominal pain, weight loss, diabetes, increased triglycerides, increased cholesterol
Saquinavir (Invirase, Fortovase) **Protease inhibitor (Roche)**	Diet interactions: Take with high-calorie, high-fat meal unless combined with ritonavir; grapefruit juice increases retention Potential side effects: nausea, diarrhea, constipation, abdominal pain, taste changes, impaired glucose tolerance
Stavudine (Zerit) **NRTI (Bristol-Myers Squibb)**	Diet interactions: Take with or without food; avoid alcohol Potential side effects: nausea/vomiting, diarrhea, anorexia, weight loss, abdominal pain, peripheral neuropathy
Tenofovir (Viread) **NRTI (Gilead)**	Diet interactions: Take with food Potential side effects: nausea/vomiting, diarrhea, abdominal pain, lactic acidosis (rare)
Zalcitabine (Hivid) **NRTI (Roche)**	Diet interactions: Take without food on an empty stomach; avoid alcohol Potential side effects: anorexia, oral/esophageal ulcers, nausea/vomiting, diarrhea, constipation, weight loss, abdominal pain, dry mouth, peripheral neuropathy, lactic acidosis (rare), pancreatitis (rare), increased triglycerides, impaired glucose tolerance
Zidovudine (Retrovir) **NRTI (GlaxoSmithKline)**	Diet interactions: Take with or without food, preferably not with high-fat meal; may require zinc, copper supplementation Potential side effects: anorexia, nausea/vomiting, upset stomach, constipation, anemias

NNRTI, Nonnucleoside Reverse Transcriptase Inhibitor; NRTI, Nucleoside Reverse Transcriptase Inhibitor.

in part by nutritional interventions.[62] Research is continuing to explore the possible advantages and disadvantages of planned treatment interruptions.[63,64]

b) Specific ARVs are associated with glucose intolerance, insulin resistance, dyslipidemia, and a variety of anemias.[65–68] See Table 10-1 for potential nutrient interactions reported with ARV medications.
   (1) Protease inhibitors have been associated with glucose intolerance or insulin resistance.
   (2) Nucleoside reverse transcriptase inhibitors have been associated with anemias.

c) Treatment recommendations for these problems are outlined by the Adult and Pediatric AIDS Clinical Trials Groups and others.[69,70]

d) Many ARVs are associated with anorexia, nausea and vomiting, diarrhea, constipation, abdominal pain, dry mouth, taste changes, and other potential interactions that can reduce food intake, absorption, and increase losses.[20]

E. Nutritional compromise in pediatric patients

1. Nutritional compromise in the forms of stunting, weight loss, failure to thrive, gastrointestinal dysfunction, and developmental delay are among the problems commonly seen in pediatric patients with HIV disease.
2. Subclinical hypothyroidism has been documented and has the potential to lead to developmental abnormalities.[71] Thyroid function monitoring has been suggested.
3. Children with growth failure may have altered levels of thyroid and insulin-like growth factor.[72]

III. Nutritional Assessment in HIV Infection

A. Specific nutrition-related assessment factors are strong predictors of morbidity and mortality. Weight loss and wasting as indicated by loss of weight, fat-free mass, body cell mass (BCM), and fat tissues are strong predictors of mortality in persons with HIV infection. Despite the use of effective ARV therapies, the incidence of wasting may be on the rise.[73]

B. General assessment for adults will include the evaluation criteria for other patients as described in the general nutrition assessment chapter.

1. Nutrition assessment includes basic evaluation of
   a) Physical findings
      (1) Anthropometry to evaluate weight for height, weight changes, changes in or high-risk patterns of body dimensions, and body composition evaluation
         (a) While the numbers of AIDS cases reported has been reduced, the relative numbers of cases that are defined by wasting continues to hover around 20%. Current research suggests that wasting episodes continue to occur regardless of the use of ARVs in as many as 40% of HIV-infected patients.[27]
         (b) Indicators of wasting in chronic HIV infection include[74]
            i) Weight decrease of more than 10% over a 6-month period
            ii) Loss from baseline or expected values of 5% BCM
            iii) Body mass index of <20
         (c) Additional measures of body dimensions and fat folds may help to characterize altered body shape and fat deposition associated with chronic HIV infection, treatment, and nontreatment host factors.[75–77]
      (2) Commonly reported altered body shape changes have been related to both chronic infection and medications used to treat HIV infection.
         (a) Subcutaneous fat losses can occur all over the body but are most noticeable in peripheral limbs and facial areas. Consequences of subcutaneous fat loss can include the initiation or exacerbation of insulin resistance and a reduced substrate for maintenance of sex hormones and normal bone metabolism. Subcutaneous fat losses can be assessed through anthropometric measures as well as dual energy x-ray absorptiometry of soft tissues in peripheral limbs.
         (b) Fat deposition is generally centrally located in the abdomen, chest, back, and nape of neck areas. Central fat deposition, sometimes known as central obesity, is associated with insulin resistance and altered fat metabolism. Central fat deposition can be assessed through anthropometric measures, magnetic resonance imaging, or computed tomography scans of an abdominal cross-section at the L4–L5 level.
   b) Bioelectrical impedance analysis (BIA)
      (1) BIA evaluation should use equations validated for use in HIV infection.[78]
      (2) BIA can be compared to expected or functional levels of BCM (muscle and organ tissue estimate), extracellular tissue (bone, collagen, and extracellular fluid estimate), and fat (both stored and essential functional fat tissues).
      (3) A 5% loss of BCM from function levels or baseline indicates wasting and risk for functional loss of tissues and increased risk of mortality.
      (4) An increase in extracellular tissue can indicate an active inflammatory process in normally hydrated persons.
      (5) A decrease in fat stores indicates a calorie imbalance and can also reflect peripheral fat losses. This problem may feed a cycle of insulin resistance, leading to additional peripheral fat losses and alterations in other hormonal balances.
   c) Other physical examination findings include
      (1) General appearance
      (2) Signs and symptoms of nutrient deficiency and excess (see Chapter 1 for more detail)
   d) Food and other nutrient intake compared to estimated needs and anticipated contraindications, upper limits, and other limitations due to organ dysfunction, inflammatory processes, and other conditions the patient experiences
      (1) Ability to eat, gastrointestinal function, and risk or indication of altered nutrient metabolism should be reviewed to determine the appropriate mode of nutrition intervention and support.
      (2) Included in this evaluation are physical activity levels, psychosocial and economic limitations, and other factors that can affect nutritional intake and nutrition security (the ability to maintain a steady and adequate supply of required nutrients).
      (3) Specific evaluation of dietary intake along with physical and laboratory evaluation can be used to determine potential deficiencies and toxicities (see Chapter 1).
         (a) Several nutrient deficiencies or metabolism alterations may be seen. Most commonly, nutrients associated with inflammation, including iron, zinc, and antioxidants, may be altered.
         (b) Supplementation to overcome reduced levels of nutrients or anticipated additional nutrient needs can increase the risk for nutrient toxicity. Nutrient supplementation should be monitored closely. In most cases, it may be better to initiate a balanced multivitamin and mineral supplement than to supplement individual nutrients.
   e) Medical history, including disease status, presence of opportunistic infections and neoplasms, existence of cofactors that can affect nutritional status, and medication history
   f) Laboratory evaluation, including disease status and markers of nutritional status
      (1) Review current and past markers of disease status, including CD4 and CD8 cell counts and viral loads. Past or current history of low T-cell counts and high viral load is associated with greater risk for adverse effects of disease and

treatments such as insulin resistance, altered body fat deposition, and osteoporosis.

(2) Note that chronic inflammatory process and dehydration may affect nutritional status markers such as albumin, prealbumin, zinc, and iron.

(3) Additional evaluation may include biochemical indices of concomitant disease such as C-reactive protein for cardiovascular disease and active inflammatory response, glycosylated hemoglobin, oral glucose tolerance tests, and C-peptide for insulin resistance.

C. Additional clinical risk factors and indicators should be assessed.

1. Other common chronic diseases that may complicate treatment of HIV infection and associated malnutrition include diabetes, cardiovascular disease, osteopenia and osteoporosis, renal dysfunction, liver disease, respiratory disease, and cancer.

2. Smoking and alcohol intake can affect nutrient intake and metabolism.

a) Alterations in organ function and greater risk for adverse effects of medications and chronic HIV infection have been suggested by cohort studies. Examples include the following:

(1) Coinfections, interactions with additional medications used to treat coinfections or neoplasms, and the long-term effects of cortisol and other hormonal changes associated with chronic inflammatory processes can contribute to changes in liver, kidney, pancreas, intestinal, and other organ systems.

(2) Liver toxicity and interactions with foods or coinfections can lead to medication intolerance in cases of medications that are heavily metabolized by the liver.

(3) Nephrotoxicity and other kidney disease can increase the potential toxicity of medications and adverse effects on nutritional status.

(4) Gastrointestinal infection by HIV and other infectious disease can reduce the absorption of both nutrients and medications.

b) Complicated interactions with medications, hormonal milieu, food intake and absorption, organ function, and cellular damage should be taken into consideration. Examples include the following:

(1) Medications can alter lipid and glucose metabolism, cause symptoms such as anorexia and diarrhea, and lead to liver and kidney cell damage.

(2) Hormonal changes associated with chronic inflammation and weight changes may include insulin resistance, hypogonadism, and growth hormone resistance. Alterations in body composition may include changes in muscle tissues, fat deposition patterns, bone tissue metabolism, and oxidative stress-related cellular damage.

D. General assessment will include items outlined in Chapter 1. Please refer to that chapter for details. Pediatric-specific nutritional assessment in HIV infection background information includes[79,80]

1. Disease process

a) Presence of HIV infection, level of immune function markers, and clinical class of disease progression are strong indicators of nutritional risk.[81]

(1) Comorbidities can include a number of opportunistic or other complications related or unrelated to HIV infection and its treatment. Examples include failure to thrive, cardiovascular disease, glucose intolerance and diabetes, renal disease, hepatic disease, pulmonary disease, a myriad of opportunist infections and neoplasms related to severe immunosuppression, neurological disorders, and developmental delay.

(2) Several common problems are specifically related to nutrition and can be treated by combinations of therapies that include nutrition-related strategies.

(a) Oral lesions are associated with CD4 counts, and gingival lesions were found to be the most common manifestations in children.[82] Dental treatment access and utilization may be underused by children with HIV infection.[83]

(b) Fever is related to opportunistic infections.

(c) Nausea, vomiting, diarrhea, malabsorption, and anorexia may be related to HIV infection, opportunistic disease, other comorbidities, or medication therapies.

(d) Folate and iron-associated anemias have been documented in children. Neurologic deficits are associated with folate deficiency, and iron-related anemia is associated with chronic disease. Additional nutrients can be lost through vomiting and diarrhea.

b) In addition to clinical problems, psychosocial and economic issues may compromise nutritional status. A child with a caretaker who is also HIV-infected may not be receiving adequate care. Additional support for nutrition may include connection with community resources and additional health care social support resources.

c) There may be nutrition-related interactions with medications.

d) Cardiovascular function may be worse in children born to women with HIV infection and especially in HIV-infected children.[84]

e) Anemia may be common in children, particularly those with prenatal exposure to ARV medications.[67]

f) Similar patterns of metabolic and body shape alterations are seen in children and adults.[85]

g) Some medications may affect children differently than adults. For instance, the protease inhibitor indinavir is associated with increased indirect bilirubin, which may be clinically inconsequential in adult patients but more threatening to health and survival in children. On the other extreme, very little pancreatitis has been reported in children taking the nucleoside reverse transcriptase inhibitor didanosine, although pancreatitis is a common occurrence in adults. Finally, while nephrolithiasis is a potential problem with both adults and children taking indinavir, it may be more difficult to ensure adequate fluid intake (estimated at 48 ounces) in small children to prevent the problem.

h) Different forms of medications are used with newborns and infants than adults. In some cases, it is a challenge to administer liquids and improve the tolerance of bad-tasting medications, such as ritonavir.

2. Physical examination

a) Anthropometry, specifically serial measures of body dimensions, which can identify particular types of problems and their severity

(1) A declining trajectory of weight for age measures may indicate calorie imbalance and is a strong indicator of risk for malnutrition-related problems and mortality.

(2) A declining trajectory of height for age measures is associated with chronic malnutrition, protein imbalance, and micronutrient deficiencies (eg, zinc) and is a strong indicator of risk of morbidity and mortality.

(3) A declining trajectory of weight for height or body mass index measures is an indicator of calorie imbalance but

may not consider existing stunting processes and is a weaker indicator of risk for malnutrition-related complications.

(4) Midarm and head circumferences can be compared to norms.

(5) Growth velocity has been correlated to survival in HIV-infected children. Best predictors of mortality were height growth, viral load, and CD4 count. Weight gain and head circumference growth may not be as well correlated with survival rates in this population.[86] Shorter survival times are associated with poor nutritional status.[87]

b) BIA

(1) Equations may be different for children.

(2) Lean body mass as expressed by BIA is a strong indicator for nutritional risk.

3. Dietary intake
4. Laboratory analysis for disease factors and nutritional indices. Nutritional indices may be affected by inflammatory processes (eg, albumin, zinc, selenium).
5. In many cases, the diagnosis of HIV infection and related disease is not disclosed to the child. In some cases, the diagnosis is disclosed to only selected caregivers. These limitations should be considered in evaluating and planning for nutrition-related interventions, especially those that support medication adherence.[88,89]

IV. Goals of Nutritional Therapy and Nutrition Decision Making

A. Primary goals for nutrition-related therapies include survival and maintenance of body and cognitive functions, growth, and development in pediatric patients.[90]

B. Medication efficacy is dependent on nutritional status and can be affected by nutrient intake. Nutrition-related interventions should support medication adherence and efficacy. Because the use of ARV therapies results in a decline in infectivity, supporting medication efficacy through nutrition education and intervention becomes of primary importance to transmission prevention efforts.[14–17]

C. Nutrition-related interventions should also aim to prevent or reduce the adverse effects of chronic HIV infection, other concomitant disease, and therapies.

1. Maintenance of nutritional status supports maintenance of immune function and resistance to opportunistic disease. Well-nourished children may respond well to ARV therapies, but response has not been tested in undernourished children.[91]
2. Education and counseling should include support for adherence to medication regimens.

V. Nutritional Management in HIV Infection

A. Alterations in nutrient requirements that may occur include the following:

1. Energy needs may increase. Increases in resting energy expenditure have been documented across the disease spectrum.[92] However, total energy expenditure depends on current nutritional status and the amount of BCM (calorie-using tissues) in the body.[93] The increase in energy needs is variable and dependent on two factors: inflammatory process and amount of metabolizing protein stores (BCM).

a) Severely wasted patients may have lower total energy expenditures and may not have the protein stores required to mount an inflammatory response. In such cases, refeeding should be implemented with extreme caution as the body may respond dramatically if there are hidden opportunistic infections.[94] Increased availability of nutrients, particularly amino acids, in a severely malnourished person with hidden infections (infections that are not accompanied by fever or other indicators because of a lack of nutritional stores to mount an adequate inflammatory response) can lead to a sudden, severe inflammatory response that increases the risk of severe reactions that can lead to multiorgan failure and death.

b) Different mechanisms for weight loss can yield differences in body composition changes during wasting, which can alter the level of nutritional risk. In most cases, opportunistic infection is associated with a cachectic form of weight loss.[95]

c) Treatment of HIV infection may alter energy expenditure and risk for malnutrition, both by decreasing energy expenditure through lowering of HIV viral burden and by increasing energy expenditure through a mechanism independent of ARV therapies.[96,97]

2. Protein turnover rates may be higher in HIV infection regardless of energy expenditure. Both calorie and protein balance appear to be important to maintaining growth in children.[98] Level of protein intake is related to the maintenance and preservation of BCM in HIV.[99] Alterations in BCM may differ in patients with coinfections.[100] Protein intake remains related to the preservation of BCM tissues.
3. Micronutrient interventions may be important to maintain adequate intake and appropriate body tissue levels.[101,102]

a) Micronutrient supplementation efforts should be approached with care due to the potential for toxic levels and the lack of knowledge about nutrient tolerance in asymptomatic and symptomatic HIV-infected individuals.

b) Antioxidant therapy using micronutrients has been explored with equivocal results. Beta-carotene supplementation has shown transient increases in CD4 cell count. Whey protein, N-acetyl cysteine, and other strategies to improve glutathione content have increased the antioxidant capacity of the body. Additional efforts to improve antioxidant status and keep oxidative stress in check with nutrient supplementation are topics of ongoing research.

B. Interventions to improve and maintain nutritional status should include education and counseling on basic nutritional principles and individualized strategies for maintaining adequate food and nutrient intake despite the challenges of disease and medications. As with other diseases, all HIV-infected patients should have access to nutrition-related care. Care should be provided in a nonjudgmental and safe environment with consideration of all the psychosocial and economic factors that can ultimately affect nutritional status and health care.[103]

1. Patient education should include basic nutrition principles, food and water safety, physical activity maintenance, and nutrition-related symptom management strategies.
2. Patient counseling should be tailored to specific risk factors and nutritional needs.

a) Weight loss and wasting should be prevented whenever possible and reversed as soon as feasible. Nutrition-related interventions can improve important nutrition-related markers of weight, fat-free mass, and body mass index.[73,104,105]

b) Symptoms of HIV infection, opportunistic disease, and medication interactions should be addressed, and nutrition should be tailored to the patient's food preferences and tolerances.[106] Care should be taken to anticipate the potential adverse effects of disease and treatments. The patient's diet plan may include contingent dietary alterations related to anticipated problems. Past concepts of palliative care should be integrated into primary care for HIV-infected patients at all points in chronic HIV disease.[107]

(1) A strong emphasis on palliative care has previously been reserved for hospice patients. With longer-term survival in HIV, symptom management and coping skills to maintain nutritional status become important in chronic HIV infection across the spectrum of disease.

(2) A patient interview might include questions about symptoms that may require palliation, such as diarrhea, nausea/vomiting, anorexia, pain, and fatigue, and other symptoms that may interfere with health maintenance, medication adherence, and quality of life.

c) Specific diets may be used to address chronic disease cofactors such as insulin resistance and diabetes, cardiovascular disease, renal dysfunction, and liver disease [108]

3. Oral nutrient supplementation may be required if it is determined that foodstuffs will not meet extraordinary requirements related to disease, gastrointestinal dysfunction, or neurologic dysfunction.

a) Nutrients lost through fever, diarrhea, and vomiting should be replaced. Oral rehydration therapy in addition to macronutrient and micronutrient supplementation may be required.

b) Weight loss and nutrient deficits may be selectively treated with supplemental nutrients.

(1) Care should be taken to ensure that supplemental nutrients do not adversely interact with medications and other dietary nutrients.

(2) Nutrient supplementation should be tailored according to patient risk factors and needs. High-protein supplementation may not be advisable in populations at high risk for renal insufficiency.

(3) Limitations of effectiveness may be related to metabolic alterations that produce an anabolic block.[109]

c) Multi-micronutrient supplements have been investigated and show some promise for slowing the progression of HIV infection to AIDS.[110,111] Caution is suggested for iron supplementation in patients with a low serum iron level, owing to the potential for toxicity and the increased risk for bacterial infections.

d) Complementary and alternative medicine may include nutrient-based therapy.

(1) Both nutrient and nonnutrient therapies in doses higher than in common food intake may be categorized as pharmaceutical therapies.

(2) Care should be taken to consider the potential for nutrient-drug interactions.[112]

C. HIV-specific considerations in enteral nutrition support (adult and pediatric) include the following:

1. Standard indications for enteral nutrition can be used in adults and children with HIV infection and immune compromise.

a) Children who fail oral supplementation, have severe growth and development failure, or have neurologic dysfunction that prevents adequate oral nutrient intake should be considered for enteral nutrition.[113]

b) Severe malabsorption and/or gastrointestinal infections may require special formulations or consideration for parenteral nutrition.[114]

c) Immune-enhancing formulas may or may not provide added benefit.[115,116]

2. In both adults and children, enteral nutrition support presents challenges for the HIV-infected patient with immune compromise (CD4 cell counts of <200/uL in adults, adolescents, and children older than 6 years, or <500/uL in children aged 1 to 5 years, or <750/uL in children under 1 year old), but standard practice guidelines should be sufficient to provide safe and effective enteral nutrition therapy options.[117]

a) The standard of care for other tube-fed adult and pediatric patients applies, with special attention to sterile/aseptic techniques and methods. The use of ready-to-feed or prepared powder products depends on the level of immune compromise as indicated by CD4 cell counts and the potential for infection in the particular setting (eg, acute care, home care).

b) The fact that several organ systems may be affected with severe immune compromise should be considered in tailoring therapy. Plans should include strategies to maintain gut mucosa and immunity.

c) Close monitoring for infection and other complications will be required.

D. HIV-specific considerations in parenteral nutrition support (adult and pediatric) include the following:

1. In both adults and children, parenteral nutrition support presents challenges for the HIV-infected patient with severe immune compromise.

a) The standard of care for other parenterally fed adult and pediatric patients applies, with special attention to sterile/aseptic techniques and methods. With appropriate care, line sepsis may or may not be more common in immune compromise.[118,119] While treatment for HIV infection has reduced the risk of catheter-associated infection rates by improving immune competence, close monitoring for infectious complications is required.[120]

b) The fact that several organ systems may be affected with severe immune compromise should be considered in tailoring therapy. Alterations in liver, pancreas, or kidney functions, for instance, may require altered formulations, rates of infusion, and methods of delivery. See chapter 11 for cancer, chapter 15 for pancreatitis, chapter 17 for liver disease, and chapter 23, 24 and 30 for kidney failure for more tailored feeding strategies.

c) Opportunistic infection treatment is essential to achieving nutritional repletion using parenteral nutrition.[121]

E. Nonnutrient adjunctive therapies to achieve nutrition-related goals may include treatment for nutrition-related symptoms, anemias and other altered laboratory values, wasting, altered body fat deposition, osteopenia and osteoporosis, altered organ functions, altered hormonal milieu, inflammatory processes, anabolic blocks, and reduced levels of physical activity. Examples include the following:

1. Chronic diarrhea may benefit from a full evaluation to identify the cause, to match appropriate treatment with antidiarrheal medications, enteric-coated pancrelipase, and hydration strategies (oral or intravenous rehydration therapy).

2. Appetite loss may benefit from medications that stimulate the appetite, such as dronabinol or megestrol acetate, or strategies to overcome anabolic blocks, such as testosterone replacement or growth hormone therapy.

3. Chronic anemias may be treated with medications to improve red blood cell production.

4. Hypogonadism, anemia, muscle wasting, and bone losses may benefit from testosterone replacement or supplemental anabolic steroids.

5. Muscle wasting, bone losses, altered fat deposition, and growth hormone resistance may benefit from varying levels of growth hormone or anticytokine medication.
6. Dyslipidemia may benefit from lipid-lowering medications.
7. Insulin resistance may benefit from oral antidiabetic agents.
8. Muscle wasting, dyslipidemia, insulin resistance, and recovery from fatigue may benefit from exercise therapy.

F. All A.S.P.E.N. standards, guidelines, and pathways can be tailored and applied to persons living with chronic HIV infection.

(HIV/AIDS material in the 1st edition was contributed by Virginia Herrmann, M. Patricia Fuhrman, Peggy R. Borum, Robin Henderson, Jose M. Saavedra, and Lynn E. Mattis)

REFERENCES

1. Joint United Nations Programme on HIV/AIDS and World Health Organization. AIDS epidemic update. December 2003. Available at: http://www.unaids.org/NetTools/Misc/DocInfo.aspx?href=http%3A%2F%2Fgva%2Ddoc%2Dowl%2FWEBcontent%2FDocuments%2Fpub%2FPublications%2FIRC%2Dpub06%2FJC943%2DEpiUpdate2003%5Fen%2Epdf. Accessed April 5, 2004.
2. Centers for Disease Control and Prevention and Department of Health and Human Services. HIV/AIDS surveillance report. Volume 14, 2002. Available at: http://www.cdc.gov/hiv/stats/hasr1402/2002SurveillanceReport.pdf. Accessed April 5, 2004.
3. Centers for Disease Control and Prevention. Increases in HIV diagnoses—29 states, 1999–2002. *MMWR.* 2003;52(47):1145–1148.
4. Wade NA, Zielinski MA, Butsashvili M, et al. Decline in perinatal HIV transmission in New York State (1997–2000). *J Acquir Immune Defic Syndr.* 2004;36(5):1075–1082.
5. Lindegren ML, Byers RH, Thomas P, et al. Trends in perinatal transmission of HIV/AIDS in the United States. *JAMA.* 1999;282(6):531–538.
6. Karon JM, Fleming PL, Steketee RW, DeCock KM. HIV in the United States at the turn of the century: an epidemic in transition. *Am J Public Health.* 2001;91(7):1060–1068.
7. DelValle S, Morales Evangelista A, Velasco MC, Kribs-Zaleta CM, Hsu Schmitz SF. Effects of education, vaccination and treatment on HIV transmission in homosexuals with genetic heterogeneity. *Math Biosci.* 2004;187(2):111–133.
8. Singh KK, Barroga CF, Hughes MD, et al. Genetic influence of CCR5, CCR2, and SDF1 variants on human immunodeficiency virus 1 (HIV-1)-related disease progression and neurological impairment, in children with symptomatic HIV-1 infection. *J Infect Dis.* 2003;188(10):1461–1472.
9. Gilad J, Walfisch A, Borer A, Schlaeffer F. Gender differences and sex-specific manifestations associated with human immunodeficiency virus infection in women. *Eur J Obstet Gynecol Reprod Biol.* 2003;109(2): 199–205.
10. Hunt R. Human immunodeficiency virus and AIDS: components and life cycle of HIV. Microbiology and Immunology On-line. University of South Carolina School of Medicine. Available at: http://www.med.sc.edu:85/lecture/hiv7.htm. Accessed April 6, 2004.
11. Moylett EH, Shearer WT. HIV: clinical manifestations. *J Allergy Clin Immunol.* 2002;110(1):3–16.
12. United States Public Health Services and Infectious Diseases Society of America. 2001 Guidelines for the Prevention of Opportunistic Infections in Persons Infected with Human Immunodeficiency Virus. Available at: http://aidsinfo.nih.gov/guidelines/op_infections/OI_112801.pdf. Accessed April 6, 2004.
13. Arendt G, vonGiesen HJ. Antiretroviral therapy regimens for neuro-AIDS. *Curr Drug Targets Infect Disord.* 2002;2(3):187–192.
14. Velasco-Hernandez JX, Gershengorn HB, Blower SM. Could widespread use of combination antiretroviral therapy eradicate HIV epidemics? *Lancet Infect Dis.* 2002;2(8):487–493.
15. Blower S, Ma L, Farmer P, Koenig S. Predicting the impact of antiretrovirals in resource-poor settings: preventing HIV infections whilst controlling drug resistance. *Curr Drug Targets Infect Disord.* 2003;3(4):345–353.
16. Clements MS, Prestage G, Grulich A, VanDeVen P, Kippax S, Law MG. Modeling trends in HIV incidence among homosexual men in Australia 1995–2006. *J Acquir Immune Defic Syndr.* 2004;35(4):401–406.
17. Porco TC, Martin JN, Page-Shafer KA, et al. Decline in HIV infectivity following the introduction of highly active antiretroviral therapy. *AIDS.* 2004;18(1):81–88.
18. Department of Health and Human Services. Guidelines for the use of antiretroviral agents in HIV-1-infected adults and adolescents. March 23, 2004. Available at: http://aidsinfo.nih.gov/guidelines/default_db2.asp?id=50. Accessed April 6, 2004.
19. Centers for Disease Control and Prevention. 1994 revised classification system for human immunodeficiency virus infection in children less than 13 years of age. *MMWR.* 1994;43(No RR-12):1–10.
20. Pronsky Z, Meyer SA, Fields-Gardner C. *HIV Medications Food Interactions.* 2nd ed. Birchrunville, PA: Food-Medications Interactions 2001.
21. Asch SM, Fremont AM, Turner BJ, et al. Symptom-based framework for assessing quality of HIV care. *Int J Qual Health Care.* 2004;16(1):41–50.
22. Ott M, Fischer H, Polat H, et al. Bioelectrical impedance analysis as a predictor of survival in patients with human immunodeficiency virus infection. *J Acquir Immune Defic Syndr Hum Retrovirol.* 1995;9(1):20–25.
23. Salomon J, deTruchis P, Melchior JC. Body composition and nutritional parameters in HIV and AIDS patients. *Clin Chem Lab Med.* 2002;40(12):1329–1333.
24. Knox TA, Spiegelman D, Skinner SC, Gorbach S. Diarrhea and abnormalities of gastrointestinal function in a cohort of men and women with HIV infection. *Am J Gastrol.* 2000;95(12):3482–3489.
25. Kotler DP, Tierney AR, Wang J, Pierson RN. Magnitude of body-cell-mass depletion and the timing of death from wasting in AIDS. *Am J Clin Nutr.* 1989;50(3):444–447.
26. Alfaro MP, Siegel RM, Baker RC, Heubi JE. Resting energy expenditure and body composition in pediatric HIV infection. *Pediatr AIDS HIV Infect.* 1995;6(5):276–280.
27. Wanke CA, Silva M, Knox TA, Forrester J, Speigelman D, Gorbach SL. Weight loss and wasting remain common complications in individuals infected with human immunodeficiency virus in the era of highly active antiretroviral therapy. *Clin Infect Dis.* 2000;31(3):803–805.
28. Jacobson DL, Bica I, Knox TA, et al. Difficulty swallowing and lack of receipt of highly active antiretroviral therapy predict acute weight loss in human immunodeficiency virus disease. *Clin Infect Dis.* 2003;37(10): 1349–1356.
29. Macallan DC, Noble C, Baldwin C, et al. Energy expenditure and wasting in human immunodeficiency virus infection. *N Engl J Med.* 1995;333(2): 83–88.
30. Poles MA, Fuerst M, McGowan I, et al. HIV-related diarrhea is multifactorial and fat malabsorption is commonly present, independent of HAART. *Am J Gastroenterol.* 2001;96(6):1831–1837.
31. Carroccio A, Guarino A, Zuin G, et al. Efficacy of oral pancreatic enzyme therapy for the treatment of fat malabsorption in HIV-infected patients. *Aliment Pharmacol Ther.* 2001;15(10):1619–1625.
32. Roubenoff R, Grinspoon S, Skolnik PR, et al. Role of cytokines and testosterone in regulating lean body mass and resting energy expenditure in HIV-infected men. *Am J Physiol Endocrinol Metab.* 2002;283(1):E138–E145.
33. Batterham MJ, Garsia R, Greenop P. Prevalence and predictors of HIV-associated weight loss in the era of highly active antiretroviral therapy. *Int J STD AIDS.* 2002;13(11):744–747.
34. Salomon J, deTruchis P, Melchior JC. Body composition and nutritional parameters in HIV and AIDS patients. *Clin Chem Lab Med.* 2002;40(12): 1329–1333.
35. Gasparis AP, Tassiopoulos AK. Nutritional support in the patient with HIV infection. *Nutrition.* 2001;17(11–12):981–982.
36. Baeten JM, Richardson BA, Bankson DD, et al. Use of serum retinol-binding protein for prediction of vitamin A deficiency: effects of HIV-1 infection, protein malnutrition, and the acute phase response. *Am J Clin Nutr.* 2004;79(2):218–225.
37. Melchior JC, Niyongabo T, Henzel D, Durack-Bown I, Henri SC, Boulier A. Malnutrition and wasting, immunodepression, and chronic inflammation

as independent predictors of survival in HIV-infected patients. *Nutrition.* 1999;15(11–12):865–869.

38. Raguso CA, Dupertuis YM, Pichard C. The role of visceral proteins in the nutritional assessment of intensive care unit patients. *Curr Opin Clin Nutr Metab Care.* 2003;6(2):211–216.
39. Manelli JC, Badetti C, Botti G, Golstein MM, Bernini V, Bernard D. A reference standard for plasma proteins is required for nutritional assessment of adult burn patients. *Burns.* 1998;24(4):337–345.
40. Wieringa FT, Dijkhuizen MA, West CE, et al. Estimation of the effect of the acute phase response on indicators of micronutrient status in Indonesian infants. *J Nutr.* 2002;132(10):3061–3066.
41. Strand TA, Adhikari RK, Chandyo RK, Sharma PR, Sommerfelt H. Predictors of plasma zinc concentrations in children with acute diarrhea. *Am J Clin Nutr.* 2004;79(3):451–456.
42. Shell-Duncan B, McDade T. Use of combined measures from capillary blood to assess iron deficiency in rural Kenyan children. *N Nutr.* 2004; 134(2):384–387.
43. Asobayire FS, Adou P, Davidsson L, Cook JD, Hurrell RF. Prevalence of iron deficiency with and without concurrent anemia in population groups with high prevalences of malaria and other infections: a study in Cote d'Ivoire. *Am J Clin Nutr.* 2001;74(6):776–782.
44. Smith PD, Meng G, Salazar-Gonzalez JF, Shaw GM. Macrophage HIV-1 infection and the gastrointestinal tract reservoir. *J Leukoc Biol.* 2003; 74(5):642–649.
45. Smith PD, Mai UE. Immunopathophysiology of gastrointestinal disease in HIV infection. *Gastroenterol Clin North Am.* 1992;21(2):331–345.
46. Becker S. Liver toxicity in epidemiological cohorts. *Clin Infect Dis.* 2004;38(suppl 2):S49–S55.
47. Qurishi N, Kreuzberg C, Luchters G, et al. Effect of antiretroviral therapy on liver-related mortality in patients with HIV and hepatitis C virus coinfection. *Lancet.* 2003;362(9397):1708–1713.
48. Butt AA, Fultz SL, Kwoh CK, Kelley D, Skanderson M, Justice AC. Risk of diabetes in HIV infected veterans pre- and post-HAART and the role of HCV coinfection. *Hepatology.* 2004;40(1):115–119.
49. Poizot-Martin I, Marimoutou C, Benhaim S, et al. Efficacy and tolerance of HCV treatment in HIV-HCV coinfected patients: the potential interaction of PI treatment. *HIV Clin Trials.* 2003;4(4):262–268.
50. Currier JS, Havlir DV. Complications of HIV disease and antiretroviral therapy. Highlights of the 11th Conference on Retroviruses and Opportunistic Infections. *Top HIV Med.* 2004;12(1):31–45.
51. Sentongo TA, Rutstein RM, Stettler N, Stallings VA, Rudy B, Mulberg AE. Association between steatorrhea, growth, and immunologic status in children with perinatally acquired HIV infection. *Arch Pediatr Adolesc Med.* 2001;155(2):149–153.
52. Carroccio A, Fontana M, Spagnuolo MI, et al. Pancreatic dysfunction and its association with fat malabsorption in HIV infected children. *Gut.* 1998;43(4):558–563.
53. Sellmeyer DE, Grunfeld C. Endocrine and metabolic disturbances in human immunodeficiency virus infection and the acquired immune deficiency syndrome. *Endocr Rev.* 1996;17(5):518–532.
54. Freda PU, Bilezikian JP. The hypothalamus-pituitary-adrenal axis in HIV disease. *AIDS Read.* 1999;9(1):43–50.
55. Hoshino Y, Yamashita N, Nakamura T, Iwamotot A. Prospective examination of adrenocortical function in advanced AIDS patients. *Endocr J.* 2002;49(6):641–647.
56. Collazos J, Mayo J, Martinez E, Ibarra S. FERUM cortisol in HIV-infected patients with and without highly active antiretroviral therapy. *AIDS.* 2003;17(1):123–126.
57. Huang JS, Wilkie SJ, Dolan S, et al. Reduced testosterone levels in human immunodeficiency virus-infected women with weight loss and low weight. *Clin Infect Dis.* 2003;36(4):499–506.
58. Rietschel P, Hadigan C, Corcoran C, et al. Assessment of growth hormone dynamics in human immunodeficiency virus-related lipodystrophy. *J Clin Endocrinol Metab.* 2001;86(2):504–510.
59. Beltran S, Lescure FX, Desailloud R, et al. Increased prevalence of hypothyroidism among human immunodeficiency virus-infected patients: a need for screening. *Clin Infect Dis.* 2003;37:579–583.
60. Collazos J, Ibarra S, Mayo J. Thyroid hormones in HIV-infected patients in the highly active antiretroviral therapy era: evidence of an interrelation between the thyroid axis and the immune system. *AIDS.* 2003;17(5): 763–765.
61. Amati L, Cirimele D, Pugliese V, Covelli V, Resta F, Jirillo E. Nutrition and immunity: laboratory and clinical aspects. *Curr Pharm Des.* 2003; 9(24):1924–1931.
62. Trotta MP, Ammassari A, Melzi S, et al. Treatment-related factors and highly active antiretroviral therapy adherence. *J Acquir Immune Defic Syndr.* 2002;31(suppl 3):S128–S131.
63. Maggiolo F, Ripamonti D, Gregis G, Quinzan G, Callegaro A, Suter F. Effect of prolonged discontinuation of successful antiretroviral therapy on CD4 T cells: a controlled, prospective trial. *AIDS.* 2004;18(3):439–446.
64. Alexander TH, Ortiz GM, Wellons MF, et al. Changes in CD4+ T-cell differentiation phenotype during structured treatment interruption in patients with chronic HIV-1 infection. *J Acquir Immune Defic Syndr.* 2003;34(5):475–481.
65. Bitnun A, Sochett E, Babyn P, et al. Serum lipids, glucose homeostasis and abdominal adipose tissue distribution in protease inhibitor-treated and naïve HIV-infected children. *AIDS.* 2003;17(9):1319–1327.
66. Wills TS, Nadler JP, Somboonwit C, et al. Anemia prevalence and associated risk factors in a single-center ambulatory HIV clinical cohort. *AIDS Read.* 2004;14(6):305–310, 313–315.
67. Bellon Cano JM, Sanchez-Ramon S, Ciria L, et al. The effects on infants of potent antiretroviral therapy during pregnancy: a report from Spain. *Med Sci Monit.* 2004;10(5):CR179–184.
68. Chironi G, Escaut L, Gariepy J, et al. Brief report: carotid intima-media thickness in heavily pretreated HIV-infected patients. *J Acquir Immune Defic Syndr.* 2003;32(5):490–493.
69. Adult AIDS clinical trials group metabolic complications guides. Available at: http://aactg.s-3.com/metabolic/. Accessed April 6, 2004.
70. Mooser V. Atherosclerosis and HIV in the highly active antiretroviral therapy era: towards an epidemic of cardiovascular disease? *AIDS.* 2003;17(suppl 1):S65–S69.
71. Vigano A, Riboni S, Bianchi R, et al. Thyroid dysfunction in antiretroviral treated children. *Pediatr Infect Dis J.* 2004;23(3):235–239.
72. Panamonta O, Kosalaraksa P, Thinkhamrop B, Kirdpon W, Ingchanin C, Lumbiganon P. Endocrine function in Thai children infected with human immunodeficiency virus. *J Pediatr Endocrinol Metab.* 2004;17(1):33–40.
73. Tang AM. Weight loss, wasting, and survival in HIV-positive patients: current strategies. *AIDS Read.* 2003;13(12 suppl):S23–S27.
74. Polsky B, Kotler D, Steinhart C. HIV-associated wasting in the HAART era: guidelines for assessment, diagnosis, and treatment. *AIDS Patient Care STDS.* 2001;15(8):411–423.
75. Fields-Gardner C. Anthropometric measures: anthropometric changes in chronic disease. Available at http://www.hi-r-ed.org. Accessed April 5, 2004.
76. Andrade S, Lan SJ, Engelson ES, et al. Use of a Durnin-Womersley formula to estimate change in subcutaneous fat content in HIV-infected subjects. *Am J Clin Nutr.* 2002;75(3):587–592.
77. McComsey G, Maa JF. Host factors may be more important than choice of antiretrovirals in the development of lipoatrophy. *AIDS Read.* 2003;13(11):539–542.
78. Kotler DP, Burastero S, Wang J, Pierson RN. Prediction of body cell mass, fat free mass, and total body water with bioelectrical impedance analysis: effects of race, sex, and disease. *Am J Clin Nutr.* 1996;64 (suppl):489S–497S.
79. Heller L, Fox S, Hell KJ, Church JA. Development of an instrument to assess nutritional risk factors for children infected with human immunodeficiency virus. *J Am Diet Assoc.* 2000;100(3):323–329.
80. Miller TL. Nutritional aspects of HIV-infected children receiving highly active antiretroviral therapy. *AIDS.* 2003;17(suppl 1):S130–S140.
81. Barker D, Younger N, MooSang M, McKenzie CA. HIV serostatus and recovery from severe childhood malnutrition. A retrospective matched case-control study. *West Indian Med J.* 2004;53(2):89–94.
82. Okunseri C, Badner V, Wiznia A, Rosenberg M. Prevalence of oral lesions and percent CD4+ T-lymphocytes in HIV-infected children on antiretroviral therapy. *AIDS Patient Care STDS.* 2003;17(1):5–11.

83. Okunseri C, Badner V, Wiznia A, Rosenberg M. Dental visits by pediatric HIV-infected medical patients. *NY State Dent J.* 2003;69(7):26–29.
84. Lipshultz SE, Easley KA, Orav EJ, et al. Cardiovascular status of infants and children of women infected with HIV-1 (P(2)C(2) HIV): a cohort study. *Lancet.* 2002;360(9330):368–373.
85. Kino T, Chrousos GP. AIDS-related insulin resistance and lipodystrophy syndrome. *Curr Drug Targets Immune Endocr Metabol Disord.* 2003;3(2):111–117.
86. Chantry CJ, Byrd RS, Englund JA, Baker CJ, McKinney RE, PACTG 152 Study Team. Growth, survival and viral load in symptomatic childhood human immunodeficiency virus infection. *Pediatr Infect Dis J.* 2003;22(12):1033–1039.
87. Hsu HW, Pelton S, Williamson JM, et al. Survival in children with perinatal HIV infection and very low CD4 lymphocyte counts. *J Acquir Immune Defic Syndr.* 2000;25(3):269–275.
88. Blasini I, Chantry C, Cruz C, et al. Disclosure model for pediatric patients living with HIV in Puerto Rico: design, implementation, and evaluation. *J Dev Behav Pediatr.* 2004;25(3):181–189.
89. Gerson AC, Joyner M, Fosarelli P, et al. Disclosure of HIV diagnosis to children: when, where, why, and how. *J Pediatr Health Care.* 2001;15(4):161–167.
90. American Dietetic Association. Nutrition management of HIV infection and AIDS. In: Williams CP, ed. *Pediatric Manual of Clinical Dietetics.* Chicago, IL: American Dietetic Association, 1998.
91. Benjamin KD, Miller WC, Ryder RW, Weber DJ, Walter E, McKinney RE. Growth patterns reflect response to antiretroviral therapy in HIV-positive infants: potential utility in resource-poor settings. *AIDS Patient Care STDS.* 2004;18(1):35–43.
92. Hamamoto LA, Cardoso AL, Marques HH, Gomes C. Energy balance in infants born from HIV seropositive mothers. *J Pediatr (Rio J).* 2000;76(2):119–124.
93. Grinspoon S, Corcoran C, Miller K, et al. Determinants of increased energy expenditure in HIV-infected women. *Am J Clin Nutr.* 1998;68(3):720–725.
94. Kotler D, Heymsfield SB. HIV infection: a model chronic illness for studying wasting diseases. *Am J Clin Nutr.* 1998;68(3):519–520.
95. Sharpstone D, Phelan M, Gazzard B. Differential metabolic response in AIDS-related chronic protozoal diarrhea. *HIV Med.* 2000;1(2):102–106.
96. Pernerstorfer-Schoen H, Schindler K, Parschalk B, et al. Beneficial effects of protease inhibitors on body composition and energy expenditure: a comparison between HIV-infected and AIDS patients. *AIDS.* 1999;13(17):2389–2396.
97. Shevitz AH, Knox TA, Spiegelman D, Roubenoff R, Gorback SL, Skolnik PR. Elevated resting energy expenditure among HIV-seropositive persons receiving highly active antiretroviral therapy. *AIDS.* 1999;13(11):1351–1357.
98. Henderson RA, Talusan K, Hutton N, Yolken RH, Caballero B. Whole body protein turnover in children with human immunodeficiency virus (HIV) infection. *Nutrition.* 1999;15(3):189–194.
99. Williams SB, Bartsch G, Muurahainen N, Collins G, Raghavan SS, Wheeler D. Protein intake is positively associated with body cell mass in weight-stable HIV-infected men. *J Nutr.* 2003;133(4):1143–1146.
100. Shah S, Whalen C, Kotler DP, et al. Severity of human immunodeficiency virus infection is associated with decreased phase angle, fat mass and body cell mass in adults with pulmonary tuberculosis infection in Uganda. *J Nutr.* 2001;131(11):2843–2847.
101. Wellinghausen N, Kern WV, Jochle W, Kern P. Zinc serum level in human immunodeficiency virus-infected patients in relation to immunological status. *Biol Trace Elem Res.* 2000;73(2):139–149.
102. Tang AM, Graham NM, Saah AJ. Effects of micronutrient intake on survival in human immunodeficiency virus type 1 infection. *Am J Epidemiol.* 1996;143(12):1244–1256.
103. Fields-Gardner C, Fergusson P. Position of the American Dietetic Association and Dietitians of Canada: nutrition intervention in the care of persons with human immunodeficiency virus infection. *J Am Diet Assoc.* In press.
104. Grinspoon S, Mulligan K. Weight loss and wasting in patients infected with human immunodeficiency virus. *Clin Infec Dis.* 2003;36(suppl 2):S69–S78.
105. Rabeneck L, Palmer A, Knowles JB, et al. A randomized controlled trial evaluating nutrition counseling with or without oral supplementation in malnourished HIV-infected patients. *J Am Diet Assoc.* 1998;98(4):434–438.
106. Norval DA. Symptoms and sites of pain experienced by AIDS patients. *S Afr Med J.* 2004;94(6):450–454.
107. Selwyn PA, Rivard M. Palliative care for AIDS: challenges and opportunities in the era of highly active anti-retroviral therapy. *J Palliat Med.* 2003;6(3):475–487.
108. Hadigan C. Dietary habits and their association with metabolic abnormalities in human immunodeficiency virus-related lipodystrophy. *Clin Infect Dis.* 2003;37(suppl 2):S101–S104.
109. Hoh R, Pelfini A, Neese RA, et al. De novo lipogenesis predicts short-term body-composition response by bioelectrical impedance analysis to oral nutritional supplements in HIV-associated wasting. *Am J Clin Nutr.* 1998;68(1):154–163.
110. Abrams B, Duncan D, Hertz-Picciotto I. A prospective study of dietary intake and acquired immune deficiency syndrome in HIV-seropositive homosexual men. *J Acquir Immune Defic Syndr.* 1993;6(8):949–958.
111. Fawzi WW, Msamanga GI, Spiegelman D, et al. A randomized trial of multivitamin supplements and HIV disease progression and mortality. *N Engl J Med.* 2004;351(1):2332.
112. deVisser R, Grierson J. Use of alternative therapies by people living with HIV/AIDS in Australia. *AIDS Care.* 2002;14(5):599–606.
113. Miller TL, Awnetwant EL, Evans S, Morris VM, Vazquez IM, McIntosh K. Gastrostomy tube supplementation for HIV-infected children. *Pediatrics.* 1995;96(4 pt 1):696–702.
114. Kotler DP, Fogleman L, Tierney AR. Comparison of total parenteral nutrition and an oral, semielemental diet on body composition, physical function, and nutrition-related costs in patients with malabsorption due to acquired immunodeficiency syndrome. *J Parenter Enteral Nutr.* 1998;22(3):120–126.
115. Keithley JK, Swanson B, Zeller JM, et al. Comparison of standards and immune-enhancing oral formulas in asymptomatic HIV-infected persons: a multicenter randomized controlled clinical trial. *J Parenter Enteral Nutr.* 2002;26(1):6–14.
116. de Luis Roman DA, Bachiller P, Izaola O, et al. Nutritional treatment for acquired immunodeficiency virus infection using an enterotropic peptide-based formula enriched with n-3 fatty acids: a randomized prospective trial. *Eur J Clin Nutr.* 2001;55(12):1048–1052.
117. Ockenga J, Suttmann U, Selberg O, et al. Percutaneous endoscopic gastrostomy in AIDS and control patients: risks and outcome. *Am J Gastroenterol.* 1996;91(9):1817–1822.
118. Moore DA, Gazzard BG, Nelson MR. Central venous line infections in AIDS. *J Infect.* 1997;34(1):35–40.
119. Tumbarello M, Tacconelli E, Donati KG, et al. HIV-associated bacteremia: how it has changed in the highly active antiretroviral therapy (HAART) era. *J Acquir Immune Defic Syndr.* 2000;23(2):145–151.
120. Nicastri E, Petrosillo N, Viale P, Ippolito G. Catheter-related bloodstream infections in HIV-infection patients. *Ann NY Acad Sci.* 2001;946:274–290.
121. Kotler DP. Human immunodeficiency virus-related wasting: malabsorption syndromes. *Semin Oncol.* 1998;25(2 suppl 6):70–75.

SUGGESTED READING

American Dietetic Association and Dietitians of Canada. Nutrition intervention in the care of persons with human immunodeficiency virus infection. *J Am Diet Assoc.* 2004;104(9):1425–1441.

Panel on Clinical Practices for Treatment of HIV Infection. CDC guidelines for HIV and opportunistic infection treatment. Available at: http://aidsinfo.nih.gov/guidelines/default_db2.asp?id=50 and http://aidsinfo.nih.gov/guidelines/op_infections/OI_112801.pdf. Accessed April 6, 2004.

World Health Organization. Guidelines for HIV treatment. Available at: http://www.who.int/3by5/publications/guidelines/en/arv_guidelines.pdf. Accessed April 6, 2004.

Elaine B. Trujillo, MS, RD;
Sara L. Bergerson, MS, RD;
Jennifer C. Graf, MS, RD;
Madeline Michael, MPH, RD

11 Cancer

Introduction

Cachexia is often observed in patients with cancer and is associated with increased morbidity and decreased quality of life and survival. The etiology of weight loss and cachexia in cancer patients includes decreased intake, altered metabolism, and increased catabolism. This chapter addresses pediatric and adult nutritional issues and adjuvant therapy for patients with cancer, along with education for patients and caregivers.

I. Background. More than 1 million Americans are diagnosed with cancer each year. Cancer is the second leading cause of death after heart disease, claiming 23% of total deaths in the United States. Although overall cancer death rates and incidence rates have remained stable over the past few years, mortality rates of the four most common cancers (lung, colorectal, breast, and prostate) have continued to decline.[1] The leading cancers affecting men and women of all races are prostate cancer and breast cancer, respectively.

A. Adults—Cancer types more likely to result in nutritional alterations
   1. There is a relation between malnutrition/weight loss and tumor type.[2] Generally, malnutrition is more prevalent in patients with cancer of the proximal gastrointestinal (GI) tract.[3]
   2. Patients with pancreatic or gastric cancer had the highest prevalence of weight loss (83%–87%).[4]
   3. Patients with non-Hodgkin's lymphoma with less favorable outcomes, colon cancer, prostate cancer, and lung cancer had a 48% to 61% prevalence of weight loss.[4]
   4. Weight loss occurs in 43% to 61% of patients with lung cancer, depending on the stage of the disease.[5]
   5. Patients with subtypes of non-Hodgkin's lymphomas with more favorable outcomes, breast cancer, acute non-lymphocytic leukemia, and sarcomas had the lowest prevalence of weight loss (31%–41%) in this study.[4]

B. Pediatrics
   1. Cancer among children ages 0 to 19 years
      a) The most common childhood cancers are leukemias, followed by cancer of the central nervous system, lymphomas, and reticuloendothelial neoplasms for all races.
      b) Leukemias are more common among 1- to 4-year-olds, whereas lymphomas are more common among 15- to 19-year-olds.
   2. Cancer trends[6]
      a) The incidence of all childhood cancers has fluctuated but has generally increased over the period 1975–2000 for 0- to 19-year-olds.
      b) The largest increase in incidence for all cancers occurred during 1975–1986.
      c) Hepatic tumors had the largest percent increase in incidence for 1975–2000, followed by soft-tissue sarcomas and renal tumors.
      d) Mortality from cancer has steadily decreased over the period 1975–2000.
      e) The 5-year survival rates for all cancers steadily increased from 1975 to 1995.
      f) The 5-year survival rates from 1985 to 1999 were highest for retinoblastoma, followed by renal tumors, germ-cell trophoblastic and other gonadal neoplasms, and carcinomas and other malignant epithelial neoplasms. Hepatic tumors had the lowest 5-year survival rate during the period.
   3. Cancer types more likely to result in nutritional alterations
      a) At diagnosis
         (1) Children have lower energy reserves and higher metabolic demands than adults and are therefore more likely to experience nutritional depletion, particularly during growth spurts.[7–10]
         (2) At presentation, patients with sarcomas frequently have compromised nutritional status.[11] Patients with intra-abdominal solid tumors were significantly more malnourished than patients with leukemia or extra-abdominal solid tumors at diagnosis.[12]
         (3) Nutritional status may be related to the length of time until diagnosis. Patients with prolonged time to diagnosis may experience more nutritional compromise.
         (4) Patients with acute lymphoblastic leukemia (ALL), high-risk malignant disease, or various solid tumors had documented increases in catabolism prior to therapy, with protein breakdown significantly greater than protein synthesis.[13]
      b) After therapy
         (1) The frequency, intensity, and type of chemotherapy regimens may affect nutritional status. Patients with soft-tissue sarcomas and osteosarcomas had greater decreases in weight-for-height compared to patients with other types of cancer, which may be attributed to aggressive and frequent chemotherapy.[11] Steroid use in the treatment of other cancers (eg, ALL) may have prevented this decrease in weight-for-height. However, height-for-age *Z* scores decreased after therapy in patients with ALL, with a corresponding decrease in lean body mass and increase in body fat.[14] Survivors of ALL were shown to have decreased

height-for-age standard deviation scores during treatment and up to 20 years postdiagnosis, while their body mass index (BMI) standard deviation significantly increased during the period from diagnosis to final height.[15,16] This tendency toward overweight in ALL survivors may be related in part to decreases in physical activity.[16–18]

(2) There are inconsistent results regarding metabolic rate before and after chemotherapy in patients with ALL.[19–22] The difference in results may be related to the tumor burden prior to chemotherapy.[20] ALL patients with a greater tumor burden had higher resting energy expenditures than those with lower tumor burden initially. This difference disappeared after 1 to 2 weeks of chemotherapy, because the resting energy expenditure decreased in the group that had a high tumor burden.[20]

(3) Patients with cancers of the central nervous system tend to require enteral nutrition or parenteral nutrition (PN) for greater lengths of time than do lymphoma, leukemia, and bone marrow transplant patients (but not patients with solid tumors), likely owing to the effect of the disease on neurological processes involved with eating.[23]

II. Nutritional Alterations in Patients With Cancer

Cachexia comes from the Greek words *kakos hexos,* which literally means "bad condition of the body." It is estimated to affect more than 80% of patients with advanced malignant disease. It is defined as a state of malnutrition characterized by anorexia, weight loss, muscle wasting, asthenia, depression, chronic nausea, and anemia and results in psychological distress, changes in body composition, and alterations in carbohydrate, lipid and protein metabolism.[24,25] Alterations may occur in tissue water content, in acid-base balance, and in the concentrations of electrolytes, vitamin or mineral concentrations. These metabolic abnormalities may impair nutritional status and contribute to cachexia through the depletion of fat, protein, water, and mineral stores.[26] The degree of cachexia is inversely correlated with the survival time of the patient, and it implies a poor prognosis.[27]

A. Weight loss and cachexia

1. Altered intake

a) Anorexia or the loss of appetite and early satiety is present in up to one half of newly diagnosed cancer patients.[4,28] Anorexia results in decreased food intake and weight loss and may lead to the development of malnutrition. Symptoms that interfere with food intake and are likely to be related to anorexia include early satiety, taste alterations, smell alterations, meat aversion, and nausea/vomiting.[29] The pathogenesis of cancer anorexia is multifactorial and is associated with disturbances of the central physiological mechanisms controlling food intake. Several factors that appear to play key roles in the development of cancer anorexia include hormones (leptin), neuropeptides (neuropeptide Y), cytokines (interleukin-1 and -6, tumor necrosis factor [TNF]), and neurotransmitters (serotonin and dopamine).[29]

b) Cancer treatment modalities, such as chemotherapy and radiotherapy, may cause nausea, vomiting, diarrhea, mucositis, and taste alterations. These side effects ultimately may decrease food intake and cause learned food aversions.

(1) Nausea and vomiting are the most feared side effects of cancer treatment. Acute nausea and vomiting occurs during the first 24 hours after treatment. Highly emetogenic chemotherapy, such as cisplatin and cyclophosphamide, may cause nausea and vomiting after 24 hours.[30]

(2) Mucositis, a result of the effect of cancer therapy on rapidly dividing cells, can occur along the GI tract but occurs more often in the mouth. Mucositis often occurs 5 to 7 days after chemotherapy and generally persists with bone marrow suppression from the treatment. Clinical manifestations include erythema, dryness, ulcers, bleeding, and pain. It is estimated to occur in 40% of cancer patients, and the incidence is the highest in bone marrow transplant patients.[30]

(3) Radiotherapy has direct short- and long-term effects on olfactory and secretory function, the digestive tract, and the mucous membranes. Long-term bone, dental, olfactory, secretory, and digestive sequelae can lead to reduced food intake and/or malabsorption of nutrients.[3]

c) Operative therapy may result in altered intake. Surgery of the head and neck may result in dysphagia. Pre- and postoperative nil per os and restrictive diets such as clear liquids further affect nutrient intake.

d) Biotherapy is associated with decreased appetite and fatigue.[30] Biotherapy, also known as biologic therapy or immunotherapy, is intended to strengthen the immune system's ability to recognize and attack cancer cells. Biotherapy is a diverse group of therapeutic strategies for cancer and includes immunotherapy, agents that inhibit angiogenesis or invasion, growth factor modulation, and small molecules (inhibitors of signal transduction).[31] Although some of these treatments stimulate immune reactions against cancer cells, they sometimes interfere with immunity against infections. People who receive biological therapies may be at risk for immunosuppression and neutropenia.[32]

e) Physical obstruction of the GI tract (stomach, small intestine, or colon) is generally associated with decreased intake or emesis after intake. Intestinal obstruction is well recognized in patients with progressive advanced gynecological and GI cancers, especially those with colon cancer or with metastasis from ovarian cancer.[33,34]

f) Dysphagia, especially due to head and neck cancer, leads to significant weight loss even in the presence of reported normal appetite.[35]

g) Depression, feelings of overwhelming sadness, and the fear and anxiety that accompany a diagnosis of cancer may lead to decreased intake. In the Psychosocial Collaborative Oncology Group Study, in which 215 adults with various types of cancers were studied, 47% of the subjects had a clinically apparent psychological disorder. Two thirds had either reactive anxiety or depressed mood, and 13% had major depression.[36] Depression has been associated more commonly with pancreatic cancer than with most other cancers.[37]

2. Energy expenditure

a) Tremendous variability in resting energy expenditure measurements has been reported in malnourished patients with cancer, ranging from hypometabolism to hypermetabolism.[38]

b) Elevated resting energy expenditure was reported in pancreatic and lung cancer patients and unchanged in patients with gastric and colorectal cancer.[28,39]

c) Hypermetabolism and weight loss are significant predictors of decreased survival.[38]

d) In a group of almost 300 patients with various types of cancer, about one half had elevated resting energy expenditures. The increase in energy expenditure was not associated with a different dietary intake compared to normometabolic patients.[40] Feedback regulation of dietary intake in relation to energy expenditure is frequently lost in patients with cancer, so that hypermetabolism is not compensated for by an increase in spontaneous food intake as it is in normometabolism.[38,40]

3. Decreased absorption[41]
   a) Treatment modalities, such as surgery, chemotherapy, and radiotherapy, may result in malabsorption.
      (1) Operative therapy may result in intestinal ileus and stasis of bowel contents, which adversely affects absorption. Pancreatic resection may be associated with malabsorption of fat and protein. Gastric resection may lead to dumping syndrome. Large segment resection of the small bowel or colon may affect absorption of nutrients, fluid, and electrolytes and sometimes results in long-term PN dependency.
      (2) Chemotherapeutic agents often cause severe GI symptoms, such as mucositis and diarrhea, which may result in malabsorption.
      (3) Radiotherapy causes both acute and delayed reactions that affect intestinal absorption. Acute reactions usually occur within days to weeks of therapy and include enteritis, diarrhea, and decreased production of saliva with consequently reduced enzymes. Late reactions to radiation therapy include persistent mucosal inflammation, intestinal fibrosis, and stricture.[42]
   b) Tumor involvement of the GI tract may result in mechanical obstruction, with decreased absorption and diarrhea. Serosal involvement of the bowel may cause functional malabsorption, pseudo-obstruction, or intestinal ileus, precluding optimal absorption.
   c) Stasis of bowel contents from partial or complete intestinal obstruction may lead to bacterial overgrowth and interfere with absorption of nutrients.
4. Changes in the immune system
   a) It is now established that nutritional deficiency is commonly associated with impaired immune responses, particularly cell-mediated immunity, phagocyte function, cytokine production, secretory antibody response, antibody affinity, and the complement system.[43] Nutritional deprivation, such as protein energy malnutrition, often causes immunodeficiency, leading to increased frequency and severity of infection and an increased incidence of common infections affecting the upper and lower respiratory, urinary, and genital tracts.[44] In a study that examined the relationship between nutritional status as indicated by the presence or absence of the cutaneous delayed hypersensitivity response and treatment-related morbidity, disease recurrence, and survival at 2 years in 67 head and neck patients, survival was improved in patients whose cell-mediated immunity was preserved compared with those who were anergic at completion of treatment. Morbidity due to surgical therapy and tumor recurrence rates were also higher in the anergic group.[35]
   b) Immunodeficiency may result from treatment. Operative intervention, radiation therapy, and chemotherapeutic agents all affect cell-mediated immunity, even in well-nourished subjects.[41,45]
   c) T-cell function is also altered with certain hematologic malignancies, whereas humoral (B-cell) immunity is affected in chronic lymphocytic leukemia and multiple myeloma.[41]
   d) Immunoglobulin A deficiency, noted in many malnourished patients, may play a role in facilitating bacterial translocation and absorption of endotoxin into the circulation.[41]
5. Hormones and cytokines
   a) Cytokines and other mediators play a major role in the complex cascade of biological responses leading to the wasting associated with cancer cachexia. Cytokines are a diverse group of soluble glycoproteins and low–molecular weight peptides that mediate interactions between cells and regulate cell and tissue functions.[46] In relation to cancer cachexia, they modulate gastric motility and emptying, either in the GI tract or via the brain, by altering efferent signals that regulate satiety.[47] Although elevated levels of numerous cytokines were found in the blood and urine of cancer patients, the absence of clinically detectable cytokine levels does not exclude the idea that cytokines play a role in systemic effects.[46,48]
      (1) TNF was one of the first cytokines thought to play a role in cancer cachexia. Early studies found that mice with tumors producing TNF also developed cachexia and that weight loss was reversed with TNF-neutralizing antibodies.[46,49] TNF also suppresses lipoprotein lipase activity in adipocytes.[50]
      (2) Interleukin-1 (IL-1) is associated with the initiation of anorexia by blocking neuropeptide Y (NPY)–induced feeding.[47,51]
      (3) TNF and IL-1 may increase the levels of corticotropin-releasing hormone, which is a central nervous system neurotransmitter that suppresses food intake and the release of glucose-sensitive neurons and ultimately decreases food intake.[47,52,53]
      (4) Interleukin-6 (IL-6) and leukemia inhibitor factor (LIF) are produced by some cancers and may contribute to cachexia.[46,50,54] Ciliary neurotropic factor, which is a member of the family of cytokines that includes IL-6 and LIF, is expressed in skeletal muscle and induces potent cachectic effects and acute-phase proteins in tumor-bearing mice.[47,50,55]
      (5) Interferon (IFN)-γ may be involved in cancer cachexia. In animals, the provision of antibodies against IFN-γ reversed the wasting syndrome, which clarified that there was an endogenous production of IFN-γ.[47,56]
      (6) Lipid-mobilizing factor induces lipolysis and correlates with weight loss.[57]
      (7) Proteolysis-inducing factor induces protein degradation in skeletal muscle by upregulating the ubiquitin-proteasome proteolytic pathway and by decreasing protein synthesis.[28,58] This factor also may increase cytokines and acute-phase proteins.[28,59,60]
   b) Leptin, neuropeptides, and uncoupling proteins
      (1) Leptin acts to control food intake and energy expenditure via neuropeptideric effector molecules within the hypothalamus.[61] TNF, IL-1, and LIF increase plasma levels of leptin, despite a decrease in food intake that would normally suppress leptin expression.[62–64] Increased leptin levels may contribute to anorexia by preventing the normal compensatory mechanisms in light of decreased food intake. Results on leptin levels are not consistent. Leptin levels were not elevated in tumor-bearing rats and in patients with cancer cachexia.[65–67] On the other hand, very low levels of leptin with high levels of inflammatory cytokines were found in patients with advanced-stage cancer.[68]
      (2) NPY is the most potent feeding-stimulatory peptide activated by the fall of leptin. NPY is thought to restore normal energy balance and body fat stores under conditions of energy deficit, the signals of which are falling leptin and/or insulin.[62]
      (3) Uncoupling protein (UPC) 1, 2, and 3 may be involved in the control of energy metabolism. They are mitochondr-

ial membrane proteins that mediate proton leakage and decrease the coupling of respiration to adenosine diphosphate phosphorylation, resulting in the generation of heat instead of adenosine triphosphate. UPC 1 is expressed only in brown adipose tissue, which in adult humans is very scarce and probably not functional.[69] UPC 2 is distributed and expressed in most tissues. UPC 3 is expressed in brown adipose tissue and skeletal muscle and may be of significant importance in energy expenditure. Changes in UPC expression may be induced by tumor products of cytokines.[28]

B. Metabolic alterations. Although altered nutrient intake and anorexia contribute to cancer cachexia, decreased food intake alone does not entirely account for the weight loss seen in cancer patients.[70] This is evident in studies in which the loss of muscle and adipose tissue precedes the fall in food intake and the provision of extra calories does not result in weight gain.[70,71] It is clear that the cachectic cancer patient uses nutrients ineffectively and seems unable to adapt to the malnourished state as normal humans do by conserving lean body mass.[72]

1. Glucose homeostasis
   a) There is an elevation in Cori cycle activity in malnourished cancer patients, and this increased activity accounts for approximately 300 kcal per day loss of energy.[28,73] The demand for glucose carbons by the tumor tissue can increase demand for glucose production by the liver, especially if glucose cannot be fully oxidized by the tumor tissue itself. The inability to effectively oxidize glucose may explain why some cancer patients exhibit an increase in Cori cycle activity and elevated glucose production.[73]
   b) Increased lactate levels and production rates in cancer patients are due to increased glycolysis and lactate release by the tumor tissue and skeletal muscle tissue. Glucose is the main energy source of most solid tumors, and it is highly used by the tumor and host, with an associated release of substantial amounts of lactate. Lactate is then regenerated into glucose by the liver through the Cori cycle.[70]
   c) Gluconeogenesis is increased to maintain glucose homeostasis in the cancer patient. Amino acids and glycerol from muscle and fat breakdown, respectively, are used as the main substrates in gluconeogenesis.[70] The reduced plasma levels of alanine, glycine, and glutamine seen in cachectic cancer patients may be caused by an increase in their use by the liver for glucose production.[74]
   d) Glucose production, glucose intolerance, and insulin resistance often are increased in cancer patients. Glucose use by skeletal muscle is reduced due to insulin resistance. The counter regulatory hormones, such as glucocorticoids and glucagons, increase and may contribute to insulin resistance.[52]
2. Protein metabolism
   a) Increased muscle catabolism. Muscle wasting is common in cancer patients and contributes to the asthenia, or lack of strength, seen in these patients. It is caused by an increase in protein breakdown and, to a lesser extent, a decrease in protein synthesis.[70]
   b) Negative nitrogen balance may be present, whole body protein turnover is increased, and amino acid turnover is altered.[58,75]
   c) Decreased muscle protein synthesis and increased liver and tumor protein synthesis occur. There is a shift from normal muscle protein and other tissue protein synthesis to increased hepatic protein synthesis, which is reprioritized with an increased production of acute-phase proteins.[50,58,76]
3. Lipid metabolism
   a) Patients with cancer cachexia have a profound loss of adipose tissue due to an increase in lipolysis and a reduction in lipogenesis.[28,50,52]
   b) Cancer patients with weight loss have a higher turnover of both glycerol and free fatty acids.[28]
   c) Patients with cancer have been shown to have significantly reduced levels of lipoprotein lipase, the enzyme responsible for triglyceride clearance from plasma.[50,52]
   d) The lipid profile in cancer patients is characterized by decreased high-density lipoproteins, decreased low-density lipoproteins, and relatively high serum triglycerides.[77,78] Hypertriglyceridemia is a consequence of the decreased lipoprotein lipase activity, which results in a decrease in the plasma clearance of both endogenous and exogenous triglycerides.[52]

C. Micronutrient deficiencies. Dietary compounds may affect cancer development through several mechanisms, including the alteration of carcinogen metabolism, antioxidation, enhancement of differentiation and growth inhibition, and immunologic modulation.[79]

1. Vitamins
   a) Vitamin C and Vitamin E act as antioxidants, stimulate the immune system, and reduce nitrite, which prevents the formation of nitrosamine and nitrosamine compounds known to induce tumor formation in experimental animals and humans.[79]
   b) Studies on vitamins reveal reduced levels associated with different malignancies. Reduced levels of vitamins and minerals were found in the following cancer sites:
      (1) Vitamin A levels in colorectal cancer and esophageal cancer[80,81] and in pretreatment pediatric leukemia and lymphoma[82]
      (2) Beta-carotene in lung cancer, gastric cancer, pancreatic cancer, oral cancer, and thyroid cancer[83–87] and in pediatric leukemia, lymphoma, and malignant bone tumors[82]
      (3) Vitamin E in lung cancer, gastric cancer, pancreatic cancer, prostate cancer, and gallbladder cancer[79,83–85,88] and in pediatric leukemia, lymphoma, malignant bone tumors, and central nervous system tumors[82]
      (4) Vitamin C in lung cancer, gastric cancer, pancreatic cancer, esophageal cancer, colon cancer, and prostate cancer[81,83–85,88,89]
      (5) Vitamin D (and calcium) in colon cancer[89]
   c) A multivitamin and mineral supplement may be recommended for patients with an inadequate nutrient intake. Further evaluation of vitamin and mineral status may be indicated if deficiencies are suspected, such as in patients with prolonged poor nutrient intake and/or with malabsorption, and repletion may be warranted.
2. Trace elements
   a) Selenium, zinc, manganese, and copper are cofactors for various antioxidant enzymes such as glutathione peroxidase, RNA polymerase, superoxide dismutase, and diamine oxidase.[79]
   b) Metabolism of metals, especially zinc, is affected in patients with cancer. There is an increase in urinary zinc with a variety of tumors, such as melanoma, gynecologic malignancies, and lung cancer. Low zinc levels were reported in the serum and tissues of cervical cancer patients[90] and in patients with prostate cancer and breast cancer,[88,91,92] as well as in pediatric patients with leukemia, lymphoma, malignant bone tumors, and tumors of the central nervous system.[82] Zinc is released during protein catabolism bound to amino acids and may pass the glomerular

membrane.[80] Zinc deficiency may occur if nutrient intake is poor or GI losses are great.

c) Copper functions as a cofactor in metabolic substrate pathways and nucleic acid synthesis. Levels may be low secondary to chronic decreased intake and absorption.

d) Selenium deficiency has been reported in cancer patients, particularly those who are chronically malnourished or dependent on home nutrition support. Low serum and tissue selenium levels were reported in patients with cervical cancer.[90] Reduced levels of serum selenium were found in patients with hepatocellular carcinoma and breast cancer.[91–93]

e) Selenium deficiency is common among newly diagnosed pediatric cancer patients, even in the absence of malnutrition.[94]

f) Low serum, biliary, and tissue concentrations of selenium and zinc were reported in patients with carcinoma of the gallbladder as compared to patients with cholelithiasis.[79]

g) The copper-to-zinc ratio was demonstrated to be useful as a diagnostic tool in GI, lung, and gallbladder cancer and may contribute to an early diagnosis of these cancers.[79,95,96]

D. Electrolyte disturbances

1. Hypercalcemia, hyperphosphatemia, hypocalcemia, and hyperkalemia are associated with tumor lysis syndrome (TLS).[97] TLS frequently occurs in patients with lymphoma and is defined as the metabolic derangements produced by rapid tumor breakdown, which can occur either spontaneously from rapid tumor growth followed by spontaneous tumor cell death or as a consequence of therapy. It is characterized by hyperuricemia due to DNA breakdown, hyperkalemia related to cytosol breakdown, hyperphosphatemia due to protein breakdown, and hypocalcemia secondary to the hyperphosphatemia. As phosphate levels rise, serum calcium decreases.[97]

2. Hypocalcemia, hypomagnesemia, and hypophosphatemia are often observed in association with the use of platinum-containing therapy, and hyponatremia often accompanies treatment with cyclophosphamide and vincristine.[97]

III. Nutritional Assessment of Patients With Cancer

A. Adults

1. Screening

a) Early assessment of nutritional risk and serial reassessments throughout a cancer patient's course are necessary to ensure that interventions are timely and effective.[98] The focus of nutritional assessments varies depending on a patient's situation and needs.

b) The Patient-Generated Subjective Global Assessment (PG-SGA), a modification of the Subjective Global Assessment, is an outcome-based assessment tool developed specifically for cancer patients (see Figure 11-1). It is applicable in varied health care settings and can be used to identify and prioritize nutritional risk and capture short-term changes in nutritional status.[98,99] The PG-SGA is formatted so that components of the medical history can be completed first by the patient using a check-box format. This segment includes four sections: short-term weight status, food intake change, nutrition impact symptoms, and functional capacity. A three-part physical assessment section evaluating metabolic demand of underlying disease and degree of metabolic stress, and a subjective evaluation of fat stores, muscle status, and fluid status, are then completed by the clinician. In addition to a global rating of nourishment status, the scored PG-SGA incorporates a numerical score. The numerical score of the completed PG-SGA can guide the nutrition intervention pathway and assist in determining effective strategies, such as patient education, symptom management, aggressive oral nutrition, and enteral/parenteral support. An observational study of cancer patients demonstrated that the scored PG-SGA is a simple, valid, and reliable assessment tool.[100] The scored PG-SGA was adopted by the Oncology Nutrition Dietetic Practice Group of the American Dietetic Association as the standard for nutrition assessment of cancer patients.

2. History and medication use

a) A detailed nutritional focused history should supplement other parts of the nutritional evaluation. In cancer patients, a focused history should evaluate for any impediments to food intake and tolerance, including previous medical conditions or surgeries, taste alterations and food aversions, complementary and alternative therapies (including supplements, herbs, and botanicals), rigid or restrictive dietary habits, food allergies, and oral or dental disease. Family members and significant others may provide useful information in the assessment.

b) A history should be used to assess the impact that a medical condition, medication, and/or modified diet may have on nutritional care during treatment. If a patient has difficulty eating during cancer treatment, it may be appropriate to liberalize or discontinue a previously prescribed diet. A history of GI surgery might necessitate an adjustment in a patient's dietary pattern or consideration for nutrition support.

3. Physical examination and functional assessment. A physical examination and functional evaluation are incorporated in the PG-SGA.

a) Body weight is the most basic anthropometric measure. Body weight evaluation provides a simple, dependable, and proven measure of nutritional risk. More than 45% of hospitalized adult cancer patients have been identified as having significant (>10%) weight loss (from usual weight).[101] Unlike people experiencing starvation who lose fat while lean body mass is preserved, cancer patients lose both fat and lean body mass.[28] Percent body weight loss from usual weight correlates with complications and mortality.[102] Multiple factors (eg, location and stage of tumor, cancer treatment) affect weight status.[102] Since weight loss may be masked by altered fluids (eg, edema, ascites), hydration status should be taken into consideration. Timely intervention for weight loss is essential, since weight loss may be stabilized or reversed in some cancer patients if quickly identified.[98] When body weight is being evaluated, a comparison should be made to usual or normal weight, not a reference standard. Accurate body weight may be needed to calculate a treatment dose.

b) The physical examination should evaluate for muscle wasting and edema or ascites. A decrease in protein and fat stores and an associated increase in extracellular fluid accounts for the changes in body composition observed in cancer patients.[41] Peripheral edema suggests increased extracellular fluid or decreased visceral protein stores.[41] Temporal wasting is a hallmark of cachexia that is seen in patients with depleted lean body mass. However, muscle mass in cachectic cancer patients may be underestimated, limiting the usefulness of this measurement.[41] While muscle wasting is apparent in cachectic patients, it may be more subtle in obese patients.

c) A functional assessment should determine a patient's ability to perform activities of daily living. This evaluation should

FIGURE 11-1.

Scored Patient-Generated Subjective Global Assessment (PG-SGA)

Patient ID Information

History (Boxes 1-4 are designed to be completed by the patient.)

1. Weight *(See Worksheet 1)*

In summary of my current and recent weight:

I currently weigh about _______ pounds
I am about _________ feet _________ tall

One month ago I weighed about _________ pounds
Six months ago I weighed about _________ pounds

During the past two weeks my weight has:
☐ decreased (1) ☐ not changed (0) ☐ increased (0)

Box 1 ☐

2. Food Intake: As compared to my normal intake, I would rate my food intake during the past month as:

☐ unchanged (0)
☐ more than usual (0)
☐ less than usual (1)

I am now taking:

☐ *normal food* but less than normal amount (1)
☐ little solid food (2)
☐ only liquids (3)
☐ only nutritonal supplements (3)
☐ very little of anything (4)
☐ only tube feedings or only nutrition by vein (0)

Box 2 ☐

3. Symptoms: I have had the following problems that have kept me from eating enough during the past two weeks (check all that apply):

☐ no problems eating (0)
☐ no appetite, just did not feel like eating (3)
☐ nausea (1) ☐ vomiting (3)
☐ constipation (1) ☐ diarrhea (3)
☐ mouth sores (2) ☐ dry mouth (1)
☐ things taste funny or have no taste (1) ☐ smells bother me (1)
☐ problems swallowing (2) ☐ feel full quickly (1)
☐ pain; where? (3)__________
☐ other** (1) ____________________________

** Examples: depression, money, or dental problems

Box 3 ☐

4. Activities and Function: Over the past month, I would generally rate my activity as:

☐ normal with no limitations (0)
☐ not my normal self, but able to be up and about with fairly normal activities (1)
☐ not feeling up to most things, but in bed or chair less than half the day (2)
☐ able to do little activity and spend most of the day in bed or chair (3)
☐ pretty much bedridden, rarely out of bed (3)

Box 4 ☐

Additive Score of the Boxes 1-4 ☐ A

The remainder of this form will be completed by your doctor, nurse, or therapist. Thank you.

5. Disease and its relation to nutritional requirements *(See Worksheet 2)*

All relevant diagnoses (specify) ____

Primary disease stage (circle if known or appropriate) I II III IV Other ________________

Age ________

Numerical score from Worksheet 2 ☐ **B**

6. Metabolic Demand *(See Worksheet 3)*

Numerical score from Worksheet 3 ☐ **C**

7. Physical *(See Worksheet 4)*

Numerical score from Worksheet 4 ☐ **D**

Global Assessment *(See Worksheet 5)*

☐ Well-nourished or anabolic (SGA-A)
☐ Moderate or suspected malnutrition (SGA-B)
☐ Severely malnourished (SGA-C)

Total PG-SGA score

(Total numerical score of A+B+C+D above) ☐

(See triage recommendations below)

Clinician Signature ____________________________ RD RN PA MD DO Other ___ Date ________

Nutritional Triage Recommendations: Additive score is used to define specific nutritional interventions including patient & family education, symptom management including pharmacologic intervention, and appropriate nutrient intervention (food, nutritional supplements, enteral, or parenteral triage). First line nutrition intervention includes optimal symptom management.

0-1	No intervention required at this time. Re-assessment on routine and regular basis during treatment.
2-3	Patient & family education by dietitian, nurse, or other clinician with pharmacologic intervention as indicated by symptom survey (Box 3) and laboratory values as appropriate.
4-8	Requires intervention by dietitian, in conjunction with nurse or physician as indicated by symptoms survey (Box 3).
≥9	Indicates a critical need for improved symptom management and/or nutrient intervention options.

FIGURE 11-2.

Worksheets for PG-SGA Scoring

© FD Ottery, 2001

Boxes 1-4 of the PG-SGA are designed to be completed by the patient. The PG-SGA numerical score is determined using 1) the parenthetical points noted in boxes 1-4 and 2) the worksheets below for items not marked with parenthetical points. Scores for boxes 1 and 3 are additive within each box and scores for boxes 2 and 4 are based on the highest scored item checked off by the patient.

Worksheet 1 - Scoring Weight (Wt) Loss

To determine score, use 1 month weight data if available. Use 6 month data only if there is no 1 month weight data. Use points below to score weight change and add one extra point if patient has lost weight during the past 2 weeks. Enter total point score in Box 1 of the PG-SGA.

Wt loss in 1 month	Points	Wt loss in 6 months
10% or greater	4	20% or greater
5-9.9%	3	10 -19.9%
3-4.9%	2	6 - 9.9%
2-2.9%	1	2 - 5.9%
0-1.9%	0	0 - 1.9%

Score for Worksheet 1 ☐
Record in Box 1

Worksheet 2 - Scoring Criteria for Condition

Score is derived by adding 1 point for each of the conditions listed below that pertain to the patient.

Category	Points
Cancer	1
AIDS	1
Pulmonary or cardiac cachexia	1
Presence of decubitus, open wound, or fistula	1
Presence of trauma	1
Age greater than 65 years	1

Score for Worksheet 2 = ☐
Record in Box B

Worksheet 3 - Scoring Metabolic Stress

Score for metabolic stress is determined by a number of variables known to increase protein & calorie needs. The score is additive so that a patient who has a fever of > 102 degrees (3 points) and is on 10 mg of prednisone chronically (2 points) would have an additive score for this section of 5 points.

Stress	none (0)	low (1)	moderate (2)	high (3)
Fever	no fever	>99 and <101	≥101 and <102	≥102
Fever duration	no fever	<72 hrs	72 hrs	> 72 hrs
Corticosteroids	no corticosteroids	low dose (<10mg prednisone equivalents/day)	moderate dose (≥10 and <30mg prednisone equivalents/day)	high dose steroids (≥30mg prednisone equivalents/day)

Score for Worksheet 3 = ☐
Record in Box C

Worksheet 4 - Physical Examination

Physical exam includes a subjective evaluation of 3 aspects of body composition: fat, muscle, & fluid status. Since this is subjective, each aspect of the exam is rated for degree of deficit. Muscle deficit impacts point score more than fat deficit. Definition of categories: 0 = no deficit, 1+ = mild deficit, 2+ = moderate deficit, 3+ = severe deficit. Rating of deficit in these categories are *not* additive but are used to clinically assess the degree of deficit (or presence of excess fluid).

Fat Stores:				
orbital fat pads	0	1+	2+	3+
triceps skin fold	0	1+	2+	3+
fat overlying lower ribs	0	1+	2+	3+
Global fat deficit rating	**0**	**1+**	**2+**	**3+**
Muscle Status:				
temples (temporalis muscle)	0	1+	2+	3+
clavicles (pectoralis & deltoids)	0	1+	2+	3+
shoulders (deltoids)	0	1+	2+	3+
interosseous muscles	0	1+	2+	3+
scapula (latissimus dorsi, trapezius, deltoids)	0	1+	2+	3+
thigh (quadriceps)	0	1+	2+	3+
calf (gastrocnemius)	0	1+	2+	3+
Global muscle status rating	**0**	**1+**	**2+**	**3+**

Fluid Status:				
ankle edema	0	1+	2+	3+
sacral edema	0	1+	2+	3+
ascites	0	1+	2+	3+
Global fluid status rating	**0**	**1+**	**2+**	**3+**

Point score for the physical exam is determined by the overall subjective rating of total body deficit.

No deficit	score = 0 points
Mild deficit	score = 1 point
Moderate deficit	score = 2 points
Severe deficit	score = 3 points

Score for Worksheet 4 = ☐
Record in Box D

Worksheet 5 - PG-SGA Global Assessment Categories

	Stage A	**Stage B**	**Stage C**
Category	Well-nourished	Moderately malnourished or suspected malnutrition	Severely malnourished
Weight	No wt loss **OR** Recent non-fluid wt gain	~5% wt loss within 1 month (or 10% in 6 months) **OR** No wt stabilization or wt gain (i.e., continued wt loss)	> 5% wt loss in 1 month (or >10% in 6 months) **OR** No wt stabilization or wt gain (i.e., continued wt loss)
Nutrient Intake	No deficit **OR** Significant recent improvement	Definite decrease in intake	Severe deficit in intake
Nutrition Impact Symptoms	None **OR** Significant recent improvement allowing adequate intake	Presence of nutrition impact symptoms (Box 3 of PG-SGA)	Presence of nutrition impact symptoms (Box 3 of PG-SGA)
Functioning	No deficit **OR** Significant recent improvement	Moderate functional deficit **OR** Recent deterioration	Severe functional deficit **OR** recent significant deterioration
Physical Exam	No deficit **OR** Chronic deficit but with recent clinical improvement	Evidence of mild to moderate loss of SQ fat &/or muscle mass &/or muscle tone on palpation	Obvious signs of malnutrition (e.g., severe loss of SQ tissues, possible edema)

Global PG-SGA rating (A, B, or C) = ☐

determine and then compare preexisting abilities and deficits to those after diagnosis and treatment. The Karnofsky Performance Status Scale can classify a patient's functional impairment. This scale may be used to compare the effects of varied treatments and to assess the prognosis in individual patients. Generally, the lower the Karnofsky score, the poorer the survival prognosis for cancer patients.[103]

d) Functional limitations may affect a patient's ability to purchase, prepare, and eat food without assistance.[104] A rehabilitation therapy referral may be appropriate if the patient has significant deficits.

e) Assessment of muscle function using tests such as grip strength, respiratory muscle function, and electrical stimulation of specific muscles has effectively detected malnutrition-related changes before biochemical levels fall.[105]

f) Pain in cancer patients may be related to physical factors, such as the disease itself, cancer treatment, or psychological variables.[106] Since uncontrolled pain may affect a patient's appetite and ability to eat, an assessment of pain should be an integral part of a nutrition assessment of cancer patients.

4. Biochemical and laboratory tests

a) A measure of visceral proteins is used to judge protein status and effectiveness of nutritional repletion. Although serum albumin is commonly used to evaluate nutritional status, its ability to reflect nutritional status is questionable, however it is considered predictive of morbidity and mortality. Prealbumin, with its shorter half-life, provides a better indication of nutritional status and nutritional recovery during nutritional support, and also serves as a prognostic indicator of outcome.[107]

b) A low albumin, and to a lesser extent a lowered prealbumin, may reflect poor nutrition but may also indicate infection, over hydration, and decreased synthesis due to cytotoxic agents.[107]

c) Laboratory tests to identify micronutrient deficiencies may be appropriate in limited circumstances when other areas of assessment suggest deficits.

d) Objective parameters, such as anthropometrics and biochemical and immunological measures, support other aspects of the nutritional assessment. However, their validity and predictive capability as sole measures have been questioned since non-nutritional factors may skew results.

5. Quality of life (QOL)

a) Disease- and treatment-related symptoms affect a cancer patient's ability to eat and, therefore, are important aspects of a patient's QOL. A patient's willingness to eat also can be negatively affected by financial constraints, depressed psychological state, and poor attitude. Ultimately, disinterest in eating can lead to social isolation and conflict with caregivers and friends.

b) Weakness and fatigue, resulting from poor nutritional status and treatment side effects, may limit a patient's ability to work and carry out activities of daily living, thereby compromising QOL.[108]

c) A patient's well-being is composed of a physical component and a spiritual, psychological, and emotional component; both components are crucial to a patient's QOL and should be addressed in assessment.[106,109]

d) In a study of patients with head and neck cancer receiving radiation treatment, individualized nutrition counseling for symptom management not only improved nutrient intake but positively influenced QOL.[110]

B. Pediatrics

1. Screening

a) A PG-SGA for pediatric oncology has yet to be validated. However, many of the areas covered by the adult PG-SGA may also be applied to pediatrics, with some additions.

b) These additions include current height-for-age and weight-for-height or BMI-for-age as well as recent growth trends; food intake change; nutrition impact symptoms (nausea, vomiting, diarrhea, constipation); and functional capacity.

2. History and medication use

a) A diet history similar to that described for adults should be performed with the child and family. It should also include assessment of feeding behavior and skills. In addition, the family's viewpoints about nutrition and the child's level of understanding of the importance of nutrition should be assessed. These factors may have an impact on the child's motivation to eat when not feeling well, to try oral nutritional supplements, and to tolerate specialized nutrition support.

b) A medical history, including medication use, should be used when establishing the nutrition care plan and interpretating nutrition laboratory tests. Numerous medications often needed during disease and treatment, including antibiotics and diuretics, can alter vitamin, mineral, and electrolyte status. Certain medications may have greater nutritional impact in children. For example, glucocorticoids, which are often used chronically in leukemia and lymphoma treatment, interfere with bone metabolism, causing decreased bone mineral density.[111] Supplementation with calcium and vitamin D has been shown to significantly reduce the effects of corticosteroids on bone mineral density in adults,[112] and supplementation with calcium and vitamin D should be seriously considered in children receiving chronic steroids to ensure appropriate bone mineral accretion during childhood. However, recommended doses of calcium and vitamin D in children receiving steroids are not clear, so children who are taking calcium and vitamin D supplements should be closely monitored for the development of hypercalcemia and hypercalciuria.

3. Physical examination and functional assessment

a) Anthropometrics

(1) Weight and height are essential tools in assessing acute and chronic nutritional status and changes in nutritional status in children. Height-for-age is a measure of chronic or long-term nutrition in children. Weight-for-height or BMI-for-age can be used to assess acute or recent nutritional status. The criteria for poor growth or malnutrition in children have included any of the following: weight-for-height or height-for-age that is 2 standard deviations below the mean for sex and age[113]; the downward crossing of more than 2 major percentile markings on the National Center for Health Statistics (NCHS) growth charts from a child's established growth curve[114]; or the stages of acute and chronic malnutrition described by the Waterlow criteria.[115] The validity of specific cutoffs based on the 2000 NCHS pediatric BMI-for-age data as a screen for underweight has yet to be assessed. However, the World Health Organization defines BMI below the 5th percentile as an indication of underweight.[113] Meeting any of these criteria indicates the need for nutrition assessment. Keep in mind that serial measurements of growth over time provide much more information regarding the individual's nutritional status than a single point on the growth chart. A patient who has a decrease in

height-for-age or weight-for-age or BMI-for-age from the patient's established curve can cause greater concern (even if the patient's current point is above the 10th percentile) than a child who is below the 5th percentile but following his or her established curve. Overweight and its comorbidities can also be problematic in children with cancer. BMI-for-age is used to classify adolescents as at risk for overweight if between the 85th and 95th percentile and as overweight if at the 95th percentile or greater.[116,117] Recommendations for appropriate nutrition intervention as well as referral for additional medical workup have been described for healthy children over 2 years of age with elevated BMIs based on their age and their BMI-for-age percentile.[116,117] These recommendations can be applied to cancer survivors. However, weight maintenance and weight loss recommendations for patients currently battling cancer are not appropriate except in extreme cases, as the patient is likely to experience unintentional weight loss.

(2) When interpreting weight and height, one should bear in mind that other factors such as tumor size and hydration status can affect weight. Medication and length and type of treatment can affect growth. These factors should be considered when evaluating growth and determining the cause of growth delays in children.

b) Body composition

(1) Caliper skinfold and circumference measurements should be used as part of a complete nutritional assessment and can be especially useful in situations where loss of lean body mass may not be apparent because of overall body weight maintenance due to edema. Triceps skinfold thickness, mid–upper arm circumference, mid–upper arm muscle area, and subscapular skinfold thickness are common anthropometric measurements. Caliper skinfold measurements and circumference measurements can be compared to reference tables based on the age and sex of the child to determine relative fat and lean body mass composition.[118] Typically, values less than the 5th percentile for sex and age are consistent with acute malnutrition.[119] A triceps skinfold thickness greater than the 95th percentile in a child with a BMI-for-age above the 85th percentile can confirm that the child's BMI is elevated due to excessive fat rather than substantial lean body mass or frame size.[116] Skinfold and circumference measurements can be used to track changes in an individual patient over time when collected serially (every 3–6 months). The methodology for performing anthropometrics is described elsewhere.[120]

(2) Bioelectrical impedance analysis can be used in older children to determine total body composition. This is a quick, noninvasive tool and also can be used to track changes over time. However, factors such as fluid status may affect the validity of results. This tool has been validated in well-nourished and malnourished children.[121]

(3) A physical exam should involve assessment of muscle or fat depletion, fluid status, gastrointestinal symptoms, and pain. Edema may manifest as a clinical symptom of hypoalbuminemia, in which case aggressive protein repletion measures are often indicated. In some cases, severe hypoalbuminemia is due to protein losses via gut or capillary leakage, and increases in visceral protein levels may be limited by the rate of synthesis by the liver rather than by protein consumption. The liver may not be able to synthesize albumin at a rate that surpasses loss. Knowledge of the patient's hydration status is also important for accurate interpretation of body weight. Pain assessment is included in the physical evaluation as a factor that may reduce a child's appetite or capacity to eat.

(4) Functional assessment should determine the patient's ability to perform activities of daily living as compared to pretreatment capacity as well as to developmental stage. Having enough strength and energy to play is important psychosocially in children and should be considered as part of the functional assessment.

4. Biochemical and laboratory tests

a) As in adults, serum albumin and prealbumin[122] can be useful tools to assess the visceral protein status of children. A Prealbumin in Nutritional Care Consensus Group[123] developed the following levels of nutritional risk based on prealbumin levels: Less than 5 mg/dL indicates a poor prognosis; 5.0 to 10.9 mg/dL indicates significant risk and calls for aggressive nutrition support; and 11.0 to 15.0 mg/dL suggests increased risk with recommendation for close monitoring. When using this scale, bear in mind that each medical institution has its own normal standards for laboratory values based on analytical methods used, so that the values listed above may not exactly reflect the values in a given institution. In addition to indicating current nutritional status, prealbumin, with its rapid 2-day turnover rate, is useful in early assessment of the effectiveness of nutrition repletion regimens. A 1 mg/dL increase in prealbumin per day indicates adequate nutrition support in malnourished patients.[123,124] Increasing trends in prealbumin suggest that at least 65% of energy and protein needs are being met.[123] However, numerous non nutrition factors may affect interpretations of both albumin and prealbumin levels. Infection, extremes in hydration, liver synthetic function, protein-losing enteropathies, corticosteroid therapy, surgery, and impaired renal function may alter albumin and/or prealbumin levels.[125]

b) Absolute neutrophil count is important to monitor, as neutropenic patients must be especially careful to avoid food-borne pathogens.

c) Electrolyte and mineral wasting can be due to medications used in cancer treatment and management or to side effects of cancer therapy, such as diarrhea and vomiting. Serum potassium, magnesium, calcium, and phosphorous levels should be monitored regularly and replaced, if low. Note that total serum calcium and magnesium levels underestimate true status when albumin is low. Serum ionized calcium and magnesium levels more accurately reflect true calcium and magnesium status when albumin is decreased.

d) Glucose and lipids may be elevated with some commonly used medications, such as corticosteroids, and should be monitored regularly.

5. QOL

a) A poor QOL can affect a patient's nutritional status. Children may be physically and socially isolated due to infection or risk of infection. Long-term isolation may cause them to become bored, anxious, and depressed, leading to poor intake. Recreation therapists, psychiatrists/psychologists, and spiritual advisors can be consulted to help in these situations.

b) Conversely, poor nutrition may lead to a poor QOL. Undernourished patients are likely to feel fatigued and weak, which can affect their ability to play and enjoy life.

c) Poor intake by the child may also affect the parent's QOL. Parents often equate good eating with good health, so poor intake can cause them much distress.

d) QOL is an important issue to be assessed periodically as children undergo therapy or to evaluate when assessing the effectiveness of a palliative treatment in children who are at the end of life, but QOL is difficult to measure in children.[126] First, children pass through numerous developmental stages of physical, emotional, cognitive, and social functioning, meaning that no single measure can appropriately assess children of all ages.[127] Assessment tools must consider the developmental stage of the child being evaluated in terms of the child's ability to use the tool (Likert scale vs yes/no options) as well as the tool's ability to address the factors that may affect the child's QOL (fear of pain vs concern about appearance).[126] Longitudinal assessment of children may require use of different tools as they develop. Second, a proxy respondent is necessary for assessment of very young children who are unable to express their feelings in the structured manner of an assessment tool. However, proxy respondents may not accurately represent the child's perceptions or priorities. In a systematic review of studies examining proxy reports of QOL, children with chronic illness and their parents were found to have good agreement for domains reflecting physical activity, physical symptoms, and somatic distress but poor agreement for domains reflecting social and emotional issues.[128] Parents have been found to rate their children's functioning in certain categories and overall QOL as lower than the children's ratings, possibly due to differences in perception of the situation.[128,129] For example, parents may be considering long-term outcomes such as future fertility or compromised education, while a young child may be concerned with immediate consequences, such as missing friends.[129] This is not to say, however, that parental concerns are not important.

e) Specific QOL assessment tools for use during cancer therapy in children include the Miami Pediatric Quality of Life Questionnaire,[130] the Pediatric Oncology Quality of Life Scale,[131] and the Behavioral, Affective, and Somatic Experiences Scale.[132] A common modular instrument (which combines generic as well as disease-specific scales) is the Pediatric Quality of Life Inventory.[133] Tools used to assess QOL of childhood cancer survivors include the Minneapolis-Manchester Quality of Life Instruments for both youth and adolescents.[134,135] Other tools have also been used to measure the QOL of pediatric cancer patients after treatment.[136–140]

IV. Criteria for Intervention and Goals of Therapy

A. Nutritional considerations for specific cancer treatments
  1. Nutritional considerations for chemotherapy
    a) Nausea and vomiting
    b) Mucositis
    c) Constipation
    d) Diarrhea
    e) Neutropenia
    f) Changes in taste
    g) Loss of appetite
  2. Nutritional considerations for radiation therapy
    a) Mucositis
    b) Diarrhea, nausea, vomiting if the GI tract is in the radiation field
    c) Changes in taste
    d) Dry mouth
    e) Fatigue
    f) Endocrinological effects (adverse endocrinological effects of cranial radiation have been reviewed)[141–143]
  3. Nutritional considerations for immunotherapy
    a) Nausea, vomiting
    b) Mucositis
    c) Diarrhea
    d) Changes in taste
    e) Dry mouth
  4. Nutritional considerations for surgery
    a) One week before an operative procedure, patients should stop all herbal products or supplements (eg, borage or fish oil, vitamin E) that may affect blood thinning, unless otherwise advised by their physician.[144]
    b) Nutritional considerations vary depending on type and degree of surgical intervention. Potential issues depend on the patient's mechanical and physical impairment and ability to ingest, digest, and absorb adequate nutrients.
    c) The patient's perioperative and long-term nutritional needs should be taken into account and planned for from the onset.

B. Adults
  1. Criteria for intervention[145]
    a) Preoperative tube-feeding or PN support provided for at least 7 to 14 days preoperatively may benefit moderately and severely malnourished cancer patients, but the potential benefits of nutrition support should be appraised against the inherent risks of nutrition support and the delay in surgery.
    b) Specialized nutrition support should not be used routinely in well-nourished or mildly malnourished patients receiving surgery, chemotherapy, or radiation therapy when reasonable oral intake is anticipated.
    c) Specialized nutrition support is indicated in selected patients who are receiving cancer treatment and who are either severely malnourished or unable to consume and/or absorb an adequate oral diet for an extended period of time.
    d) Palliative specialized nutrition support is seldom indicated in patients with terminal cancer that is unresponsive to conventional therapy.
  2. Goals
    a) Maintenance of nutritional status or reversal of protein-calorie malnutrition
      (1) The caloric needs of cancer patients depend on the tumor type and other medical factors such as fever or infection. Caloric needs are not static and can vary with medical changes throughout the treatment course.
      (2) Nutrition support should provide calories sufficient to meet a cancer patient's needs by minimizing body catabolism without overfeeding. A variety of empiric formulas are available to estimate energy needs. See Chapter 2. However, ongoing monitoring is essential to ensure that the caloric estimate is appropriate. Providing most cancer patients with 25 to 35 kcal/kg per day is a reasonable estimate.[106] Although not routine and felt by some to be controversial, the use of indirect calorimetry to measure resting energy expenditure in the clinical setting may be of value.
      (3) A cancer patient's degree of catabolism will dictate protein requirements. Generally, an intake of 1.2 to 1.5 g/kg/d protein is adequate,[106] although hypermetabolic or extremely wasted patients may have higher requirements.

(4) Although visceral proteins are influenced by non nutritional factors, monitoring them may provide an indication of a patient's protein status, and a nitrogen balance evaluation may be appropriate in selected cases.

b) Decreased morbidity, improved survival, and improved QOL

(1) There is no definitive evidence that specialized nutrition support in cancer patients increases treatment tolerance, decreases treatment complications, or extends survival; therefore, the effects of nutrition support in this regard remain controversial.[146,147]

(2) Provision of nutrition support to selected patients with cancer may improve QOL. As expectations of quality vary with individual patients, decision making requires multidisciplinary assessment and should be addressed on a case-by-case basis.

(3) Use of home PN in a group of appropriately selected cancer patients resulted in improved performance status and reported improved QOL (judged as returning to work or previous activity level).[98]

(4) There is no conclusive evidence in humans that feeding cancer patients to replete the host will stimulate further tumor growth.[148,149]

(5) In head and neck cancer, preexisting poor intake commonly results from alcohol and nicotine abuse and difficulty swallowing due to obstruction from tumor. Multiple treatment modalities—such as surgery, radiation, and chemotherapy—may be employed and may affect diet tolerance and adequacy of intake. Multiple studies show that early enteral feeding with percutaneous endoscopic gastrostomy (PEG) or surgical jejunostomy before or during cancer treatment can minimize weight loss, dehydration, and interruptions in treatment and can limit hospital admissions.[147,150–153] Prospective, randomized clinical trials (PRCTs) have failed to show improved survival in patients receiving parenteral or tube-feeding support with their cancer treatment.[154]

(6) Some nutrients, such as glutamine, arginine, essential fatty acids, and nucleic acids, were evaluated as having specific biologic effects on the tumor and the host. The potential benefits of these specific nutrients, individually or combined, in enhancing immune function, lessening the inflammatory response, and enabling recovery from surgery are inconclusive.[145,151,155]

C. Pediatrics

1. Criteria for intervention

a) Nutritional status is related to relapse rates and survival as well as to tolerance of treatment in pediatric oncology. This relationship varies based on the type and stage of cancer.

(1) The cancer relapse rate has been shown to be increased in patients who are malnourished at diagnosis or referral in ALL[156,157] and in solid tumors.[158] Five-year disease-free survival was significantly greater for patients with ALL who were well nourished compared to patients with ALL who were malnourished at diagnosis.[157] The time to relapse or death was significantly longer in patients with Stage IV neuroblastoma who were well nourished at diagnosis compared to those who were malnourished at diagnosis and received PN.[159] However, nutritional status was not related to survival in these patients, in a group of pediatric patients in El Salvador and Brazil that included various types of cancer,[159,160] or in two large retrospective studies in pediatric ALL.[161,162] Conversely, patients with pediatric lymphoma and solid tumor with localized disease and with good nutritional status at time of referral had significantly improved likelihood of survival compared to patients with poor nutritional status at referral. This significance did not hold true for patients with regional and metastatic disease.[158]

(2) Tolerance to treatment and treatment delays varies with type of cancer. Patients with ALL and Wilms' tumor who were malnourished at diagnosis required a reduction in drug therapy compared to patients who were well nourished at diagnosis, owing to poor tolerance of drug therapy.[9,157] Treatments were delayed in significantly more patients with Stage IV neuroblastoma who were malnourished at diagnosis or who had early decrease in nutritional status than in patients who were well nourished at diagnosis or who had early improvement in their nutritional status.[159]

(3) Nutritional status may serve as a marker, rather than a cause, of a particular outcome in cancer patients. There is insufficient evidence to support the assertion that improvements in nutritional status will result in improved patient outcomes.

b) Indications for nutrition support

(1) Specialized nutrition support and dietary interventions must be implemented to support normal growth and development and to provide the energy needed in patients who cannot meet requirements via oral intake.[99]

(2) Palliative specialized nutrition support in terminally ill children with cancer is rarely indicated.[99]

(3) Newly diagnosed pediatric cancer patients tend to consume 90% or less of the recommended dietary allowance for calories but have adequate protein intake.[12,163] However, disease progression plus side effects from therapy may result in decreased oral consumption and the need for nutrition support.[164]

(4) A task force formed by the American Academy of Pediatrics developed criteria for nutrition intervention in pediatric cancer patients.[8] Andrassy and Chwals[165] and Ollenschlager et al[166] slightly modified and contributed to the criteria, which include

(a) Weight loss of more than 5% of preillness body weight

(b) Weight less than 90% of ideal body weight (IBW) or weight-for-height less than 10th percentile on NCHS growth curves.[167] The NCHS growth chart showing BMI-for-age can be used for older children.

(c) Serum albumin less than 3.2 mg/dL (barring acute metabolic stress within the last 14 days)

(d) Triceps skinfold less than the 5th percentile for age and sex

(e) Decrease of weight- and/or height-for-age across 2 percentile increments on the NCHS growth curves

(f) Oral intake less than 70% of that needed for growth for more than 5 days in well-nourished patients

(g) Expected GI dysfunction for more than 5 days in well-nourished patients

(h) High risk for malnutrition based on type of tumor and cancer therapy

(i) Delayed cutaneous hypersensitivity anergy in children over 2 years old prior to treatment

(5) Oral intake

(a) Numerous studies show that pediatric cancer patients tend to experience significant weight loss and have decreases in arm muscle area and triceps skinfold measurements on an oral diet.[10,168,169]

(b) Patients who experienced intervention by a registered dietitian while on an oral diet had significantly more weeks at a stable weight than did patients who did not receive intensive nutritional intervention.[166]

(c) Counseling must be individualized to the type and stage of cancer, the degree of disease, symptoms, and the type and stage of treatment.

(6) Enteral nutrition support

(a) Indications for enteral support in children are similar to those in adults. In addition, children who fail to gain weight should be considered for nutrition support.

(b) Studies reveal that pediatric cancer patients significantly increase their body weight after 1, 3, and 4 months of tube feeding.[168,170,171]

(c) In malnourished cancer patients, 60% of the patients reached 95% of their IBW in a mean of 4.9 months of tube feeding, and the remaining patients gained at least 7% of their IBW in that time.[172]

(d) Lack of randomized studies has hampered the ability to determine the effectiveness of enteral nutrition support in pediatric cancer patients.

(7) PN support

(a) Indications for PN in children are similar to those in adults.

(b) Numerous PRCTs have examined the effectiveness of PN at nutritionally repleting pediatric cancer patients and improving their clinical outcome.

(c) PRCTs in primarily well-nourished cancer patients demonstrate that PN given for 17 to 104 days is able to significantly increase weight and nitrogen balance and results in increases in arm muscle area and triceps skinfold measurements. In addition, PN promotes maintenance of total leukocyte and absolute granulocyte counts compared to those of control groups.[169,173,174]

(d) Other PRCTs in primarily well-nourished patients who were given PN through the first cycle of chemotherapy until recovery from myelosuppression showed no difference in survival rates, tumor response, or duration of myelosuppression and actually showed shorter remission in patients with parenteral nutrition (PN) than in controls.[174,175]

(e) Nonrandomized studies that administered PN for approximately 4 weeks showed a significant increase from baseline in arm muscle area, triceps skinfold measurements, subscapular skinfold measurements, and percentage of diagnosis weight. Serum transferrin, albumin, prealbumin, and retinol-binding protein levels were increased. In addition, there was a significant decrease in treatment delays compared to those in nourished patients receiving enteral nutrition.[10,176–179]

(f) Overall, PN seems to improve nutritional status but not clinical outcome.

(g) The duration of PN provision necessary to achieve nutritional repletion is difficult to predict. Nine to 14 days of PN resulted in a slight weight gain and a significant increase in serum transferrin levels, but only 9 of 15 subjects repleted their weight, whereas all but 1 subject repleted their weight on 28 days of PN.[10]

(h) The beneficial nutritional effects of PN fail to persist once PN is discontinued if the patient's clinical situation has not improved.[173]

(i) Comparing results from different studies is difficult because of variability in the type and stage of cancer, the type of therapy, the stage of treatment, and nutritional status. Furthermore, small sample sizes may prevent detection of differences between groups.

2. Goals

a) Growth and/or maintenance of nutritional status or reversal of protein-calorie malnutrition

(1) Body weight should be greater than IBW.[8]

(2) Arm fat area should be greater than the 10th percentile for age and sex.[8]

(3) Serum albumin should be greater than 3.2 mg/dL.[8]

(4) Calorie and protein needs vary with age, disease state, type of treatment, presence of fever, infection, wound status, activity level, and individual needs. See Chapter 2 for help with determining calorie and protein needs.

(5) Fluid balance is important. See Chapter 2 for help with determining fluid requirements.

(6) Vitamin and mineral deficiency should be prevented. Monitor mineral and electrolyte levels regularly and other vitamins and minerals when deficiency or toxicity is suspected. For example, vitamin K levels may decrease with long-term antibiotic therapy, and copper and manganese levels may exceed normal levels when provided in TPN during cholestasis.[180,181]

b) Decreased morbidity, improved survival, and improved QOL

(1) Improvement in nutritional status has not clearly been shown to increase the survival or treatment tolerance in pediatric oncology patients.

(2) Improvement in nutritional status can theoretically enhance QOL by increasing energy level and wound healing and reducing risk of infection. However, the inconvenience of some nutrition interventions (eg, time-consuming tube-feeding regimen that interferes with play time) may outweigh the potential benefits. The pros and cons should be presented to the child and family, allowing them to make the final decision.

V. Nutritional Management

A. Management for specific cancer treatments

1. Pharmacological

a) Commonly used antiemetics include [182]

(1) Serotonin-receptor antagonists (eg, ondansetron, granisetron)

(2) Phenothiazines (eg, promethazine, chlorpromethazine)

(3) Antihistamines (eg, diphenhydramine, hydroxyzine)

(4) Benzodiazepines (eg, lorazepam)

(5) Steroids (eg, dexamethasone)

(6) Cannabinoids

b) Prevention/treatment of mucositis[182]

(1) Salt, soda rinse

(2) Chlorhexidine

(3) Mouthwash consisting of diphenhydramine, antacid, and lidocaine

c) Bowel medications

(1) Stool softeners (docusate)

(2) Bulk laxatives (psyllium, calcium polycarbophil, methylcellulose)

(3) Lubricants (mineral oil)
(4) Osmotic agents (glycerin, lactulose)
(5) Saline laxatives (magnesium salts, sodium biphosphate/phosphate)
(6) Stimulants (bisacodyl, cascara sagrada, senna)
(7) Antidiarrheals (bismuth subsalicylate, difenoxin, kaolin/pectin, loperamide, opium tincture)

2. Nutritional
   a) Nausea and vomiting
      (1) Consume small, frequent meals or snacks.
      (2) Eat slowly.
      (3) Choose cold, nonodorous foods.
      (4) Select light, starchy, low-fat foods.
      (5) Avoid very sweet or spicy foods.
      (6) Save favorite foods for periods without nausea or vomiting.
      (7) Rest and sit up after eating.
      (8) Refrain from eating prior to therapies that cause nausea or vomiting.
   b) Mucositis
      (1) Choose bland, cold, soft foods.
      (2) Moisten dry foods.
      (3) Cut food into small pieces or puree.
      (4) Use a straw with fluids.
      (5) Coordinate eating with analgesic use.
   c) Constipation
      (1) Obtain adequate fluid intake.
      (2) Increase insoluble fiber consumption.
      (3) Drink hot beverages prior to the usual time of bowel movements.
      (4) Incorporate physical activity as permitted by the medical team.
   d) Diarrhea
      (1) Consume extra fluid and potassium-rich food sources.
      (2) Increase intake of soluble fiber and reduce insoluble fiber consumption.
      (3) Avoid lactose and sugar alcohols.
      (4) Select low-fat foods.
      (5) Consume foods and beverages at room temperature.
   e) Neutropenia
      (1) Choose foods less likely to contain a high bacterial load.
         (a) Wash raw fruits and vegetables well and reject any that have indications of damage or spoilage.
         (b) Avoid unpasteurized products and ripened, soft cheeses.
      (2) Follow safe handling, storage, thawing, and cooking procedures for meat, fish, poultry, and eggs.
         (a) Keep raw meat, fish, and poultry separated from other foods to prevent cross-contamination.
         (b) Store frozen foods at 0°F and refrigerated foods at 35 to 40°F.
         (c) Thaw foods in the refrigerator, in the microwave, or in cold water that is changed every 30 minutes.
         (d) Cook meat (including deli meats), fish, poultry, and eggs until well done (160°F).
         (e) Do not leave perishable foods unrefrigerated for more than 2 hours. Dispose of leftovers after 2 to 3 days.
   f) Taste changes. Choose flavorful foods as tolerated, such as sour, seasoned, and spicy foods.
   g) Loss of appetite
      (1) Consume small, frequent meals.
      (2) Save beverages for the end of meals.
      (3) Give priority to high-calorie and protein- and nutrient-dense foods.
      (4) Do not force children to eat if they refuse.
   h) Dry mouth
      (1) Select sweet or sour foods.
      (2) Moisten or puree dry foods.
      (3) Sip water frequently.
   i) Fatigue
      (1) Consume small, frequent meals.
      (2) Choose high-calorie and protein- and nutrient-dense foods.

3. Complementary and alternative approaches
   a) Although gaps still exist, research is growing that indicates that complementary and alternative medicine (CAM) therapies can be effectively integrated into conventional medicine. Current evidence indicates that CAM usage is more effective in relieving cancer-related symptoms than in slowing disease progression.[183]
   b) CAM therapies commonly used by cancer patients that can be recommended for use[183] include acupuncture for chemotherapy-related nausea and vomiting or for pain, massage (except deep tissue or forceful) for anxiety or pain, moderate exercise to minimize fatigue, psychological and mind-body techniques (eg support groups, relaxation training, imagery), reduction of animal and saturated fat, and addition of soy in the diet of well-nourished men with prostate cancer.
   c) Some CAM therapies should be discouraged in cancer patients.[183] These include very restrictive diets in patients with poor nutritional status; antioxidants in patients undergoing radiation or chemotherapy; supplements with anticoagulant effects in patients with thrombocytopenia, patients undergoing anticoagulation therapy, and postoperatively; acupuncture in patients with thrombocytopenia and anticoagulation therapy; and high-dose vitamin A and vitamin C in all cancer patients.
   d) Any CAM therapy should be discouraged if any of the following apply:
      (1) It delays conventional treatment.
      (2) It has not been scientifically proven to be efficacious.
      (3) It is provided by an unlicensed practitioner.
      (4) It requires injection of substances not approved by the US Food and Drug Administration.[183]

B. Adults

1. Special aspects of diet and nutritional supplements
   a) Aggressive strategies to optimize oral intake and tolerance should be instituted early, especially for patients with preexisting nutritional problems. A patient's calorie and protein needs should be determined, diet strategies and oral supplements should be instituted, unnecessary diet restrictions should be eliminated, and eating times should be planned to be separated from treatment sessions.[98]
   b) Physiological and mechanical considerations of the disease and/or treatment may necessitate an alteration in the cancer patient's diet.[184] These considerations include the following:
      (1) Multiple feedings and postgastrectomy diet after gastric resection
      (2) A soft diet for esophageal strictures
      (3) A low-fat diet with or without enzyme supplementation for improved absorption in patients with pancreatic insufficiency
      (4) Low fiber and lactose for radiation enteritis
   c) Oral supplements are a valuable addition to the diets of cancer patients. The use of oral supplements resulted in significantly increased protein and calorie intake without reducing foods consumed in a group of cancer patients counseled to use nutrition

supplements between meals and at bedtime.[185] A limitation of oral supplementation use is taste fatigue; therefore, ongoing evaluation of acceptance is necessary, as are plans to provide varied alternatives for patients with anticipated long-term needs.

d) There is evidence from animal studies that polyunsaturated fatty acids can promote cell growth by stimulating cell proliferation and by inhibiting apoptosis. Fish oil, on the other hand, can reduce the tumor growth rate and decrease host body weight loss in animals. In humans, a small, pilot trial of 20 patients with pancreatic cancer was conducted in which patients were given an eicosapentaenoic acid (EPA)–enriched supplemented oral diet.[186] Cachexia was reversed, and body weight was increased at 3 and 7 weeks. However, these results could not be replicated in a follow-up study of 200 patients with pancreatic cancer, possibly because several patients in the control group were taking EPA.[187]

e) Cancer patients can benefit from nutrition counseling not only before and during treatment but also later in their course. Cancer survivors are interested in making lifestyle changes to improve their diet and physical activity level. According to a survey, approximately 66% of survivors reported making lifestyle changes, 40% made one or more dietary changes, 21% started a new physical activity, and 48% started taking dietary supplements.[188]

f) Information on food safety issues should be incorporated into the nutrition education provided to neutropenic patients.

2. Special aspects of enteral nutrition
   a) Indications and goals
      (1) Aggressive nutritional support with enteral nutrition should be considered in selected instances in cancer patients who are unable to attain adequate oral intake. Patients with small-bowel resections and patients with mucosal injury from chemotherapy or radiation who are unable to ingest and/or digest nutrients may benefit from enteral feeding. Critically ill cancer patients may also benefit from enteral nutrition.[150]
      (2) The aim of enteral feeding is to meet macronutrient, micronutrient, and fluid needs with acceptable GI tolerance.
      (3) Cycled and intermittent feedings may be well tolerated, allow patients more mobility, and encourage some oral intake. The ultimate goal is to transition to an oral diet as soon as the patient is able to attain adequate intake by mouth.
   b) Monitoring
      (1) Cancer patients should be monitored for aspiration risk and GI tolerance. Preexisting treatment-related side effects, such as nausea or diarrhea, may be exacerbated during enteral feeds. In postoperative patients, ileus may preclude tolerance; and in critically ill patients who are receiving mechanical ventilation, poor perfusion may limit ability to maintain enteral feeds.
      (2) Nasoenteric feeding tubes may be contraindicated in patients with severe thrombocytopenia, significant mucositis, or recent extensive neck resection.
      (3) Immune-suppressed patients should be educated regarding careful tube-feeding technique to minimize the risk of feeding-related infection.
3. Special aspects of PN
   a) Indications and goals
      (1) PN is recommended in appropriately chosen cancer patients who need aggressive nutrition support when tube feeding has been unsuccessful or when use of the GI tract is not appropriate (eg, obstruction, high-output fistula).
      (2) In cachectic cancer patients, given the metabolic alterations from advanced or untreated disease, the goal of nutrition support may be to minimize wasting rather than to nutritionally replete the patient.
   b) Monitoring (see Chapter 8 for PN monitoring)
4. CAM aspects. Cancer patients may use a variety of CAM therapies in conjunction with or as a substitute for conventional treatment.[189] Many cancer patients are motivated to seek CAM therapies as a means of self-healing and of maintaining optimism when faced with the uncertainty of their disease.[190] Patients should be questioned about possible use of CAM therapies throughout treatment. Clinicians need to communicate openly and without judgment so patients feel comfortable disclosing CAM usage. Reputable and up-to-date Web sites and resources are available, so clinicians have access to reliable information describing the growing number of CAM therapies and detailing some dangerous interactions between these therapies and allopathic medicines.
5. Ethical issues
   a) The goals of nutritional care in the framework of cancer treatment should be discussed with patients and their caregivers proactively in an open, straightforward, supportive manner. Patients should recognize the short- and long-term nutritional consequences of their treatments. For example, certain GI surgeries may necessitate long-term nutrition support or special diet modifications. Radiation treatment may cause lasting mucosal damage that affects diet tolerance. Patients requiring massive surgery and tube feeding, such as head and neck patients, have unique ethical issues related to disfigurement and dysfunction.[33,98,191]
   b) Transitioning a patient from active nutritional care to end-of-life care can present numerous challenges. The provision or withdrawal of nutrition support to patients with advanced disease is an issue that evokes medical, emotional, ethical, and legal considerations. Ethical decision making should involve the multidisciplinary team, including the patient and caregivers, and should account for patient needs for autonomy, QOL, and a holistic structure. While there may be facility guidelines to help decision making, ultimately decisions need to be made on an individualized, case-by-case basis.[191–196]
   c) Given that cancer patients are interested in CAM therapies, it is crucial for clinicians to recognize their ethical obligation when recommending, allowing, and guiding patients to these therapies and modalities. It is necessary to keep in mind the risk-to-benefit ratio when determining the appropriateness of any therapy, especially when there is limited or no scientific evidence to support it.[197]
6. Patient and caregiver education
   a) Review all drug-nutrient interactions that apply to the patient.
   b) Educate the patient and family about the nutrition side effects commonly experienced with the cancer therapy being used and how to maximize calorie and protein intake when the patient faces these side effects.
   c) Teach the patient and caregivers the principles of the neutropenic diet and when it is to be followed.
   d) When implementing specialized nutrition support, help the patient and family to understand the reason it is being used, how the nutrients are being delivered, and the risks and benefits associated with the feeding method.
   e) Share the known effects of the CAMs being used with the patient and family, being sure to emphasize, when appropriate, the possible unknown effects due to lack of controlled studies.

f) As long-term effects become known, patients with good outcomes to therapy should be educated on nutrition-related problems they may face later in life and the need for follow-up.

C. Pediatrics

1. Special aspects of diet and nutritional supplements
   a) When the appetite is at a preillness level, follow a well-balanced diet with a variety of foods according to the Food Guide Pyramid and Dietary Guidelines.
   b) If appetite or intake is compromised, make high-calorie, high-protein, and nutrient-dense foods a priority in the diet. A multivitamin/multimineral supplement may be indicated. However, extra iron should be avoided in patients who undergo numerous blood transfusions, and folate supplements should not be given with methotrexate therapy.
   c) Avoid favorite foods during periods of nausea and vomiting or therapies that lead to GI upset in order to minimize learned aversions to those foods.
   d) Oral supplements may be used to increase nutrient intake.
      (1) Pediatric supplements are designed to meet the nutrient needs of children aged 1 to 10 years.
      (2) Modular supplements (protein, carbohydrate, lipid) may be given to increase intake of a particular macronutrient.
      (3) In cases of diarrhea or malabsorption, low osmolar nutritional supplements that contain hydrolyzed carbohydrate and protein and a higher percentage of medium-chain triglycerides may be appropriate. These supplements should be flavored when taken orally.
      (4) The safety of fish oil supplementation in children has not been well studied.
2. Special aspects of enteral nutrition
   a) Goals
      (1) Growth. Provide adequate calories, protein, and micronutrients to support growth along the NCHS growth curves.
      (2) Tolerance of feeds. The type of formula, concentration, and rate must be well tolerated by the patient to promote optimal absorption of the nutrients provided.
      (3) Minimization of the burden associated with tube feeding. Cycle the tube feeding, as tolerated, overnight, so that days are free for eating and playing, and so feedings are less often interrupted by medical procedures performed during the day. If the patient is unable to take anything by mouth, then provide boluses, as tolerated, to mimic meals during the day.
      (4) Prealbumin. Increase prealbumin by 1 mg/dL per day.[123,124]
   b) Monitoring
      (1) The most common complications associated with nasogastric tubes (NGTs) in pediatric cancer patients are tube dislodgment due to vomiting and feeding intolerances (diarrhea, nausea, vomiting).[198,199] Diarrhea can often be controlled by adjusting the rate, strength, or osmolarity of feeds.[172,198] Nausea and vomiting are well managed pharmacologically.[199] No episodes of epistaxis, sinusitis, or GI bleeding were reported,[198,199] even in patients who had NGTs placed during thrombocytopenia and neutropenia.[198]
      (2) Minor complications associated with PEGs and gastrostomy tubes (GTs) are common and primarily include insertion site inflammation.[170,172,200–202] Other complications include feeding discharge from the GT site and GT occlusion.[170,172,200–202]
      (3) Major complications included systemic infection and peritonitis. The rate of these ranged from 3% to 7%,[170,200] 1.58 episodes/1000 days of GT use,[172] or 4.5 episodes/1000 days of PEG use[201] in pediatric cancer patients.
3. Special aspects of PN
   a) Goals
      (1) Growth. Adequate calories, protein, and micronutrients should be provided to support growth along the NCHS growth curves.
      (2) Catch-up growth. If the patient has protein calorie malnutrition, catch-up growth and repletion of lean body mass is the goal.
      (3) Prealbumin levels and trends. These can be monitored as one measure of the adequacy of energy and protein intake. Increases of 1 mg/dL per day indicate appropriate effectiveness of the nutrition regimen.[123,124]
      (4) Replacement of any minerals and electrolytes that are being wasted, and provision of additional micronutrients at levels indicated by secondary conditions. For example, voluminous diarrhea may require the provision of additional zinc.
      (5) Minimization of metabolic disturbances associated with PN. Glucose should be maintained at less than 180 mg/dL, and triglycerides should not exceed 300 mg/dL.
      (6) Avoidance of refeeding syndrome by repleting mineral and electrolyte levels prior to starting PN and by initiating PN slowly in cases of severe malnutrition.
   b) Monitoring
      (1) Major complications with catheter insertion include hemothorax and infection at the insertion site, reported in one study to occur at a rate of 4.4%.[203] A minor complication is hematoma, which reportedly occurred at a rate of 6.7%.[203]
      (2) The most commonly reported complication with PN is sepsis. PN patients had significantly more days with fever; however, the catheter tip never cultured positively.[204] Catheter-related sepsis has been reported to occur at a rate of 3%.[205] This rate seems to vary depending on the nutritional status of the patient, with significantly more sepsis occurring in malnourished patients on PN than in well-nourished patients on PN.[205]
      (3) Metabolic complications also can develop. They include hyperglycemia, hypophosphatemia, altered electrolytes, and increases in liver function tests and bilirubin levels.
4. CAM aspects. Reports from studies conducted in 1997–2000 in the United States suggest that anywhere from 47% to 84% of pediatric cancer patients have used at least one CAM since diagnosis.[206–208] The most popular CAMs reported in these studies were faith healing, diet changes, and dietary or herbal supplements. Literature on the safety and efficacy of herbal supplements in children is lacking. In general, concerns include adverse interactions with standard medications and/or contamination of the herbal supplements with agents that can cause illness. Other CAMs include hypnosis and art therapy, the benefits of which have been reported in children.[209–211] The International Society of Pediatric Oncology (SIOP) working committee on psychosocial issues in pediatric oncology developed guidelines for the use of nonconventional therapies in childhood cancer.[212] The committee recommended that the health care team not automatically discourage the use of CAM therapies if they are deemed nonharmful, even if the patient or family benefits only psychologically.[212] On the other hand, the health care team should attempt to maintain open communication with the patient and family about use of nonconventional therapies and should be vigilant about discouraging therapies that may be harmful, either

physically or psychologically.[212] The committee also warned that parents should be wary of therapies that have the following characteristics: the therapy is a secret that is known only by the promoter of the therapy; the therapy is touted as a cure for a wide range of cancers; the promoter attacks the medical community or claims to be persecuted by it; or treatment with the therapy requires a large sum of money to be paid up front.[212]

5. Ethical issues
   a) The same ethical considerations that exist for adult cancer patients exist for pediatric cancer patients.
   b) The use of specialized nutrition support in terminally ill patients is controversial but should be considered if it may improve QOL.
   c) Discontinuance of nutritional support can be the factor that transitions the parents/caregivers to acceptance of the end-of-life status of their child. Sensitivity to the significance of nutrition to the family and caregivers in this regard is very important.
6. Patient and caregiver education
   a) The same topics should be covered with pediatric patients that are covered with adults (see Section V.B.6).
   b) With increasing survival of pediatric cancer patients, the long-term effects of cancer treatments must be considered. Long-term gastrointestinal toxicity may be one adverse effect of cancer therapy in patients who survive into adolescence and adulthood.[213] Survivors of ALL tend to become overweight by the time they reach their final height,[15,16] and decreased physical activity has been purported to be a likely cause.[17,18] Survivors of brain tumors may also experience intractable weight gain if the hypothalamus is damaged during therapy.[214] Numerous long-term health-related issues secondary to radiotherapy and chemotherapy have been reviewed.[140–142] As long-term effects continue to become known, patients with good outcomes to therapy should be educated on possible nutrition-related problems they may face later in life and the need for follow-up.

VI. Patient and Caregiver Education Internet Resources

A. Internet resources for the patient and caregiver
1. American Cancer Society, www.cancer.org
   a) Contains information for patients, family and friends, survivors, health information seekers, American Cancer Society supporters, and professionals.
   b) The health information section contains information about food and fitness, such as guidelines for eating well and being active, cooking smart, and taking control of one's weight; the power of fruits and vegetables; recipes; and nutrition during treatment.
2. American Institute for Cancer Research, www.aicr.org
   a) AICR is the cancer charity that fosters research on diet and cancer prevention and educates the public about the results.
   b) The site contains information for survivors and health professionals.
   c) The nutrition information includes eating healthier with the new American plate, a recipe corner, strategies for cooking for lower cancer risk, and special featured topics
3. Cancer Centers, www.cancerlinksusa.com
   a) This is the Web site of the Cancer Information Network. A newsletter is also available.
   b) The site provides information about various types of cancers and discusses a wide array of topics.
4. Cancer Research and Prevention Foundation, www.preventcancer.org
   a) The mission of the Cancer Research and Prevention Foundation is the prevention and early detection of cancer through scientific research and education. It focuses on cancers that can be prevented through lifestyle changes or early detection followed by prompt treatment. These include breast, cervical, colorectal, lung, oral, prostate, skin, and testicular cancers.
   b) The Web site spotlights topics and discusses cancer prevention in the news. There is information for patients and researchers.
5. Diet Guidelines for Immunosuppressed Patients, www.fhcrc.org/clinical/ltfu/
   a) The Web site of the Fred Hutchinson Cancer Research Center in Seattle, Washington.
   b) The site provides guidelines for adult and pediatric patients, including a patient and caregiver resource manual with guidelines on food and water safety, diet, adult nutrition, pediatric nutrition, and GI diets.
6. National Cancer Institute, www.cancer.gov
   a) A comprehensive site that includes information on cancer topics, clinical trials, cancer statistics, research and funding, and news.
   b) Eating Hints for Cancer Patients, http://www.cancer.gov/cancertopics/eatinghints, provides nutritional advice for before treatment begins, advice on managing eating problems during treatment, special notes for caregivers, discussion of the posttreatment period, recipes, and more.
7. OncoLink, http://www.oncolink.upenn.edu/
   a) The Web site of the Abramson Cancer Center of the University of Pennsylvania.
   b) This site highlights daily and weekly cancer-related news and offers a newsletter. There are sections on types of cancer, treatment options, coping with cancer, clinical trials, cancer resources, and expert advice.
8. Oncology Nutrition Dietetic Practice Group, www.oncologynutrition.org
   a) The Oncology Nutrition Dietetic Practice Group is a dietetic practice group of the American Dietetic Association. Its mission is to provide direction and leadership for quality oncology nutrition practice through education and research. It is a national organization with over 1200 members.
   b) The practice of oncology nutrition covers research, prevention, treatment, recovery, palliative care, and hospice. Oncology nutritionists provide dietetic professionals with resources and networking opportunities to deal with the complexities of oncology practice. Members work in clinical, public health, education, and research settings.

(Cancer chapters from the 1st edition were contributed by Virginia Hermann, Patricia Fuhrman, Peggy Borum, Karyl Rickard, Barbara Godshall, Angelita Lopez, and Robert Weetman)

REFERENCES

1. Weir HK, Thun MJ, Hankey BF, et al. Annual report to the nation on the status of cancer, 1975–2000, featuring the uses of surveillance data for cancer prevention and control. *J Natl Cancer Inst.* 2003;95(17):1276–1299.
2. Bozzetti F. Rationale and indications for preoperative feeding of malnourished surgical cancer patients. *Nutrition.* 2002;18(11–12):953–959.
3. Duguet A, Bachmann P, Lallemand Y, Blanc-Vincent MP. Summary report of the Standards, Options and Recommendations for malnutrition and nutritional assessment in patients with cancer (1999). *Br J Cancer.* 2003; 89(suppl 1):S92–97.

4. Dewys WD, Begg C, Lavin PT, et al. Prognostic effect of weight loss prior to chemotherapy in cancer patients. Eastern Cooperative Oncology Group. *Am J Med.* 1980;69(4):491–497.
5. Gail MH, Eagan RT, Feld R, et al. Prognostic factors in patients with resected stage I non-small cell lung cancer. A report from the Lung Cancer Study Group. *Cancer.* 1984;54(9):1802–1813.
6. Surveillance, epidemiology, and end results cancer statistics review. Available at: http://seer.cancer.gov/csr/1975_2000/. Accessed August 21, 2004
7. Han-Markey T. Nutritional considerations in pediatric oncology. *Semin Oncol Nurs.* 2000;16(2):146–151.
8. Mauer AM, Burgess JB, Donaldson SS, et al. Special nutritional needs of children with malignancies: a review. *J Parenter Enteral Nutr.* 1990;14(3): 315–324.
9. Lahorra JM, Ginn-Pease ME, King DR. The prognostic significance of basic anthropometric data in children with advanced solid tumors. *Nutr Cancer.* 1989;12(4):361–369.
10. Rickard KA, Grosfeld JL, Kirksey A, Ballantine TV, Baehner RL. Reversal of protein-energy malnutrition in children during treatment of advanced neoplastic disease. *Ann Surg.* 1979;190(6):771–781.
11. Carter P, Carr D, van Eys J, Coody D. Nutritional parameters in children with cancer. *J Am Diet Assoc.* 1983;82(6):616–622.
12. Smith DE, Stevens MC, Booth IW. Malnutrition at diagnosis of malignancy in childhood: common but mostly missed. *Eur J Pediatr.* 1991;150(5): 318–322.
13. Attard-Montalto SP, Hadley J, Kingston JE, Eden OB, Saha V. Ongoing assessment of nutritional status in children with malignant disease. *Pediatr Hematol Oncol.* 1998;15(5):393–403.
14. Halton JM, Atkinson SA, Barr RD. Growth and body composition in response to chemotherapy in children with acute lymphoblastic leukemia. *Int J Cancer Suppl.* 1998;11:81–84.
15. Birkebaek NH, Clausen N. Height and weight pattern up to 20 years after treatment for acute lymphoblastic leukaemia. *Arch Dis Child.* 1998;79(2): 161–164.
16. Didi M, Didcock E, Davies HA, Ogilvy-Stuart AL, Wales JK, Shalet SM. High incidence of obesity in young adults after treatment of acute lymphoblastic leukemia in childhood. *J Pediatr.* 1995;127(1):63–67.
17. Warner JT, Bell W, Webb DK, Gregory JW. Daily energy expenditure and physical activity in survivors of childhood malignancy. *Pediatr Res.* 1998;43(5):607–613.
18. Reilly JJ, Ventham JC, Ralston JM, Donaldson M, Gibson B. Reduced energy expenditure in preobese children treated for acute lymphoblastic leukemia. *Pediatr Res.* 1998;44(4):557–562.
19. Vaisman N, Stallings VA, Chan H, Weitzman SS, Clarke R, Pencharz PB. Effect of chemotherapy on the energy and protein metabolism of children near the end of treatment for acute lymphoblastic leukemia. *Am J Clin Nutr.* 1993;57(5):679–684.
20. Stallings VA, Vaisman N, Chan HS, Weitzman SS, Hahn E, Pencharz PB. Energy metabolism in children with newly diagnosed acute lymphoblastic leukemia. *Pediatr Res.* 1989;26(2):154–157.
21. Bond SA, Han AM, Wootton SA, Kohler JA. Energy intake and basal metabolic rate during maintenance chemotherapy. *Arch Dis Child.* 1992; 67(2):229–232.
22. Delbecque-Boussard L, Gottrand F, Ategbo S, et al. Nutritional status of children with acute lymphoblastic leukemia: a longitudinal study. *Am J Clin Nutr.* 1997;65(1):95–100.
23. Tyc VL, Vallelunga L, Mahoney S, Smith BF, Mulhern RK. Nutritional and treatment-related characteristics of pediatric oncology patients referred or not referred for nutritional support. *Med Pediatr Oncol.* 1995;25(5):379–388.
24. Emery PW. Cachexia in experimental models. *Nutrition.* 1999;15(7–8): 600–603.
25. Bruera E, Sweeney C. Cachexia and asthenia in cancer patients. *Lancet Oncol.* 2000;1:138–147.
26. Bloch A. Cancer. In: Matarese L, Gottschlich M, eds. *Contemporary Nutrition Support Practice.* 1st ed. Philadelphia: W. B. Saunders Company; 1998:475–495.
27. Argiles JM, Moore-Carrasco R, Fuster G, Busquets S, Lopez-Soriano FJ. Cancer cachexia: the molecular mechanisms. *Int J Biochem Cell Biol.* 2003;35(4):405–409.
28. Tisdale MJ. Cachexia in cancer patients. *Nat Rev Cancer.* 2002;2(11): 862–871.
29. Laviano A, Meguid MM, Rossi-Fanelli F. Cancer anorexia: clinical implications, pathogenesis, and therapeutic strategies. *Lancet Oncol.* 2003; 4(11):686–694.
30. Finley JP. Management of cancer cachexia. *AACN Clin Issues.* 2000;11(4): 590–603.
31. Khanna C, the Perseus Foundation. Biotherapy of cancer. Available at: http://www.perseusfoundation.org/page33.html. Accessed August 24, 2004.
32. American Cancer Society. Infections in individuals with cancer. Available at: www.cancer.org/docroot/ETO/content/ETO_1_2X_Infections_in_Individuals_with_Cancer.asp. 2004. Accessed August 24, 2004.
33. Echenique M, Correia MI. Nutrition in advanced digestive cancer. *Curr Opin Clin Nutr Metab Care.* 2003;6(5):577–580.
34. Ripamonti C, Bruera E. Palliative management of malignant bowel obstruction. *Int J Gynecol Cancer.* 2002;12(2):135–143.
35. Lopez MJ, Robinson P, Madden T, Highbarger T. Nutritional support and prognosis in patients with head and neck cancer. *J Surg Oncol.* 1994; 55(1):33–36.
36. Derogatis LR, Morrow GR, Fetting J, et al. The prevalence of psychiatric disorders among cancer patients. *JAMA.* 1983;249(6):751–757.
37. Ellison NM, Chevlen E, Still CD, Dubagunta S. Supportive care for patients with pancreatic adenocarcinoma: symptom control and nutrition. *Hematol Oncol Clin North Am.* 2002;16(1):105–121.
38. Bosaeus I, Daneryd P, Lundholm K. Dietary intake, resting energy expenditure, weight loss and survival in cancer patients. *J Nutr.* 2002;132(11 suppl):3465S–3466S.
39. Guirao X. Impact of the inflammatory reaction on intermediary metabolism and nutrition status. *Nutrition.* 2002;18(11–12):949–952.
40. Bosaeus I, Daneryd P, Svanberg E, Lundholm K. Dietary intake and resting energy expenditure in relation to weight loss in unselected cancer patients. *Int J Cancer.* 2001;93(3):380–383.
41. Herrmann V, Fuhrman MP, Borum P. Wasting diseases. In: Merritt R, ed. *The A.S.P.E.N. Nutrition Support Practice Manual.* Silver Spring, MD: American Society for Parenteral and Enteral Nutrition; 1998:11/11–11/15.
42. Hunter AM. Nutrition management of patients with neoplastic disease of the head and neck treated with radiation therapy. *Nutr Clin Pract.* 1996;11(4):157–169.
43. Chandra RK. Nutrition and the immune system from birth to old age. *Eur J Clin Nutr.* 2002;56(suppl 3):S73–76.
44. Marcos A, Nova E, Montero A. Changes in the immune system are conditioned by nutrition. *Eur J Clin Nutr.* 2003;57(suppl 1):S66–69.
45. Miller JS. Biology of natural killer cells in cancer and infection. *Cancer Invest.* 2002;20(3):405–419.
46. Dunlop RJ, Campbell CW. Cytokines and advanced cancer. *J Pain Symptom Manage.* 2000;20(3):214–232.
47. Argiles JM, Moore-Carrasco R, Busquets S, Lopez-Soriano FJ. Catabolic mediators as targets for cancer cachexia. *Drug Discov Today.* 2003;8(18): 838–844.
48. Todorov P, Cariuk P, McDevitt T, Coles B, Fearon K, Tisdale M. Characterization of a cancer cachectic factor. *Nature.* 1996;379:739–742.
49. Yoneda T, Alsina M, Chavez J, Bonewals L, Nishimura R, Mundy G. Evidence that tumor necrosis factor plays a pathogenetic role in the paraneoplastic syndrome of cachexia, hypercalcaemia, and leucocytosis in a human tumor in nude mice. *J Clin Invest.* 1991;87:977–985.
50. Barber MD, Ross JA, Fearon KC. Cancer cachexia. *Surg Oncol.* 1999; 8(3):133–141.
51. Plata-Salaman C. Central nervous system mechanisms contributing to the cachexia-anorexia syndrome. *Nutrition.* 2000;16(10):1009–1012.
52. Argiles JM, Lopez-Soriano FJ. New mediators in cancer cachexia. *Nestle Nutr Workshop Ser Clin Perform Programme.* 2000;4:147–162; discussion 163–165.
53. Argiles JM, Busquets S, Lopez-Soriano FJ. Cytokines in the pathogenesis of cancer cachexia. *Curr Opin Clin Nutr Metab Care.* 2003;6(4):401–406.
54. Yasumoto K, Mukaida N, Harada A, et al. Molecular analysis of the cytokine network involved in cachexia in colon 26 adenocarcinoma-bearing mice. *Cancer Res.* 1995;55(4):921–927.

55. Wang M, Forsberg N. Effects of ciliary neurotrophic factor (CNTF) on protein turnover in cultured muscle cells. *Cytokine.* 2000;12(1):41–48.
56. Matthys P, Heremans H, Opdenakker G, Billiau A. Anti-interferon-gamma antibody treatment, growth of Lewis ling tumours in mice and tumour-associated cachexia. *Eur J Cancer.* 1991;27(2):182–187.
57. Islam-Ali B, Khan S, Price SA, Tisdale MJ. Modulation of adipocyte G-protein expression in cancer cachexia by a lipid-mobilizing factor (LMF). *Br J Cancer.* 2001;85(5):758–763.
58. Strasser F, Bruera ED. Update on anorexia and cachexia. *Hematol Oncol Clin North Am.* 2002;16(3):589–617.
59. Watchorn TM, Waddell I, Dowidar N, Ross JA. Proteolysis-inducing factor regulates hepatic gene expression via the transcription factors NF-(kappa)B and STAT3. *FASEB J.* 2001;15(3):562–564.
60. Lorite MJ, Smith HJ, Arnold JA, Morris A, Thompson MG, Tisdale MJ. Activation of ATP-ubiquitin-dependent proteolysis in skeletal muscle in vivo and murine myoblasts in vitro by a proteolysis-inducing factor (PIF). *Br J Cancer.* 2001;85(2):297–302.
61. Mantovani G, Maccio A, Massa E, Madeddu C. Managing cancer-related anorexia/cachexia. *Drugs.* 2001;61(4):499–514.
62. Inui A. Cancer anorexia-cachexia syndrome: are neuropeptides the key? *Cancer Res.* 1999;59(18):4493–4501.
63. Sarraf P, Frederich RC, Turner EM, et al. Multiple cytokines and acute inflammation raise mouse leptin levels: potential role in inflammatory anorexia. *J Exp Med.* 1997;185(1):171–175.
64. Finck BN, Kelley KW, Dantzer R, Johnson RW. In vivo and in vitro evidence for the involvement of tumor necrosis factor-alpha in the induction of leptin by lipopolysaccharide. *Endocrinology.* 1998;139(5):2278–2283.
65. Chance WT, Sheriff S, Moore J, Peng F, Balasubramaniam A. Reciprocal changes in hypothalamic receptor binding and circulating leptin in anorectic tumor-bearing rats. *Brain Res.* 1998;803(1–2):27–33.
66. Jensen PB, Blume N, Mikkelsen JD, et al. Transplantable rat glucagonomas cause acute onset of severe anorexia and adipsia despite highly elevated NPY mRNA levels in the hypothalamic arcuate nucleus. *J Clin Invest.* 1998;101(2):503–510.
67. Wallace AM, Sattar N, McMillan DC. Effect of weight loss and the inflammatory response on leptin concentrations in gastrointestinal cancer patients. *Clin Cancer Res.* 1998;4(12):2977–2979.
68. Mantovani G, Maccio A, Mura L, et al. Serum levels of leptin and proinflammatory cytokines in patients with advanced-stage cancer at different sites. *J Mol Med.* 2000;78(10):554–561.
69. Klaus S. Adipose tissue as a regulator of energy balance. *Curr Drug Targets.* 2004;5(3):241–250.
70. Cravo ML, Gloria LM, Claro I. Metabolic responses to tumour disease and progression: tumour-host interaction. *Clin Nutr.* 2000;19(6):459–465.
71. Ovesen L, Allingstrup L, Hannibal J, Mortensen EL, Hansen OP. Effect of dietary counseling on food intake, body weight, response rate, survival, and quality of life in cancer patients undergoing chemotherapy: a prospective, randomized study. *J Clin Oncol.* 1993;11(10):2043–2049.
72. Heslin MJ, Brennan MF. Advances in perioperative nutrition: cancer. *World J Surg.* 2000;24(12):1477–1485.
73. Eden D, Edstrom S, Bennegard K, Schersten T, Lundholm K. Glucose flux in relation to energy expenditure in malnourished patients with and without cancer during periods of fasting and feeding. *Cancer Res.* 1984;44(4):1718–1724.
74. Burt ME, Aoki TT, Gorschboth CM, Brennan MF. Peripheral tissue metabolism in cancer-bearing man. *Ann Surg.* 1983;198(6):685–691.
75. Argiles JM, Busquets S, Lopez-Soriano FJ. Metabolic interrelationships between liver and skeletal muscle in pathological states. *Life Sci.* 2001;69(12):1345–1361.
76. Wigmore SJ, McMahon AJ, Sturgeon CM, Fearon KC. Acute-phase protein response, survival and tumour recurrence in patients with colorectal cancer. *Br J Surg.* 2001;88(2):255–260.
77. Fiorenza AM, Branchi A, Sommariva D. Serum lipoprotein profile in patients with cancer. A comparison with non-cancer subjects. *Int J Clin Lab Res.* 2000;30(3):141–145.
78. Halton JM, Nazir DJ, McQueen MJ, Barr RD. Blood lipid profiles in children with acute lymphoblastic leukemia. *Cancer.* 1998;83(2):379–384.
79. Shukla VK, Adukia TK, Singh SP, Mishra CP, Mishra RN. Micronutrients, antioxidants, and carcinoma of the gallbladder. *J Surg Oncol.* 2003;84(1):31–35.
80. Hronek M, Zadak Z, Solichova D, Jandik P, Melichar B. The association between specific nutritional antioxidants and manifestation of colorectal cancer. *Nutrition.* 2000;16(3):189–191.
81. Brown LM, Blot WJ, Schuman SH, et al. Environmental factors and high risk of esophageal cancer among men in coastal South Carolina. *J Natl Cancer Inst.* 1988;80(20):1620–1625.
82. Malvy DJ, Arnaud J, Burtschy B, et al. Antioxidant micronutrients and childhood malignancy during oncological treatment. *Med Pediatr Oncol.* 1997;29(3):213–217.
83. Yong LC, Brown CC, Schatzkin A, et al. Intake of vitamins E, C, and A and risk of lung cancer. The NHANES I epidemiologic followup study. First National Health and Nutrition Examination Survey. *Am J Epidemiol.* 1997;146(3):231–243.
84. Choi MA, Kim BS, Yu R. Serum antioxidative vitamin levels and lipid peroxidation in gastric carcinoma patients. *Cancer Lett.* 1999;136(1):89–93.
85. Woutersen RA, Appel MJ, Van Garderen-Hoetmer A. Modulation of pancreatic carcinogenesis by antioxidants. *Food Chem Toxicol.* 1999;37(9–10):981–984.
86. Gupta PC, Hebert JR, Bhonsle RB, Murti PR, Mehta H, Mehta FS. Influence of dietary factors on oral precancerous lesions in a population-based case-control study in Kerala, India. *Cancer.* 1999;85(9):1885–1893.
87. D'Avanzo B, Ron E, La Vecchia C, Francaschi S, Negri E, Zleglar R. Selected micronutrient intake and thyroid carcinoma risk. *Cancer.* 1997;79(11):2186–2192.
88. Kristal AR, Stanford JL, Cohen JH, Wicklund K, Patterson RE. Vitamin and mineral supplement use is associated with reduced risk of prostate cancer. *Cancer Epidemiol Biomarkers Prev.* 1999;8(10):887–892.
89. La Vecchia C, Braga C, Negri E, et al. Intake of selected micronutrients and risk of colorectal cancer. *Int J Cancer.* 1997;73(4):525–530.
90. Cunzhi H, Jiexian J, Xianwen Z, Jingang G, Shumin Z, Lili D. Serum and tissue levels of six trace elements and copper/zinc ratio in patients with cervical cancer and uterine myoma. *Biol Trace Elem Res.* 2003;94(2):113–122.
91. Huang YL, Sheu JY, Lin TH. Association between oxidative stress and changes of trace elements in patients with breast cancer. *Clin Biochem.* 1999;32(2):131–136.
92. Borella P, Bargellini A, Caselgrandi E, Piccinini L. Observations on the use of plasma, hair and tissue to evaluate trace element status in cancer. *J Trace Elem Med Biol.* 1997;11(3):162–165.
93. Yu MW, Horng IS, Hsu KH, Chiang YC, Liaw YF, Chen CJ. Plasma selenium levels and risk of hepatocellular carcinoma among men with chronic hepatitis virus infection. *Am J Epidemiol.* 1999;150(4):367–374.
94. Postovsky S, Arush MW, Diamond E, Elhasid R, Shoshani G, Shamir R. The prevalence of low selenium levels in newly diagnosed pediatric cancer patients. *Pediatr Hematol Oncol.* 2003;20(4):273–280.
95. Poo JL, Romero RR, Robles JA, et al. Diagnostic value of the copper/zinc ratio in digestive cancer: a case control study. *Arch Med Res.* 1997;28(2):259–263.
96. Ferrigno D, Buccheri G, Camilla T. Serum copper and zinc content in non-small cell lung cancer: abnormalities and clinical correlates. *Monaldi Arch Chest Dis.* 1999;54(3):204–208.
97. Cabanillas F. Metabolic abnormalities in lymphoma. *Clin Lymphoma.* 2002;3(suppl 1):S32–36.
98. Ottery F. Nutritional oncology: a proactive, integrated approach to the cancer patient. In: Shikora S, Blackburn G, eds. *Nutrition Support: Theory and Therapeutics.* New York, NY: Chapman and Hall; 1997:394–409.
99. Ferguson M. Patient-generated subjective global assessment. *Oncology (Huntingt).* 2003;17(2 suppl 2):13–14; discussion 14–16.
100. Bauer J, Capra S, Ferguson M. Use of the scored Patient-Generated Subjective Global Assessment (PG-SGA) as a nutrition assessment tool in patients with cancer. *Eur J Clin Nutr.* 2002;56(8):779–785.
101. Shils ME. Principles of nutritional therapy. *Cancer.* 1979;43(5 suppl):2093–2102.
102. Whitman MM. The starving patient: supportive care for people with cancer. *Clin J Oncol Nurs.* 2000;4(3):121–125.

103. Karnofsky DA, Abelman WH, Craver LF, et al. The use of nitrogen mustards in the palliative treatment of carcinoma. *Cancer.* 1948;1:634–656.
104. Bloch A, Charuhas P. Cancer and cancer therapy. In: Gottschlich MM ed. *The Science and Practice of Nutrition Support: A Core-Based Curriculum 2001.* Dubuque, IA: American Society for Parenteral and Enteral Nutrition (A.S.P.E.N.), Kendall/Hunt Publishing; 2001:643–662.
105. Jeejeebhoy KN. Nutritional assessment. *Gastroenterol Clin North Am.* 1998;27(2):347–369.
106. Turk DC, Monarch ES, Williams AD. Cancer patients in pain: considerations for assessing the whole person. *Hematol Oncol Clin North Am.* 2002;16(3):511–525.
107. Robinson MK, Trujillo EB, Mogensen KM, Rounds J, McManus K, Jacobs DO. Improving nutritional screening of hospitalized patients: the role of prealbumin. *J Parenter Enteral Nutr.* 2003;27(6):389–395; quiz 439.
108. Capra S, Ferguson M, Ried K. Cancer: impact of nutrition intervention outcome—nutrition issues for patients. *Nutrition.* 2001;17(9):769–772.
109. Berger A, Baker K, Bolle J, Pereira D. Establishing a palliative care program in a research center: evolution of a model. *Cancer Invest.* 2003;21(2): 313–320.
110. Ravasco P, Monteiro Grillo I, Marques Vidal P, Camilo M. Nutritional counselling vs supplements: A prospective randomised controlled trial in head-neck cancer patients undergoing radiotherapy. *Clin Nutr.* 2003; 22(S1):S63–64.
111. Schimmer BP, Parker KL. Adrenocorticotropic hormone; adrenocortical steroids and their synthetic analogs; inhibitors of the synthesis and actions of adrenocortical hormones. In: Hardman JG, Limbird LE, Molinoff PB, Ruddon TW, Goodman Gilman A, eds. *Goodman and Gilman's The Pharmacological Basis of Therapeutics.* 9th ed. New York, NY: McGraw-Hill; 1996
112. Amin S, LaValley MP, Simms RW, Felson DT. The role of vitamin D in corticosteroid-induced osteoporosis: a meta-analytic approach. *Arthritis Rheum.* 1999;42(8):1740–1751.
113. *Physical Status: The Use and Interpretation of Anthropometry.* WHO Technical Support Series 854. Geneva, Switzerland: World Health Organization; 1995.
114. Corrales KM, Utter SL. Failure to thrive. In: Samour PQ, Helm KK, Lang CE, eds. *Handbook of Pediatric Nutrition.* 2nd ed. Boston, MA: Jones and Bartlett Publishers; 2004:395–412.
115. Waterlow JC. Classification and definition of protein-calorie malnutrition. *Br Med J.* 1972;3(826):566–569.
116. Barlow SE, Dietz WH. Obesity evaluation and treatment: Expert Committee recommendations. The Maternal and Child Health Bureau, Health Resources and Services Administration and the Department of Health and Human Services. *Pediatrics.* 1998;102(3):E29.
117. Himes JH, Dietz WH. Guidelines for overweight in adolescent preventive services: recommendations from an expert committee. The Expert Committee on Clinical Guidelines for Overweight in Adolescent Preventive Services. *Am J Clin Nutr.* 1994;59(2):307–316.
118. Frisancho AR. *Anthropometric Standards for the Assessment of Growth and Nutritional Status.* Ann Arbor, MI: University of Michigan Press; 1990.
119. Motil KJ. Sensitive measures of nutritional status in children in hospital and in the field. *Int J Cancer Suppl.* 1998;11:2–9.
120. Lohman TG, Roche AF, Martorell R. *Anthropometric Standardization Reference Manual.* Champaign, IL: Human Kinetics Books; 1988.
121. Fjeld CR, Freundt-Thurne J, Schoeller DA. Total body water measured by 18-O dilution and bioelectrical impedance in well and malnourished children. *Pediatr Res.* 1990;27(1):98–102.
122. Elhasid R, Laor A, Lischinsky S, Postovsky S, Weyl Ben Arush M. Nutritional status of children with solid tumors. *Cancer.* 1999;86(1):119–125.
123. Measurement of visceral protein status in assessing protein and energy malnutrition: standard of care. Prealbumin in Nutritional Care Consensus Group. *Nutrition.* 1995;11(2):169–171.
124. Spiekerman AM. Nutritional assessment (protein nutriture). *Anal Chem.* 1995;67(12):429R–436R.
125. Beck FK, Rosenthal TC. Prealbumin: a marker for nutritional evaluation. *Am Fam Physician.* 2002;65(8):1575–1578.
126. Nathan PC, Furlong W, Barr RD. Challenges to the measurement of health-related quality of life in children receiving cancer therapy. *Pediatr Blood Cancer.* 2004;43(3):215–223.
127. Rosenbaum P, Cadman D, Kirpalani H. Pediatrics: assessing quality of life. In: Spilker B, ed. *Quality of Life Assessments in Clinical Trials.* New York, NY: Raven Press; 1990:205–215.
128. Eiser C, Morse R. Can parents rate their child's health-related quality of life? Results of a systematic review. *Qual Life Res.* 2001;10(4):347–357.
129. Vance YH, Morse RC, Jenney ME, Eiser C. Issues in measuring quality of life in childhood cancer: measures, proxies, and parental mental health. *J Child Psychol Psychiatry.* 2001;42(5):661–667.
130. Armstrong FD, Toledano SR, Miloslavich K, et al. The Miami Pediatric Quality of Life Questionnaire: Parent Scale. *Int J Cancer Suppl.* 1999; 12:11–17.
131. Boggs SR, Durning P. The Pediatric Oncology Quality of Life Scale: development and validation of a disease-specific quality of life measure. In: Drotar D, ed. *Measuring Health-Related Quality of Life in Children and Adolescents: Implications for Research and Practice.* Mahwah, NJ: Lawrence Erlbaum Associates; 1998:187–202.
132. Phipps S, Hinds PS, Channell S, Bell GL. Measurement of behavioral, affective, and somatic responses to pediatric bone marrow transplantation: development of the BASES scale. *J Pediatr Oncol Nurs.* 1994;11(3): 109–117; discussion 118–119.
133. Varni JW, Burwinkle TM, Katz ER, Meeske K, Dickinson P. The PedsQL in pediatric cancer: reliability and validity of the Pediatric Quality of Life Inventory Generic Core Scales, Multidimensional Fatigue Scale, and Cancer Module. *Cancer.* 2002;94(7):2090–2106.
134. Bhatia S, Jenney ME, Bogue MK, et al. The Minneapolis-Manchester Quality of Life Instrument: reliability and validity of the Adolescent Form. *J Clin Oncol.* 2002;20(24):4692–4698.
135. Bhatia S, Jenney ME, Wu E, et al. The Minneapolis-Manchester Quality of Life Instrument: reliability and validity of the Youth Form. *J Pediatr.* 2004;145(1):39–46.
136. Eiser C, Havermans T, Craft A, Kernahan J. Development of a measure to assess the perceived illness experience after treatment for cancer. *Arch Dis Child.* 1995;72(4):302–307.
137. Feeny D, Furlong W, Barr RD, Torrance GW, Rosenbaum P, Weitzman S. A comprehensive multiattribute system for classifying the health status of survivors of childhood cancer. *J Clin Oncol.* 1992;10(6):923–928.
138. Barr RD, Furlong W, Dawson S, et al. An assessment of global health status in survivors of acute lymphoblastic leukemia in childhood. *Am J Pediatr Hematol Oncol.* 1993;15(3):284–290.
139. Barr RD, Simpson T, Whitton A, Rush B, Furlong W, Feeny DH. Health-related quality of life in survivors of tumours of the central nervous system in childhood—a preference-based approach to measurement in a cross-sectional study. *Eur J Cancer.* 1999;35(2):248–255.
140. Barr RD, Chalmers D, De Pauw S, Furlong W, Weitzman S, Feeny D. Health-related quality of life in survivors of Wilms' tumor and advanced neuroblastoma: a cross-sectional study. *J Clin Oncol.* 2000;18(18): 3280–3287.
141. Moshang T Jr, Grimberg A. The effects of irradiation and chemotherapy on growth. *Endocrinol Metab Clin North Am.* 1996;25(3):731–741.
142. DeLaat CA, Lampkin BC. Long-term survivors of childhood cancer: evaluation and identification of sequelae of treatment. *CA Cancer J Clin.* 1992;42(5):263–282.
143. Gleeson HK, Shalet SM. Endocrine complications of neoplastic diseases in children and adolescents. *Curr Opin Pediatr.* 2001;13(4):346–351.
144. Norred C. Hot topics in healthcare. Thomson American Health Consultants. Available at: http://www.ahcpub.com/ahc root html/hot/archive/atwh042001.html. Accessed August 24, 2004.
145. A.S.P.E.N. Board of Directors and The Clinical Guidelines Task Force. Guidelines for the use of parenteral and enteral nutrition in adult and pediatric patients. *J Parenter Enteral Nutr.* 2002;26(1 suppl):83SA.
146. A.S.P.E.N. Board of Directors and The Clinical Guidelines Task Force. Guidelines for the use of parenteral and enteral nutrition in adult and pediatric patients. *J Parenteral Enteral Nutr.* 2002;26(1 suppl):82SA.

147. Barrera R. Nutritional support in cancer patients. *J Parenter Enteral Nutr.* 2002;26(5 suppl):S63–71.
148. Laviano A, Meguid MM. Nutritional issues in cancer management. *Nutrition.* 1996;12(5):358–371.
149. Archer SB, Burnett RJ, Fischer JE. Current uses and abuses of total parenteral nutrition. *Adv Surg.* 1996;29:165–189.
150. Flynn MB, Leightty FF. Preoperative outpatient nutritional support of patients with squamous cancer of the upper aerodigestive tract. *Am J Surg.* 1987;154(4):359–362.
151. Wong PW, Enriquez A, Barrera R. Nutritional support in critically ill patients with cancer. *Crit Care Clin.* 2001;17(3):743–767.
152. Fietkau R, Iro H, Sailer D, Sauer R. Percutaneous endoscopically guided gastrostomy in patients with head and neck cancer. *Recent Results Cancer Res.* 1991;121:269–282.
153. Nayel H, el-Ghoneimy E, el-Haddad S. Impact of nutritional supplementation on treatment delay and morbidity in patients with head and neck tumors treated with irradiation. *Nutrition.* 1992;8(1):13–18.
154. Klein S, Koretz RL. Nutrition support in patients with cancer: what do the data really show? *Nutr Clin Pract.* 1994;9(3):91–100.
155. Klein S, Kinney J, Jeejeebhoy K, et al. Nutrition support in clinical practice: review of published data and recommendations for future research directions. Summary of a conference sponsored by the National Institutes of Health, American Society for Parenteral and Enteral Nutrition, and American Society for Clinical Nutrition. *Am J Clin Nutr.* 1997;66(3):683–706.
156. Reilly JJ, Odame I, McColl JH, McAllister PJ, Gibson BE, Wharton BA. Does weight for height have prognostic significance in children with acute lymphoblastic leukemia? *Am J Pediatr Hematol Oncol.* 1994;16(3):225–230.
157. Lobato-Mendizabal E, Ruiz-Arguelles GJ, Marin-Lopez A. Leukaemia and nutrition, I: malnutrition is an adverse prognostic factor in the outcome of treatment of patients with standard-risk acute lymphoblastic leukaemia. *Leuk Res.* 1989;13(10):899–906.
158. Donaldson SS, Wesley MN, DeWys WD, Suskind RM, Jaffe N, vanEys J. A study of the nutritional status of pediatric cancer patients. *Am J Dis Child.* 1981;135(12):1107–1112.
159. Rickard KA, Detamore CM, Coates TD, et al. Effect of nutrition staging on treatment delays and outcome in Stage IV neuroblastoma. *Cancer.* 1983;52(4):587–598.
160. Pedrosa F, Bonilla M, Liu A, et al. Effect of malnutrition at the time of diagnosis on the survival of children treated for cancer in El Salvador and Northern Brazil. *J Pediatr Hematol Oncol.* 2000;22(6):502–505.
161. Weir J, Reilly JJ, McColl JH, Gibson BE. No evidence for an effect of nutritional status at diagnosis on prognosis in children with acute lymphoblastic leukemia. *J Pediatr Hematol Oncol.* 1998;20(6):534–538.
162. Ringwald-Smith K, Todd J, Liu A, Hancock M, Pui C-H. Nutritional status: potential impact on survival in children with acute lymphoblastic leukemia [abstract]. *J Am Diet Assoc.* 1998;98(suppl):A-107.
163. Carter P, Carr D, van Eys J, Ramirez I, Coody D, Taylor G. Energy and nutrient intake of children with cancer. *J Am Diet Assoc.* 1983;82(6):610–615.
164. Skolin I, Axelsson K, Ghannad P, Hernell O, Wahlin YB. Nutrient intake and weight development in children during chemotherapy for malignant disease. *Oral Oncol.* 1997;33(5):364–368.
165. Andrassy RJ, Chwals WJ. Nutritional support of the pediatric oncology patient. *Nutrition.* 1998;14(1):124–129.
166. Ollenschlager G, Thomas W, Konkol K, Diehl V, Roth E. Nutritional behaviour and quality of life during oncological polychemotherapy: results of a prospective study on the efficacy of oral nutrition therapy in patients with acute leukaemia. *Eur J Clin Invest.* 1992;22(8):546–553.
167. Kuczmarski RJ, Ogden CL, Grummer-Strawn LM, et al. CDC growth charts: United States. *Adv Data.* 2000(314):1–27.
168. Bakish J, Hargrave D, Tariq N, Laperriere N, Rutka JT, Bouffet E. Evaluation of dietetic intervention in children with medulloblastoma or supratentorial primitive neuroectodermal tumors. *Cancer.* 2003;98(5):1014–1020.
169. Hays DM, Merritt RJ, White L, Ashley J, Siegel SE. Effect of total parenteral nutrition on marrow recovery during induction therapy for acute nonlymphocytic leukemia in childhood. *Med Pediatr Oncol.* 1983;11(2):134–140.
170. Barron MA, Duncan DS, Green GJ, et al. Efficacy and safety of radiologically placed gastrostomy tubes in paediatric haematology/oncology patients. *Med Pediatr Oncol.* 2000;34(3):177–182.
171. den Broeder E, Lippens RJ, van't Hof MA, et al. Effects of naso-gastric tube feeding on the nutritional status of children with cancer. *Eur J Clin Nutr.* 1998;52(7):494–500.
172. Aquino VM, Smyrl CB, Hagg R, McHard KM, Prestridge L, Sandler ES. Enteral nutritional support by gastrostomy tube in children with cancer. *J Pediatr.* 1995;127(1):58–62.
173. Donaldson SS, Wesley MN, Ghavimi F, Shils ME, Suskind RM, DeWys WD. A prospective randomized clinical trial of total parenteral nutrition in children with cancer. *Med Pediatr Oncol.* 1982;10(2):129–139.
174. Shamberger RC, Brennan MF, Goodgame JT Jr, et al. A prospective, randomized study of adjuvant parenteral nutrition in the treatment of sarcomas: results of metabolic and survival studies. *Surgery.* 1984;96(1):1–13.
175. Shamberger RC, Pizzo PA, Goodgame JT Jr, et al. The effect of total parenteral nutrition on chemotherapy-induced myelosuppression. A randomized study. *Am J Med.* 1983;74(1):40–48.
176. Rickard KA, Foland BB, Detamore CM, et al. Effectiveness of central parenteral nutrition versus peripheral parenteral nutrition plus enteral nutrition in reversing protein-energy malnutrition in children with advanced neuroblastoma and Wilms' tumor: a prospective randomized study. *Am J Clin Nutr.* 1983;38(3):445–456.
177. Rickard KA, Godshall BJ, Loghmani ES, et al. Integration of nutrition support into oncologic treatment protocols for high and low nutritional risk children with Wilms' tumor. A prospective randomized study. *Cancer.* 1989;64(2):491–509.
178. Rickard KA, Becker MC, Loghmani E, et al. Effectiveness of two methods of parenteral nutrition support in improving muscle mass of children with neuroblastoma or Wilms' tumor. A randomized study. *Cancer.* 1989;64(1):116–125.
179. Rickard KA, Loghmani ES, Grosfeld JL, et al. Short- and long-term effectiveness of enteral and parenteral nutrition in reversing or preventing protein-energy malnutrition in advanced neuroblastoma. A prospective randomized study. *Cancer.* 1985;56(12):2881–2897.
180. Leung FY. Trace elements in parenteral micronutrition. *Clin Biochem.* 1995;28(6):561–566.
181. Helphingstine CJ, Bistrian BR. New Food and Drug Administration requirements for inclusion of vitamin K in adult parenteral multivitamins. *J Parenter Enteral Nutr.* 2003;27(3):220–224.
182. Bryant R. Managing side effects of childhood cancer treatment. *J Pediatr Nurs.* 2003;18(2):113–125.
183. Weiger WA, Smith M, Boon H, Richardson MA, Kaptchuk TJ, Eisenberg DM. Advising patients who seek complementary and alternative medical therapies for cancer. *Ann Intern Med.* 2002;137(11):889–903.
184. Rivadeneira DE, Evoy D, Fahey TJ 3rd, Lieberman MD, Daly JM. Nutritional support of the cancer patient. *CA Cancer J Clin.* 1998;48(2):69–80.
185. McCarthy D, Weihofen D. The effect of nutritional supplements on food intake in patients undergoing radiotherapy. *Oncol Nurs Forum.* 1999;26(5):897–900.
186. Barber MD, Ross JA, Voss AC, Tisdale MJ, Fearon KC. The effect of an oral nutritional supplement enriched with fish oil on weight-loss in patients with pancreatic cancer. *Br J Cancer.* 1999;81(1):80–86.
187. Fearon KC, Von Meyenfeldt MF, Moses AG, et al. Effect of a protein and energy dense N-3 fatty acid enriched oral supplement on loss of weight and lean tissue in cancer cachexia: a randomised double blind trial. *Gut.* 2003;52(10):1479–1486.
188. Patterson RE, Neuhouser ML, Hedderson MM, Schwartz SM, Standish LJ, Bowen DJ. Changes in diet, physical activity, and supplement use among adults diagnosed with cancer. *J Am Diet Assoc.* 2003;103(3):323–328.
189. Eisenberg DM, Davis RB, Ettner SL, et al. Trends in alternative medicine use in the United States, 1990–1997: results of a follow-up national survey. *JAMA.* 1998;280(18):1569–1575.

190. Ritvo P, Irvine J, Katz J, Matthew A, Sacamano J, Shaw BF. The patient's motivation in seeking complementary therapies. *Patient Educ Couns.* 1999;38(2):161–165.
191. Schenck DP. Ethical considerations in the treatment of head and neck cancer. *Cancer Control.* 2002;9(5):410–419.
192. Breier-Mackie S, Newell CJ. Home parenteral nutrition: an ethical decision making dilemma. *Aust J Adv Nurs.* 2002;19(4):27–32.
193. Chiu TY, Hu WY, Chuang RB, Chen CY. Nutrition and hydration for terminal cancer patients in Taiwan. *Support Care Cancer.* 2002;10(8):630–636.
194. Eberhardie C. Nutrition support in palliative care. *Nurs Stand.* 2002;17(2): 47–52; quiz 54–55.
195. Angus F, Burakoff R. The percutaneous endoscopic gastrostomy tube: medical and ethical issues in placement. *Am J Gastroenterol.* 2003;98(2): 272–277.
196. Daugherty CK. Examining ethical dilemmas as obstacles to hospice and palliative care for advanced cancer patients. *Cancer Invest.* 2004;22(1): 123–131.
197. Adams KE, Cohen MH, Eisenberg D, Jonsen AR. Ethical considerations of complementary and alternative medical therapies in conventional medical settings. *Ann Intern Med.* 2002;137(8):660–664.
198. Pietsch JB, Ford C, Whitlock JA. Nasogastric tube feedings in children with high-risk cancer: a pilot study. *J Pediatr Hematol Oncol.* 1999;21(2): 111–114.
199. Deswarte-Wallace J, Firouzbakhsh S, Finklestein JZ. Using research to change practice: enteral feedings for pediatric oncology patients. *J Pediatr Oncol Nurs.* 2001;18(5):217–223.
200. Mathew P, Bowman L, Williams R, et al. Complications and effectiveness of gastrostomy feedings in pediatric cancer patients. *J Pediatr Hematol Oncol.* 1996;18(1):81–85.
201. Skolin I, Hernell O, Larsson MV, Wahlgren C, Wahlin YB. Percutaneous endoscopic gastrostomy in children with malignant disease. *J Pediatr Oncol Nurs.* 2002;19(5):154–163.
202. Pedersen AM, Kok K, Petersen G, Nielsen OH, Michaelsen KF, Schmiegelow K. Percutaneous endoscopic gastrostomy in children with cancer. *Acta Paediatr.* 1999;88(8):849–852.
203. van Eys J, Wesley MN, Cangir A, et al. Safety of intravenous hyperalimentation in children with malignancies: a cooperative group trial. *J Parenter Enteral Nutr.* 1982;6(4):291–294.
204. Ghavimi F, Shils ME, Scott BF, Brown M, Tamaroff M. Comparison of morbidity in children requiring abdominal radiation and chemotherapy, with and without total parenteral nutrition. *J Pediatr.* 1982;101(4):530–537.
205. van Eys J, Copeland EM, Cangir A, et al. A clinical trial of hyperalimentation in children with metastatic malignancies. *Med Pediatr Oncol.* 1980;8(1):63–73.
206. Kelly KM, Jacobson JS, Kennedy DD, Braudt SM, Mallick M, Weiner MA. Use of unconventional therapies by children with cancer at an urban medical center. *J Pediatr Hematol Oncol.* 2000;22(5):412–416.
207. Neuhouser ML, Patterson RE, Schwartz SM, Hedderson MM, Bowen DJ, Standish LJ. Use of alternative medicine by children with cancer in Washington state. *Prev Med.* 2001;33(5):347–354.
208. McCurdy EA, Spangler JG, Wofford MM, Chauvenet AR, McLean TW. Religiosity is associated with the use of complementary medical therapies by pediatric oncology patients. *J Pediatr Hematol Oncol.* 2003;25(2): 125–129.
209. Liossi C, Hatira P. Clinical hypnosis versus cognitive behavioral training for pain management with pediatric cancer patients undergoing bone marrow aspirations. *Int J Clin Exp Hypn.* 1999;47(2):104–116.
210. Liossi C, Hatira P. Clinical hypnosis in the alleviation of procedure-related pain in pediatric oncology patients. *Int J Clin Exp Hypn.* 2003;51(1):4–28.
211. Aasgaard T. An ecology of love: aspects of music therapy in the pediatric oncology environment. *J Palliat Care.* 2001;17(3):177–181.
212. Jankovic M, Spinetta JJ, Martins AG, et al. Non-conventional therapies in childhood cancer: guidelines for distinguishing non-harmful from harmful therapies: a report of the SIOP Working Committee on Psychosocial Issues in Pediatric Oncology. *Pediatr Blood Cancer.* 2004;42(1):106–108.
213. Bottomley SJ, Kassner E. Late effects of childhood cancer therapy. *J Pediatr Nurs.* 2003;18(2):126–133.
214. Lustig RH, Post SR, Srivannaboon K, et al. Risk factors for the development of obesity in children surviving brain tumors. *J Clin Endocrinol Metab.* 2003;88(2):611–616.

Mary Kramlich, MS, RD, LD, CNSD;
Angie Iverson, RD, LMNT;
Vincent Armenti, MD, PhD;
Jeanette Hasse, PhD, RD, LD, FADA, CNSD

12

Solid Organ Transplantation

Introduction

Solid organ transplantation outcomes may be influenced by nutritional factors such as preoperative malnutrition or obesity. Postoperative immunosuppressive medication regimens often affect nutritional management along with growth and development in pediatric patients. Nutrition-related medication side effects, oral nutrition therapy, and enteral and parenteral nutrition management will be addressed in this chapter.

I. Indications for Transplantation.

Organ transplantation is indicated for individuals who have organ failure that is no longer "curable" with current medical and surgical therapies. See Table 12-1 for specific disease states that may lead to organ transplantation.

II. Immunosuppression

A. Organ transplant recipients are maintained on immunosuppressive regimens to prevent rejection.
B. Immunosuppression is designed to disable or destroy various components of the immune response; this is typically achieved with multiple drug therapy. Regimens fall into three categories:
  1. Induction regimens
    a) The aim of these regimens is to avoid rejection and establish good graft function within the early postoperative course.
    b) Induction regimens usually involve biologic agents, including antilymphocyte sera (polyclonal or monoclonal antibodies) or interleukin-2 receptor blockade.
    c) Examples include Thymoglobulin, ATGAM, basiliximab, daclizumab, and muromonab CD3 (Table 12-2)
  2. Antirejection regimens
    a) Antirejection regimens are high-dose, short-term treatments aimed at reversing acute rejection.
    b) Agents include corticosteroids, Thymoglobulin, or muromonab CD3 (Table 12-2).
  3. Maintenance regimens
    a) Maintenance regimens are designed to provide long-term immunosuppression to prevent rejections.
    b) These regimens are typically initiated soon after transplantation and include one or two drugs often combined with a corticosteroid.
    c) Recent attempts have been designed to withdraw corticosteroids over some period or even avoid corticosteroids completely.
    d) Maintenance therapy agents include combinations of cyclosporine or tacrolimus with either mycophenolate mofetil or sirolimus.
    e) Two new immunosuppressive agents on the horizon are myfortic (Novartis Pharmaceutical Corporation, East Hanover, NJ) and Certican (Novartis Pharmaceutical Corporation), which have mechanisms of action similar to mycophenolate mofetil and sirolimus, respectively.
C. There is potential for drug-nutrient interactions (Table 12-2).

III. Nutritional Factors Influencing Postoperative Outcomes

A. Malnutrition
  1. Malnutrition reduces posttransplant survival.
    a) Malnutrition increased risk for morbidity and mortality post liver transplant in several studies,[18–23] although findings by Figueiredo et al and Stephenson et al did not support this correlation.[24,25]
    b) Madill et al reported that lung transplant recipients with a body mass index (BMI) <17 kg/m^2 had a 4-fold greater risk of dying within 90 days posttransplant compared with a normal weight group, although the finding was not statistically significant.[16]
    c) Frazier et al reported that mortality was increased in heart transplant recipients who were malnourished.[26]
    d) Becker et al showed that hypoalbuminemia in kidney transplant recipients increased rates of cytomegalovirus infection and graft failure and was associated with a trend for reduced survival.[27]
  2. Malnutrition increases blood loss and use of blood products during liver transplant surgery.[24,25,28]
  3. Malnutrition increases length of intensive care unit (ICU)[22,24] and hospital stay after liver transplant.[22,25,29]
  4. Malnutrition impairs wound healing.
  5. Physical deconditioning, associated with malnutrition, may also increase length of hospital stay and rehabilitation.
B. Obesity
  1. Lung. Madill et al reported that lung transplant patients with a BMI >27 kg/m^2 had an increased mortality within 90 days posttransplant as well as an increased length of ICU stay.[16]
  2. Kidney and kidney/pancreas

<table>
<tr><th colspan="3">TABLE 12-1. Common Diagnoses Leading to Organ Transplantation</th></tr>
<tr><th>Organ</th><th>Adult</th><th>Pediatric</th></tr>
<tr><td>Liver transplant[1–4]</td><td>• Alcoholic cirrhosis
• Viral hepatitis—hepatitis B and C (fulminant and chronic)
• Cholestatic disease—primary biliary cirrhosis, primary sclerosing cholangitis
• Metabolic disease—hemochromatosis, Wilson's disease, alpha 1-antitrypsin deficiency, glycogen storage disease
• Nonalcoholic steatohepatitis
• Autoimmune disease
• Miscellaneous—cryptogenic liver failure, polycystic liver disease, hepatocellular carcinoma, Budd-Chiari syndrome, sarcoidosis</td><td>• Pediatric
• Acute and chronic hepatitis—fulminant hepatic failure, chronic viral hepatitis with cirrhosis
• Intrahepatic cholestasis—idiopathic neonatal hepatitis, Alagille's syndrome, familial intrahepatic cholestasis (Byler's disease)
• Cholestatic disease—extrahepatic biliary atresia, sclerosing cholangitis
• Metabolic disease—alpha-1-antitrypsin deficiency, tyrosinemia, Wilson's disease, perinatal hemochromatosis, glycogen storage disease</td></tr>
<tr><td>Kidney transplant[3,5,6]</td><td>• Diabetes mellitus
• Hypertension
• Chronic glomerulonephritis
• Systemic lupus erythematosus
• Chronic pyelonephritis
• Polycystic kidney disease
• Hyperoxaluria
• Vasculitis
• Nephritis</td><td>• Obstructive uropathy
• Aplastic/hypoplastic/dysplastic kidneys
• Focal segmental glomerulosclerosis
• Reflux nephropathy
• Chronic glomerulonephritis
• Syndrome of agenesis of abdominal musculature
• Medullary cystic disease/juvenile nephronophthisis
• Hemolytic uremic syndrome
• Congenital nephritic syndrome
• Polycystic kidney disease</td></tr>
<tr><td>Pancreas transplant[3,7,8]</td><td>• Type 1 diabetes mellitus is the indication for 99% of pancreas transplants
• Islet cell transplantation is another option for patients with type 1 diabetes mellitus</td><td>• Pancreas transplantation is uncommon in pediatric patients
• A pancreas graft is sometimes included in a multivisceral transplant</td></tr>
<tr><td>Small-bowel transplant[3,9–13]</td><td colspan="2">• Indicated for patients with irreversible intestinal failure who cannot tolerate parenteral nutrition due to life-threatening complications such as cholestatic liver disease, loss of venous access, repeated central line sepsis
• Causes of intestinal failure include mesenteric thrombosis, necrotizing enterocolitis, Crohn's disease, desmoid tumor, Gardner's syndrome, ischemia, pseudo-obstruction, trauma, intestinal volvulus, radiation enteritis</td></tr>
<tr><td>Heart transplant[3,14,15]</td><td>• Primary cardiomyopathy
• Coronary artery disease
• Inoperable ischemic coronary disease</td><td>• Complex congenital heart disease
• Primary cardiomyopathy
• Hypoplastic left heart syndrome
• Endocardial fibroelastosis
• Acquired heart disease</td></tr>
<tr><td>Lung transplant[3,14,16,17]</td><td>• Cystic fibrosis
• Chronic obstructive pulmonary disease
• Pulmonary hypertension
• Bronchiectasis
• Pulmonary fibrosis
• Emphysema
• Eisenmenger's syndrome
• Bronchiolitis obliterans
• Alpha-1-antitrypsin deficiency
• Scleroderma</td><td>• Cystic fibrosis
• Primary pulmonary hypertension
• Chronic obstructive pulmonary disease
• Alpha-1-antitrypsin deficiency
• Idiopathic pulmonary fibrosis
• Interstitial lung disease
• Congenital heart disease
• Bronchiolitis obliterans
• Desquamative interstitial pneumonitis</td></tr>
</table>

TABLE 12-2. Immunosuppressant Drugs, Nutritional Side Effects, and Interventions

Drug	Activity	Nutritional side effects	Suggested nutrition therapy
Antilymphocyte serum (ATGAM, Thymoglobulin)	Binds with lymphocytes, resulting in phagocytosis Inhibits and destroys lymphocytes	Fever and chills Increased risk of infection, profound leukopenia	Provide nutrient-dense foods patient will eat Ensure that patient is receiving adequate protein
Azathioprine (Imuran)	Inhibits purine nucleotide synthesis, blocking T- and B-lymphocyte proliferation	Nausea, vomiting Diarrhea Sore throat/mucositis Altered taste acuity Macrocytic anemia Pancreatitis	Try antiemetic medications; if vomiting does not subside, consider tube feeding or PN Review drugs and substitute for those that may be causing diarrhea; make sure that patient is receiving adequate fluid to replace losses Provide foods that will not irritate throat Offer a variety of foods with different tastes Make sure folate intake is adequate Initiate EN or PN if pancreatitis is severe
Basiliximab (Simulect)	Acts against the interleukin-2R-alpha chain (CD25) on activated T-lymphocytes and inhibits interleukin-2-mediated activation of lymphocyte	None reported	
Corticosteroids (methyl-prednisone, prednisone, prednisolone, Solu-Medrol, Solu-Cortef)	Anti-inflammatory properties Inhibits cell-mediated—and, to a lesser degree, humoral—immunity Inhibits lymphocyte proliferation Inhibits lymphokine production	Hyperglycemia Sodium retention Ulcers Osteoporosis Hyperphagia Impaired wound healing and increased infection risk Hypertension Pancreatitis	Monitor blood sugar and need for long-term diabetes diet and hypoglycemic agents Avoid high-sodium foods Avoid foods that irritate stomach Ensure adequate calcium and vitamin D intake; consider need for calcitriol, fluoride, or estrogen Behavior modification to prevent overeating Ensure adequate protein intake; consider need for vitamins A or C or zinc Avoid high-sodium foods, maintain healthy weight Initiate EN or PN if pancreatitis is severe
Cyclosporine (Neoral, Sandimmune)	Inhibits cell-mediated immunity; inhibits T-cell proliferation Suppresses interleukin-2 production Prevents gamma-interferon release	Hyperkalemia Hypomagnesemia Hypertension Hyperglycemia Hyperlipidemia	Restrict high-potassium foods Supplement with high-magnesium foods or supplements Avoid high-sodium foods, maintain healthy weight Monitor blood sugar and need for long-term diabetes diet and hypoglycemic agents Limit fat intake to <30% calories during long-term phase; maintain healthy weight
Daclizumab (Zenapax)		None reported	

TABLE 12-2. Immunosuppressant Drugs, Nutritional Side Effects, and Interventions (*Continued*)

Drug	Activity	Nutritional Side Effects	Suggested Nutrition Therapy
Muromonab-CD3 (OKT3)	Blocks T3 antigen recognition and T-cell effector function Causes T-cell lysis	Nausea, vomiting Diarrhea Anorexia	Try antiemetic medications; if vomiting does not subside, consider tube feeding or PN Review drugs and substitute for those that may be causing diarrhea; make sure that patient is receiving adequate fluid to replace losses Offer frequent meals of nutrient-dense foods
Sirolimus (Rapamycin, Rapamune)	Blocks the response of T- and B-cell activation by cytokines, which prevents cell-cycle progression and proliferation	Hyperlipidemia Gastrointestinal disorders (constipation, diarrhea, nausea/ vomiting, dyspepsia)	Limit fat intake to <30% calories during long-term phase; maintain healthy weight Monitor for adequate nutrient intake
Tacrolimus (Prograf, FK506)	Suppresses T cell-mediated immunity and interleukin-2 production	Nausea, vomiting Hyperkalemia Hyperglycemia Abdominal distress	Try antiemetic medications; if vomiting does not subside, consider tube feeding or PN Avoid high-potassium foods Monitor blood sugar and need for long-term diabetes diet and hypoglycemic agents Monitor oral intake; consider alternate methods of nutrition support if intake is suboptimal
Mycophenolate mofetil (CellCept)	Inhibits DNA synthesis and mixed lymphocyte production Inhibits antibody formation	Diarrhea	Review drugs and substitute for those that may be causing diarrhea; make sure that patient is receiving adequate fluid to replace losses

EN, enteral nutrition; PN, parenteral nutrition.

Reprinted from Hasse JM. Solid organ transplantation. In: Matarese LE, Gottschlich MM, eds. *Contemporary Nutrition Support Practice: A Clinical Guide,*. 2nd ed. Philadelphia, PA: Elsevier; 2003:560–573 with permission from Elsevier.

a) Obesity may increase the risk of delayed renal graft function.[30–33]
b) Obesity has been shown to adversely affect graft survival in some[31,32,34–37] but not all studies.[33,38]

3. Liver. Obesity may delay wound healing, prolong ventilator time, and increase postoperative infections.[39–41]

IV. Nutrition Assessment.

A combination of objective and subjective parameters form the basis of a comprehensive nutrition assessment (see Table 12-3 for assessment guidelines specific to transplant recipients).

V. Nutrient Requirements

A. Pretransplant
1. Adult. See Table 12-4; review other chapters on nutritional care of adult patients with specific organ failure
2. Pediatric. See Tables 12-5 and 12-6; review other chapters on nutritional care of pediatric patients with specific organ failure

B. Postoperative
1. Adult
a) Table 12-7 highlights postoperative nutrient requirements.
b) Table 12-8 summarizes nutrition considerations associated with common posttransplant complications.
2. Pediatric. See Table 12-7.

VI. Nutrition Goals for Posttransplant Maintenance Phase

A. Adult
1. Attain/maintain appropriate weight.
a) Excess weight gain posttransplant has been well documented.[52,59–64]
b) Posttransplant obesity is attributed to numerous factors, including the side effects of corticosteroids (hyperphagia, increase in adipose stores), pretransplant obesity, improved gastrointestinal (GI) absorption, limited exercise, and noncompliance with dietary recommendations.[5,42,65,66]
c) Regular exercise is encouraged for weight maintenance as well as promotion of lean muscle tissue; posttransplant patients are at risk for increased muscle loss due to the side effects of corticosteroids.
d) Weight loss recommendations posttransplant are similar to general population guidelines (ie, exercise, diet modifications).[67]

TABLE 12-3. Nutrition Assessment Criteria for Organ Transplant Patients[5,9,14,42–48]

Components of an assessment	Assessment parameters	
Medical history	• Patient age • Etiology, duration, and severity of organ failure prior to transplantation • Time since transplant and current transplant function • Other organ damage (eg, renal insufficiency, diabetes, cardiovascular disease) • GI conditions (eg, nausea, vomiting, diarrhea, GI bleeding) or diseases (eg, Crohn's disease, celiac sprue, gastroesophageal reflux)	• Previous surgeries (other than transplant) such as GI surgeries (eg, noting location and extent of intestinal resections in small-bowel transplant recipients) • Other supportive therapies (eg, hemodialysis, oxygen, heart assist devices if pretransplant) • History of diabetes mellitus and level of glucose control • Functional ability, energy level, attendance at work or school • Current diet prescription
Nutrition history	• Diet history to assess quality and quantity of intake • Medication history to identify drug-nutrient interactions • Previous enteral or parenteral nutrition support; type and amount of formula • For infants, consideration of route of feeding and type of formula if bottle-fed • Fluid and electrolyte supplementation	• Use of nutrition supplements, including vitamin, mineral, and herbal preparations • Psychosocial and economic conditions to determine patient's or caregiver's ability to obtain/prepare food and comply with diet • Changes in appetite, taste acuity, satiety • Dietary restrictions • Food allergies and intolerances • Religious or cultural food preferences
Physical examination	• Mental status • Muscle and fat stores • Edema or ascites	• Skin color, dryness, turgor, and integrity • Oral/dental health
Anthropometric measurements	• Height or length • For children, weight and percentile for age, weight for length percentile, head circumference and percentile for age • Weight history (to assess degree of fluid retention and weight loss)	• Tricep skinfold and midarm muscle circumference measurements may be helpful if measured serially over time • Hand grip strength may be an indirect measure of muscle stores
Laboratory tests	• Tests to evaluate transplant graft function • Serum electrolytes • Serum glucose and, if indicated, hemoglobin A1c and C-peptide levels • Tests to evaluate renal function, such as blood urea nitrogen and creatinine	• Hepatic transport proteins: not especially helpful in the postoperative period because concentrations are affected by fluid status, liver and kidney function, and vitamin status • Iron studies • Serum lipid levels • Fat-soluble vitamin levels (for patients with malabsorption)
Other tests	• Subjective global assessment may be helpful as an initial assessment tool • Bioelectrical impedance is probably not an accurate measure of protein calorie malnutrition in fluid-overloaded patients • Creatinine-height index is influenced by renal function • Dual-energy x-ray absorptiometry can accurately measure bone density and body fat • Indirect calorimetry can accurately determine resting energy expenditure	• The D-xylose test is recommended for small-bowel transplant recipients 30 days posttransplant and then weekly to evaluate intestinal graft function and carbohydrate absorption

GI, gastrointestinal

TABLE 12-4. Pretransplant Calorie and Protein Goals for Solid Organ Transplant Candidates

Nutrition Goal	
	Calorie Needs
Weight maintenance	1.2 to 1.3 x basal energy expenditure (by Harris-Benedict equation), depending on activity level 30 kcal/kg
Weight gain	1.5 x basal energy expenditure 35 to 40 kcal/kg
Weight loss	Deficit of 500 to 1000 kcal/day, depending on current intake, anticipated time until transplant, and ability to exercise
	Protein Needs
Maintenance	0.8 to 1.2 g/kg/d
Repletion	1.3 to 2.0 g/kg/d
Dialysis	Hemodialysis: 1.2 to 1.5 g/kg/d Peritoneal: 1.5 g/kg/d

Adapted from Hasse JM. Solid organ transplantation. In: Matarese LE, Gottschlich MM, eds. *Contemporary Nutrition Support Practice: A Clinical Guide.* 2nd ed. Philadelphia, PA: Elsevier; 2003:560–573 with permission from Elsevier.

e) Although limited data are available, small-bowel transplant patients appear to be at low risk for posttransplant obesity due to decreased intestinal absorption.[9]

2. Optimize diabetes management.
   a) Transplant patients are at higher risk of developing diabetes[68–72] due to immunosuppressive medications (eg, corticosteroids, tacrolimus, cyclosporine); the incidence of diabetes may lower as corticosteroid doses are reduced.[73]
      (1) Cyclosporine and tacrolimus inhibit insulin secretion, increase insulin resistance, and exert a direct toxic effect on beta cells[74]; tacrolimus may be more diabetogenic than cyclosporine.[75]
      (2) Corticosteroids cause insulin resistance, increase gluconeogenesis and glucagon production, and antagonize peripheral glucose uptake.[74,76,77]
   b) Other risk factors for the development of diabetes include heredity, obesity, and renal insufficiency.
   c) Diabetes treatment should include an appropriate carbohydrate-controlled diet, self-monitoring of blood glucose, and medication as needed (insulin or oral agents).[70–72]
   d) Weight management, lipid control, and exercise are stressed for patients with diabetes.
3. Prevent and treat bone mass loss.
   a) Posttransplant patients are at increased risk for bone loss[78–81] due to
      (1) Osteopenic effects of immunosuppressive drugs (specifically, corticosteroids and cyclosporine)
      (2) Pretransplant risk factors such as type of pretransplant disease, vitamin D deficiency, hypogonadism, impaired absorption or inadequate intake of calcium, reduced physical activity, and preexisting bone disease
   b) Treatment includes
      (1) Adequate calcium intake (1500 mg per day) with vitamin D
      (2) Regular resistance exercise to improve bone density[82]
      (3) Smoking avoidance
      (4) Annual bone density testing to monitor bone health
      (5) Treatment with estrogen and/or bisphosphonates (indicated for certain patients)[83–85]
4. Achieve normal serum lipid levels.
   a) Risk factors for posttransplant hyperlipidemia include immunosuppressive medications (especially sirolimus, corticosteroids, and cyclosporine)[52,86–88] as well as obesity, genetic predisposition, diabetes mellitus, sedentary lifestyle, renal dysfunction, high-fat diet, antihypertensive drugs, and proteinuria.
   b) Treatment of hyperlipidemia includes
      (1) Dietary changes
      (2) Lipid-lowering agents
      (3) Fish oil supplementation, whose benefits are being studied
5. Achieve normal blood pressure.
   a) Transplant patients are at risk for increased blood pressure caused by corticosteroids and cyclosporine.
   b) Treatment includes weight management, antihypertensive medications, and a dietary restriction of 2 to 4 g sodium per day.
6. Wean nutrition support.
   a) Patients should achieve adequate intake with oral diet.
   b) Small-bowel transplant recipients may require a period of nutrition support and/or intravenous (IV) fluids.

B. Pediatric
1. Obtain adequate calories and protein; needs reflect recommended daily allowance (RDA) for age if there is good graft function, minimal complications, and appropriate growth since transplant.
2. Achieve appropriate catch-up and long-term growth (Table 12-9).
   a) Growth retardation often occurs in pediatric patients prior to transplantation.
   b) The use of corticosteroids after transplantation can compound this problem; however, the use of alternate-day prednisone can reduce the growth-depressing effects of steroids[89]; withdrawal of corticosteroids can also result in improved catch-up growth.
   c) Liver and heart recipients normally experience catch-up growth during the first posttransplant year if chronic rejection is absent[90]; however, patients with poor graft function, those requiring high-dose corticosteroids due to rejection, or those requiring multiple operations are more likely to continue to experience poor linear growth.[89]
   d) Children with renal failure have short stature for multiple reasons. Optimizing nutrition support, supplementing with oral bicarbonate, preventing renal osteodystrophy, and treating anemia prior to transplantation can help stabilize growth.[91]
      (1) The use of recombinant human growth hormone before transplant in patients with chronic renal failure has been shown to result in improved growth.[91]
      (2) Some studies indicate that catch-up growth occurs in only 30% to 50% of children after renal transplantation; it occurs most often in children less than 6 years old rather

TABLE 12-5. Nutrition Considerations for Pediatric Transplant Candidates[10,45,48–50]

	Considerations
Diet factors	• Oral intake can be maximized by concentrating infant formulas • Modular protein, fat, and carbohydrate components can be added to food or formulas to increase nutrient density • If early satiety or tiring while feeding occur, offer patients small, frequent meals • If an infant is breast-feeding, continue as long as he or she gains weight and grows well; increased calorie and protein needs may make it difficult to meet 100% of nutritional needs with breast milk unless the mother is willing to pump and additives are added to the milk • Most intestinal transplant candidates will have oral aversions; patients should receive as much oral stimulation as possible: bottles should be offered to children <1 year of age and solid food should be introduced at normal developmental milestones
Nutrition support considerations	• Tube feeding is indicated if patients are severely malnourished or unable to achieve adequate nutrient intake by mouth; when possible, tube feedings should be administered nocturnally or with a nipple/bolus schedule during the day to preserve as much oral intake as possible and prevent development of oral aversions • If a patient is not growing adequately despite tube feedings, PN is indicated to maximize nutritional status prior to transplant • Patients awaiting heart transplantation or requiring extracorporeal membrane oxygenation may also require PN • Patients with severe esophagitis or gastric varices secondary to liver disease may require PN if oral intake is inadequate and placing a nasogastric tube is contraindicated due to bleeding risk

Pre-liver transplant	• Biliary atresia is the most common cause of liver disease in pediatric patients
	  ○ Calorie requirements may be as high as 180% of the RDA for calories and up to 4 g protein per kg per day due to malabsorption of nutrients
	  ○ Malabsorption of fat and fat-soluble vitamins also occurs; fat-soluble vitamin supplementation is frequently required (see TABLE 12-6)
	  ○ Infant formulas high in medium-chain triglycerides are helpful in reducing steatorrhea and improving growth
	• Patients with noncholestatic liver disease require 100% to 120% of the RDA for calories, 2.2 to 2.5 g protein per kg per day for infants, and the RDA for protein for children ages 1 year to 18 years

Pre-intestinal transplant	• Patients awaiting intestinal transplant are dependent upon PN • Calorie needs are normally less than the RDA • If the patient is stable, 70 to 80 calories per kg per day are adequate for growth • Protein requirements are 1.8 to 2.5 g per kg per day • Hypertriglyceridemia occurs frequently in patients awaiting combined liver and intestinal transplantation • Adequate fat (0.5 g/kg/day) should be provided to prevent essential fatty acid deficiency
Pre-kidney transplant	• Calorie and protein requirements vary depending on need for dialysis and type of dialysis • Electrolyte requirements need to be individualized based on serum levels
Pre-heart transplant	• Calorie needs vary greatly • Infants and children requiring ventricular assist devices or extracorporeal membrane oxygenation prior to transplantation are often dependent upon PN • Calorie requirements are typical for other children requiring PN, approximately 80% to 85% of the RDA • Calorie needs for children with congenital heart disease vary widely but may be 150 calories per kg per day or higher • Children with less advanced heart disease will have calorie and protein needs similar to the RDA for their age
Pre-lung transplant	• Most children requiring lung transplantation have CF; this population has specific nutrient requirements • Because the degree of lung disease is quite advanced in many patients with CF awaiting lung transplantation, tube feeding may be required to meet nutrient needs

CF, cystic fibrosis; PN, parenteral nutrition; RDA, recommended daily allowance.

TABLE 12-6. Fat-Soluble Vitamin Recommendations for Pediatric Liver Transplant Candidates[45]

Vitamin	Daily Recommended Amount
Vitamin A, emulsified A	5000 to 15 000 International Units
Vitamin D, 25 (OH) D	5 to 7 mcg/kg
Vitamin E, D-alpha-tocopherol	15 to 25 International Units/kg
Vitamin K	2.5 to 5 mg

than older children[92]; however, there are reports of significant catch-up growth in children of pubertal age.

e) Lung and intestinal transplant recipients require more immunosuppression than other organ transplant recipients.
  (1) Antirejection medications, specifically corticosteroids, can result in additional growth delay.
  (2) After 5 years post small-bowel transplant, it appears that children do begin to experience catch-up growth in the absence of renal failure or chronic rejection.[93]

3. Overcome oral aversions.
   a) This is primarily a complication in intestinal transplant recipients; these children have not developed normal oral motor skills due to long-term dependence on parenteral nutrition (PN).
   b) Most small-bowel transplant recipients will require intensive posttransplant feeding therapy to achieve adequate nutritional intake by mouth.[10]
   c) Patients with a long dependence on tube feedings or PN prior to transplantation will require feeding therapy to meet nutritional needs orally.
4. Achieve normal blood pressure.
   a) A sodium-restricted diet is recommended for patients who have posttransplant hypertension (HTN).
   b) HTN is common after pediatric kidney transplantation and can be associated with graft failure; higher systolic blood pressure in the first few posttransplant months is associated with decreased renal allograft function in children 1 year after transplantation.[94]
   c) By 1 year after liver or heart transplantation, most patients are normotensive and do not require antihypertensive therapy.[95]
   d) HTN is also common in lung transplant recipients; patients with cystic fibrosis should restrict dietary sodium with caution.
5. Prevent and treat bone loss.
   a) Long-term corticosteroid use can lead to bone loss over time.[96]
   b) Corticosteroids are often discontinued or changed to alternate-day dosing in the first 6 to 12 posttransplant months to maximize long-term growth and minimize bone loss.[97]
   c) Calcium intake should meet the RDA for age.
   d) Vitamin D levels should be monitored and supplemented with 400 to 1000 International Units per day if needed.
   e) Daily exercise is recommended to minimize bone disease.
6. Achieve and maintain normal serum lipid levels.
   a) Elevated serum cholesterol and triglyceride levels can occur in children posttransplantation, most commonly in renal and heart transplant recipients.[98]
   b) Family history of hyperlipidemia correlates with increased risk.
   c) Complete serum lipid profiles should be performed, counseling regarding dietary changes provided, and lipid-lowering agents prescribed as needed.[99]
7. Treat posttransplant diabetes mellitus (PTDM).
   a) The incidence of hyperglycemia and PTDM ranges from 4% to 41%.
   b) Significant risk factors for the development of PTDM include first-degree family history of type 2 DM, second-degree family history of type 2 DM, tacrolimus use, and hyperglycemia occurring in the 2 weeks after transplantation.
   c) Patients with family history of DM or hyperglycemia may benefit from the avoidance of tacrolimus in the immediate posttransplant period.[100]
   d) If PTDM develops, patients and families will need in-depth dietary counseling to learn management principles.
8. Avoid obesity.
   a) Corticosteroids, inactivity, and poor dietary habits can contribute to the development of obesity in children after transplantation.
   b) Patients and families should be counseled on healthy eating habits and the importance of daily exercise.

VII. Enteral Nutrition

A. Indications

1. Advantages of early posttransplant enteral nutrition have been documented in adults.[101–106]
   a) Benefits include promotion of protein metabolism, improvement in wound healing, maintenance of gut immunity, and prevention of infectious complications.
   b) The use of probiotics in early enteral nutrition to reduce bacterial translocation and decrease the risk of infections is being studied in posttransplant populations.[107]
2. If a feeding tube is not placed at the time of transplantation, indications for enteral nutrition include
   a) Prolonged ventilator requirements
   b) Postsurgical complications
   c) Failure to eat adequately when an oral diet is initiated
   d) Severe malnutrition
   e) Physical deconditioning or overall weakness and failure to thrive
   f) Gastroparesis
   g) Oral aversion
   h) Growth failure in children
3. A transplant recipient who develops a critical illness at any time posttransplant should be assessed for nutritional risk, and nutrition support should be considered (Figure 12-1).
4. Following small-bowel transplantation, enteral nutrition is not initiated until approximately 1 to 2 weeks after transplantation, when the postoperative ileus is resolved and it is verified that there is no anastomotic leakage; the patient is gradually weaned off PN as enteral nutrition tolerance is established (meeting 50% of needs).[9]

B. Route of feeding

1. Small bowel
   a) Nasoenteral—indicated for postoperative feedings if gastric emptying is delayed and possibly to reduce risk of aspiration.
   b) Jejunostomy—indicated for longer-term feedings. These tubes have a higher complication rate and risk compared with nasoenteral tubes and may be placed during small-bowel transplantation.
2. Gastric
   a) Nasogastric—indicated for patients in whom aspiration risk is reduced and gastric emptying is normal.

TABLE 12-7. Nutrient Recommendations for Organ Transplant Recipients During Postoperative Stage or Subsequent Critical Illness

Nutrient	Adult recommendations[5,9,14,42,44]	Pediatric recommendations[10,43,46–48,51]
Calories	130% to 150% of calculated basal energy expenditure or measure with indirect calorimetry • Calorie needs are individualized considering pretransplant nutritional status, postoperative stress factors, and presence of steatorrhea • Adjustments may be made for obese patients	• Needs vary depending upon clinical status • Up to 130 kcal/kg for patients with open wounds, sepsis, preexisting malnutrition, history of growth failure, cardiac failure, or respiratory distress • 80 to 90 kcal/kg for infants and preschoolers without complications • 50 to 60 kcal/kg for adolescents • Ventilator dependence decreases calorie needs due to decreased respiratory effort and inactivity • Research indicates that the increase in energy expenditure associated with surgery lasts only 24 hours
Protein	1.5 to 2 g/kg • Protein catabolism is increased owing to surgical stress and high-dose corticosteroids • Adjust for nitrogen balance studies, decubitus, wounds, fistulas, dialysis, and additional posttransplant surgeries	2 times the RDA for age during the recovery period • Protein needs are elevated in the first 2 weeks posttransplant to account for protein catabolism from corticosteroids and increased needs for wound healing • If renal function is poor (without dialysis), decrease protein intake to 0.75 to 1.25 x the RDA
Carbohydrate	50% to 70% of nonprotein calories • Hyperglycemia may occur as a result of immunosuppressive medications (corticosteroids, tacrolimus, cyclosporine), metabolic stress, or infection • Hyperglycemia may be a risk factor for infection • Treat hyperglycemia with short-acting and long-acting insulin as indicated; consider insulin drip during critical conditions • For small-bowel transplant recipients, limit lactose for postoperative secondary lactase deficiency	50% to 60% of calories • Hyperglycemia may occur as a result of immunosuppressive medications (corticosteroids, tacrolimus, cyclosporine), metabolic stress, or infection • Hyperglycemia may be a risk factor for infection • Insulin may be required • Glucose should not be overfed; doing so could create more problems with hyperglycemia or hypercapnia
Fat	30% of calories • Monitor serum triglyceride and cholesterol levels • Sirolimus (an immunosuppressant) can cause significant hyperlipidemia • Fish oil (n-3 fatty acids) may reduce the nephrotoxic effects of cyclosporine • For small-bowel transplant recipients, initially provide medium-chain triglycerides	30% of calories • Medications, sepsis, and liver or kidney dysfunction can increase the incidence of hypertriglyceridemia • Despite much research studying the effects of intravenous fat on immune function and pulmonary function, there are not enough data suggesting that lipids should be held for these reasons • Discontinue intravenous lipids if serum triglyceride levels exceed 400 mg/dL

Fluid	30 mL/kg; adjust based on output
	• Adjust intake based on output from urine, drains, wounds, diarrhea, nasogastric tube suction, fistulas, and para- or thoracentesis
	• In pancreas transplant recipients with urinary drainage of exocrine secretions, losses can be as high as 2 to 3 L/day
	• In small-bowel transplant recipients, ostomy output can be as high as 4 L/day
		Daily maintenance needs for pediatric patients:
		• mL/kg
		  ○ 1 to 10 kg: 100 mL/kg
		  ○ 11 to 20 kg: 1000 mL plus 50 mL for every kg >10
		  ○ 21 to 40 kg: 1500 mL plus 20 mL for every kg >20
		• Body surface area: 1500 to 2000 mL/m2
		• Fluid may be restricted to less than maintenance if there is edema, congestive heart failure, or renal failure

TABLE 12-7. Nutrient Recommendations for Organ Transplant Recipients During Postoperative Stage or Subsequent Critical Illness (*Continued*)

Nutrient	Adult recommendations[5,9,14,42,44]	Pediatric recommendations[10,43,46–48,51]
Fluid (*Continued*)		• Fluid needs may be increased with fever, diarrhea, or vomiting; high volumes of gastric output need to be replaced; kidney recipients often require additional fluid to replace urine output • Intestinal transplant patients will require intravenous replacement fluids for ileostomy output >35 to 40 mL/kg/day
Electrolytes	• Hypernatremia may require additional free water administration • Hyponatremia may require fluid restriction • Hyperkalemia may occur with tacrolimus, cyclosporine, potassium-sparing diuretics, renal insufficiency, or metabolic acidosis • Hypokalemia may be caused by potassium-wasting diuretics, amphotericin, refeeding syndrome, diarrhea, and fistulas • Hyperphosphatemia may occur with renal insufficiency • Hypophosphatemia may occur with refeeding syndrome or administration of corticosteroids • Hypermagnesemia may occur with renal insufficiency • Hypomagnesemia may be caused by cyclosporine, tacrolimus, diuretics, refeeding syndrome, diabetic ketoacidosis, and diarrhea; oral magnesium supplements may cause diarrhea • Bicarbonate loss may occur with urinary diversion of transplanted pancreas exocrine secretions or ostomy output in small-bowel transplantation	
Vitamins and minerals	• A multivitamin/mineral supplement is recommended • Adequate calcium for age is needed for bone health and prevention of osteopenia • Vitamin C and B6 may be low in post–kidney transplant patients[31] • Hyperhomocysteinemia is correlated in renal transplant recipients with renal function and status of vitamin B_6, B12, and folate[53–58] • Patients with cystic fibrosis need water-miscible forms of fat-soluble vitamins • Zinc and vitamin C may help with wound healing • Zinc levels may be decreased in small-bowel transplant recipients due to high stomal losses requiring supplementation of zinc	

RDA, recommended daily allowance.

b) Gastrostomy—indicated for long-term feedings when aspiration risk is reduced and gastric emptying is normal. Gastrostomy tubes may be contraindicated if posttransplant ascites is present.

C. Indications for formula selection

1. Adults

a) Protein content

(1) A high-nitrogen formula may be indicated for postoperative recovery and in situations such as critical illness or sepsis in which protein needs are increased; a modular protein may be used to meet needs.

(2) Glutamine-enhanced, small-peptide formulas may be advantageous for small-bowel transplant recipients receiving early feedings following transplantation.

b) Calorie contribution

(1) Enteral nutrition may be required to meet all or part of the patient's estimated needs, depending on oral intake.

(2) Calorie-dense formulas are indicated when patients are unable to tolerate high infusion rates to meet needs.

c) Electrolyte content

(1) Immunosuppressive medications can affect potassium, magnesium, phosphorous, and calcium levels.

(2) Formulas with reduced potassium and/or phosphorus may be helpful for patients with renal failure with hyperkalemia and hyperphosphatemia

d) Fluid content

(1) Calorie-dense formulas may be indicated for patients with fluid overload or reduced urine output.

(2) Fluid should be increased for patients with hypernatremia, fever, increased losses via drains, wounds, nasogastric tube, or diarrhea.

(3) IV fluids may be required for small-bowel transplant recipients when PN is discontinued.

2. Children

a) Age of patient

(1) Children should be given age-appropriate formulas.

(2) Infants can normally resume breast-feeding or feeding with formulas they were receiving prior to transplantation.

(3) Liver recipients requiring a hydrolyzed-protein formula pretransplant for malabsorption will usually tolerate an intact-protein formula after transplantation.

TABLE 12-8. Nutrition Support Considerations for Specific Posttransplant Complications

Transplant complication	Nutrition considerations	
Rejection	• Rejection rates are reduced in malnourished patients • Antirejection medications have many nutritional side effects • Corticosteroids increase protein catabolic rate and effects are dose dependent; protein catabolism increases during rejection treatment	• If muromonab-CD3 is used to treat rejection, nausea, vomiting, diarrhea, and headache, it may prevent adequate dietary intake
Infection	• Immunosuppressed patients are at increased risk of infection • Malnutrition also increases the rate of infection	• Antimicrobial agents may cause gastrointestinal upset and affect dietary intake or cause diarrhea
Wound healing	• Severely malnourished or obese patients are at increased risk of wound complications	
Renal insufficiency	• If renal replacement therapy is required, 5–10 g amino acids may be lost in dialysate • During hemofiltration, 300 g glucose can be absorbed over 24 hours from glucose-rich replacement fluids	• 43%–45% of glucose is absorbed from dialysate with continuous hemodialysis
Hyperglycemia	• Hyperglycemia is common due to metabolic stress, insulin resistance caused by corticosteroids, and inhibition of islet cell function and insulin release by cyclosporine and tacrolimus	• Infection rates are higher in diabetic patients than in nondiabetic patients
Surgical complications	• Vascular complications, postoperative bleeding, or complications requiring further surgery will delay oral intake • Severe pancreatitis or ileus may be indications for nutrition support	• Edema and ascites may respond to sodium restriction • Intestinal complications (diarrhea, ulcers, etc) may require that the route of feeding or type of food be altered

Adapted from Hasse JM. Nutrition assessment and support of organ transplant recipients. *J Parenter Enteral Nutr.* 2001;25(3):120–131 with permission from A.S.P.E.N.

b) Calorie content
   (1) Infant formulas provide 20 kcal/oz, and most children's formulas provide 30 kcal/oz; these are normally adequate to meet posttransplant requirements.
   (2) Occasionally, 1.5 and 2.0 kcal/mL formulas are used for pediatric transplant recipients if a severe fluid restriction is required due to a complication such as renal failure.

c) Osmolality
   (1) Isotonic formulas can be initiated full strength at low rates and advanced as tolerated.
   (2) Small-bowel transplant recipients often receive a diluted formula initially, but it is concentrated as needed to meet fluid and calorie goals.

d) Protein content
   (1) Protein content should be adequate to meet posttransplant needs.
   (2) For patients with reduced calorie needs due to intubation, pretransplant obesity, and so on, protein modulars can be added to formulas to meet protein needs.
   (3) Small-bowel transplant recipients should receive a hydrolyzed, low-osmolality formula containing medium-chain triglycerides (MCTs) for the first 4 to 6 weeks following transplantation; tube feedings should be initiated slowly (eg, 5 mL/hour) and advanced gradually (eg, 5 mL/hour per day).[108]

e) Fat content. A low-fat formula containing MCT oil may be prescribed if a patient develops chylothorax. If the condition does not resolve, PN with bowel rest is prescribed.[109]

D. Complications. Posttransplant enteral complications for organ transplant patients are similar to those of postsurgical patients. See Chapter 5. In addition, the following should be done:
1. Monitor stomal output and absorption in small-bowel transplant patients.
2. Evaluate potential causes of diarrhea, commonly found in transplant recipients:
   a) Cytomegalovirus invasion of the intestine
   b) *Clostridium difficile*
   c) High levels of tacrolimus
   d) Mycophenolate mofetil
3. Gastroparesis may be present posttransplant[110]; patients may require a prokinetic agent to tolerate tube feeds.

E. Home enteral nutrition
1. Patients may be sent home with tube feedings when the only factor keeping them hospitalized is inadequate oral intake; most

TABLE 12-9. Estimation of Catch-up Requirements

1. Plot the child's height and weight on the National Center for Health Statistics growth chart
2. Determine the child's recommended calories for age (recommended daily allowance [RDA])
3. Determine the ideal weight (50th percentile) for the child's height
4. Multiply the RDA calories by ideal body weight for height (kg)
5. Divide this value by the child's actual weight

Catch-up growth requirement = Calories required for weight

$$\frac{\text{RDA calories for age (kcal/kg/day)} \times \text{Ideal weight for height (kg)}}{\text{Actual weight (kg)}}$$

Protein requirement = Protein required for weight

$$\frac{\text{RDA protein for age} \times \text{Ideal weight for height (kg)}}{\text{Actual weight (kg)}}$$

Adapted from Peterson K, Washington JS, Rathburn J. Team management of failure-to-thrive. *J Am Diet Assoc.*1984;84:810–815 with permission from the American Dietetic Association.

pediatric intestine recipients will require tube feeding after hospital discharge.

2. Usually, nocturnal tube feedings are recommended for home enteral nutrition; limiting factors include the inability to control blood sugars with nocturnal tube feeds or intolerance of the higher tube feed rate required to meet calorie/protein needs.
3. Appetite enhancers (eg, megestrol acetate) may stimulate appetite and oral intake in adults.
4. Patients should be encouraged to try oral nutrition supplements and/or between-meal snacks to improve intake.
5. Outpatient calorie count records should be kept by the patient or family members and reviewed 1 to 2 times per week by a dietitian to determine when enteral nutrition can be discontinued.

VIII. Parenteral Nutrition

A. Indications
1. Prolonged ileus
2. Fistula or intestinal perforations
3. Bowel obstruction
4. GI bleed
5. Pancreatitis (when tube feeding is not tolerated)
6. Severe malabsorption or diarrhea

FIGURE 12-1. Algorithm for Providing Nutrition Support to a Critically Ill Organ Transplant Recipient

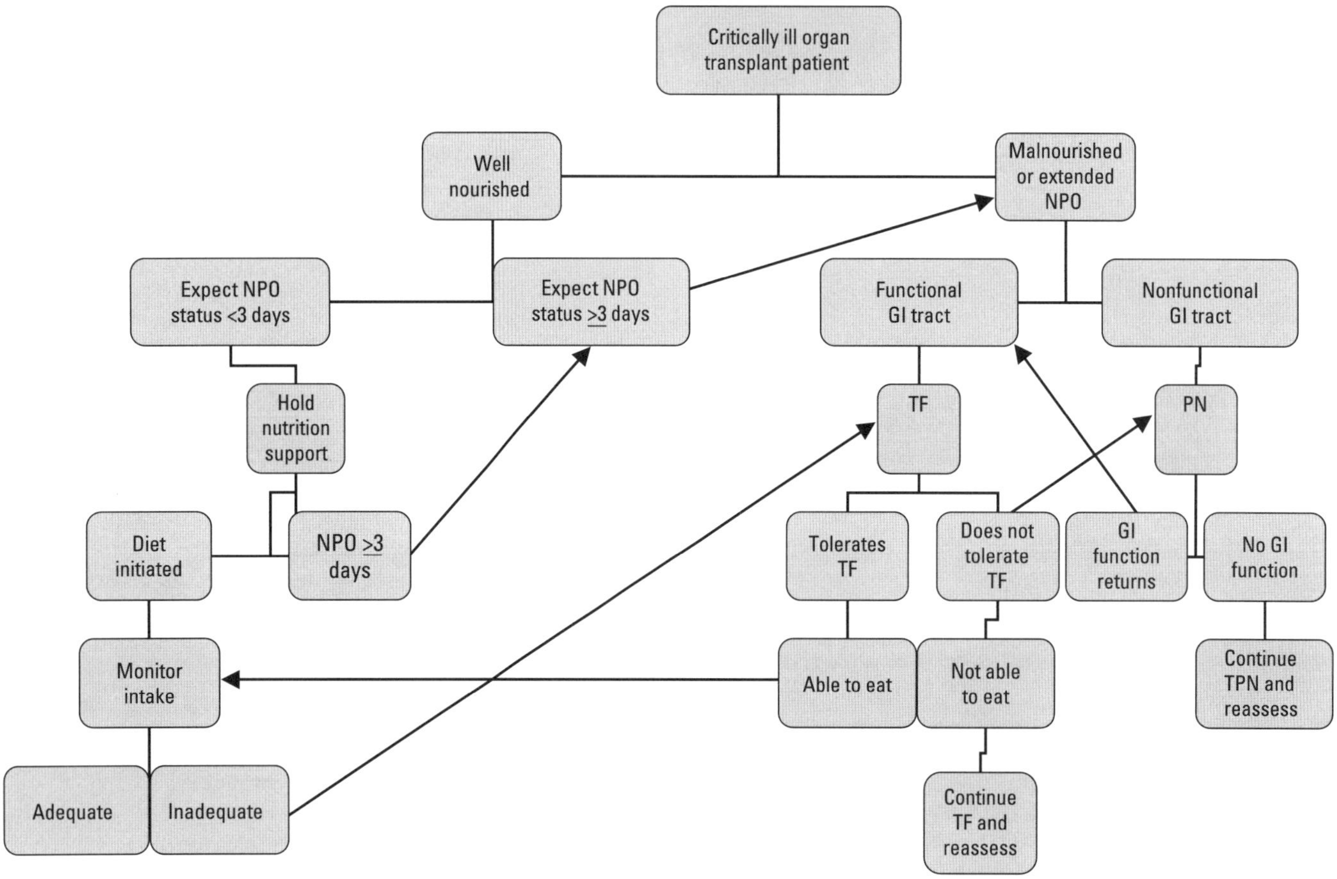

Reprinted with permission from Hasse JM, Chinnakotla S. Solid organ transplantation. In: Cresci G, ed. *Nutrition Support for the Critically Ill Patient: A Guide to Practice.* Boca Raton, FL: CRC Press; in press.

7. Severe esophagitis (when tube feeding or oral diet is not tolerated)
8. Small-bowel transplantation[9,43]
   a) PN is usually initiated within 24 to 48 hours posttransplant when the patient and his or her electrolyte and fluid status are stable.
   b) PN is continued until the patient can meet about 50% of estimated needs with enteral nutrition.
   c) PN may need to be resumed if the patient experiences severe rejection or infection.

B. Formula selection
1. Provide solution that most closely meets needs and is tolerated.
2. For small-bowel transplant patients, providing glutamine supplement may improve repair of small-bowel mucosa.[111,112]

C. Complications
1. See Chapter 8. In addition, consider hydration and weight; fluid balance and weight should be closely monitored, noting edema and ascites and losses (urine, stool, ostomy, drains).
2. Posttransplant patients may be at greater risk for hyperglycemia and hypertriglyceridemia secondary to immunosuppressive medications.

D. Home PN
1. Adult small-bowel transplant recipients may require home PN to provide all or part of their nutrition needs.
2. Most pediatric intestinal transplant recipients are weaned from PN prior to discharge from the hospital.

IX. Oral Nutrition

A. Diet initiation
1. Adult—varies among transplant type
   a) Heart, lung. Diet is usually initiated within 24 to 48 hours posttransplant.
   b) Kidney. Diet is usually initiated within 24 hours posttransplant; diet is restricted as needed (ie, fluid, potassium, sodium, phosphorus, and concentrated carbohydrates).
   c) Liver. Diet is usually initiated within 48 to 72 hours posttransplant; most frequent diet restriction is concentrated carbohydrates for hyperglycemia.
   d) Pancreas. Diet is usually initiated within 5 days posttransplant when nasogastric decompression is discontinued; a prokinetic agent may be needed for gastroparesis.
   e) Small-bowel transplant[9]
      (1) Oral diet is not initiated until tube feeding tolerance has been established, about 1 to 2 weeks posttransplant.
      (2) Low-fat, lactose-free, no-caffeine diet is provided (lymphatics and lacteals are severed at time of transplant; a lactase deficiency may exist); the low-fat and lactose-free restrictions should be continued for 4 to 6 weeks posttransplant.
      (3) A prokinetic agent or antidiarrheal may be indicated depending on GI motility.
2. Pediatric
   a) Oral diets are initiated 3 to 4 days posttransplant if the patient is extubated and bowel function has returned.
   b) A clear liquid is usually initiated; the diet is advanced to a regular diet as tolerated.

B. Oral supplements. Use of oral nutrition supplements is encouraged to improve calorie and protein intake. Select a supplement on the basis of patient age, diet restrictions, and preference.

C. Monitoring and intervention
1. Patients frequently complain of decreased appetite, dysgeusia, early satiety, abdominal fullness, bloating, or food aversions.
2. Monitor patients for vomiting, diarrhea, abdominal distension, or other GI complications.
3. Initiate calorie counts to monitor the transition from parenteral or enteral nutrition to oral intake.
4. Appetite enhancers (eg, megestrol acetate) can be considered for adult patients with loss of appetite and without functional swallow problems.
5. Dysphagia
   a) Dysphagia frequently occurs in posttransplant patients who require prolonged intubation, who have tracheostomies, and/or who have physical deconditioning.
   b) Swallow evaluations and/or dysphagiagrams are indicated to evaluate patients' capacity for oral intake and safe progression of diet.

X. Patient Education

A. Discuss nutrient intake goals with patients and caregivers to achieve improvement in nutritional status (and growth in children). Goals are individualized and should be reassessed during follow-up visits.

B. Maintenance needs for adults:
1. Calories: 1.2 to 1.3 × basal energy expenditure (BEE) to maintain weight; small-bowel transplant patients may need higher calorie amounts at 1.3 to 1.5 × BEE.
2. Protein: 0.8 to 1.3 g/kg (depends partly on maintenance corticosteroid dose); small-bowel recipients require 1.0 to 1.5 g/kg.
3. Carbohydrate: 50% to 60% of calories adjusting for hyperglycemia control; 20 g to 30 g fiber per day; small-bowel transplants should include lactose as tolerated.
4. Fat: 25% to 35% total calories, 10% to 15% of calories as monounsaturated fat, <300 mg cholesterol; for small-bowel transplants, reintroduce long-chain triglycerides as tolerated.

C. Instruct the patient and caregivers about individualized diet modifications for
1. Weight control—calorie-controlled diet, behavior control related to eating habits and hyperphagia from corticosteroids, daily activity, and exercise
2. Diabetes mellitus—carbohydrate-controlled diet, self-monitoring of blood glucose, medication administration, daily activity, and exercise
3. Dyslipidemia—low saturated fat, low simple carbohydrate, calorie-controlled diet; weight maintenance; possibly drug therapy and/or fish oil therapy; daily activity; and exercise
4. HTN—2 to 4 g per day sodium diet, weight maintenance, possibly drug therapy, daily activity, and exercise
5. Electrolyte balance—monitoring of potassium, phosphorus, and magnesium; restricting or supplementing as needed
6. Vitamin/mineral supplementation—daily multivitamin and mineral supplement; consideration of need for additional calcium and vitamin D for osteopenia

D. Food safety[113]
1. Adequately cook all animal foods.
   a) No raw seafood (eg, sushi, raw oysters, ceviche)
   b) No raw eggs
2. Wash fresh fruits and vegetables with a scrub brush, even when the outer covering will not be consumed.
3. Certain foods are prohibited:
   a) Grapefruit, grapefruit juice—contain flavonoids, naringin, and aglycone naringenin, which inhibit cytochrome P450 enzymes and increase serum concentrations of cyclosporine and tacrolimus

b) Herbal supplements—may affect levels of immunosuppressive drugs
c) Alcohol—usually discouraged. Each transplant center has its own guidelines regarding alcohol consumption.

REFERENCES

1. Facts on liver transplantation. Available at: http://www.liverfoundation.org. Accessed March 1, 2004.
2. Rosen HR, Shackleton CR, Martin P. Indications for and timing of liver transplantation. *Med Clin North Am.* 1996;80:1069–1101.
3. Scientific Registry of Transplant Recipients. Available at: http://www.ustransplant.org. Accessed April 1, 2004.
4. Whitington P, Alonso E. General criteria for pediatric transplantation. In: Busuttil RW, Klintmalm GB, eds. *Transplantation of the Liver.* Philadelphia, PA: W. B. Saunders; 1996:159–175.
5. Blue LS. Adult kidney transplantation. In: Hasse JM, Blue LS, eds. *Comprehensive Guide to Transplant Nutrition.* Chicago, IL: American Dietetic Association; 2002:44–57.
6. Seikaly M, Ho PL, Emmett L, Tejani A. The 12th annual report of the North American Pediatric Renal Transplant Cooperative Study: renal transplantation from 1987 through 1998. *Pediatr Transplant.* 2001;5:215–231.
7. Gruessner A, Sutherland DER. Pancreas transplantation in the United States (US) and non-US as reported to the United Network for Organ Sharing (UNOS) and the International Pancreas Transplant Registry (IPTR). In: Cecka JM, Teraksi PI, eds. *Clinical Transplantation 1998.* Los Angeles, CA: UCLA Tissue Typing Laboratory; 1999:53–71.
8. Markmann JF, Deng S, Huang X, et al. Insulin independence following isolated islet transplantation and single islet infusions. *Ann Surg.* 2003;237(6):741–750.
9. Weseman R. Adult small bowel transplantation. In: Hasse JM, Blue LS, eds. *Comprehensive Guide to Transplant Nutrition.* Chicago, IL: American Dietetic Association; 2002:106–122.
10. Iyer KR, Iverson AK, DeVoll-Zabrocki A, Buckman S, Horslen S, Langnas A. Pediatric intestinal transplantation: review of current practice. *NCP Bull.* 2002;17:350–360.
11. Dionig P, Alessiani M, Ferrez A. Irreversible intestinal failure, nutrition support, and small bowel transplantation. *Nutrition.* 2001;17:747–750.
12. Kumar N, Grant D. Gastrointestinal transplantation: an update. *Liver Transpl.* 2000;6(4):515–519.
13. Nishidi S, Levi D, Kato T, et al. Ninety-five cases of intestinal transplantation at the University of Miami. *J Gastrointest Surg.* 2002;6(2):233–239.
14. Pahwa N, Hedberg AM. Adult heart and lung transplantation. In: Hasse JM, Blue LS, eds. *Comprehensive Guide to Transplant Nutrition.* Chicago, IL: American Dietetic Association; 2002:31–43.
15. Berg A. Pediatric heart transplantation: a clinical overview. *Crit Care Nurs.* 2002;25(3):79–87.
16. Madill J, Gutierrez C, Grossman J, et al. Nutrition assessment of the lung transplant patient: body mass index as a predictor of 90-day mortality following transplantation. *J Heart Lung Transplant.* 2001;20(3):288–296.
17. Boucek M, Edwards L, Keck B, et al. The Registry of the International Society for Heart and Lung Transplantation: Fifth Official Pediatric Report—2001 to 2002. *J Heart Lung Transplant.* 2002;21(8):827–840.
18. Selberg O, Bottcher J, Tusch G, Pichlmayer R, Henkel E, Muller M. Identification of high- and low-risk patients before liver transplantation: a prospective cohort study of nutritional and metabolic parameters in 150 patients. *Hepatology.* 1996;25(3):652–657.
19. Porayko MK, DiCecco S, O'Keefe SJ. Impact of malnutrition and its therapy on liver transplantation. *Semin Liver Dis.* 1991;11(4):305–314.
20. Lautz H, Selberg O, Körber M, Bürger M, Müller MJ. Protein-calorie malnutrition in liver cirrhosis. *Clin Invest.* 1992;70:478–486.
21. Harrison J, McKiernan J, Neuberger JM. A prospective study on the effect of recipient nutritional status on outcome in liver transplantation. *Transpl Int.* 1997;10:369–374.
22. Pikul J, Sharpe MD, Lowndes R, Ghent CN. Degree of preoperative malnutrition is predictive of postoperative morbidity and mortality in liver transplant recipients. *Transplantation.* 1994;57(3):469–472.
23. Hasse JM, Gonwa TA, Jennings LW, et al. Malnutrition affects liver transplant outcomes [abstract]. *Transplantation.* 1998;66:S53.
24. Figueiredo F, Dickson ER, Pasha T, et al. Impact of nutritional status on outcomes after liver transplantation. *Transplantation.* 2000;70(9):1347–1352.
25. Stephenson GR, Moreth EW, El-Moalem H, Clavien PA, Tuttle-Newhall JE. Preoperative subjective global assessment is predictive of outcome after liver transplantation. *Transplantation.* 2001;72(4):666–670.
26. Frazier OH, Van Buren CT, Poindexter SM, Waldenberger F. Nutritional management of the heart transplant recipient. *Heart Transplant.* 1985;4(4):450–452.
27. Becker BN, Becker YT, Heisey DM, et al. The impact of hypoalbuminemia in kidney-pancreas transplant recipients. *Transplantation.* 1999;68(1):72–75.
28. Ricci P, Therneau T, Malinchoc M, et al. A prognostic model for the outcome of liver transplantation in patients with cholestatic liver disease. *Hepatology.* 1997;25(3):672–677.
29. Hade AM, Shine AM, Kennedy NP, McCormick PA. Both under-nutrition and obesity increase morbidity following liver transplantation. *Ir Med J.* 2003;97(5):140–142.
30. Moreso F, Serón D, Anunciada AI, et al. Recipient body surface area as a predictor of posttransplant renal allograft evolution. *Transplantation.* 1998;65(5):671–676.
31. Pirsch JD, Armbrust MJ, Knechtle SJ, et al. Obesity as a risk factor following renal transplantation. *Transplantation.* 1995;59(4):631–633.
32. Holley JL, Shapiro R, Lopatin WB, Tzakis AG, Hakala TR, Starzl TE. Obesity as a risk factor following cadaveric renal transplantation. *Transplantation.* 1990;49(2):387–389.
33. Drafts HH, Anjum MR, Wynn JJ, Mulloy LL, Bowley JN, Humphries AL. The impact of pretransplant obesity on renal transplant outcomes. *Clin Transplant.* 1997;11:493–496.
34. Baumgardner GL, Henry ML, Elkhammas E, et al. Obesity as a risk factor after combined pancreas/kidney transplantation. *Transplantation.* 1995;60(12):1426–1430.
35. Gill IS, Hodge EE, Novick AC, Steinmuller DR, Garred D. Impact of obesity on renal transplantation. *Transplant Proc.* 1993;25:1047–1048.
36. Wilson GA, Bumbgardner GL, Henry ML, et al. Decreased graft survival rate in obese pancreas/kidney recipients. *Transplant Proc.* 1995;27:3106–3107.
37. Halme L, Eklund B, Kyllönen L, Salmela K. Is obesity still a risk factor in renal transplantation? *Transpl Int.* 1997;10:284–288.
38. Meier-Kriesche HU, Vaghela M, Thambuganipalle R, Friedman G, Jacobs M, Kaplan B. The effect of body mass index on long-term renal allograft survival. *Transplantation.* 1999;68(9):1294–1297.
39. Testa G, Hasse JM, Jennings LW, et al. Morbid obesity is not an independent risk factor for liver transplantation [abstract]. *Transplantation.* 1998;66:S53.
40. Braunfeld MYY, Chan S, Pregler J, et al. Liver transplantation in the morbidly obese. *J Clin Anesth.* 1996;8:585–590.
41. Sawyer RG, Pelletier SJ, Pruett TL. Increased early morbidity and mortality with acceptable long-term function in severely obese patients undergoing liver transplantation. *Clin Transplant.* 1999;13:126–130.
42. Hasse JM. Adult liver transplantation. In: Hasse JM, Blue LS, eds. *Comprehensive Guide to Transplant Nutrition.* Chicago, IL: American Dietetic Association; 2002:58–89.
43. Strohm S, Reyes J, Koehler AN. Pediatric small bowel transplantation. In: Hasse JM, Blue LS, eds. *Comprehensive Guide to Transplant Nutrition.* Chicago, IL: American Dietetic Association; 2002:216–225.
44. Obayashi PAC. Adult pancreas transplantation. In: Hasse JM, Blue LS, eds. *Comprehensive Guide to Transplant Nutrition.* Chicago, IL: American Dietetic Association; 2002:90–105.
45. Becht MB, Pedersen S, Ryckman F, Balistreri W. Growth and nutritional management of pediatric patients after orthotopic liver transplantation. *Gastroenterol Clin North Am.* 1993;22:367–380.
46. Fulton JA, McKenna A. Pediatric lung transplantation. In: Hasse JM, Blue LS, eds. *Comprehensive Guide to Transplant Nutrition.* Chicago, IL: American Dietetic Association; 2002:153–171.
47. Connolly C. Pediatric kidney transplantation. In: Hasse JM, Blue LS, eds. *Comprehensive Guide to Transplant Nutrition.* Chicago, IL: American Dietetic Association; 2002:172–181.

48. Sutton MM. Pediatric liver transplantation. In: Hasse JM, Blue LS, eds. *Comprehensive Guide to Transplant Nutrition.* Chicago, IL: American Dietetic Association; 2002:182–215.
49. Ford EG. Nutrition support of pediatric patients. *Nutr Clin Pract.* 1996;11: 183–191.
50. Smith P. Primary care in children with congenital heart disease. *J Pediatr Nurs.* 2001;16(5):308–319.
51. Shulman R, Phillips S. Parenteral nutrition in infants and children. *J Pediatr Gastroenterol Nutr.* 2003;36:587–607.
52. du Plessis AS, Randall H, Escreet E, et al. Nutritional status of renal transplant patients. *S Afr Med J.* 2002;92(1):68–74.
53. Arnadottir M, Hultberg B, Vladov V, Nilsson-Ehle P, Thysell H. Hyperhomocysteinemia in cyclosporine-treated renal transplant recipients. *Transplantation.* 1996;61(3):509–512.
54. Arnadottir M, Hultberg B, Wahlberg J, Fellström B, Dimény E. Serum total homocysteine concentration before and after renal transplantation. *Kidney Int.* 1998;54:1380–1384.
55. Huh W, Kim B, Kim SJ, et al. Changes of fasting plasma total homocysteine in the early phase of renal transplantation. *Transplant Proc.* 2000;32: 2811–2813.
56. Fonseca I, Queirós JM, Satos JM, et al. Hyperhomocysteinemia in renal transplantation: preliminary results. *Transplant Proc.* 2000;32:2602–2604.
57. Kim SI, Yoo TH, Song HY, et al. Hyperhomocysteinemia in renal transplant recipients with cyclosporine. *Transplant Proc.* 2000;32:1878–1879.
58. Stein G, Muller A, Busch M, Fleck C, Sperschneider H. Homocysteine, its metabolites, and B-group vitamins in renal transplant patients. *Kidney Int.* 2001;59(suppl 78):262–265.
59. Trust NHS. The effect of dietary intervention on weight gain after renal transplantation. *J Ren Nutr.* 1998;8:137–141.
60. Mor E, Facklam D, Hasse J, et al. Weight gain and lipid profile changes in liver transplant recipients. long term results of the American FK506 multi center study. *Transplant Proc.* 1995;27:1126.
61. Everhart JE, Lombardero J, Lake JR, Wiesner RH, Zetterman RK, Hoofnagle JH. Weight change and obesity after liver transplantation: incidence and risk factors. *Liver Transplant Surg.* 1998;4:285–296.
62. Ragsdale D. Nutritional program for heart transplantation. *J Heart Transplant.* 1987;6(4):228–233.
63. Hussaini SH, Oldroyd B, Stewart SP, et al. Effects of orthotopic liver transplantation on body composition. *Liver.* 1998;18(3):173–179.
64. Pischon T, Sharma AM. Obesity as a risk factor in renal transplant patients. *Nephrol Dial Transplant.* 2001;16:14–17.
65. Lopes IM, Martin N, Errasti P, Martinez JA. Benefits of a dietary intervention on weight loss, body composition and lipid profile after renal transplantation. *Nutrition.* 1999;15:7–10.
66. Hines L. Can lowfat/cholesterol nutrition counseling improve food intake habits and hyperlipidemia of renal transplant patients? *J Ren Nutr.* 2000;10:30–35.
67. Munoz SJ. Long term management of the liver transplant recipient. *Med Clin North Am.* 1996;80:1103–1120.
68. Navasa M, Bustamante J, Morroni C, et al. Diabetes mellitus after liver transplantation: prevalence and predictive factors. *J Hepatol.* 1996;65: 64–71.
69. Weir MR, Fink JC. Risk for posttransplant diabetes mellitus with current immunosuppressive medications. *Am J Kidney Dis.* 1999;34:1–13.
70. Obayashi PAC. Posttransplant diabetes mellitus: cause, impact, and treatment options. *Nutr Clin Pract.* 2004;19:165–171.
71. Davidson J, Wilkinson A, Dantal J, et al. New-onset diabetes after transplantation: 2003 international consensus guidelines. *Transplantation.* 2003;75(10, suppl):SS3–SS24.
72. Marchetti P. New-onset diabetes after transplantation. *J Heart Lung Transplant.* 2004;23:S194–S201.
73. Gentile S, Turco S, Torella R. Diabetes mellitus after liver transplantation: a possible relation with the nutritional status. *Diabetes Res Clin Pract.* 1998;41:203–205.
74. Jindal RM, Sidner RA, Milgrom ML. Post-transplant diabetes mellitus: the role of immunosuppression. *Drug Saf.* 1997;16(4):242–257.
75. Heisel O, Heisel R, Balshaw R, Keown P. New onset diabetes mellitus in patients receiving calcineurin inhibitors: a systematic review and meta-analysis. *Am J Transplant.* 2004;4:583–595.
76. Silva F, Queirós J, Vargas G, Henriques A, Sarmento A, Guimarãs S. Risk factors for posttransplant diabetes mellitus and impact of this complication after renal transplantation. *Transplant Proc.* 2000;32:2609–2610.
77. Jawad F, Rizvi SAH. Posttransplant diabetes mellitus in live-related renal transplantation. *Transplant Proc.* 2000:32:1888.
78. Ulivieri FM, Piodi LP, Aroldi A, Cesana BM. Effect of kidney transplantation on bone mass and body composition in males. *Transplantation.* 2002;73(4):612–615.
79. Aroldi A, Tarantino A, Montagnino G, Cesana B, Cocucci C, Ponticelli C. Effects of three immunosuppressive regimens on vertebral bone density in renal transplant recipients. *Transplantation.* 1997;63:380–386.
80. Kwan JTC, Almond MK, Evans K, Cunningham J. Changes in total body bone mineral content and regional bone mineral density in renal patients following renal transplantation. *Miner Electrolyte Metab.* 1992;18:166–168.
81. Epstein S, Shane E, Bilezikian JP. Organ transplantation and osteoporosis. *Curr Opin Rheumatol.* 1995;7:255–261.
82. Braith RW, Mills RM, Welsch MA, Keller JW, Pollock ML. Resistance exercise training restores bone mineral density in heart transplant recipients. *J Am Coll Cardiol.* 1996;28(6):1471–1477.
83. Isoniemi H, Appelberg J, Nilsson C-G, Makela P, Risteli J, Hockerstedt K. Transdermal oestrogen therapy protects postmenopausal liver transplant women from osteoporosis. A 2-year follow-up study. *J Hepatol.* 2001;34: 299–305.
84. Reeves HL, Francis RM, Mana DM, Hudson M, Day CP. Intravenous bisphosphonate prevents symptomatic osteoporotic vertebral collapse in patients after liver transplantation. *Liver Transpl Surg.* 1998;4(5):404–409.
85. Ninkovic M, Love S, Tom BDM, Bearcroft PW, Alexander GJ, Compston JE. Lack of effect of intravenous pamidronate on fracture incidence and bone mineral density after orthotopic liver transplantation. *J Hepatol.* 2002;37:93–100.
86. Kasiske BL, Uman AJ. Persistent hyperlipidemia in renal transplant patients. *Medicine.* 1987;66:309–316.
87. Baumgardner GL, Wilson GA, Tso PL, et al. Impact of serum lipids on long term graft and patient survival after renal transplantation. *Transplantation.* 1995;60:1418–1421.
88. Eich D, Thompson JA, Ko D, et al. Hypercholesterolemia in long-term survivors of heart transplantation: an early marker of accelerated coronary artery disease. *J Heart Lung Transplant.* 1991;10(1 pt 1):45–49.
89. Balistreri W, Bucuvalas J, Ryckman F. The effect of immunosuppression on growth and development. *Liver Transplant Surg.* 1995;1(5, suppl 1):64–73.
90. Fine RN. Growth following solid-organ transplantation. *Pediatr Transplant.* 2002;6:47–52.
91. Furth S, Hwang W, Yang C, Neu A, Fivush B, Powe N. Growth failure, risk of hospitalization and death for children with end-stage renal disease. *Pediatr Nephrol.* 2002;17:450–455.
92. Simon D, Rosilio M, Maisin A, et al. Post graft development of short children treated with growth hormone before kidney graft. *Pediatr Nephrol.* 1999;13:723–729.
93. Iverson AK. Long term growth and nutritional status in pediatric small bowel transplant [abstract]. *Nutr Clin Pract.* 2002;17:56.
94. Mitsnefes MM, Omoloja A, McEnery PT. Short-term pediatric renal transplant survival: blood pressure and allograft function. *Pediatr Transplant.* 2001;5:160–165.
95. Atkison P, Ross C, Williams S, et al. Long-term results of pediatric liver transplantation in a combined pediatric and adult transplant program. *CMAJ.* 2002;166(13):1663–1671.
96. Sprague S. Mechanism of transplantation-associated bone loss. *Pediatr Nephrol.* 2002;14:650–653.
97. Guest JE, Hasse J. Nutritional aspects of pediatric liver transplantation. In: Busuttil RW, Klintmalm GB, eds. *Transplantation of the Liver.* Philadelphia, PA: W. B. Saunders; 1996:227–235.
98. Silverstein D, Palmer J, Polinsky M, Braas C, Conley S, Baluarte HJ. Risk factors for hyperlipidemia in long-term pediatric renal transplant recipients. *Pediatr Nephrol.* 2000;14:105–110.

99. Chin C, Rosenthal D, Bernstein D. Lipoprotein abnormalities are highly prevalent in pediatric heart transplant recipients. *Pediatr Transplant.* 2000;4:193–199.
100. Greenspan L, Gitelman S, Leung MA, Glidden D, Mathias R. Increased incidence in post-transplant diabetes mellitus in children: a case-control analysis. *Pediatr Nephrol.* 2002;17:1–5.
101. Hasse JM, Blue LS, Liepa GU, et al. Early enteral nutrition support in patients undergoing liver transplantation. *J Parenter Enteral Nutr.* 1995; 19:437–443.
102. Sekido H, Matsuo K, Takeda D, et al. Impact of early enteral nutrition after liver transplantation for acute hepatic failure: report of four cases. *Transplant Proc.* 2003;35:369–371.
103. Anbar R, Lipa R, Zinger P, Mor E. The role of nutritional support in transplant recipients: two case reports. *Transplant Proc.* 2003;35:614–616.
104. Wicks C, Somasundaram S, Bjarnason I, et al. Comparison of enteral feeding and total parenteral nutrition after liver transplantation. *Lancet.* 1994; 344:837–840.
105. Mehta PL, Alaka KJ, Filo RS, Leapman SB, Milgrom ML, Pescovitz MD. Nutrition support following liver transplantation: a comparison of jejunal versus parenteral routes. *Clin Transplant.* 1995;344:837–840.
106. Pescovitz MD, Mehta PL, Leapman SB, Milgrom ML, Jindal RM, Filo RS. Tube jejunostomy in liver transplant recipients. *Surgery.* 1995;117:642–647.
107. Rayes N, Seehofer D, Hansen S, et al. Early enteral supply of lactobacillus and fiber versus selective bowel decontamination: a controlled trial in liver transplant recipients. *Transplantation.* 2002;74(1):123–128.
108. Strohm S, Koehler A, Mazariegos G, Reyes J. Nutrition management in pediatric small bowel transplant. *Nutr Clin Pract.* 1999;14(2):58–63.
109. Buttiker V, Fanconi S, Burger R. Chylothorax in children: guidelines for diagnosis and management. *Chest.* 1999;116:682–687.
110. Sodhi S, Guo JP, Maurer A, O'Brien G, Srinivasan R, Parkman H. Gastroparesis after combined heart and lung transplantation. *J Clin Gastroenterol.* 2002;34(1):34–39.
111. Nemoto A, Krajack A, Suzuki T, et al. Glutamine metabolism of intestine grafts: influence of mucosal injury by prolonged preservation and transplantation. *Transplant Proc.* 1996;28:2545–2546.
112. Schroeder P, Schweizer E, Blomer A, Deltz E. Glutamine prevents mucosal injury after small bowel transplantation. *Transplant Proc.* 1992; 24:1104.
113. Cabelof D. Preventing infection from foodborne pathogens in liver transplant patients. *J Am Diet Assoc.* 1994;94(10):1140–1144.

Paula M. Charuhas, MS, RD, FADA, CNSD;
Ann Lipkin, MS, RD, CNSD;
Polly Lenssen, MS, RD, FADA;
Kerry McMillen, MS, RD

13

Hematopoietic Stem Cell Transplantation

Introduction

Hematopoietic stem cell transplantation (HSCT) is an accepted therapeutic modality for many diseases, including hematologic malignancies, some malignant solid tumors, immunodeficiency syndromes, nonmalignant hematologic disorders of the bone marrow, inherited storage diseases, and some autoimmune disorders. The objective is to replace the malignant or defective marrow to restore hematopoietic and immunologic function. While the diversity of applications for and approaches to HSCT has expanded significantly in the last decade, it remains a highly morbid treatment in terms of potentially fatal toxicities, nutrition implications, and, among children, developmental sequelae. This chapter reviews the nutritional consequences of HSCT and offers guidelines for nutrition management of transplant-related complications and nutrition support practices.

I. Overview of Diseases and Conditions Treated by HSCT[1]

A. Hematologic malignancies: acute leukemias; chronic leukemias; lymphomas; multiple myeloma; myelodysplastic syndromes (ie, refractory anemias)
B. Malignant solid tumors: advanced-stage neuroblastoma; refractory Ewing's sarcoma; ovarian cancer; prostate cancer; testicular cancer; renal cell carcinoma
C. Immunologic disorders: severe combined immunodeficiency disease; Wiskott-Aldrich syndrome; other cellular immunodeficiencies
D. Nonneoplastic disorders of hematopoiesis: severe aplastic anemia; β-thalassemia major; Fanconi's anemia; paroxysmal nocturnal hemoglobinuria
E. Nonmalignant congenital disorders: storage diseases (ie, Gaucher's disease); lysosomal diseases (ie, Lesch-Nyhan syndrome); mucopolysaccharidoses (ie, Hurler's syndrome; Hunter's disease); mucolipidoses (ie, metachromatic leukodystrophy; Niemann-Pick disease); infantile osteopetrosis
F. Autoimmune disorders: multiple sclerosis; systemic lupus erythematosus; systemic sclerosis

II. Types of Transplants

A. The objective of HSCT is to replace the malignant or defective bone marrow to restore hematopoietic and immunologic function.
B. The preparative conditioning regimen consists of cytotoxic chemotherapy directed at eradicating the malignancy or defective stem cells with or without total body irradiation (TBI) and possibly local irradiation.
    1. Myeloablative conditioning regimens deliver high-dose chemotherapy and radiation to eliminate disease and ablate bone marrow.
    2. Some myeloablative regimens use reduced conditioning to reduce toxicity.
    3. Nonmyeloablative conditioning regimens deliver low-dose chemotherapy and radiation to develop a mixed immune system or chimera. Candidates for nonmyeloablative conditioning regimens include
        a) Older patients
        b) Patients with relapsed malignancy following myeloablative HSCT
        c) Patients with pretransplant comorbidities (ie, hepatic compromise) that make them ineligible for conventional transplant
        d) Patients with nonmalignant disorders in which it is not necessary to ablate diseased tissues
C. An infusion of hematopoietic stem cells follows the conditioning regimen.
D. Sources for new stem cells are
    1. Bone marrow
    2. Peripheral blood
    3. Umbilical cord blood
E. Three types of HSCT[1]
    1. Autologous: patient receives stem cells from him- or herself
    2. Syngeneic: patient receives stem cells from a genetically identical twin
    3. Allogeneic: patient receives stem cells from a related or unrelated donor

III. Nutritional Aspects of HSCT

A. Multiple oral and gastrointestinal (GI) toxicities
    1. Mucositis and esophagitis
        a) These involve an inflammation of the epithelial tissue that may vary in severity from cracked and painful lips and mouth sores (ulcers on tongue/cheek) to bleeding mucosa with epithelial loss. The mucositis may be present throughout the entire GI tract.
        b) They are an expected complication of myeloablative conditioning regimens; often, oral or intravenous (IV) opioids are needed for pain management.
        c) Methotrexate, used to prevent graft-versus-host disease (GVHD), aggravates ulceration and thinning of the oral mucosa.
        d) Symptoms may develop as early as 4 days after chemotherapy and several days after TBI starts.

e) Healing begins with marrow engraftment (absolute neutrophil count >500/cm^3).

f) Oral glutamine supplementation has not been effective in decreasing the incidence or severity of mucositis.[2]

2. Altered salivation
   a) Xerostomia (oral dryness) is associated primarily with TBI but also with antiemetics, antidepressants, and opiate-containing pain medications.
   b) Saliva production diminishes and saliva becomes thick and viscous.
3. Taste alterations
   a) Dysgeusia (impaired taste) and hypogeusia (diminished taste) are primarily an effect of TBI.
   b) Medications such as morphine and antibiotics may induce taste changes.
   c) Altered salivation and dry mouth affect taste due to decreased saliva production. Saliva is essential for taste perception, as food particles must be in solution to stimulate taste bud receptor cells.[3] Taste loss is temporary, with recovery between 30 and 50 days posttransplant.[4]
   d) Sweet is the first taste to return, followed by bitter, sour, and salty.[4]
4. Nausea and vomiting
   a) These are associated with the preparative conditioning regimen, such as myeloablative agents (alkylating agents, TBI); other supportive care medications (antibiotics, cyclosporine, interleukin-2, trimethoprim-sulfamethoxazole, and mycophenolate mofetil); GI infections (eg, cytomegalovirus, *Helicobacter pylori*); intestinal GVHD; and fluid and electrolyte imbalances.
   b) Antiemetics are routinely administered to prevent and control symptoms. Initially, postablation symptoms are severe and patients often require regularly scheduled IV antiemetics. IV antiemetics are changed to oral forms with symptom improvement.
5. Anorexia
   a) Anorexia has a multifactorial etiology.
   b) Loss of appetite during and immediately postconditioning therapy may be related to mouth pain, nausea and vomiting, electrolyte imbalances, psychological factors, and medications. After engraftment, loss of appetite may stem from these factors as well as ongoing delayed gastric emptying, taste alterations, GI infections, esophageal ulcers, or upper intestinal GVHD.
   c) Prolonged use of parenteral nutrition (PN) post-HSCT has been associated with anorexia and delayed resumption of oral intake.[5]
6. Diarrhea and steatorrhea
   a) Diarrhea is associated with high-dose cytoreductive therapy, oral antibiotics, intestinal infections, GI GVHD, lactose intolerance, gastric motility agents, and magnesium salts.
   b) Liver and intestinal GVHD may produce steatorrhea and fat malabsorption.
7. Dietary guidelines for managing oral and GI toxicities associated with HSCT are shown in Table 13-1.[6]

B. Sinusoidal obstructive syndrome (SOS) (also known as hepatic veno-occlusive disease)

1. SOS is the leading cause of morbidity and mortality in the first 2 months posttransplant.
   a) The incidence varies from 1% to 2% in some conditions (ie, thalassemia) but may be as high as 50% in patients with preexisting hepatic compromise.[7]
   b) Patients with a history of hepatitis and second transplants are at increased risk of developing SOS.
   c) SOS is characterized by subendothelial edema, endothelial cell damage with microthrombosis, fibrin deposition, and expression of factor VIII and von Willebrand's factors within venular walls. Hepatic necrosis follows these events in severe SOS, with a reported survival of 38%.[8]
   d) Clinical symptoms associated with SOS:
      (1) Weight gain with concomitant ascites
      (2) Increased serum bilirubin and jaundice
      (3) Hepatomegaly
      (4) In severe cases, hepatorenal failure and encephalopathy
2. Nutrition management of SOS
   a) Minimize fluid retention by concentrating PN fluids.
   b) Eliminate sodium from PN and diet.
   c) Remove or reduce copper and manganese from PN for persistent hyperbilirubinemia (ie, serum bilirubin >10.0 mg/dL). Ensure that patient continues to receive adequate zinc.
   d) Monitor serum triglyceride levels. If fasting serum levels are >500 mg/dL, provide a minimal amount of IV fat emulsion (ie, 4%–8% of total energy support).
   e) Consider obtaining indirect calorimetry measurements to ensure that the patient is not being overfed, and adjust energy support as appropriate.

C. GVHD

1. GVHD is a T-cell–mediated immunologic reaction of engrafted lymphoid cells against the tissues of the host.
2. The incidence increases in mismatched and unrelated donor transplants.[9]
3. The major target organs affected are the skin, mouth, GI tract, and liver. Ocular and pulmonary symptoms have also been described.[9]
   a) Skin GVHD is characterized by a pruritic, maculopapular, and erythematous rash. In severe cases, it may evolve into ulcerations, blisters, and desquamation that necessitates burn care. Chronic skin GVHD can result in pigment changes, contracture, and scleroderma.
   b) Oral GVHD is associated with pain, ranging from mild sensitivity to frank mucosal ulceration. Oral GVHD may also cause xerostomia.
   c) Gastrointestinal GVHD
      (1) Esophageal complications associated with GVHD include dysphagia with esophageal webbing or strictures.
      (2) Intestinal complications are characterized by anorexia, nausea, vomiting, severe abdominal pain/cramping, and high-volume watery diarrhea. In severe cases, the disease may be life-threatening, with mucosal ulceration, extensive bleeding, and mucosal sloughing. Mucosal degeneration associated with GVHD also induces fat malabsorption and intestinal protein losses (ie, protein-losing enteropathy). Upper-gut GVHD is characterized by anorexia, nausea, and vomiting.
   d) Liver GVHD presents as cholestasis, elevated alkaline phosphatase and serum bilirubin levels, jaundice, hepatomegaly, and, in severe cases, encephalopathy and hepatorenal failure.
4. Nutritional consequences associated with GVHD can be extensive. Hypermetabolism, tissue damage, fluid and electrolyte imbalances, and medication-induced effects all affect nutritional status.
5. GVHD can be hyperacute, acute, and/or chronic.
   a) Hyperacute GVHD generally occurs before engraftment and primarily affects the skin.[9]
   b) Acute GVHD develops posttransplant and is graded by several criteria (Table 13-2).[10]

TABLE 13-1. Dietary Guidelines for Managing Common Nutrition Problems Associated With HSCT

Oral and esophageal mucositis

- Try soft/puree-textured or blenderized liquid diet.
- Try smooth, bland, moist foods (custard, cream soups, mashed potatoes).
- Offer soft, nonirritating, cold foods (popsicles, ice cream, frozen yogurt, slushes).
- Encourage frequent mouth rinsing to remove food and bacteria and promote healing.

Xerostomia (oral dryness)

- Offer moist foods (stews, casseroles, canned fruit) and liquids.
- Add extra sauces, gravies, margarine, butter, and broth to foods.
- Encourage liquids with meals.
- Add vinegar or pickles to foods.
- Offer lemon-flavored, sugarless candy to help stimulate saliva.
- Encourage good oral hygiene.
- Try commercial saliva substitutes.

Thick, viscous saliva and mucous

- Encourage adequate fluid intake.
- Offer clear liquids (tea, popsicles, slushes, warm broth).
- Encourage good oral hygiene.

Dysgeusia (impaired taste)

- Flavor poultry, fish, eggs, and dairy products.
- Enhance food taste with herbs, spices, flavor extracts, and marinades.
- Offer cold, nonodorous foods.
- Offer fruit-flavored beverages.
- Try highly aromatic foods.
- Try tart foods like oranges or lemonade, which may have more taste.
- Offer fluids with meals to help take away bad tastes in the mouth.
- Encourage good oral hygiene.

Anorexia

- Offer small, frequent meals of nutrient-dense foods.
- Use carbohydrate supplements and protein powders.
- Create a pleasant mealtime atmosphere by enhancing food aromas, using colorful place settings, and offering foods with varied colors and textures.
- Involve the patient in grocery shopping, meal planning, and simple meal preparation.
- Encourage relaxation techniques and light exercise before meals, which may help improve food intake.

Nausea and vomiting

- Try high-carbohydrate foods and fluids (crackers, toast, gelatin) as well as nonacidic juices.
- Try small, frequent feedings.
- Offer cold, clear liquids and solids.
- Avoid overly sweet or high-fat foods.
- Avoid feeding in a stuffy, too-warm room or one filled with cooking odors or other potentially disagreeable odors.
- Encourage the patient to drink or sip liquids frequently throughout the day; having the patient use a straw may help.
- Encourage rest periods after meals (but discourage reclining).
- Avoid offering favorite foods when the patient is nauseated; it may cause a permanent dislike of the food.
- Observe whether there is a pattern to when nausea occurs or what causes it (specific foods, events, surroundings); suggest appropriate changes in diet or schedule.

Diarrhea

- Try a low fat, low fiber diet.
- Avoid caffeine.
- Offer cold or room-temperature foods and beverages, which may be better tolerated.
- Offer low lactose intake.
- Encourage adequate fluids to prevent dehydration.
- Avoid excessive fruit juice ingestion.

Constipation

- Encourage fluids.
- Offer a hot beverage in the morning or evening to help stimulate a bowel movement.
- Offer high-fiber foods.

Adapted with permission from Charuhas PM. Introduction to marrow transplantation. *Oncol Nutr Diet Pract Group Newsletter.* 1994;2:2–9.

c) Chronic GHVD generally develops 4 to 7 months posttransplant but has been found to occur as early as 2 months or as late as 2 years after transplant from nonidentical related and unrelated donors. The greatest risk factor for development of chronic GVHD is the prior development of acute GVHD.[11]

(1) Nutrition problems reported at 1 year post transplant in patients with chronic GVHD include weight gain, weight loss, oral sensitivity, xerostomia, stomatitis, anorexia, reflux, diarrhea, malabsorption, and osteoporosis.[12]

(2) Community-based nutrition monitoring is necessary for patients with chronic GVHD after discharge from the transplant center.

d) Table 13-3 discusses the dietary management of intestinal GVHD.[13]

e) Medications and therapy may have significant nutritional consequences (Table 13-4).[14]

D. Renal complications

1. Multifactorial etiology

a) Chemotherapeutic agents and TBI, which may cause kidney damage

b) Medications such as cyclosporine, tacrolimus, amphotericin, aminoglycosides, vancomycin, and trimethoprim-sulfamethoxazole, which are associated with renal damage and renal insufficiency

TABLE 13-2. Clinical Manifestations and Staging of Acute GVHD

Organ	Clinical manifestations	Differential	Histology	Staging
Skin	Erythematous, maculo-papular rash often involving palms and soles; may become confluent; severe disease: bullae described as tender, like a sunburn, pruritic	Chemo/radiotherapy effect, drug allergy, viral exanthem, infection	Basal vaculopathy dyskeratosis, exocytosis of lymphocytes, edema, dermal-epidermal separation	Stage 1: <25% rash Stage 2: 25% to 50% rash Stage 3: generalized erythroderma Stage 4: bullae
Liver	Painless jaundice with conjugated hyperbilirubinemia and increased alkaline phosphatase	Veno-occlusive disease, drug toxicity, viral infection, sepsis	Lymphocytic infiltration of bile ducts, bile duct damage with epithelial cell dropout	Stage 1: bili 2 to 3 mg/dL Stage 2: bili 3.1 to 6 mg/dL Stage 3: bili 6.1 to 15 mg/dL Stage 4: bili >15 mg/dL
GI tract	Upper: nausea, vomiting anorexia. Lower: diarrhea, crampy abdominal pain, distention, ileus, GI bleeding	Infection (bacterial. viral, *C. Difficile*), toxicity from conditioning regimen	Crypt cell necrosis and dropout; mucosal separation and sloughing	Stage 1: diarrhea >500 mL/day Stage 2: diarrhea >1000 mL/day Stage 3: diarrhea >1500 mL/day Stage 4: ileus, bleeding

Bili, bilirubin; GI, gastrointestinal; GVHD, Graft Versus Host Disease.
Reprinted with permission from Vogelsang GB, Lee L, Bensen-Kennedy DM. Pathogenesis and treatment of graft-versus-host disease after bone marrow transplant. *Ann Rev Med.* 2003;54:29–52.

c) Radiocontrast agents
d) Intravascular volume depletion
e) Tumor lysis syndrome
f) Sepsis
g) Hepatorenal syndrome
h) Thrombotic microangiopathies: hemolytic uremic syndrome and thrombotic thrombocytic purpura[15,16]
   (1) These are associated with TBI and exacerbated by cyclosporine.
   (2) The common pathology is partial or complete occlusion of the arterioles and capillaries by thrombi containing multiple platelet remnants. The result is consumption of platelets, fragmentation of red cells, and diverse organ dysfunction.
   (3) HSCT nephropathy presents as nephrotic syndrome with membranous nephropathy.[17]
   (4) Diffuse proliferative glomerulonephritis has also been reported and may be an effect of GVHD.[17]

2. Nutritional management
   a) Maintain sufficient intravascular volume.
   b) Correct electrolyte imbalances.
   c) Maximize nutrition within fluid allowance.
   d) If continuous venovenous hemofiltration/hemodialysis or intermittent hemodialysis is instituted,
      (1) Assay serum vitamin A levels if the patient is to continue on therapy for an extended period (correcting for retinol-binding protein levels). For patients at high risk of toxicity at low doses of parenteral vitamin A intake (ie, those with compromised liver function, those taking high-dose vitamin A supplements preadmission, or children),[18,19] discontinue or decrease IV multivitamin if appropriate depending on vitamin A and retinol binding protein levels. Toxicity symptoms are known to occur at vitamin A levels 1½ to 2 times normal[20] in some patients who develop renal failure during hospitalization and receive PN support.
      (2) Provide a complete complex of water-soluble vitamins and folic acid to compensate for ultrafiltrate losses.[21,22] Ensure that vitamin K needs are met.
      (3) Provide additional protein supplementation (baseline needs plus 0.2 mg/kg/day) to compensate for filtered amino acid losses.[23]
      (4) Control serum glucose levels to prevent excessive glucose losses.[24] Adjusting total kilocalorie intake in nutrition support may be necessary to compensate for extra dextrose provided through continuous renal replacement therapy.
      (5) Calcium and magnesium losses are high.[25] Patients treated with citrate anticoagulation therapy are likely to require IV calcium supplementation.

E. Infection
   1. Infection can be a major source of morbidity and mortality. Patients are at risk for viral (ie, cytomegalovirus; varicella zoster; herpes simplex), bacterial (ie, coagulase-negative *Staphylococcus; Pseudomonas aeruginosa*), and fungal (ie, *Candida glabrata; Aspergillus fumigatus*) infections.
   2. Oropharyngeal, esophageal, and GI infections may influence the patient's ability to ingest and tolerate oral feedings.

TABLE 13-3. GI GVHD Diet Progression[13]

Phase	Clinical Symptoms	Diet	Nutrition Support
1. Bowel rest	GI cramping Large-volume watery diarrhea or active GI bleeding Depressed serum albumin Severely reduced transit time Small-bowel obstruction or diminished bowel sounds Nausea and vomiting	Oral: NPO	PN with supplemental zinc and possibly copper
2. Introduction of oral feeding	Minimal GI cramping Diarrhea less than 500 mL/day Guaiac-negative stools Improved transit time (minimum 1.5 hours) Infrequent nausea and vomiting	Oral: isosmotic, low- residue, low-lactose beverages, initially 60 mL every 2 to 3 hours, for several days	PN Trophic enteral feeds of semielemental formula if patient unable to eat
3. Introduction of solids	Minimal or no GI cramping Formed stool	Oral: allow introduction of solid food, once every 3 to 4 hours: minimal lactose, low fiber, low fat (20–40 g/day), low total acidity, no gastric irritants	Begin to cycle and decrease PN Advance feeds slowly (small boluses or continuous infusion) if patient unable to eat
4. Expansion of diet	Minimal or no GI cramping Formed stool	Oral: minimal lactose, low fiber, low total acidity, no gastric irritants; if stools indicate fat malabsorption: low fat	Nighttime supplemental PN if oral intake less than needs or patient unable to maintain weight owing to malabsorption Enteral feed schedule and formula dependent on any residual GI symptoms
5. Resumption of regular diet	No GI cramping Normal stool Normal transit time Normal albumin	Oral: progress to regular diet by introducing 1 restricted food per day: acid foods with meals, fiber-containing foods, lactose-containing foods; order of addition will vary depending on individual tolerances and preferences Patients no longer exhibiting steatorrhea should have the fat restriction liberalized slowly	Discontinue PN Supplemental enteral feeds if patient unable to eat adequate nutrients

GI, gastrointestinal; GVHD, graft-versus-host disease; NPO, nil per os.

3. Treatment includes antiviral, antibiotic, and/or antifungal medications, which may induce anorexia, nausea, vomiting, diarrhea, and possible nutrient malabsorption, necessitating increased fluids and electrolytes.
4. Lipids do not increase bacteremia or fungemia when provided in typical doses (25%–30% of total calories) for critically ill patients.[26]

F. Osteoporosis[27]
1. Osteoporosis is a significant cause of morbidity, with subsequent fractures and joint avascular necrosis (AVN). Osteoporosis has been reported in 8% of adult autologous HSCT patients[28] and 18% of allogeneic HSCT patients with chronic myeloid leukemia.[29]
2. The pathogenesis is complex and incompletely understood. Post-transplant steroid use is associated with an odds ratio of 14.4 for

TABLE 13-4. Therapies Used for Prophylaxis and Treatment of GVHD[14]

Medication	Nutritional Implications
Antithymocyte globulin	Nausea and vomiting; diarrhea; stomatitis
Azathioprine	Nausea and vomiting; anorexia, diarrhea; mucosal ulceration; esophagitis; steatorrhea
Beclomethasone dipropionate	Xerostomia; dysgeusia; nausea
Budesonide	None known
Corticosteroids	Sodium and fluid retention resulting in weight gain or hypertension; hyperphagia; weight gain; hypokalemia; skeletal muscle catabolism and atrophy; gastric irritation and peptic ulceration; osteoporosis; growth retardation in children; decreased insulin sensitivity and impaired glucose tolerance; hyperglycemia or steroid-induced diabetes; hypertriglyceridemia
Cyclosporine	Nausea and vomiting; renal insufficiency; magnesium wasting; potassium wasting
Extracorporeal photopheresis	IV fluid may be necessary to maintain adequate hydration status; monitor calcium status if citrate anticoagulant is used, because it may bind calcium and induce hypocalcemia
Methotrexate	Nausea and vomiting (mild to moderate); anorexia; mucositis and esophagitis; diarrhea; renal and hepatic changes; decreased absorption of vitamin B_{12}, fat, and D-xylose; hepatic fibrosis; change in taste acuity
Methoxsalen (in conjunction with psoralen + ultraviolet A light)	Nausea; hepatotoxicity
Monoclonal antibodies	Nausea and vomiting
Mycophenolate mofetil	Nausea and vomiting; diarrhea
Sirolimus	Hypertriglyceridemia
Tacrolimus	Nephrotoxicity; hyperglycemia; hyperkalemia; hypomagnesemia
Thalidomide	Constipation; nausea; xerostomia
Ursodeoxycholic acid	Nausea and vomiting; diarrhea; dyspepsia

GVHD, graft-versus-host disease; IV, intravenous

the occurrence of AVN. TBI is associated with an adjusted odds ratio of 3.2 for the occurrence of AVN.[30] It is also thought that hypogonadism plays a role.

3. Medications
   a) Furosemide and heparin have negative effects on bone mineral density.
   b) Glucocorticoids lower osteoblast levels, shorten osteoblast life span, and reduce osteoblast function. Early in the course of glucocorticoid use, there may be increased bone resorption. However, with chronic long-term use, glucocorticoids are associated with decreased bone resorption.
   c) Glucocorticoids cause decreased intestinal calcium absorption and increased renal calcium excretion.[31]
   d) Cyclosporine and tacrolimus are associated with bone loss, but the mechanisms are unclear.
4. Two main phases of bone loss exist and are distinguished from each other by the presence or absence of glucocorticoids.
   a) During the first 6 months posttransplant, serum markers of bone formation are suppressed and urinary markers show increased bone resorption.
   b) Nephrotoxic effects of cyclosporine and tacrolimus cause declines in renal function and decreased synthesis of 1,25-OH vitamin D, resulting in inhibited intestinal calcium transport. Parathyroid hormone levels increase, resulting in osteoclast-mediated bone resorption.
   c) As glucocorticoid doses are tapered to below 5 mg per day, osteoblast function recovers and the suppressive effects on bone formation are reversed. Adverse effects of cyclosporine and tacrolimus remain, both the direct effects on the skeleton and the indirect effects that occur as a result of the nephrotoxicity. Bone resorption remains elevated.
5. Prevention and management of osteoporosis[32]
   a) Baseline and serial dual-energy x-ray absorption scans are important for monitoring status.
   b) Calcium and vitamin D supplementation for patients treated with corticosteroids, based on duration of supplementation[14]:
      (1) 1 to 5 years: 600 to 800 mg calcium; 400 international units vitamin D
      (2) 6 to 8 years: 800 to 1200 mg calcium; 400 international units vitamin D
      (3) >9 years: 1500 mg calcium; 400 to 800 international units vitamin D
   c) Hormone replacement therapy (HRT) is used in postmenopausal women and in men with low levels of serum testosterone.[32]
   d) Bisphosphonates are recommended for adults when glucocorticoid therapy is initiated, for patients with documented osteoporosis, for patients who have had fractures while treated with HRT, and for patients in whom HRT is poorly tolerated.[32]
   e) Bisphosphonate use is not well studied in the pediatric population.

f) Weight-bearing and resistive exercise is also recommended.

G. Endocrine dysfunction[33]

1. Thyroid dysfunction is associated with TBI.
2. Treatment with glucocorticoids suppresses the pituitary adrenal axis. Recovery is related to the duration and intensity of glucocorticoid therapy.
3. Pancreatic function changes occur with GVHD.
   a) Insulin resistance and hyperglycemia are associated with steroid therapy for GVHD. Long-term effects include insulin resistance, impaired glucose tolerance, diabetes, and the core signs of the metabolic syndrome.
      (1) Insulin therapy and instruction related to diabetes are necessary.
      (2) Dietary management includes modification of carbohydrate intake.
      (3) Weight control is essential.
   b) Alterations in lipid metabolism may occur as a result of steroid and cyclosporine therapy.
   c) Extensive chronic GVHD can result in pancreatic scarring and reduced function, with effects on endocrine and exocrine function.
4. Reproductive failure is common following HSCT.
5. Vitamin D deficiency may occur with chronic GVHD due to diarrhea and malabsorption and decreased exposure to sunlight (patients are encouraged to apply daily sunblock therapy). Serum levels of 25-OH vitamin D should be monitored.

H. Growth and development issues[34,35]

1. Growth hormone deficiency is common in children who have received prior cranial radiation and/or been treated with TBI or busulfan plus cyclophosphamide.
2. Effects include decreased growth velocity, decreased bone mineral density, and delayed onset of puberty.
3. Regular long-term follow-up evaluations are necessary to detect occurrence of endocrine gland dysfunction.
4. If abnormal endocrine function is detected, appropriate hormonal therapy may improve growth and development.

IV. Nutrition Assessment

A. Nutrition history

1. The nutrition history should include a comprehensive evaluation of current oral and GI symptoms associated with the disease or prior therapy.
   a) Chewing or swallowing difficulties
   b) Mucositis and esophagitis
   c) Dental health, including denture fit and presence of oral abrasions
   d) Taste alterations
   e) Xerostomia
   f) Heartburn or reflux
   g) Nausea and vomiting
   h) Early satiety
   i) Anorexia
   j) Changes in bowel habits
2. Assess current dietary modifications or unproven diets.
3. Assess food allergies or intolerances.
4. Evaluate current use and dosage of vitamin and mineral supplements, herbal supplements, and other integrative medicine therapies.
5. Evaluate past or current use of nutritional supplements, enteral nutrition, PN, or fluid support.
6. Pediatric patients
   a) For infants, determine if breast-fed or formula-fed. If infant is breast-fed, encourage weaning, as breast milk contains live T-lymphocytes; if formula-fed, determine infant formula and concentration.
   b) Evaluate stage of eating development (ie, cup vs bottle; pureed vs table food; self-feeding skills).
   c) Assess for oral aversions.

B. Physical examination

1. Assess for presence of obesity, emaciation, dehydration, ascites, or edema.
2. Assess musculature, physical abilities, and activity level.
3. Evaluate for signs of vitamin or mineral deficiency (ie, eyes, mouth, hair, nails, skin).
4. Assess for presence of stomas.

C. Anthropometry

1. Obtain baseline height and weight to determine body surface area.
   a) Assess weight changes, body mass index (BMI), ideal body weight, percent ideal body weight, and if appropriate, adjusted weight.
   b) In pediatric patients, assess growth history, weight-for-age, height- or length-for-age, and weight-for-length or BMI-for-age.
   c) These measurements may be used to determine chemotherapy and other medication dosages.
   d) Chronic disease and prior treatment may affect growth, development, and physical abilities (ie, activities of daily living, exercise tolerance).
2. Obtain baseline arm circumference and skinfold measurements to assess somatic muscle protein and adipose reserves. These measurements may be helpful in further assessing the patient's nutritional status.
3. Establish baseline anthropometry, which provides landmark data for serial measurements.
4. Obtain head circumference in children less than 36 months old.

D. Laboratory parameters

1. Obtain baseline serum values of:
   a) Electrolytes
   b) Glucose
   c) Creatinine
   d) Blood urea nitrogen
   e) Calcium
   f) Magnesium
   g) Phosphate
   h) Albumin or prealbumin
   i) Liver function enzymes
   j) Cholesterol and triglyceride
2. Assay serum ferritin levels in patients with a history of multiple blood transfusions to assess for iron overload.
3. Hematologic indices such as hemoglobin, hematocrit, and total lymphocyte count are readily affected by disease and treatment, so they are not valid parameters for nutrition assessment of HSCT patients.

E. Medications

1. Medications often affect appetite or alter GI function.
2. Analgesics, narcotics, antiemetics, antacids, laxatives, antibiotics, diuretics, and corticosteroids all have nutritional implications. See Tables 13-4 and 13-5.
3. Assess for drug-nutrient interactions.

F. Quality of life

1. Assess physical strength, usual activity level, and any changes in activity level.

TABLE 13-5. Nutritional Implications of Medications Used During Hematopoietic Stem Cell Transplantation[14]

Medication	Classification	Nutritional implications
Amphotericin	Antifungal	Nephrotoxicity including azotemia; hypokalemia; hypomagnesemia; increased creatinine; anorexia; nausea and vomiting
Busulfan	Alkylating agent	Nausea and vomiting; anorexia; hepatic toxicity; absorption impaired by food
Cyclophosphamide	Alkylating agent	Nausea and vomiting
Foscarnet	Antiviral agent	Nephrotoxicity; potassium, magnesium, calcium, and phosphorus wasting; pancreatitis
Melphalan	Alkylating agent	Nausea and vomiting; anorexia; diarrhea; hepatic toxicity; metallic taste
Pamidronate	Bisphosphonate	Hypophosphatemia; hypocalcemia; hypokalemia; hypomagnesemia
Thiotepa	Alkylating agent	Nausea and vomiting; mucositis and esophagitis
Trimethoprim-sulfamethoxazole	Antibiotic	Anorexia; nausea and vomiting; stomatitis; diarrhea; nephrotoxicity; increased liver function tests; possible folate deficiency; possible decreased vitamin K absorption

2. Assess level of pain and pain control, which may interfere with oral intake.

V. Nutrition Therapy

A. Goals of nutrition support
1. To identify patients at nutritional risk early to avert morbidity associated with malnutrition[36]
2. To provide nutrition support during regimen-related toxicities, prolonged anorexia, and GVHD in order to minimize loss of lean body mass and maintain fluid and electrolyte balance

B. Nutrient requirements
1. Energy[14]
   a) Increased energy requirements due to the preparative regimen, fever, infections, acute GVHD, metabolic complications, and growth demands of children
   b) Estimating energy requirements early posttransplant
      (1) Infants and very young children: basal metabolic rate (BMR) × 1.6 to 1.8[14,37]
      (2) Children (up to 16 years of age and ≤ 75 kg): BMR × 1.6[14,37]
      (3) Older adolescents (>16 years of age or >75 kg): basal energy expenditure (BEE) × 1.5 to 1.6[14,38]
      (4) Adults: BEE × 1.5[14,38] or 30 to 35 kcal/kg/day[39,40]
      (5) Following engraftment and resolution of metabolic complications, energy needs decrease to BEE × 1.3 for adults and BMR × 1.4 to 1.6 for children and adolescents.
      (6) When possible, use metabolic chart measurements in complex patients (ie, patients on long-term nutrition support or with significant body composition changes).
2. Protein[14]
   a) Increased protein is provided for tissue repair after cytoreductive therapy and to spare breakdown of lean body mass.
   b) Guidelines for protein support
      (1) Ages 1 to 6: 2.5 to 3.0 g/kg/day
      (2) Ages 7 to 10: 2.4 g/kg/day
      (3) Ages 11 to 14: 2.0 g/kg/day
      (4) Ages 15 to 18: 1.8 g/kg/day
      (5) Adults: 1.5 g/kg/day
   c) Needs may be further increased during high-dose corticosteroid therapy and during active GVHD.
   d) If hepatic, renal, or neurologic function is altered, protein intake may need to be modified.
3. Fat
   a) Typical intake is 15% to 30% of total energy.
   b) Maximum dose of intravenous lipid must not exceed 60% of total energy intake, or no more than 3 g/kg/day.
   c) Monitor weekly serum triglyceride levels when supporting patients with >40% total energy from fat.
   d) Fat should account for a minimum of 4% to 8% of total calories, to prevent essential fatty acid deficiency.
4. Carbohydrate
   a) Carbohydrate typically comprises 50% to 60% of total energy support.
   b) Recommended carbohydrate infusion rates during PN:
      (1) Infants and children: ≤15 mg/kg/min
      (2) Adolescents: 7 to 10 mg/kg/min
      (3) Adults: <5 mg/kg/min
   c) Hyperglycemia (preexisting or induced by PN or steroids) often mandates a lower carbohydrate delivery.
5. Fluids[14]
   a) Fluid needs are dependent on clinical status.
      (1) ≤10 kg: 100 mL/kg/day
      (2) 11 to 20 kg: 1000 mL + 50 mL/kg for each kg >10 kg/day
      (3) 21 to 40 kg: 1500 mL + 20 mL/kg for each kg >20 kg/day
      (4) >40 kg: 1500 mL/m^2/day
   b) Fluid needs are increased with fever, excessive GI losses, hypermetabolism, high-output renal failure, nephrotoxic medications, and during HSCT conditioning.
   c) Fluid restrictions may be necessary during compromised organ function and iatrogenic volume overload.

6. Vitamins and minerals
   a) Specific vitamin and mineral recommendations for HSCT patients are not known.
   b) Oral multivitamin and mineral supplementation with 100% of the dietary reference intakes for age is recommended for all patients for 1 year posttransplant and longer in patients who remain on long-term immunosuppressive medications.
   c) Because patients undergoing HSCT often require administration of blood products and experience iron overload, supplemental iron is not recommended.
   d) IV vitamin and mineral recommendations are based on the American Medical Association recommendations for daily requirements.[41,42]
   e) Provide additional vitamin C in PN during HSCT to promote tissue recovery via collagen biosynthesis after cytoreductive therapy.[14]
      (1) <31 kg, additional 250 mg of vitamin C per day
      (2) ≥31 kg, additional 500 mg of vitamin C per day
      (3) Additional vitamin C, which may act as a pro-oxidant, is contraindicated in patients with serum ferritin levels >1000 mcg/L, to decrease oxidative damage from release of free iron.[43]
      (4) During hemodialysis, discontinue additional vitamin C to prevent secondary oxalosis.
   f) Malabsorptive disorders, such as with liver or intestinal GVHD or long-term oral antibiotic therapy, may precipitate a vitamin K deficiency.
      (1) Pediatric IV multivitamin preparations (used for patients <11 years old) contain vitamin K, while only some adult IV preparations (used for patients ≥11 years old) do.
      (2) For pediatric patients >11 years old, add 200 mcg/day of vitamin K.
      (3) For adults, add 10 mg/week of vitamin K.
   g) Additional zinc supplementation is indicated in patients who develop diarrhea, with a suggested replacement guideline of 1 mg/100 mL stool when volume exceeds
      (1) 250 mL for patients <20 kg
      (2) 500 mL for patients 20 to 40 kg
      (3) 1000 mL in patients >40 kg[14]
   h) In the presence of hepatic failure, eliminate the biliary excreted trace elements copper and manganese from PN solutions.
   i) Calcium and vitamin D supplementation is recommended for patients maintained on high-dose corticosteroids when dietary intake is inadequate. (See Section III.F.5.b).)
7. Electrolytes
   a) Electrolyte requirements vary widely, because medications and GI losses influence needs.
   b) Serum electrolyte levels should be closely monitored, especially for patients maintained on PN or IV hydration containing electrolyte additives.
   c) Magnesium
      (1) Hypomagnesemia: Causes include diarrhea and steatorrhea, malabsorption syndromes, medications (ie, amphotericin, cyclosporine; foscarnet; tacrolimus), refeeding syndrome, and severe malnutrition.
      (2) Hypermagnesemia: Causes include discontinuation of a magnesium-wasting medication, excessive supplementation, and renal insufficiency.
   d) Potassium
      (1) Hypokalemia: Causes include GI losses, medications (ie, amphotericin; corticosteroids; furosemide; foscarnet), refeeding syndrome, and anabolism.
      (2) Hyperkalemia: Causes include excessive supplementation, potassium-sparing diuretics, renal insufficiency, tacrolimus, and tumor lysis syndrome.
   e) Sodium
      (1) Hyponatremia: Causes include excessive GI losses, fluid retention, excessive IV or oral fluid or free water intake, hyperglycemia, medications (ie, cyclophosphamide; cyclosporine; furosemide), and syndrome of inappropriate antidiuretic hormone.
      (2) Hypernatremia: Causes include inadequate fluid replacement during GI losses, aggressive diuretic therapy, and fever.[44]
   f) Phosphorus
      (1) Hypophosphatemia: Causes include diabetes mellitus, medications (ie, corticosteroids; cyclophosphamide; foscarnet; sirolimus), refeeding syndrome, renal acidosis, and steatorrhea.
      (2) Hyperphosphatemia: Causes include excessive phosphorus intake, multiple myeloma, myelogenous leukemia, renal failure, and tumor lysis syndrome.
   g) Calcium
      (1) Hypocalcemia: Causes include medications (ie, corticosteroids; foscarnet; pamidronate) and vitamin D deficiency.
      (2) Hypercalcemia: Causes include lymphoma, metastatic breast cancer, multiple myeloma, renal failure, and tumor lysis syndrome.
8. Drug-nutrient interactions (Tables 13-4 and 13-5)[14]

VI. Nutrition Management

A. Oral feedings
1. Oral feedings are indicated for patients with a functional GI tract and good nutritional status.
2. High-calorie, high-protein intake is emphasized, supplemented by nutrient-dense snacks as necessary.
3. Liquid, blended, or soft diets may be necessary in patients with chewing or swallowing difficulties due to mucositis, esophagitis, or oral GVHD.
4. Nutrient modifications may be necessary.
   a) A lactose-restricted diet is indicated for diarrhea.
   b) A sodium-restricted diet is indicated in patients with ascites or significant edema as a result of cardiac dysfunction or medication-induced fluid retention.
   c) Potassium or phosphorus restriction is occasionally necessary in patients with renal dysfunction.
   d) If total calories and simple carbohydrate intake are greater than needs, restriction is indicated in steroid-induced hyperglycemia (>180 mg/dL). (See III.G.3.a). However, diet modifications generally do not avert the need for insulin administration (short-acting with meals and long-acting if morning blood glucose is elevated).
5. A five-phase diet regimen has been developed for patients with GI GVHD with moderate to excessive diarrhea (Table 13-3).[13]
6. Elimination of foods most commonly associated with food-borne illness as well as food and herbal sources of fungal organisms is recommended until all immunosuppressive therapy has been discontinued (Table 13-6).
   a) Safe food handling and preparation methods are probably more beneficial than restriction of individual foods.[45]
   b) There is no scientific evidence to support restricting fruits and vegetables or providing only well-cooked foods.

TABLE 13-6. Diet Guidelines for Immunosuppressed Patients

These guidelines are intended to minimize the introduction of pathogenic organisms into the gastrointestinal tract by food while maximizing healthy food options for immunosuppressed patients. The guidelines should be coupled with food safety education to ensure proper food preparation and storage in the home and hospital kitchen. High-risk foods identified as *potential* sources of organisms known to cause infection in immunosuppressed patients are restricted.

In general, autologous transplant patients follow the diet during the first 3 months after hematopoietic stem cell transplantation. Allogeneic transplant patients should follow the diet until they are off all immunosuppressive therapy (ie, cyclosporine, tacrolimus, prednisone).

Food restrictions

- Raw and undercooked meat (including wild game), fish, shellfish, poultry, eggs, sausage, bacon
- Raw tofu, unless pasteurized or aseptically packaged
- Luncheon meats (including salami, bologna, hot dogs, ham), unless heated until steaming
- Refrigerated smoked seafood typically labeled as lox; kippered, nova-style, or smoked fish; fish jerky (unless contained in a cooked dish)
- Pickled fish
- Unpasteurized milk and raw milk products, nonpasteurized cheese, and unpasteurized yogurt
- Soft and blue-veined cheeses, including brie, Camembert, feta, farmer's, blue, Gorgonzola, Roquefort, Stilton
- Mexican-style soft cheeses, including queso blanco and queso fresco
- Cheese containing chili peppers or other uncooked vegetables
- Fresh salad dressings (stored in the grocer's refrigerated case) containing raw eggs or contraindicated cheeses
- Unwashed raw vegetables and fruits and those with visible mold
- All raw vegetable sprouts (alfalfa, mung bean, all others)
- Unpasteurized commercial fruit and vegetable juices
- Raw honey; honey in the comb
- All miso products (including miso soup); tempeh; maté tea
- All moldy and outdated food products
- Raw, uncooked brewer's yeast
- Well water, unless boiled for 1 minute

Source: Courtesy of the Nutrition Program, Seattle Cancer Care Alliance, 2004.

c) The effect of these diet modifications is unknown and warrants further research.[46]

B. Enteral nutrition
1. Indications
a) Patients with a functional GI tract who are either undernourished or who have poor oral intake that is expected to continue for 1 week or longer
b) Candidates include patients who
(1) Receive nonmyeloablative or reduced-intensity conditioning regimens
(2) Fail to recover appetite and resume eating after engraftment and resolution of conditioning-related mucositis and esophagitis[45]
(3) Have chronic GVHD (ie, oral; esophageal; liver; pulmonary; weight loss; quiescent phases of GI)
(4) Have neurological complications that preclude safe swallowing
(5) Are ventilated
2. Access
a) Nasoenteric
(1) Gastric feeding may be tried initially. Postpyloric placement is sometimes necessary in patients with delayed gastric emptying and frequent emesis.
(2) Self-propelling tubes have been used with partial success in the early posttransplant period.[47]
b) Percutaneous endoscopic or surgically placed gastrostomies
(1) Platelets >50 000 units/L and absolute neutrophil count >1000 cm^2 are recommended for safe placement.
(2) Pretransplant placement needs to occur 3 to 4 weeks prior to conditioning and period of neutropenia to ensure adequate healing.
(3) Posttransplant placement is dependent on the clinical status of the patient; a trial of nasoenteral feeding is appropriate prior to placement.
3. Complications
a) Dislodgment of nasoenteral tubes, necessitating frequent replacement[47,48]
b) Delayed gastric emptying, especially among allograft recipients.[49] Prokinetic agents or jejunal feeds may ameliorate the situation[50]; however, not all patients tolerate prokinetic agents.
c) Poor tolerance of rapid advancement of feeds when transitioning from PN after myeloablative conditioning
d) Infections and gastric leakage at gastrostomy sites. Gastric leakage requires special protection of the skin during the neutropenic period to prevent breakdown.[51,52]
e) Inadequate energy intake. With a predominantly enteral approach early post-HSCT, inadequate energy intake results in weight loss, decreased body cell mass, and increased frequency of malnutrition, as it supplies on average less than 50% of needs.[47,53,54] PN[51,52] or a combination of enteral feedings and PN may be needed.[55]
f) Inadequate protein intake. In children, modular protein additives often are required to meet high protein needs.
g) Inadequate electrolyte and mineral intake, specifically inadequate magnesium, calcium, phosphorus, and zinc with enteral feeds.[53,56] IV supplementation of magnesium and phosphorus may be needed to avoid excessive diarrhea.
h) Malabsorption in patients with chronic GVHD or pancreatic insufficiency. This necessitates semi-elemental or elemental formulas with supplemental vitamins and minerals.

C. PN
1. Indications
a) PN is associated with improved long-term disease-free survival compared to hydration support in allogeneic patients receiving myeloablative conditioning regimens.[57]
b) Candidates include patients who
(1) Receive high-intensity conditioning regimens and experience severe GI toxicity that precludes adequate intake.[55] The length of time before starting PN will depend on the

nutritional status of the patient, the risk of GVHD, and the expected duration of GI toxicity.

(2) Develop severe intestinal GVHD or other GI toxicities, such as high-volume infectious diarrhea

(3) Fail to receive adequate nutrition via the enteral route, especially children who need adequate nutrition to maximize growth and development and malnourished patients with minimal reserves

2. Access

a) Most patients have dual-lumen central venous access as a standard of care for infusion of chemotherapy, blood products, and intravenous medications for several months and sometimes even years (in patients with severe chronic GVHD) post-HSCT. Occasionally, single-lumen access requires cycling of PN because of competition with other IV therapies.

b) Line infections are common, and line removal may require use of peripheral PN until central access is reestablished.

3. Complications

a) Hyperglycemia management will depend on clinical status, etiology, and institutional practice, with the goal to achieve a glucose level as close to normal as is safely possible.

(1) Patients with preexisting diabetes need insulin titrated to each advancement of dextrose toward goal dextrose (approximately 40% of total energy needs). Achieving tight control may require an insulin drip with glucose monitoring every 2 hours. If an insulin drip is not available, a base amount of insulin may be added to the PN and sliding-scale coverage provided every 4 to 6 hours to maintain a serum glucose level of <180 mg/dL. If a patient is clinically stable and needs predictable amounts of insulin, then a lower level of glucose may be safely achieved.

(2) Patients who develop hyperglycemia on PN or with the addition of corticosteroids may have partial replacement of dextrose with lipid calories (in the absence of hypertriglyceridemia) and/or insulin added. Target glucose will depend on the clinical stability of the patient and the ability to monitor glucose/adjust insulin frequently (ie, via insulin drip or base amount in PN with sliding-scale coverage as discussed above). Patients on a tapering corticosteroid schedule need to be monitored closely for decreased insulin needs; those on a stable alternate-day schedule may be managed with a base amount of insulin in PN with sliding-scale coverage for steroid days.

b) Hypertriglyceridemia (ie, serum triglyceride >500 mg/dL) due to medications or organ dysfunction requires reduction of IV lipids to 4% to 8% of total energy.

c) Essential fatty acid deficiency occurs rapidly in patients supported without lipids. Only in patients with grossly lipemic serum should lipids be withheld entirely.

d) Cholestasis and gallbladder sludge occur several weeks after HSCT in patients on PN. Specialized pediatric amino acid solutions should be used in infants and can be considered in children as a possible preventive measure. For older patients, ursodiol is recommended, along with initiation of oral or enteral feeds as soon as possible.

e) Infections are higher in patients on PN.[57,58] While bacteremia may be treatable, in allogeneic patients infections may activate life-threatening flares of GVHD. Transition to enteral feeds should be considered in patients with recurring infections.

(1) Glutamine-enriched PN solutions have been recommended to reduce infectious complications,[59] but larger, controlled clinical trials are needed to ensure that they have no adverse effect on GVHD or survival before specific recommendations can be made. Alanyl-glutamine dipeptide was associated with significantly more relapses in patients undergoing autologous HSCT in one randomized study.[60]

(2) Lipids are not associated with an increased incidence of bacteremia or fungemia.[23] (See Section III.E.4.)

D. Nutrition support monitoring

1. Monitor alterations in medical condition and nutritional status, treatment-related symptoms, and modifications in nutrient requirements.

2. Monitor weights and intake and output daily during early postgrafting period. Monitor weights weekly in patients with chronic GVHD.

3. Monitor laboratory parameters for abnormalities at least 3 times per week and in some critical cases daily in the early posttransplant period.

a) Serum glucose, creatinine, blood urea nitrogen, and electrolytes are often needed daily, with adjustments to PN required.

b) Serum phosphate, magnesium, calcium, and albumin are needed twice weekly.

c) Blood lipids are needed weekly in patients with preexisting hyperlipidemia; liver, renal, or pancreatic dysfunction; or prolonged course of medication associated with hyperlipidemia (ie, corticosteroids, sirolimus, cyclosporine).

d) Liver function tests are needed twice weekly.

e) Prealbumin is not useful in the early postgrafting period, because prealbumin parallels neutrophil count.

f) If the patient is on long-term PN, check serum zinc, copper, carnitine, selenium, manganese, and chromium.

g) If the patient is on long-term tube feeding and has chronic GVHD, check serum vitamins A and D.

4. Assess the adequacy of nutrition support daily during the early postgrafting period, while maintained on enteral feedings or PN support, and when transitioning to an oral diet.

VII. Patient and Caregiver Education

A. Discuss increased nutrient requirements during HSCT.

B. Review nutrient and fluid goals.

C. Review nutrition support feeding modalities (ie, oral, enteral, and/or parenteral).

D. Review safe food handling and high-risk foods to avoid.

E. Instruct on pertinent dietary modifications.

1. GI diets (Table 13-3)[13]

2. Corticosteroid-induced hyperglycemia (see Section III.G.3.a)

3. Osteoporosis prevention (see Section III.F.5)

F. Discuss dietary guidelines for managing common posttransplant nutrition problems (Table 13-1).[6]

G. Establish a mechanism for nutrition follow-up as needed.

REFERENCES

1. Horowitz MM. Uses and growth of hematopoietic cell transplantation. In: Blume KG, Forman SJ, Appelbaum FR, eds. *Thomas' Hematopoietic Cell Transplantation.* 3rd ed. Malden, MA: Blackwell Publishing; 2004:9–15.

2. Clarkson JE, Worthington HV, Eden OB. Interventions for preventing oral mucositis for patients with cancer receiving treatment [Cochrane Review]. *The Cochrane Library.* 2003;issue 3.

3. Pedersen AM, Bardow A, Beier Jensen S, Nauntofte B. Saliva and gastrointestinal functions of taste, mastication, swallowing and digestion. *Oral Dis.* 2002;8:117–129.

4. Barale KV, Aker SN, Martinsen CS. Primary taste thresholds in children with leukemia undergoing marrow transplantation. *J Parenter Enteral Nutr.* 1982;6:287–290.
5. Charuhas PM, Fosberg KL, Bruemmer B, et al. A double-blind randomized trial comparing outpatient parenteral nutrition with intravenous hydration: effect on resumption of oral intake after marrow transplantation. *J Parenter Enteral Nutr.* 1997;21:157–161.
6. Charuhas PM. Introduction to marrow transplantation. *Oncol Nutr Diet Pract Group Newsletter.* 1994:2:2–9.
7. Shulman HM, Hinterberger W. Hepatic veno-occlusive disease—liver toxicity syndrome after bone marrow transplantation. *Bone Marrow Transplant.* 1992;10:197–214.
8. Vogelsang GB, Dalal J. Hepatic venoocclusive disease in blood and bone marrow transplantation in children: incidence, risk factors, and outcome. *J Pediatr Hematol Oncol.* 2002;24:706–709.
9. Sullivan KM. Graft-vs-host disease. In: Blume KG, Forman SJ, Appelbaum FR, eds. *Thomas' Hematopoietic Cell Transplantation.* 3rd ed. Malden, MA: Blackwell Publishing; 2004:635–664.
10. Vogelsang GB, Lee L, Bensen-Kennedy DM. Pathogenesis and treatment of graft-versus-host disease after bone marrow transplant. *Ann Rev Med.* 2003;54:29–52.
11. Bhushan V, Collins, RH. Chronic graft-vs-host disease. *JAMA.* 2003;290: 2599–2603.
12. Lenssen P, Sherry ME, Cheney CL, et al. Prevalence of nutrition-related problems among long-term survivors of allogeneic marrow transplantation. *J Am Diet Assoc.* 1990;90:835–842.
13. Gauvreau JM, Lenssen P, Cheney CL, et al. Nutritional management of patients with intestinal graft-versus-host disease. *J Am Diet Assoc.* 1981;79:673–677.
14. Seattle Cancer Care Alliance. *Hematopoietic Stem Cell Transplantation Nutrition Care Criteria.* 2nd ed. Seattle, WA: Seattle Cancer Care Alliance; 2002.
15. Byrnes JJ, Hussein AM. Thrombotic microangiopathic syndromes after bone marrow transplantation. *Cancer Invest.* 1996;14:151–157.
16. Elliott MA, Nichols WL. Thrombotic thrombocytopenic purpura and hemolytic uremic syndrome. *Mayo Clinic Proc.* 2001;76:1154–1162.
17. Suehiro T, Masutani K, Yolotama M, et al. Diffuse proliferative glomerulonephritis after bone marrow transplantation. *Clin Nephrol.* 2002;58: 231–237.
18. Hathcock JN, Hattan DG, Jenkins MY, et al. Evaluation of vitamin A toxicity. *Am J Clin Nutr.* 1990;52:183–202.
19. Vitamin A toxicity. *Med Lett Drugs Ther.* 1980;22:19–20.
20. Gleghorn EE, Eisenberg LD, Hack S, et al. Observations of vitamin A toxicity in three patients with renal failure receiving parenteral alimentation. *Am J Clin Nutr.* 1986;44:107–112.
21. Story DA, Ronco C, Bellomo R. Trace element and vitamin concentrations and loss in critically ill patients treated with continuous venovenous hemofiltration. *Crit Care Med.* 1999;27:220–223.
22. Fortin MC, Amyot SL, Geadah D, Leblanc M. Serum concentrations and clearances of folic acid and pyridoxal—5′-phosphate during venovenous continuous renal replacement therapy. *Intensive Care Med.* 1999;25: 594–598.
23. Maxvold NJ, Smoyer WE, Custer JR, Bunchman TE. Amino acid loss and nitrogen balance in critically ill children with acute renal failure: a prospective comparison between classic hemofiltration and hemofiltration with dialysis. *Crit Care Med.* 2000;28:1161–1165.
24. Frankenfield DC, Reynolds HN. Nutritional effect of continuous hemodiafiltration. *Nutrition.* 1995;11:388–393.
25. Klein CJ, Moser-Veillon PB, Schweitzer M, et al. Magnesium, calcium, zinc, and nitrogen loss in trauma patients during continuous renal replacement therapy. *J Parenter Enteral Nutr.* 2002;26:77–93.
26. Lenssen P, Bruemmer B, Bowden RA, et al. Intravenous lipid dose and incidence of bacteremia and fungemia in patients undergoing bone marrow transplantation. *Am J Clin Nutr.* 1998;67:927–933.
27. Cohen A, Shane E. Osteoporosis after solid organ and bone marrow transplantation. *Osteoporos Int.* 2003;14:617–630.
28. Schimmer AD, Mah K, Bordeleau L, et al. Decreased bone mineral density is common after autologous blood or marrow transplantation. *Bone Marrow Transplant.* 2001;28:387–391.
29. Kiss TL, Abdolell M, Jamal N, et al. Long term medical outcomes and quality of life assessment of patients with chronic myeloid leukemia followed at least 10 years after allogeneic bone marrow transplantation. *J Clin Oncol.* 2002;20:2334–2343.
30. Fink JC, Leisenring WM, Sullivan KM, et al. Avascular necrosis following bone marrow transplantation: a case control study. *Bone.* 1998;22:67–71.
31. Zeitler PS, Travers S, Kappy MS. Advances in the recognition and treatment of endocrine complications in children with chronic illness. *Adv Pediatr.* 1999;46:101–149.
32. American College of Rheumatology Ad Hoc Committee on Glucocorticoid-Induced Osteoporosis. Recommendations for the prevention and treatment of glucocorticoid-induced osteoporosis 2001 update. *Arthritis Rheum.* 2001;44:1496–1503.
33. Brennan BM, Shalet SM. Endocrine late effects after bone marrow transplant. *Br J Haematol.* 2002;118:58–66.
34. Shalet SM, Brennan BMD. Growth and growth hormone status after a bone marrow transplant. *Hormone Res.* 2002;58(suppl 1):86–90.
35. Darzy KH, Shalet SM. Radiation induced growth hormone deficiency. *Hormone Res.* 2003;59(suppl 1):1–11.
36. Lenssen P, Aker SN. Adult hematopoietic stem cell transplantation. In: Hasse JM, Blue LS, eds. *Comprehensive Guide to Transplant Nutrition.* Chicago, IL: American Dietetic Association; 2002:123–152.
37. Altman PL, Dittmer DS. *Metabolism.* Bethesda, MD: Federation of American Societies for Experimental Biology; 1968.
38. Harris JA, Benedict FG. *Biometric Studies of Basal Metabolism in Man.* Publication 279. Washington, DC: Carnegie Institution; 1919.
39. Geibig CB, Owens JP, Mirtallo JM, et al. Parenteral nutrition for marrow transplant recipients: evaluation of an increased nitrogen dose. *J Parenter Enteral Nutr.* 1991;15:184–188.
40. Peters E, Beck J, Lemaistre C, et al. Changes in resting energy expenditure (REE) during allogeneic bone marrow transplantation (ABMT) [abstract]. *Am J Clin Nutr.* 1990;51:521.
41. American Medical Association, Department of Foods and Nutrition. Multivitamin preparations for parenteral use: a statement by the nutrition advisory group. *J Parenter Enteral Nutr.* 1979;3:258–262.
42. American Medical Association. Guidelines for essential trace element preparations for parenteral use: a statement by the nutrition advisory group. *J Parenter Enteral Nutr.* 1979;3:263–267.
43. Gordon LI, Brown SG, Tallman MS, et al. Sequential changes in serum iron and ferritin in patients undergoing high-dose chemotherapy and radiation with autologous bone marrow transplantation: possible implications for treatment-related toxicity. *Free Radic Biol Med.* 1995;18:383–389.
44. Adrogué HJ, Madias NE. Hypernatremia. *New Engl J Med.* 2000;342: 1493–1499.
45. American Society for Parenteral and Enteral Nutrition. Guidelines for the use of parenteral and enteral nutrition in adult and pediatric patients. *J Parenter Enteral Nutr.* 2002;1S:83SA–85SA; 124SA–126SA.
46. Moody K, Charlson ME, Finlay J. The neutropenic diet: what's the evidence. *J Pediatr Hematol Oncol.* 2002;24:717–721.
47. Sefcick A, Anderton D, Byrne JL, et al. Naso-jejunal feeding in allogeneic bone marrow transplant recipients: results of a pilot study. *Bone Marrow Transplant.* 2001;28:1135–1139.
48. Lenssen P, Bruemmer B, McDonald GB, Aker S. Nutrient support in hematopoietic cell transplantation. *J Parenter Enteral Nutr.* 2001;25:219–228.
49. Eagle DA, Gian V, Lauwers GY, et al. Gastroparesis following bone marrow transplantation. *Bone Marrow Transplant.* 2001;28:59–62.
50. Roberts SR, Miller JE. Success using PEG tubes in marrow transplant recipients. *Nutr Clin Pract.* 1998;13:74–78.
51. Pedersen AM, Kok K, Petersen G, et al. Percutaneous endoscopic gastrostomy in children with cancer. *Acta Paediatr.* 1999;88:849–852.
52. Barron MA, Duncan DS, Green GJ, et al. Efficacy and safety of radiologically placed gastrostomy tubes in paediatric haematology/oncology patients. *Med Pediatr Oncol.* 2000;34:177–182.

53. Langdana A, Tully N, Molloy E, et al. Intensive enteral nutrition support in paediatric bone marrow transplantation. *Bone Marrow Transplant.* 2001;27: 741–746.
54. Szeluga DJ, Stuart RK, Brookmeyer R, et al. Nutritional support of bone marrow transplant recipients: a prospective randomized clinical trial comparing total parenteral nutrition to an enteral feeding program. *Cancer Res.* 1987;47:3309–3316.
55. Hopman GD, Pena EG, Le Cessie S, et al. Tube feeding and bone marrow transplantation. *Med Pediatr Oncol.* 2003;40:375–379.
56. Papadopoulou A, MacDonald A, Williams MD, et al. Enteral nutrition after bone marrow transplantation. *Arch Dis Child.* 1997;77:131–136.
57. Weisdorf SA, Lysne J, Wind D, et al. Positive effect of prophylactic total parenteral nutrition on long-term outcome of bone marrow transplantation. *Transplantation.* 1987;43:833–838.
58. Lough M, Watkins R, Garden OJ, et al. Parenteral nutrition in bone marrow transplant recipients. *Clin Nutr.* 1986;9:97–102.
59. Murray SM, Pindoria S. Nutrition support in bone marrow transplant patients [Cochrane Review]. *The Cochrane Library,* 2002;issue 3.
60. Pytlik R, Penes P, Patorkova M, et al. Standardized parenteral alanyl-glutamine dipeptide supplementation is not beneficial in autologous transplant patients: a randomized, double-blind, placebo controlled study. *Bone Marrow Transplant.* 2002;30:953–961.

SECTION EDITOR
Mark DeLegge, MD

III

Gastrointestinal Related Conditions

Mark R. Corkins, MD, CNSP, FAAP;
James Scolapio, MD, CNSP

14

Diarrhea

Introduction

Diarrhea is a symptom of a variety of diseases. Many steps are required to break down the food we ingest into the basic building blocks that are metabolized or used by our bodies. A failure in one of the many components of the digestive process can result in malabsorption. At the most basic level, diarrhea is a reflection of malabsorption. One difficulty is that this single symptom, diarrhea, can be the result of so many different processes and that these etiologies may require dramatically different treatments and nutritional approaches.

I. General Principles

A. Epidemiology
1. The best estimate for children under age 5 years in the United States is 3.2 episodes of diarrhea a year.[1,2]
2. Because children become dehydrated more frequently than adults, the economic impact of diarrhea is also higher in children. In a survey of a large privately insured population, diarrhea accounted for 4% of all hospitalizations and 2% of all outpatient visits in children under 5 years of age.[3]
3. Acute diarrhea of short duration is not life-threatening in the United States, where good nutrition predominates. In other areas of the world, diarrhea is the leading killer of malnourished children.
4. Worldwide, diarrhea accounts for 21% of all deaths in children less than 5 years of age, which represents 2.5 million deaths a year.[1]
5. Persistent diarrhea is always a clinical concern because it can lead to malnutrition.

B. Diagnostic evaluation
1. Diarrhea is defined as 250 mL of stool per day, or ≥3 loose stools a day,[4] or total fluid loss in the stool greater than 10 mL/kg/day in children.[5]
2. Chronic diarrhea is diarrhea that lasts longer than 2 weeks.
3. Fecal urgency and incontinence are different from diarrhea.
4. Having patients chart stool frequency and volume is often a helpful start in the diagnostic process.
5. Associated symptoms are also very important in making a diagnosis. Weight loss and oily stool would suggest a malabsorptive process.
6. Other important historical data include previous gastrointestinal surgical history (eg, short-bowel syndrome, bacterial overgrowth); previous abdominal radiation treatment; and travel, sexual, medication, and family history.
7. Diarrhea can be classified as osmotic, hypersecretory, malabsorptive, inflammatory, and dysmotility related.
8. Initial examination of the stool for blood, white blood cells, and fat globules is helpful.
9. Red and white cells in the stool suggest an inflammatory process, usually of the colon. Examples include Crohn's colitis, idiopathic ulcerative colitis, and malignancy.
10. Stool samples should be tested for pathological organisms, including ova and parasites, and C diff toxin (made by the organism *Clostridium difficile*).
11. Diarrhea that is purely hypersecretory (bile salt induced, hormonally mediated); osmotic (disaccharidase deficiency, laxative abuse); dysmotility related (irritable bowel, diabetic, postsurgical); or malabsorptive (celiac disease, bacterial overgrowth, pancreatic disease, Whipple's disease, tropical sprue) usually does not present with blood or white cells in the stool.
12. Other fecal testing that is commonly done in the pediatric population includes the Clinitest for reducing substances (detects most unabsorbed dietary carbohydrates except sucrose) and stool pH to detect fermentation of unabsorbed carbohydrates.
13. Clinitest-positive stools with low pH indicate that the small intestine is not digesting and absorbing dietary carbohydrates. This can be due to a variety of causes, including viral enteritis and congenital enzyme deficiencies.
14. If malabsorption is suspected, a 72-hour collection for stool volume and fecal fat should be performed while the adult patient is on a 100-g fat diet. In children, no specific diet is recommended, but a 3-day diet record is kept. The grams of fat consumed are then calculated for the 72 hours of the collection.
15. Steatorrhea in adults is defined as fat excretion of greater than 7 grams/24 hours. If greater than 7 g of fecal fat is found, further testing is required for a specific diagnosis. In children, the grams of fat in the stool and the grams of fat consumed are used to calculate a percentage of fat lost. In children under 6 months of age, up to 15% of dietary fat can be excreted normally; after this age, the excretion should be less than 7%.[6]
16. Testing may also include an upper endoscopic small-bowel biopsy for histopathology as well as a small-bowel aspirates to rule out bacterial overgrowth.
17. If chronic pancreatic insufficiency is thought to be causing the malabsorption, a sweat chloride test (in pediatric patients) and/or a duodenal aspirate should be obtained after intravenous (IV) administration of either cholecystokinin or secretin.
18. Stool osmolality can also give a general idea of the etiology of the diarrhea. The stool cannot have an osmolality less than that of serum, even if secretory. If it does, the sample may have been tampered with in some manner. The values to use are as follows[7]:
   a) Normal: mean stool osmolality 275–290 mOsm/kg water

b) Osmotic diarrhea: mean stool osmolality 400 mOsm/kg water
c) Secretory: mean stool osmolality 280 mOsm/kg water

19. A small-bowel x-ray can reveal a number of abnormalities associated with malabsorption, such as Crohn's disease, jejunal diverticulosis, radiation enteritis, and infiltrative disease of the small intestine. A complete blood cell count and chemistry panel should also be checked in patients with chronic diarrhea. Further laboratory testing should be based on clinical suspicion of a specific disease process.
20. The role of capsule endoscopy in the workup of chronic diarrhea is not well defined.

II. Acute Diarrhea

A. Infectious diarrhea

1. By far the most common cause of acute diarrhea is viral gastroenteritis.
2. The damage to the enterocytes results in a temporary malabsorption with diarrhea.
3. The most common viral pathogens are rotavirus, enteric adenovirus, Norwalk virus, calicivirus, and astrovirus.[8] There are rapid stool antigen tests for rotavirus and adenovirus.
4. Bacterial causes are usually diagnosed by stool culture. Discovering the etiology of most viral and bacterial causes is not crucial, as the treatment is largely supportive.
5. Nutrition support of infectious diarrhea first focuses on restoring hydration.
6. Recent guidelines for treatment of children with diarrhea have been uniform in their recommendations.[4,9,10] If a child presents clinically dehydrated, the first step, if clinically reasonable, is an oral rehydration solution; hydration can usually be completed in less than 4 hours.
7. Severe dehydration should be initially treated with IV fluid replenishment, but even then, once the patient has improved, oral rehydration can be attempted.
8. Following rehydration, the recommendations in acute diarrhea are to return to a normal diet as soon as possible.[4,9,10] Breast-fed infants should continue breast-feeding. Formula-fed infants should continue to receive *full-strength* formula. In most situations, no benefit has been shown of using lactose-free formulas. Older children and adults should resume appropriate solids without restriction.[4]
9. Food-borne illnesses often present with diarrhea. These illnesses arise from consumption of raw or poorly cooked food as well as unpasteurized milk or juices, home-canned goods, fresh produce, or soft cheeses made from unpasteurized milk.[11] The diarrhea is caused by toxins produced by the bacteria in the food or by the contaminating agents themselves. The incubation time for these illnesses ranges from several hours to several days. The diagnosis is suggested by a careful history of the patient's dietary intake.
10. For the majority of these patients, the recommended treatment is supportive care to maintain hydration, usually with oral hydration.[11] The nutritional therapy is the same as for other infectious causes of diarrhea.
11. In persistent diarrhea, a parasite must be suspected and the ova and parasite screen should be performed. It is important to identify these, as treatment can prevent malnutrition and shorten the course of illness.
12. There are rapid antigen tests for Giardia and Cryptosporidia, the most common parasites. Various types of tapeworms, amoeba, and other helminths can also cause a long-standing diarrhea that will require treatment.

B. Antibiotics and drugs

1. One drug-associated cause of diarrhea is abuse of stool softeners and laxatives. Many of over-the-counter antacids can also result in diarrhea, as can promotility agents such as metoclopramide and erythromycin.
2. Osmolality is an important potential cause of diarrhea. A survey of 58 commercially available solutions and suspensions found that 56 had an osmolality greater than 1000 mOsm/kg.[12] Many pediatric suspensions are made with syrups containing sorbitol, which can lead to osmotic diarrhea. In a report of adults in an intensive care unit receiving IV aminophylline or an oral solution containing sorbitol, the IV patients had diarrhea only 4% of the hospital days compared to 43% of the patients on the oral solution.[13]
3. The common occurrence of diarrhea during antibiotic therapy is well recognized. A recent study of children on antibiotics found that 11% developed diarrhea; this increased to 18% in children less than 2 years of age.[14] It is widely believed that the antibiotics alter the natural anaerobic flora of the gastrointestinal tract.[15]
4. *C difficile* accounts for 10% to 20% of antibiotic-associated diarrhea.[15] *C diff* produces toxins that are responsible for pseudomembranous colitis, which can occur with use of both oral and IV antibiotics. Most cases are mild and resolve in 2 to 3 weeks.
5. The diagnosis is made by obtaining a stool cytotoxin test for the B toxin.
6. The first response is discontinuation of the antibiotic if possible. When symptoms are persistent or severe, metronidazole 250 to 500 mg (30 mg/kg/day in children) 3 to 4 times per day for 10 days is the drug of choice.
7. A recent meta-analysis has supported the use of probiotics to prevent antibiotic-associated diarrhea.[16]
8. A randomized trial also has suggested that adults given regular intake of yogurt (227 g twice a day) containing active cultures had a reduced incidence of antibiotic-associated diarrhea.[17] An infant formula with fiber has been used to firm up loose stools in this situation.

C. Enteral feeding

1. Diarrhea is one of the most common complications reported with enteral feeding, occurring in up to 30% of patients.
2. The causes include the concurrent use of antibiotics, *C difficile* toxin, antacids, or the use of sorbitol-based liquid medications and magnesium in the formula.
3. Prior to investigation of the cause of the diarrhea, the amount of stool volume should be determined, since stool incontinence is often reported as diarrhea even when the volume is less than 200 mL/day.
4. Two reviews of this subject found that for the overwhelming majority of patients on enteral feedings, the cause of the diarrhea was not the formula, even if the formula was hypertonic.[18,19]
5. Careful review of the patient's current medical record, including medications, is very important.
6. Bacterial contamination of the enteral formula has been reported to cause colonization of the intestinal tract and diarrhea. This problem can be minimized by proper formula handling, including limiting infusion time or hang time to 8 to 12 hours. A closed delivery system has also been shown to significantly reduce the risk of formula contamination.
7. If the formula is thought to be the culprit after other causes have been excluded, then the formula can be changed to help manage this problem.

8. Confusion still exists regarding the dilution of a hypertonic formula and the development of diarrhea. When the formula is fed into the stomach, the osmolarity of the formula should not matter. Occasionally, feeding a hypertonic formula into the small intestine may cause diarrhea.
9. Starting the infusion slowly usually suffices, and dilution of the formula is rarely needed. Changing to a different formula (ie, a fiber-based formula) may be helpful in some cases of tube feeding–related diarrhea.
10. Using antidiarrheal agents while continuing tube feeds is helpful in many cases.
11. Patients should not be switched to parenteral nutrition for tube feeding–related diarrhea unless the above-mentioned approaches fail.

D. Allergic disorders
1. Diarrhea can be one of the manifestations of food allergy.
2. The most common allergy is cow's milk allergy in infants.
3. The frequency of food allergies is highest the first several years of life, with an estimated 6% to 8% of children affected in the first year of life.[20] The incidence falls with age to the adult level of 1% to 2%.
4. In developed countries, the incidence of cow's milk allergy in infants is 2% to 5% of all infants.[21] These infants often present with other symptoms besides diarrhea, including gastroesophageal reflux, blood in the stool (visible or detected during testing), and irritability.
5. Most infants develop symptoms shortly after the introduction of cow's milk–based formula.[21] Some infants appear to be sensitized before birth and will even develop a reaction to the small quantities of milk protein present in human breast milk. Nearly 100% of infants resolve this gastrointestinal allergy by 2 years of age, and the majority do so before their first birthday.[22]
6. Therapeutically, the logical first step is a trial of soy formula.
7. Only about half of infants with cow's milk–induced enteritis or colitis will respond to soy formula.[23] The American Academy of Pediatrics (AAP) recommends that such infants be treated with a hydrolyzed cow's milk formula.
8. A small subset of infants mount an immune response even to the hydrolyzed formulas and require feedings with an amino acid–based formula.[24–26]
9. One important point is that these infants are not lactose intolerant (in the absence of severe enteropathy) and do not have an immune response to lactose.[27] A milk-based lactose-free formula contains the proteins of the standard formulas, and using this type of formula will not resolve the problem.

III. Chronic Diarrhea (Cystic fibrosis and inflammatory bowel diseases are covered in Chapters 15 and 16, respectively.)

A. Celiac disease
1. Celiac disease, also known as gluten-sensitive enteropathy, is characterized by inflammation of the small-intestine mucosa that results from a genetically based immunologic intolerance to ingested gluten.
2. This disorder is now known to arise due to a cross-reaction between the gluten protein of certain cereal grains and the human enzyme transglutaminase.[28]
3. The inflammation occurring in celiac disease typically produces a malabsorptive syndrome, with diarrhea, steatorrhea, and loss of weight or failure to thrive.
4. Deficiencies of fat-soluble vitamins A, D, E, and K; iron; folic acid; and calcium are also common.
5. This disorder is much more common in persons of Northern European extraction, who tend to carry certain human leukocyte antigen (HLA) types, including DQw2.[28] Population-based serologic surveys have noted a prevalence of celiac disease of 1 in 250 to 500 individuals in most countries studied, including the United States. Siblings who share the specific HLA type of DQw2 have a 40% likelihood of concordance for celiac disease; monozygotic twins have a 70% concordance.
6. Several other disease associations have been described, primarily with juvenile-onset diabetes, short stature, cystic fibrosis, and Down's syndrome.[29]
7. The most important environmental factor in celiac disease is gluten. The harmful proteins are gliadins (wheat), hordeins (barley), and secalins (rye).
8. This disorder can show up at any age after the introduction of gluten-containing foods, although the peak is during the first and second years of life.[30]
9. Breast-feeding may reduce the likelihood of the infant developing celiac disease at an early age.
10. Patients with celiac disease have a loss of their intestinal villi as a result of the inflammatory cross-reaction, with resultant malabsorption. The inflammatory response consists of increased numbers of T lymphocytes, plasma cells, and macrophages in the lamina propria and increased numbers of lymphocytes in the surface layer of the epithelium. The changes may be patchy and affect a variable length of small bowel.
11. The villi are shortened and flattened, and the crypts are increased in depth.
12. In addition to the malabsorptive symptoms, including diarrhea and weight loss, atypical clinical presentations of celiac disease include isolated iron deficiency anemia (with or without heme-positive stool), osteoporosis, stunting of growth in children, tetany, infertility, dementia, and dermatitis herpetiformis (bullous skin rash).
13. Although very good antibody tests are now available, the gold standard for diagnosis continues to be the histological demonstration of the characteristic lesion in the small intestine and the subsequent clinical response to a gluten-free diet.
14. Serological testing offers methods to screen individuals suspected of having celiac disease without the need for invasive endoscopy. Of the serological antibodies, the immunoglobulin A (IgA) endomysial antibody (an indirect immunofluorescent assay) is the most sensitive and specific for the diagnosis of celiac disease.
15. Endomysial IgA antibody titers diminish with the institution of a gluten-free diet, often within weeks, and by 6 months may be undetectable.
16. The therapy for celiac disease is both simple and difficult. The institution of gluten-free diets should result in prompt and often dramatic improvements in patient's symptoms. Recovery appears to be more rapid in children.
17. Dietary advice from a dietitian experienced in gluten-free diets is very important to the treatment of patients with celiac disease. Patients should also take an active role in self-education.
18. There are celiac disease support groups and volumes of information regarding celiac disease via the Internet. Patients need to understand that the disease is lifelong and requires a lifetime of avoidance of gluten protein.
19. Gluten is normally found in products containing wheat, barley, or rye.[28] Other grains are acceptable but may be contaminated

during production at facilities that also process wheat, barley, or rye (Table 14-1).

20. Secondary lactose intolerance is common but usually resolves once the damage to the small intestine is healed. Folate deficiency is also common.
21. Specific minerals such as iron, calcium, and magnesium may need to be replaced if deficient. Rarely, a celiac patient will develop refractory disease. Noncompliance with a gluten-free diet should first be considered as the cause.
22. Other causes of refractory celiac symptoms include T-cell small-bowel lymphoma, collagenous sprue, and ulcerative jejunoileitis. Endoscopic, radiographic, and surgical testing is often required to make these diagnoses.
23. Occasionally, a patient with refractory celiac disease will require parenteral nutrition (PN).

B. Irritable bowel syndrome

1. Irritable bowel syndrome (IBS) is a diagnosis of exclusion. The diagnosis can often be made on the basis of the history, physical examination, and simple blood screening.
2. Chronic, nonprogressive symptoms of abdominal pain; alternating diarrhea and constipation in the absence of nocturnal symptoms; weight loss; fever; anemia; or blood in the stool should raise the possibility of this diagnosis.
3. The etiology is unknown, but IBS is most likely related to some form of disordered gastrointestinal motility. In children, this is often associated with some dyspepsia.
4. Symptoms reported more commonly in IBS patients include relief of abdominal pain with bowel movements, increased mucus on the stool, and the sensation of incomplete evacuation of stool.
5. Psychosocial factors, including anxiety, depression, and stressors, often worsen symptoms.
6. In older patients, a colonic neoplasm must always be excluded.
7. Celiac disease should also be excluded. Many patients who are labeled as having IBS are later found to have celiac disease.
8. Dietary therapy for IBS, especially in children with dyspepsia, may be helpful. Dietary triggers, including fried foods, spicy foods, high-fat foods, and carbonated and caffeinated beverages should be avoided.[31]
9. Another dietary intervention that has been shown to be very helpful is increased dietary intake of fiber in the form of bran, or use of commercial fiber preparations such as psyllium or methylcellulose.
10. Fiber is usually prescribed based on a patient's age. The initial dosage is approximately 5 g a day, increasing to a maximum of 25 g a day in adults.[31] When starting to take fiber, patients may complain of bloating or diarrhea. This usually improves with time.
11. Foods high in undigestible carbohydrates, such as beans, cabbage, and brussels sprouts, should be avoided.
12. Because lactase deficiency may produce symptoms similar to those of IBS, a trial of lactose restriction would also be indicated. (See Section III.D.)
13. Other dietary factors may also exacerbate IBS symptoms, including excess use of alcohol or coffee, or diets that contain sorbitol.

TABLE 14-1. Celiac Disease Diet

Do Not Eat	Do Eat	Caution Advised
Wheat (all types) Barley Soy sauce (made with wheat) Licorice Prepared soups Prepared sauces and dressings	Plain rice (including wild) Tapioca Potato Legumes Soy Corn	Processed foods Oats (contaminated mills) Pharmacy products (binder) Cold cuts Caramel coloring Spice extracts

C. Toddler's diarrhea (chronic nonspecific diarrhea, irritable colon of childhood)

1. This is a common presentation to pediatric caregivers during the toddler years.
2. This is a functional disorder. The Rome criteria define it as daily passage of three or more large, unformed stools, for 4 or more weeks, with onset in infancy or preschool years. There is no evidence of poor weight gain if the diet is adequate.[32]
3. The common presentation is a toddler who has a normal to slightly increased frequency of extremely liquid stools but is otherwise normal to examination and healthy by history.
4. The child has normal growth and development despite having what the parents often describe as "explosive" stools that often contain recognizable vegetable and other food particles.[33]
5. It is believed that this diarrhea arises because meals fail to interrupt the migrating motor complex.[32]
6. Some authorities believe toddler's diarrhea is more common in patients with a family history of IBS.[33]
7. A major contributor to this disorder is the intake of fluids with a high carbohydrate level. Parents often believe that older infants and toddlers need to drink juice, and juices, soft drinks, or powdered drinks (all liked for their sweet taste) can come to replace higher-quality liquids in the diet.
8. The diagnosis is supported by a thorough dietary history, including assessment for overfeeding, fruit juice/sorbitol intake, and excessive dietary reliance on carbohydrates rather than fats.[32,34]
9. The initial dietary therapy is to eliminate these fluids completely from the toddler's diet (although it is crucial that the parents not create a highly restrictive diet).[34] Elimination normally results in a dramatic improvement in the patient's stools.
10. A high-fat, low-carbohydrate diet is recommended to reduce the intestinal motility.[33] This includes restarting whole milk, the food that has often been removed from the patient's diet. The symptoms resolve by the time the child reaches school age.[32]

D. Lactose intolerance

1. Lactase deficiency is the most common disaccharidase deficiency.
2. Because lactose cannot be hydrolyzed and absorbed, it passes into the colon, where osmotically active substances are formed that induce diarrhea.
3. Infants born at term have adequate lactase levels in the brush border cells of the small intestine to digest the lactose found in human breast milk.
4. Congenital lactase deficiency is an extremely rare autosomal recessive disease that results in severe diarrhea and weight loss in early infancy.
5. In most populations, the lactase level normally declines after infancy.
6. In some ethnic groups, this developmental lactase deficiency is more common. People of African, Asian, and South American heritage tend to exhibit lactase deficiency more often than do people from other cultures.

7. A temporary secondary lactase deficiency may occur following acute gastroenteritis in children. Secondary lactase deficiency can also occur in other disease processes of the intestinal mucosa, such as celiac disease, short-bowel syndrome, and inflammatory bowel disease.
8. Clinical symptoms following the intake of milk or milk products include abdominal bloating, increased flatus, nausea, and sometimes loose to watery stools.
9. Weight loss and wasting is not part of this clinical entity, unless associated with an underlying disorder.
10. The hydrogen breath test is the most accurate indirect method for detecting lactase deficiency. Breath hydrogen is measured at 30- to 60-minute intervals for 2 to 4 hours following a 50-gram oral lactose dose. A sustained rise in breath hydrogen of greater then 20 ppm above baseline indicates lactose malabsorption.
11. Patients may also note symptoms during lactose administration, which supports the diagnosis.
12. Lactase levels can be directly measured in small intestinal biopsy samples from patients who undergo endoscopic procedures.
13. Patients with mild symptoms can manage the condition by reducing the amount of milk products in their diets. Patients with more severe symptoms may need to ingest only milk products with enzymatic products added or to eliminate lactose from their diets.

E. Intractable/protracted diarrhea of infancy

1. There is a small subset of infants who, after a significant gastrointestinal illness, have persistent diarrhea (lasting more than 2 weeks).
2. The diffuse mucosal injury that is present is believed to arise either from formula protein intolerance or following an infectious enteritis.[33,35]
3. This injury can result in secondary formula-protein intolerance and a mild inflammation with mild malabsorption.[33,35] The malabsorption is frequently manifested by the presence of carbohydrates in the stool, noted by a positive Clinitest.
4. Once there is malabsorption, malnutrition may quickly develop. Malnutrition may place the patient at risk for infections and repeated mucosal injury, resulting in a vicious cycle.
5. This disorder has been renamed "protracted diarrhea of infancy" by some authorities to differentiate it from disorders in which infants truly have unrelenting (and thus intractable) diarrhea.[36]
6. Other disorders such as autoimmune enteropathy and congenital enterocyte disorders must be eliminated as the cause of the diarrhea.[36,37]
7. Fortunately, this disorder will usually resolve with time and good nutrition.
8. Previously, many of these infants required an extended course of PN. The development of hydrolysate and amino acid–based formulas has made this approach unnecessary for most patients.
9. PN may be required initially, but enteral feedings are crucial to speed the resolution of this disorder.[33,35] PN is sometimes used to begin reversing the general malnutrition while allowing for time to restore the normal gastrointestinal mucosa. It is important to maintain normal hydration and electrolytes, including zinc.
10. These infants are usually first tried on a lactose-free formula, most often a protein hydrolysate formula. If small amounts of this formula are tolerated, the volume is advanced as tolerated. If the hydrolysate formula is met with evidence of intolerance, then an amino acid–based formula is initiated.[35] This type of formula is usually well tolerated.
11. In some infants with more severe mucosal injury, a continuous drip of the amino acid–based formula is necessary (via nasogastric tube). The volume of drip feedings is initially low and is advanced according to patient tolerance. Tolerance can be assessed by measuring the volume of stool and the amount of carbohydrate in the stool via the Clinitest method for reducing substances.
12. In extreme cases, PN may be needed until the mucosa is able to reconstitute itself and the patient can be transitioned off PN to full-drip enteral feeds, then to intermittent bolus feedings, and eventually to completely oral intake.
13. This disorder is normally transient, with complete resolution eventually; the goal is to prescribe the least invasive therapy possible.

F. Short-bowel syndrome

1. Short-bowel syndrome is a collection of signs and symptoms occurring after intestinal resection and characterized by weight loss, malabsorption of fluids, and malabsorption of micro- and macronutrients.
   a) In adults, the most common etiologies include small-bowel resection for Crohn's disease and vascular events such as acute mesenteric ischemia.
   b) In adults, the normal small intestine is approximately 600 cm in length and the colon, approximately 150 cm.
   c) The incidence of short-bowel syndrome is split almost evenly between pediatric and adult populations.[38] The etiologies are different in pediatric cases. The leading causes in pediatric cases are intestinal volvulus, intestinal atresia, necrotizing enterocolitis, and complications of gastroschisis.[38]
   d) Patients with a preserved colon had lower fecal volumes and fecal energy loss than patients without a colon.[39]
   e) Patients with less than 150 to 200 cm of remaining small intestine without a colon may have significant energy and fluid losses and may require PN for survival.
   f) Patients with a partial or complete remaining colon in continuity with the small intestine may not have significant fluid and energy loss until less than 50 to 70 cm of the small bowel remains. With shorter lengths, patients may require PN for survival.
   g) In infants, the crucial factor determining small-bowel length needed is the ileocecal valve. If the valve is present, survival is possible with 20 to 40 cm of intestine; if not, greater than 40 cm is usually required.[38] Survival of infants with less than 20 cm of small intestinal is rare.[38]
   h) The remaining intestine can often compensate or adapt with time. The results of this compensation can be observed clinically in the form of patient weight gain, reduced intestinal fluid losses, and stabilization of micronutrients. These changes usually are clinically obvious approximately 3 months after intestinal resection and may continue for years.
2. Dietary management
   a) Specific dietary recommendations should be based on the presence or absence of a colon. Those with a colon should consume a high-carbohydrate/low-fat (HCLF) diet.
   b) The colon can convert complex carbohydrates by bacterial fermentation to short-chain fatty acids (acetate, propionate, and butyrate), which can provide a source of up to 500 calories per day.[40] Also, short-chain fatty acids stimulate colonic sodium and water absorption.
   c) In patients with a colon, an HCLF diet can reduce fecal losses of energy by 500 kcal/d compared to the low-carbohydrate/high-fat (LCHF) diet.[40] In contrast, patients with end jejunostomies excrete equal amounts of calories on both types of diets.[40–43]

d) Use of lactose in diets of patients with short-bowel syndrome should be individualized since most patients can tolerate dairy products.[44]
e) Patients with short-bowel syndrome who have had more than 60 cm of terminal ileum resected or diseased should receive vitamin B_{12}.[45] For replacement, 1000 mcg should be given intramuscularly once a month.
f) Patients with colonic continuity are at increased risk of oxalate nephropathy and should be placed on low-oxalate diets if 24-hour urinary oxalate levels are elevated. Increasing dietary calcium and using an HCLF diet may also be helpful.[46]
g) In infants, fats are better tolerated than carbohydrates and the nutritional needs for fats are higher.
h) Infants with short-bowel syndrome tend to develop formula protein allergies. The use of a hydrolysate protein formula is recommended; in rare cases, an amino acid–based formula will be required.[47] The feedings should be administered continuously to maximize absorption.
i) In infants, feeding formulas should be started as soon as possible after surgery and advanced as tolerated. The measurement of stool volume and the amount of reducing substances (Clinitest) are used to guide advancement.[47] At the developmentally appropriate time, small amounts of oral solids should be initiated to prevent the child from having a feeding aversion when he or she is older.[47]
j) Children are susceptible to the same vitamin and mineral deficiencies as adults, so vitamin and mineral levels should be monitored and supplemented at the appropriate doses.

3. Oral rehydration solutions
   a) Most of the published success with oral rehydration solutions (ORSs) has been in the context of treating patients with cholera, in which such solutions have substantially reduced mortality.
   b) Few data are available on ORS efficacy in short-bowel syndrome. The sodium concentration of the effluent is almost constant, at approximately 90 mmol/L.
   c) ORSs work by the solvent drag mechanism in the jejunum. Nutrients such as glucose promote the passive absorption of electrolytes and water. To avoid osmotically driven secretion of salt and water, solutions should be isotonic with plasma. They should also be balanced in sodium and glucose content to promote sodium and glucose cotransport. Standard "sport drinks" have a high sugar content and too little sodium. In studies in rats and in humans, the optimal ORS has a sodium concentration of at least 90 mmol/L.[48]
   d) Rice-based ORSs (such as Ceralyte [Cera Products, Columbia, MD], 40 g of rice carbohydrate; osmolality, 225 [sodium, 50 mmol/L], 235 [sodium 70], or 260 [sodium 90]) allow more glucose delivery to the small intestine without increasing the osmotic load from free glucose.
   e) The addition of glutamine to a standard rehydration formula did not enhance sodium absorption in a study of six patients with end jejunostomies.[49]
   f) Eight case reports[50–58] showed successful results (defined as discontinuation of parenteral fluids and electrolytes) of ORSs with sodium concentrations between 77 and 116 mmol/L. The mean length of jejunum in these studies was 100 cm (range, 25–180 cm). Two of the patients had parts of their colon remaining: one still had 25 cm and one had 30 cm of small intestine.
   g) Intake is often limited by palatability. Commercial products with a better taste have been marketed.
4. Octreotide
   a) Octreotide, a synthetic octapeptide analogue of somatostatin, has many effects on the gastrointestinal tract. It reduces splanchnic blood flow and inhibits gastric, pancreatic, and small-bowel secretions that inhibit intestinal adaptation and increase fecal fat losses. All of these changes can negatively affect nutrient assimilation and absorption.
   b) In perfusion studies, it has been shown that somatostatin has no effect on jejunal absorption of sodium and water. Therefore, the improved balance is most likely the result of reduced water and electrolyte secretion.
   c) A double-blind, placebo-controlled study of six TPN-dependent patients with short-bowel syndrome without a colon reported improved sodium and fluid balance with octreotide, but TPN nutrient requirements could not be reduced.[59]
   d) In another study, 10 patients who had been dependent on home PN (HPN) for 1 to 15 years and who had end jejunostomies and no colons were treated in an open-labeled trial with 100 mcg of octreotide, administered subcutaneously 3 times a day.[60] Significant improvement was noted in fluid (30%–40% reduction), sodium, potassium, and chloride balance. Despite improvement in net fluid secretion, all but one patient remained in negative balance, and HPN could not be discontinued.
   e) An open-labeled trial evaluated the effects of the long-acting release analogue of octreotide during a 15-week period in eight TPN-dependent patients with short-bowel syndrome.[61] They reported no statistically significant decrease in stool weight (despite a positive trend) or in stool sodium, potassium, or fat.
5. Growth hormone and glutamine
   a) Negative studies
      (1) In a randomized, double-blind, placebo-controlled crossover study, 10 patients with short-bowel syndrome who were treated for 8 weeks with subcutaneous human recombinant growth hormone reported no significant changes in absorptive capacity.[62]
      (2) A randomized, double-blind, placebo-controlled crossover study in eight patients with short-bowel syndrome evaluated the effects of oral administration of glutamine (0.45 g/kg per day) with a constant HCLF (60%:20%) diet. No significant changes were seen in the measured parameters.[63]
      (3) A randomized, double-blind, placebo-controlled crossover study with subcutaneous human recombinant growth hormone, oral glutamine, and a constant HCLF (60%:20%) diet for 21 days was completed in eight HPN-dependent patients who had short-bowel syndrome.[64] There was no significant improvement in fecal volume, fecal fat, nitrogen, or D-xylose absorption.
      (4) A randomized, placebo-controlled, double-blind crossover study of eight patients with short-bowel syndrome treated with their usual diets, human recombinant growth hormone, and oral and parenteral glutamine for 28 days was performed.[65] No improvement was observed in the absorption of carbohydrate, fat, or nitrogen. Stool weight and stool electrolytes were unchanged.
   b) Positive studies
      (1) An open-labeled study evaluated the effects of subcutaneous human recombinant growth hormone, parenteral glutamine or oral glutamine, and an HCLF (60%:20%, including soluble fiber) diet on eight HPN-dependent patients with short-bowel syndrome. There was a significant increase in the absorption of total calories, protein, carbohydrate, sodium, and water.[66]

(2) The open-label study of eight patients was expanded to an additional 31 HPN-dependent patients. The growth hormone dose was reduced.[67] At the end of the 21-day treatment period, 57% of patients did not require TPN, 30% had reduced TPN requirements, and 13% had no change. The side effects of the treatment were minor and consisted of fluid retention and arthralgias, both of which varied with the growth hormone dose.

(3) The latest prospective, randomized, double-blind, placebo-controlled crossover study used low-dose growth hormone alone for 3 weeks in 12 TPN-dependent patients with short-bowel syndrome.[68] This study found an increased uptake of energy, nitrogen, and carbohydrates. The increased absorption was calculated to represent 37% of the energy received from the TPN. Body weight, lean body mass, and D-xylose absorption were improved without any major side effects.

c) Conclusion

(1) The results of the current randomized, controlled studies using growth hormone or glutamine alone or in combination are inadequate to confirm a clinical benefit in patients with short-bowel syndrome both with and without colons.

(2) Given the potential side effects associated with growth hormone and glutamine, treatment should not be considered a standard of practice in short-bowel syndrome.

6. Other agents

a) Glucagon-like peptide (GLP-2) is a 33–amino acid peptide with known intestinotropic, antisecretory, and transit-modulating effects in rodents. It is excreted from the intestinal mucosa of the terminal ileum and colon after food ingestion. An open-labeled study[69] with GLP-2 was completed in eight patients with short-bowel syndrome. A significant increase was seen in absolute absorption and stool wet weight. Patients with the shortest length of small bowel tended to experience the greatest benefit. However, no significant increase occurred in the absolute absorption of total energy, carbohydrate, fat, or protein.

b) The first clinical observation of the potential trophic effect of enteroglucagon was in a patient with a renal tumor producing enteroglucagon. Hypertrophy of the small bowel was found, suggesting that this agent may be useful in short-bowel syndrome.

REFERENCES

1. Kosek M, Bern C, Guerrant RL. The global burden of diarrhoeal disease, as estimated from studies published between 1992 and 2000. *Bull World Health Organ.* 2003;81:197–204.
2. Kotloff KL, Wasserman SS, Steciak JY, et al. Acute diarrhea in Baltimore children attending an outpatient clinic. *Pediatr Infect Dis J.* 1988;7:753–759.
3. Zimmerman CM, Bresee JS, Parashar UD, et al. Cost of diarrhea-associated hospitalizations and outpatient visits in an insured population of young children in the United States. *Pediatr Infect Dis J.* 2001;20:14–19.
4. King CK, Glass RI, Bresee JS, et al. Managing acute gastroenteritis among children. *MMWR Recomm Rep.* 2003;52:1–16.
5. Guandalini S. Acute diarrhea. In: Walker WA, Durie PR, Hamilton JR, Walker-Smith JA, Watkins JB, eds. *Pediatric Gastrointestinal Disease.* 3rd ed. Hamilton, Ontario: BC Decker; 2000:28–38.
6. Huynh H, Couper R. Pancreatic function tests. In: Walker WA, Durie PR, Hamilton JR, Walker-Smith JA, Watkins JB, eds. *Pediatric Gastrointestinal Disease.* 3rd ed. Hamilton, Ontario: BC Decker; 2000:1515–1528.
7. Walker-Smith JA, Hamilton JR, Walker WA. *Practical Paediatric Gastroenterology.* London, UK: Butterworth & Co.; 1983:85.
8. Blacklow NR, Greenberg HB. Viral gastroenteritis. *N Engl J Med.* 1991;325:252–261.
9. Armon K, Stephenson T, MacFaul R, et al. An evidence and consensus based guideline for acute diarrhoea management. *Arch Dis Child.* 2001;85:132–142.
10. Sullivan PB. Nutritional management of acute diarrhea. *Nutrition.* 1998;14: 758–762.
11. Tan LJ, Lyznicki J, Adcock PM, et al. Diagnosis and management of food-borne illnesses: a primer for physicians. *MMWR Recomm Rep.* 2001;50:1–69.
12. Dickerson RN, Melnik G. Osmolality of oral drug solutions and suspensions. *Am J Hosp Pharm.* 1988;45(4):832–834
13. Hill DB, Henderson LM, McClain CJ. Osmotic diarrhea induced by sugar-free theophylline solution in critically ill patients. *J Parenter Enteral Nutr.* 1999;15:332–336.
14. Turck D, Bernet J-P, Marx J, et al. Incidence and risk factors of oral antibiotic-associated diarrhea in an outpatient pediatric population. *J Pediatr Gastroenterol Nutr.* 2003;37:22–26.
15. Bartlett JG. Antibiotic-associated diarrhea. *N Engl J Med.* 2002;346: 334–339.
16. D'Souza AL, Rajkumar C, Cooke J, et al. Probiotics in prevention of antibiotic associated diarrhoea: meta-analysis. *BMJ.* 2002;324:1361–1369.
17. Beniwal RS, Arena VC, Thomas L, et al. A randomized trial of yogurt for prevention of antibiotic-associated diarrhea. *Dig Dis Sci.* 2003;48: 2077–2082.
18. Heimburger DC, Sockwell DG, Geels WJ. Diarrhea with enteral feeding: prospective reappraisal of putative causes. *Nutrition.* 1994;10:392–396.
19. Mobarhan S, DeMeo M. Diarrhea induced by enteral feeding. *Nutr Rev.* 1995;53:67–70.
20. Wood RA. The natural history of food allergy. *Pediatrics.* 2003;111: 1631–1637.
21. Host A. Frequency of cow's milk allergy in childhood. *Ann Allergy Asthma Immunol.* 2002;89(suppl):33–37.
22. Exl B-M, Fritsché R. Cow's milk protein allergy and possible means for its prevention. *Nutrition.* 2001;17:642–651.
23. Klemola T, Vanto T, Juntunen-Backman K, et al. Allergy to soy formula and to extensively hydrolyzed whey formula in infants with cow's milk allergy: a prospective, randomized study with a follow-up to the age of 2 years. *J Pediatrics.* 2002;140:219–224.
24. de Boissieu D, Dupont C. Allergy to extensively hydrolyzed cow's milk proteins in infants: safety and duration of amino acid–based formula. *J Pediatrics.* 2002;141:271–273.
25. de Boissieu D, Matarazzo P, Dupont C. Allergy to extensively hydrolyzed cow milk proteins in infants: identification and treatment with an amino acid–based formula. *J Pediatrics.* 1997;131:744–747.
26. Vanderhoof JA, Murray ND, Kaufman SS, et al. Intolerance to protein hydrolysate infant formulas: an underrecognized cause of gastrointestinal symptoms in infants. *J Pediatrics.* 1997;131:741–744.
27. Fiocchi A, Restani P, Leo G, et al. Clinical tolerance to lactose in children with cow's milk allergy. *Pediatrics.* 2003;112:359–362.
28. Farrell RJ, Kelly CP. Celiac sprue. *N Engl J Med.* 2002;346:180–188.
29. Hill I, Fasano A, Schwartz R, et al. The prevalence of celiac disease in at-risk groups of children in the United States. *J Pediatrics.* 2000;136:86–90.
30. Pietzak MM, Catassi C, Drago S, et al. Celiac disease: going against the grains. *Nutr Clin Pract.* 2001;16:335–344.
31. Hyams JS. Chronic and recurrent abdominal pain. In: Hyman PE, ed. *Pediatric Functional Gastrointestinal Disorders.* New York, NY: Academy Professional Information Services; 1999:7.1–7.21.
32. Rasquin-Weber A, Hyman PE, Cucchiara S, et al. Childhood functional gastrointestinal disorders. *Gut.* 1999;45(suppl 2):1160–1168.
33. Vanderhoof JA. Chronic diarrhea. *Pediatr Rev.* 1998;19:418–422.
34. Hyams JS. Diet and gastrointestinal disease. *Curr Opin Pediatr.* 2002; 14:567–569.
35. Walker-Smith JA. Nutritional management of enteropathy. *Nutrition.* 1998; 14:775–779.
36. Goulet O. Intractable diarrhea of infancy. In: Walker WA, Durie PR, Hamilton JR, Walker-Smith JA, Watkins JB, eds. *Pediatric Gastrointestinal Disease.* 3rd ed. Hamilton, Ontario: BC Decker; 2000:762–772.
37. Sherman PM, Mitchell DJ, Cutz E. Neonatal enteropathies: defining the causes of protracted diarrhea of infancy. *J Pediatr Gastroenterol Nutr.* 2004;38:16–26.

38. Sigalet DL. Short bowel syndrome in infants and children: an overview. *Semin Pediatr Surg.* 2001;10:49–55.
39. Nordgaard I, Hansen BS, Mortensen PB. Importance of colonic support for energy absorption as small-bowel failure proceeds. *Am J Clin Nutr.* 1996;64:222–231.
40. Nordgaard I, Hansen BS, Mortensen PB. Colon as a digestive organ in patients with short bowel. *Lancet.* 1994;33:373–376.
41. Woolf GM, Miller C, Kurian R, et al. Diet for patients with short bowel: high fat or high carbohydrate? *Gastroenterology.* 1983;84:823–828.
42. McIntyre PB, Fitchew M, Lennard-Jones JE. Patients with a high jejunostomy do not need a special diet. *Gastroenterology.* 1986;91:25–33.
43. Jeppesen PB, Mortensen PB. The influence of a preserved colon on the absorption of medium chain fat in patients with small bowel resection. *Gut.* 1998;43:478–483.
44. Marteau P, Messing B, Arrigoni E, et al. Do patients with short-bowel syndrome need a lactose-free diet? *Nutrition.* 1997;13:13–16.
45. Behrend C, Jeppesen PB, Mortensen PB. Vitamin B12 absorption after ileorectal anastomosis for Crohn's disease: effect of ileal resection and time span after surgery. *Eur J Gastroenterol Hepatol.* 1995;7:397–400.
46. Dobbins JW, Binder HJ. Effect of bile salts and fatty acids on the colonic absorption of oxalate. *Gastroenterology.* 1976;70:1096–1100.
47. Vanderhoof JA, Young RJ. Enteral nutrition in short bowel syndrome. *Semin Pediatr Surg.* 2001;10:65–71.
48. Lennard-Jones JE. Oral rehydration solutions in short bowel syndrome. *Clin Ther.* 1990;12(suppl A):129–137.
49. Beaugerie L, Carbonnel F, Hecketsweiler B, et al. Effects of an isotonic oral rehydration solution, enriched with glutamine, on fluid and sodium absorption in patients with a short-bowel. *Aliment Pharmacol Ther.* 1997; 11:741–746.
50. Newton CR, Gonvers JJ, McIntyre PB, et al. Effect of different drinks on fluid and electrolyte losses from a jejunostomy. *J Royal Soc Med.* 1985;78:27–34.
51. Rodriguez-Iturbe B, Herrera J, Garcia R. Relationship between glomerular filtration rate and renal blood flow at different levels of protein-induced hyperfiltration in man. *Clin Sci (Lond).* 1988;74:11–15.
52. Crow M, Meyer GW. "Cholera solution" in short bowel syndrome. *South Med J.* 1978;71:1303.
53. Griffin GE, Fagan EF, Hodgson HJ. Enteral therapy in the management of massive gut resection complicated by chronic fluid and electrolyte depletion. *Dig Dis Sci.* 1982;27:902–908.
54. Laustsen J, Fallingborg J. Enteral glucose-polymer-electrolyte solution in the treatment of chronic fluid and electrolyte depletion in short-bowel syndrome. *Acta Chir Scand.* 1983;149:787–788.
55. MacMahon RA. The use of the World Health Organization's oral rehydration solution in patients on home parenteral nutrition. *J Parenter Enteral Nutr.* 1984;8:720–721.
56. Ward K, Murray B, Neale G. Treatment of salt losing ileostomy diarrhoea with an oral glucose polymer electrolyte solution. *Ir J Med Sci.* 1984;153:77–78.
57. Camilleri M, Prather CM, Evans MA, et al. Balance studies and polymeric glucose solution to optimize therapy after massive intestinal resection. *Mayo Clin Proc.* 1992;67:755–760.
58. Beaugerie L, Cosnes J, Verwaerde F, et al. Isotonic high-sodium oral rehydration solution for increasing sodium absorption in patients with short-bowel syndrome. *Am J Clin Nutr.* 1991;53:769–772.
59. Ladefoged K, Christensen KC, Hegnhoj J, et al. Effect of a long acting somatostatin analogue SMS 201-995 on jejunostomy effluents in patients with severe short bowel syndrome. *Gut.* 1989;30:943–949.
60. O'Keefe SJ, Peterson ME, Fleming CR. Octreotide as an adjunct to home parenteral nutrition in the management of permanent end-jejunostomy syndrome. *J Parenter Enteral Nutr.* 1994;18:26–34.
61. Nehra V, Camilleri M, Burton D, et al. An open trial of octreotide long-acting release in the management of short bowel syndrome. *Am J Gastroenterol.* 2001;96:1494–1498.
62. Ellegard L, Bosaeus I, Nordgren S, et al. Low-dose recombinant human growth hormone increases body weight and lean body mass in patients with short bowel syndrome. *Ann Surg.* 1997;225:88–96.
63. Scolapio JS, McGreevy K, Tennyson GS, et al. Effect of glutamine in short-bowel syndrome. *Clin Nutrition.* 2001;20:319–323.
64. Scolapio JS, Camilleri M, Fleming CR, et al. Effect of growth hormone, glutamine, and diet on adaptation in short-bowel syndrome: a randomized, controlled study. *Gastroenterology.* 1997;113:1074–1081.
65. Szkudlarek J, Jeppesen PB, Mortensen PB. Effect of high dose growth hormone with glutamine and no change in diet on intestinal absorption in short bowel patients: a randomized, double blind, crossover, placebo controlled study. *Gut.* 2000;47:199–205.
66. Byrne TA, Morrissey TB, Nattakom TV, et al. Growth hormone, glutamine, and a modified diet enhance nutrient absorption in patients with severe short bowel syndrome. *J Parenter Enteral Nutr.* 1995;19:296–302.
67. Byrne TA, Persinger RL, Young LS, et al. A new treatment for patients with short-bowel syndrome. Growth hormone, glutamine, and a modified diet. *Ann Surg.* 1995;222:243–255.
68. Seguy D, Vahedi K, Kapel N, et al. Low-dose growth hormone in adult home parenteral nutrition-dependent short bowel syndrome patients: a positive study. *Gastroenterology.* 2003;124:293–302.
69. Jeppesen PB, Hartmann B, Thulesen J, et al. Glucagon-like peptide 2 improves nutrient absorption and nutritional status in short-bowel patients with no colon. *Gastroenterology.* 2001;120:806–815.

Maria R. Mascarenhas, MBBS;
Donna Divito, RD, CNSD;
Stephen A. McClave, MD

15

Pancreatic Disease

Introduction

This chapter focuses on nutritional aspects of acute and chronic pancreatitis in adults and children and on cystic fibrosis (CF), the most common cause of pancreatic insufficiency. While CF is genetic in origin, pancreatitis may be related to predisposing genes and congenital structural abnormalities as well as infectious and inflammatory etiologies.

I. Background: Acute Pancreatitis
II. Nutritional Aspects of Acute Pancreatitis
III. Nutritional Alterations in Acute Pancreatitis
IV. Focused Assessment
V. Goals of Therapy
VI. Management
VII. Background: Chronic Pancreatitis
VIII. Nutritional Aspects of Chronic Pancreatitis
IX. Focused Assessment
X. Goals of Therapy
XI. Management
XII. Background: Pancreatic Insufficiency, Including Cystic Fibrosis
XIII. Nutritional Aspects of Pancreatic Insufficiency
XIV. Nutritional Alterations in Pancreatic Insufficiency
XV. Focused Assessment
XVI. Goals of Therapy
XVII. Management
References

I. Background: Acute Pancreatitis

A. Definitions
  1. Pancreatitis is a diffuse inflammatory process of the pancreas with variable involvement of other regional tissues and/or remote organ systems.[1,2]
  2. Eighty percent of hospital admissions for pancreatitis are mild in severity.[3] Most patients experience a self-limited hospital course, can be supported with intravenous (IV) fluid resuscitation and analgesia, and rapidly return to an oral diet.
  3. Severe pancreatitis (20% of hospital admissions for pancreatitis)[3] is characterized by organ failure, peripancreatic fluid collection, or evidence of necrosis on dynamic computed tomography (CT) scans. These patients tend to have a longer hospital stay, with higher mortality, and are more likely to require nutrition support. Recurrent acute pancreatitis involves flare-ups of pancreatic inflammation with abdominal pain and elevated amylase and lipase concentrations. The gland returns to normal function and anatomy between bouts.

B. Pathophysiology
  1. The exocrine pancreas secretes amylase, lipase, carboxypeptidase, phospholipase A, chymotrypsinogen, aminopeptidase, trypsinogen, and cholesterase.
  2. Autodigestion of the gland by these enzymes is normally prevented by storage of these lytic enzymes in a precursor form and by synthesis of protease inhibitors, which rapidly inactivate the enzymes.[4]
  3. Pancreatitis is caused either by premature (intrapancreatic) activation of these lytic enzymes or by disruption of the balance between the activated protease enzymes and protease inhibitors.[5]

C. Etiology
  1. In adults, acute pancreatitis involves long-term ethanol abuse in >75% of patients.[5] Fifteen percent of cases are idiopathic or due to gallstones.[5] The remaining 10% are related to pancreas divisum, trauma, hyperparathyroidism and hypercalcemia, hyperlipidemia, post–endoscopic retrograde cholangiopancreatography (post-ERCP), medications, and biliary dyskinesia.
  2. In children, acute pancreatitis is caused by trauma, viral infections, multisystem disease (systemic lupus erythematosus, Kawasaki disease, hemolytic uremic syndrome, and inflammatory bowel disease), congenital anomalies of the ducts, or medications, or is idiopathic.

II. Nutritional Aspects of Acute Pancreatitis

A. Factors promoting nutritional deterioration
  1. Protein and energy requirements increase because of the physiologic stress of acute pancreatitis.
  2. Reduced oral intake occurs because of abdominal pain with food ingestion, nausea and vomiting, gastric atony and paralytic ileus, or partial duodenal obstruction from pancreatic enlargement, or in association with ethanol addiction.
  3. Increased nutrient losses result from maldigestion and reduced absorption of luminal nutrients, excessive loss of protein because of inflammation of peritoneal and retroperitoneal surfaces, diarrhea, or formation of pancreatic fistulas.

B. Concept of pancreatic rest
  1. An ongoing precept of management that has not changed over the years is the concept of pancreatic rest. Reducing pancreatic exocrine secretion and diminishing stimulation of the gland has been found to allow resolution of the inflammatory process when mild.
  2. What has changed is the understanding of what pancreatic rest means. In the past it was felt that enzyme output from the pancreas had to be reduced to basal unstimulated levels; it is now understood that reducing secretion may be sufficient to allow resolution of inflammation.
  3. Previous prospective randomized controlled trials of severe pancreatitis in which the sole management strategy was putting the pancreas to rest (using cimetidine, nasogastric aspiration, somatostatin, etc) all failed to show an impact on patient outcome.[6]

4. Putting the pancreas to rest and using the gut are not incompatible concepts; both can be accomplished simultaneously.
5. Fortunately for the clinician, management may be guided by the patient's symptoms; placing a tube in the duodenum and monitoring enzyme output from the pancreas is not required.

C. Stimulation of pancreatic secretion

1. Multiple factors are involved in stimulation of the pancreas, including neural stimulants (the vagus nerve), chemical stimulants (luminal protein, fat, and gastric acid), mechanical stimulants (distension of the gastric wall), and hormonal stimulants (gastrin, secretin, vasoactive intestinal peptide, and cholecystokinin [CCK]).[7]
2. Stimulants may act directly or indirectly on pancreatic secretion.[7] Pancreatic secretion involves gut luminal stimulants, and the evidence that similar stimulation can occur from IV nutrients is controversial.[8]
3. Effect of IV nutrients on pancreatic secretion
   a) Animal studies on the effect of IV nutrients are inconclusive.[9–18]
   b) Among human studies, while one report in a single patient showed stimulation of pancreatic secretion from IV fat emulsion (but not IV amino acid and glucose),[19] seven other studies in patients with pancreatitis,[20–22] postoperative patients with surgically created pancreatic fistulas,[23,24] or healthy volunteers[25,26] showed no effect of IV nutrients on pancreatic secretion.
   c) There is controversy over IV fat emulsion. The consensus opinion from available studies is that hypertriglyceridemia resulting from infusion of fat is the most likely cause of an exacerbation of pancreatitis; a flare of pancreatitis resulting from IV fat infusion in the absence of hypertriglyceridemia is unlikely.[4,27–32] Multiple studies with more than 100 pancreatitis patients have shown IV fat emulsion to be a safe component of parenteral nutrition (PN).[33]
4. Effect of enteral nutrients on pancreatic inflammation
   a) It appears from a large prospective case series that the worst effect of early advancement to oral diet or use of the gut is an uncomplicated exacerbation of symptoms, which was shown to occur in approximately 21% of patients.[34]
   b) A true exacerbation of the disease process of pancreatitis occurred in only 4.3% of cases.[34] Prolongation of hospitalization and length of stay in the intensive care unit (ICU) was seen in those patients who experienced a symptomatic relapse compared to patients who did not.[34] However, early use of the gut did not prolong hospitalization.
   c) Exacerbation of symptoms appears to be simply a sign that inflammation within the gland has not resolved and the patient is not ready for dietary advancement. Ranson's warning 25 years ago[35] that early oral intake would induce late complications (specifically, abdominal abscess) has not been corroborated.
5. Evidence for the safety of early enteral nutrition (EN) in acute pancreatitis was first established by a prospective randomized trial comparing EN with PN therapy in 1997.[36] No significant difference in medical outcome parameters between the two groups was shown, including days to normalization of amylase, days to oral diet, length of hospitalization, length of time in the ICU, percent nosocomial infections, and mortality.[36]
   a) There are three phases of stimulation of pancreatic secretory output: the cephalic, gastric, and intestinal phases.[7] At each level, multiple stimulatory factors are invoked.
   b) Feeding lower in the gastrointestinal (GI) tract, especially at or below the ligament of Treitz, tends to invoke fewer stimulatory factors. The few stimulatory factors invoked at this level may be offset by the stimulation of inhibitory factors such as pancreatic inhibitory polypeptide, pancreatic polypeptide YY and bile salts.[7]
   c) There is evidence for a beneficial effect of stimulation of the GI tract at this level. In a study by McClave et al, three patients randomized to EN had resolution of symptoms and normalization of amylase on jejunal feeds.[36] Upon advancement to clear liquids by mouth, there was an exacerbation of symptoms and development of hyperamylasemia. Placing the patients back on jejunal feeds resolved symptoms and normalized amylase until efforts to advance diet could be tried again at a later date.[36] In a fourth patient, after amylase/lipase levels normalized and abdominal pain resolved on jejunal feeds, a dramatic exacerbation of the systemic inflammatory response syndrome (SIRS) occurred a week later, when the tube was found to be displaced from the jejunum into the stomach. Replacing the tube in the jejunum allowed resolution of the SIRS response, and eventually the patient was advanced successfully to oral diet and discharged.[36]
6. A second factor in the safety of EN in pancreatitis involves the content of the formula infused into the GI tract. At any given level of the GI tract, infusion of protein or fat causes greater stimulation of pancreatic exocrine output than infusion of carbohydrate.[7,37]
   a) Intact protein and individual amino acids may cause greater stimulation than small-chain oligopeptides.[37] Long-chain fat causes greater stimulation than medium-chain triglycerides (MCTs).[7]
   b) Evidence for the effect of diet content on pancreatic enzyme output was shown by Grant et al in a postoperative patient receiving jejunal feeds.[38] Switching from a nearly fat-free, elemental formula to a standard formula containing long-chain fat led to a statistically significant increase in lipase output (but no change in fluid volume, bicarbonate, or amylase output).[38]
   c) In a prospective series of patients with acute pancreatitis, patients treated with oral fat-free, elemental formula (all of whom had resolution of symptoms and normalization of serum amylase) developed an exacerbation of symptoms and hyperamylasemia when advanced to a full oral diet.[37] Placing the patients back on the oral fat-free, elemental formula resolved symptoms and normalized amylase again.
7. Tolerance of EN is variable, not an "all or nothing" phenomenon, and may be envisioned as a balance on a graded scale. The biggest factor determining tolerance is disease severity, which in turn is related to the presence or absence (and degree) of pancreatic necrosis.
   a) With greater degree of necrosis, disease severity is increased, the enteral formula may need to be infused lower in the GI tract, and the standard enteral formula may need to be replaced by either a nearly fat-free, elemental formula or a semielemental, small-peptide formula with MCT oil.
   b) While a recent study by O'Keefe et al made clear that patients randomized to EN have significantly greater increases in trypsin, amylase, and lipase output than similar patients randomized to PN,[39] the degree of stimulation is tolerated in most patients, and resolution of inflammation within the gland still occurs.

D. Role of gut integrity. For years, emphasis on pancreatic rest deterred recognition of the role of gut integrity in critical illness. The gut is the largest immune organ in the body and has been described as the motor of the multiorgan failure sepsis syndrome. The degree to which gut integrity is maintained in the critical care setting affects patient outcome.

1. Effects of enteral feeding
   a) EN maintains gut integrity by sustaining closure of the paracellular channels between the intraepithelial cells of the intestinal mucosa. It also stimulates immunoglobulin A and bile salts, which coat bacteria within the lumen of the gut. Peristalsis helps wash the bacteria downstream, and thus the overall number of enteric bacteria is held in check.
   b) EN stimulates blood flow to the gut, which helps prevent ischemia/reperfusion injury.[40]
   c) EN helps maintain the mass of gut-associated lymphoid tissue and mucosal-associated lymphoid tissue at distant sites such as the lungs, liver, and kidneys.[40,41]
   d) Whether or not EN is provided helps set the tone for the systemic immune response at the level of the gut. EN stimulates the proliferation of CD_4 helper T-cell lymphocytes in the lamina propria of the gut to proliferate down a Th2 and Th3 pathway generating interleukin-4, interleukin-10, and transforming growth factor β, all of which serve to downregulate GI inflammation.[40]
2. Effects of starvation
   a) Failure to provide EN leads to increased gut permeability (opening of the paracellular channels between the intraepithelial cells) and increased systemic bacterial challenge to the patient (with increased circulating systemic endotoxemia).
   b) Patients with severe pancreatitis and multiorgan failure have a 16-fold increase in gut permeability beyond that found in mild pancreatitis.[42] Following major insult or injury, a starved gut becomes a proinflammatory organ.
      (1) Activation of macrophages at the level of the gut by either increased permeability/bacterial challenge or subclinical ischemia/reperfusion injury leads to priming of neutrophils, which in turn circulate out to distant organ sites.
      (2) Subsequent activation of these neutrophils by hypotension or hypoxemia leads to release of superoxide radicals and exacerbation of systemic oxidative stress.[40,43]
3. Stress responses in pancreatitis
   a) Prospective randomized controlled trials of patients with acute pancreatitis placed on EN have shown patients with EN to have less stress-induced hyperglycemia, reduced use of antioxidant defenses, faster decline in C-reactive protein levels, faster resolution of SIRS, and less disease severity compared to similar patients receiving PN.[44–46]
   b) The greater the degree of severity of acute pancreatitis, the greater the importance of maintaining gut integrity and the more likely the outcome parameters will be affected by the route of nutritional support.[36,44,46,47]

III. Nutritional Alterations in Acute Pancreatitis

A. Metabolic stress state-. The metabolism of acute pancreatitis involves a classic stress state very similar to that in sepsis,[48,49] with measured resting energy expenditure as high as 139% of the value predicted by the Harris-Benedict equation.[50] More patients with acute pancreatitis are hypermetabolic than patients with chronic pancreatitis (61% vs 33%, respectively).[50] When pancreatitis is complicated by sepsis, energy expenditure may be increased by as much as 15%.[50]

B. Changes in substrate metabolism
1. Changes in carbohydrate metabolism[4,30] caused by increased cortisol and catecholamine secretion, increased glucagon/insulin ratio, impaired β-cell function, and insulin resistance lead to evidence of glucose intolerance in 40% to 90% of patients,[4,30] and insulin is required in as many as 81% of patients who were not diabetic before the onset of pancreatitis.[30] Carbohydrate intolerance has been shown to increase mortality by up to 15%.[51]
2. Changes in fat metabolism occur in only 12% to 15% of patients[30,52,53] (particularly hypertriglyceridemia) and have been shown to increase mortality by up to 33%.[51] Chronic pancreatitis causes steatorrhea once about 90% of the gland is destroyed and may result in weight loss and associated fat-soluble vitamin deficiencies.

C. Micronutrient deficiencies
1. Hypocalcemia occurs in 25% of patients[52] because of decreased parathyroid hormone secretion, increased calcitonin, hypomagnesemia, hypoalbuminemia, and saponification of calcium with free fatty acids.[30]
2. Long-term ethanol abuse predisposes patients to hypomagnesemia, decreased zinc concentrations, and deficiencies of thiamine and folate.
3. Clinical vitamin B_{12} deficiency may result from a deficiency of the pancreatic protease required to degrade the binding of the R protein with vitamin B_{12}.[5]

IV. Focused Assessment

A. History and physical exam
1. Etiologic clues that should be elicited from the interview with the patient include long-term excess ethanol use, symptoms referable to gallbladder disease or gallstones, prescription and over-the-counter medicines, and history of remote trauma (in which the pancreas might have been injured by a steering wheel or bicycle handlebars).
2. Symptoms that should be elucidated in the history include the character and time course of the abdominal pain, the presence of nausea and vomiting, weight loss, diarrhea, new onset of abdominal distension (which may indicate pancreatic ascites), muscle cramps (related to electrolyte disturbances), and easy bruising (reflecting vitamin K insufficiency).
3. The physical exam must carefully evaluate fluid status and abdominal tenderness or mass and should document any findings of xanthomas as a result of hyperlipidemia, jaundice as a result of extrinsic common bile duct compression from an enlarged pancreas, bruising around the umbilicus or flanks from retroperitoneal bleeding, Chvostek's sign (hypocalcemia), or subcutaneous nodules from fat necrosis.[54]

B. Determination of disease severity
1. An APACHE II score of ≥10 and Ranson criteria of ≥3 identify patients with severe pancreatitis who are likely to have pancreatic necrosis on CT scan, a 38% rate of complications, and an associated 19% mortality rate.[54–56] These patients represent 20% of hospital admissions for pancreatitis, have almost no likelihood of successfully advancing to oral diet within 7 days,[54–56] and are favorably affected by the use of EN rather than PN.
2. Patients with lower scores (APACHE II ≤9, Ranson criteria ≤2) have mild to moderate pancreatitis, are unlikely to have necrosis on CT scan, and have a very low complication rate (6%) and close to no mortality. They have over an 81% chance of advancing to oral diet successfully within 7 days and thus may be supported with IV fluid resuscitation and analgesia alone without nutritional support.[54–56]
3. If there is a discrepancy between the two scoring systems, patients with severe pancreatitis may be identified by a tendency for the APACHE II score to increase by 3 points over the first 48 hours,

whereas patients with mild to moderate disease severity demonstrate a decrease in the APACHE II score by 1 point over the same period.[54–56]

4. Admission bedside judgment and its associated clinical assessment have been shown to have a 34% to 44% sensitivity for identifying patients with severe pancreatitis, which is significantly less than the sensitivity of 63% seen for the APACHE II score.[56,57] After 48 to 72 hours, the sensitivity of clinical assessment increases to 44% to 66%, but this is significantly less than the increased sensitivity of 75% to 82% seen with either the APACHE II score or the Ranson criteria.[56,57]

V. Goals of Therapy

A. EN versus PN

1. Six prospective randomized trials have now shown a number of significant benefits and an overall favorable impact on patient outcome from use of EN, compared to use of PN, in patients with severe acute pancreatitis.[36,42,45,47,58,59]
2. McClave et al showed a fivefold reduction in the cost of nutritional support with EN compared to PN.[36]
3. Abou-Assi et al showed faster time to resolution of the disease process (defined by resolution of abdominal pain, near normalization of amylase, and successful advancement to clear liquid diet) by nearly 1 full week in the EN group compared to the PN group (6.2 vs 11.8 days, respectively, $P < .05$).[46]
4. Kalfarentzos et al showed a reduction in overall complications from 75% in patients receiving PN to 45% in those receiving EN ($P < .05$). Septic complications were cut nearly in half, from 50% to 28%, comparing patients receiving PN to those receiving EN ($P < .03$).[47]
5. Olah et al similarly showed a reduction in septic complications, again by half, from 27% to 12%, comparing those patients receiving PN to those receiving EN, respectively ($P = .08$).[58]
6. Two meta-analyses aggregating the data from these six prospective randomized trials have now been performed.
   a) S. A. McClave et al (unpublished data), showed that infectious complications were reduced by half with use of EN (RR = 0.52, $P < .05$), compared to use of PN.
   b) P. Marik and G. Zaloga (oral communication, January 2004) showed that the need for surgical intervention was also reduced by half in patients receiving EN (RR = 0.48, $P < .05$) compared to those receiving PN. Marik also showed a significant reduction in hospital length of stay by a mean of nearly 3 days in those patients receiving EN, compared to those placed on PN. Marik and Zaloga found trends in reduced mortality and noninfectious complications in the group receiving EN compared to patients receiving PN, but the differences did not reach statistical significance.
7. Two studies have compared EN with no nutritional therapy in patients with acute pancreatitis.[60,61]
   a) Pupelis et al showed that markers of systemic inflammation and oxidative stress (TNF, interleukin-6, and C-reactive protein levels) were all lower in a small group of patients randomized to EN compared to those patients receiving conventional therapy with no nutritional support.[60]
   b) Powell et al showed that overall complications were reduced by half, from 29% to 15%, and mortality was cut to one third, from 28% to 9%, in a small group of patients receiving EN, compared to conventional therapy with no nutritional support.[61]
   c) The nonsignificant trends seen in these small studies suggest that the issue of gut integrity and EN versus starvation is a much more important clinical factor than some negative effect from PN.

B. Tolerance of EN

1. Clinical experience with EN and expertise in placing and maintaining feeding tubes low in the GI tract vary among institutions.
   a) In one center in Great Britain, there were minimal problems involving tolerance of EN in acute pancreatitis. Out of 16 patients randomized to EN, 5 showed some degree of ileus requiring only a decrease in the infusion rate for 2 to 4 days (before resuming the full rate of feeding).[62]
   b) In contrast, a separate group from Great Britain attempted to place all patients with acute pancreatitis on EN and was successful in only 53%; 47% of patients ultimately received total parenteral nutrition (TPN) alone or no nutritional therapy.[63]
2. Duration of ileus is important. In a prospective, nonrandomized consecutive case series, duration of ileus was a factor in whether patients tolerated EN.[63] No patients in whom the duration of ileus was ≥6 days tolerated advancement to EN. If duration of ileus was limited to ≤5 days, 50% of those patients tolerated EN. However, if the nutrition support team was aggressive in placing tubes and was able to minimize the duration to <2 days, 92% of the patients tolerated EN.[63]
3. While there is wide individual enteral feeding tolerance, most patients tolerate enteral feeding below the ligament of Treitz.
   a) Eatock et al randomized patients with acute, severe pancreatitis to nasogastric or nasojejunal feeds[64]; the groups behaved indistinguishably.
   b) In contrast, two patients[39] demonstrated intolerance to infusion of nasojejunal feeds, with exacerbation of pain and elevation of serum amylase levels, in a situation where the tubes were documented to be 10 cm or more below the ligament of Treitz.

C. Methods to enhance efficacy of EN

1. Immunonutrition. In other disease processes, such as major elective surgery, burns, and trauma, immune-enhanced diets have shown even greater benefits on patient outcome than use of standard enteral formulas.[65]
   a) Concern has been raised that in an acute stress state such as pancreatitis, stimulation of interferon-gamma receptors would cause macrophages to take up arginine and produce nitric oxide, a compound that can lead to hypotension, vasodilation, and clinical shock.[66]
   b) Only one small study has compared a high arginine-supplemented immune formula to a standard enteral formula in acute pancreatitis. It showed a reduction in ICU length of stay from 34.8 to 8.6 days and hospital length of stay from 38.4 to 27.2 days (comparing controls on standard formula and those receiving immunonutrition, respectively, P = nonsignificant [*ns*]).[67]
2. Probiotics. In a small study, *Lactobacillus* added to an enteral formula infused into patients with acute pancreatitis resulted in a reduction in intra-abdominal abscess and infected pancreatic necrosis from 30.4% to 4.5% ($P = 0.023$) and a reduction in hospital length of stay from 21.4 to 13.7 days ($P = ns$), compared to similar patients receiving an enteral formula with heat-inactivated *Lactobacillus*.[68]

D. Role of PN

1. Early PN studies
   a) Early, nonrandomized, poorly controlled retrospective and prospective studies suggested that early use of PN, even with

lipids, was safe in patients with pancreatitis,[4,69–71] reduced the overall complication rate by up to 60%,[72] and reduced mortality by 8% to 25%.[51,72–74]

b) In contrast, two early retrospective reviews showed no effect of PN on the clinical course or rate of complications in pancreatitis.[22,75]

2. Prospective randomized trials with PN. Only one prospective randomized trial compared patients with mild to moderate pancreatitis placed on early PN with a control group of patients who received only IV fluid resuscitation, nasogastric decompression, and analgesia.[55]
   a) Compared with the control group, the early PN patients had a significantly longer length of hospitalization and a higher catheter sepsis rate.
   b) There was no difference in days to advancement to clear liquids, return of amylase to normal levels, or overall complications.
   c) The study concluded that widespread use of PN might not be warranted in pancreatitis.[55]
3. Timing of PN
   a) Based on the limited experience of comparing PN with no nutritional therapy, and the more extensive experience of comparing PN with EN, the timing of PN becomes important in patients with severe acute pancreatitis in whom EN is not feasible. In these patients, initiating PN within 48 hours of admission to the ICU may exacerbate the stress response and worsen outcome. It may be prudent to withhold nutrition support for 5 to 7 days, until the peak of systemic inflammation has passed, before initiating PN.
   b) In one study, an effort was made to enhance the efficacy of PN in pancreatitis by adding IV glutamine to the PN. Patients receiving PN with glutamine compared to those receiving PN alone saw a reduction in hospital length of stay by 4 days (from 25 to 21 days, $P = .07$), a reduction in sepsis from 36% to 21% ($P = ns$), and a reduction in the duration of nutritional therapy from 16 to 10 days ($P = .03$).[76]

VI. Management

A. Determining the severity of pancreatitis
   1. An APACHE II score of ≤9 with ≤2 Ranson criteria identifies patients with mild pancreatitis, who are not likely to need nutrition support, should progress to an oral diet within 7 days, and should show rapid resolution of their disease process.
   2. An APACHE II score of ≥10 with ≥3 Ranson criteria identifies patients with severe pancreatitis, who are at higher risk for complications and will require (aggressive) nutrition support. These patients should be evaluated for evidence of multiple organ failure and pancreatic necrosis.

B. Initiating EN
   1. Enteral access should be achieved fluoroscopically or endoscopically with a nasoenteric tube placed at or below the ligament of Treitz.
   2. Enteral infusion may be started with a standard enteral formula. If there is added concern in a particular patient about potential intolerance, a low-fat elemental formula or a small peptide semielemental formula (which should cause less stimulation of pancreatic exocrine secretion) may be used.

C. Monitoring. Patients should be watched closely for the possibility of tube migration and for evidence of intolerance (eg, nausea/vomiting, increasing abdominal pain, worsening fever, sudden elevations in serum amylase/lipase).

D. Using adjunctive therapy. Patients should receive aggressive fluid resuscitation, repletion of electrolytes and micronutrients, adequate analgesia to control pain, and a broad-spectrum antibiotic (eg, imipenem) to reduce septic complications.[77]

E. Using PN
   1. Progression to PN should be entertained only in patients who demonstrate clear-cut intolerance to enteral feeding or who show increasing pain with increases in amylase and lipase on EN.
   2. PN should not be initiated until after 5 to 7 days.
   3. Slightly underfeeding (providing 80% of requirements) and advancing slowly (only as control of serum glucose between 80 and 110 mg/dL will allow) may enhance the efficacy of PN.
   4. A mixed-fuel regimen should be used and patients should be watched closely for evidence of hypertriglyceridemia and hypercalcemia (either of which can exacerbate pancreatitis).

F. Watching for development of complications
   1. Failure of patients with mild pancreatitis to improve within 48 to 72 hours of admission should prompt further evaluation for evidence of complications, pancreatic necrosis, or organ failure.[1]
   2. Patients with protracted complications, such as pancreatic fistulas, ascites, or pseudocyst, still may be placed on jejunal feeding as long as there is no evidence for increasing inflammation, significant increases in serum amylase and lipase, or worsening of the complicating process.

G. Treating pediatric patients. Treatment of pediatric patients is mainly supportive and consists of hydration maintenance, pain control, and control of vomiting. Nutritional therapy is mainly via PN, since there are few studies showing the efficacy of enteral feeds in pediatric patients.

VII. Background: Chronic Pancreatitis

A. Definition. Chronic pancreatitis (CP) is a persistent inflammatory condition of the pancreas characterized by progressive, irreversible damage to the pancreas, leading to extensive fibrosis and the destruction of both exocrine and endocrine tissue.
   1. Several retrospective studies reported that the annual incidence of CP ranges from 3.5 to 10 cases per 100 000.[78]
   2. As CP is seen mainly in adults, most of the discussion in this section will focus on the care of adults with this disorder.
   3. Management in pediatric patients is similar to that in adults, with the exception of alcohol abstinence. Alcohol ingestion is not an etiologic factor in pediatric patients.
   4. CP is a common and debilitating disorder with high morbidity.
   5. Complications include malnutrition, pain, poor quality of life (QOL), diabetes mellitus, and malabsorption.
   6. The most common clinical presentation in these patients is abdominal pain, diarrhea, and weight loss.
   7. Most patients present with a variable course of intermittent acute flares of abdominal pain that become constant as the disease evolves.
   8. With destruction of the gland, diarrhea due to fat malabsorption develops, leading to progressive weight loss.
   9. The natural history of the disease and the prognosis in these patients is somewhat variable, being associated with a high morbidity rate and a mortality rate of up to 50% over 20 years.[79]
   10. Patients who continue to consume alcohol are more likely to develop complications, such as acute episodes of pancreatitis, formation of pseudocysts, duodenal obstruction, splenic vein thrombosis, and biliary strictures. These complications lead to surgical intervention in approximately 50% of patients.[80]

11. At the end stage of disease, diabetes mellitus and malnutrition are common.

B. CP is differentiated from acute pancreatitis by evidence of permanent damage to the anatomy or function of the gland, documented by calcifications on abdominal radiographic film, ductal changes on ERCP, and evidence of endocrine insufficiency (diabetes) or exocrine insufficiency (steatorrhea).

C. Causes
1. Multiple etiologies are involved in the pathogenesis of CP. They include alcohol ingestion, pancreatic duct obstruction, acute pancreatitis, pancreas divisum, CF, hereditary pancreatitis, idiopathic pancreatitis, autoimmune disorders, metabolic disorders (hypertriglyceridemia and hyperparathyroidism), trauma, and nutritional causes in tropical Africa and Asia.
2. In Western countries, alcohol consumption is the main cause in 70% to 90% of cases.[81–85]
   a) For the disease process to develop, consumption of 150 to 175 grams of alcohol per day is required for a duration ranging from 5 years up to 18 years for men and up to 11 years for women.[86]
   b) At this level of consumption, however, only 10% to 15% of patients will develop CP.
3. CP involves virtually the same etiologic possibilities as acute pancreatitis, with two exceptions: gallstone disease and biliary dyskinesia (which cause only acute pancreatitis and not CP).
4. CP is rare in children and is due to hereditary causes, congenital anomalies, and CF.

D. Pathophysiology
1. CP is an inflammatory disorder of the pancreas resulting in anatomic changes that include the infiltration of chronic inflammatory cells and fibrosis of the gland. Depending on the stage of disease, patients may present with or without functional abnormalities and abdominal pain.
2. CP starts with pancreatic injury and is characterized by loss of endocrine and exocrine function due to destruction of the acinar and islet cells and replacement of the gland by fibrous tissue.
3. Clinical presentation correlates with the severity of the histologic abnormalities.
4. Loss of exocrine function leads to malabsorption, maldigestion, steatorrhea, weight loss, and malnutrition. Pancreatic function has to fall below 10% for this to occur.[87]
5. Initially, histologic changes are patchy. These changes often progress to replacement of a large part of the gland by fibrous scar tissue.
6. CP differs from acute pancreatitis in that fibrosis and loss of exocrine tissue are present before and after an acute exacerbation.

VIII. Nutritional Aspects of Chronic Pancreatitis

A. Factors causing nutritional abnormalities
1. Malnutrition is a multifactorial process in CP and is commonly a later manifestation of the disease. A multitude of factors, ranging from poor oral intake and hypermetabolism to maldigestion and endocrine dysfunction, predispose the patient with CP to protein-calorie malnutrition.
2. There is stepwise deterioration as the disease progresses, leading to protein-calorie malnutrition.[88]
3. The major events that lead to malnutrition include poor oral intake, maldigestion resulting in malabsorption, hypermetabolism, and endocrine dysfunction.
4. The main reason for poor oral intake is persistent epigastric abdominal pain (90% of patients), which is exacerbated by eating and often accompanied by nausea and vomiting.
5. The exact cause of the pain is unknown.
   a) It is theorized that oral intake stimulates exocrine secretion of pancreatic juices released through scarred abnormal ducts, which in turn causes an increase in ductal pressure, a decrease in blood flow, and possible ischemic injury to the gland.
   b) Poor outflow of digestive enzymes may trigger autodigestion of pancreatic tissue and subsequent inflammation.
6. Poor nutritional intake may also be related to continued ethanol consumption and associated poor diet.
7. Gastroparesis has been noted in 44% of patients with exocrine insufficiency due to small-duct CP.[89]
8. A subset of patients, usually with more advanced disease, may develop gastroduodenal obstruction.
9. A large pseudocyst or diffuse inflammation of the pancreatic head may cause gastric outlet obstruction, resulting in nausea and vomiting.
10. Another component of malnutrition in these patients results from advanced destruction of the pancreas due to maldigestion and steatorrhea; this occurs in 25% to 45% of patients.[88,90–92]
   a) Patients usually have three to four loose, bulky, greasy, foul-smelling stools per day and often mention having oil droplets in the stools that are difficult to flush.
   b) Symptoms differ from those of patients with a classic malabsorptive process, which is typically characterized by watery diarrhea, abdominal bloating, and cramping.
   c) This difference in symptomatology is due to better preservation of carbohydrate absorption in the patients with maldigestion from CP.
11. The exocrine pancreas also produces bicarbonate, which is secreted with digestive enzymes in response to a meal.
   a) The bicarbonate helps neutralize gastric acid in the duodenum, which would otherwise cause breakdown of pancreatic enzymes and bile salts.
   b) Without bicarbonate present, both bile salts and enzymes are inactivated by the gastric acid, which worsens maldigestion.[93]
12. It has been shown that protein malabsorption is less than fat malabsorption because trypsin is less vulnerable to acid destruction than is lipase.[94]
13. Patients with CP and maldigestion are at risk for deficiencies of vitamins and trace elements.
   a) Vitamin B_{12} concentrations are low in an estimated 10% to 15% of patients with CP, but hematologic and neurologic complications are rare.[95] When present, the deficiency may be corrected either by supplementing B_{12} with monthly injections or by administrating pancreatic enzymes.
   b) Patients with CP are at significant risk for malabsorption of fat-soluble vitamins (A, D, E, and K), but only very rarely does it lead to overt clinical deficiency in specific vitamins.
   c) Compared to a healthy control population, these patients have been shown to have lower plasma levels of antioxidants, such as selenium, vitamins A and E, xanthine, beta-carotene, beta-cryptoxanthine, and lycopene.[96,97]
   d) Hemorrhagic complications from vitamin K deficiency are sporadic.
   e) Once thought to be insignificant, vitamin D malabsorption leading to secondary hyperparathyroidism and either osteomalacia or osteoporosis has been documented in 20% of patients with CP. A study by Haaber et al showed that approx-

imately half of patients with CP and up to 69% of those with documented steatorrhea had bone-mineral density Z scores <1, with mean 25 (OH)D and 1,25 (OH)-2D serum levels below normal.[98]

14. Up to one third of patients have chronic persistent pancreatic inflammation that causes a continuous hypermetabolic state, which plays a role in the development of malnutrition in these patients.
    a) Hypermetabolism (with a resting energy expenditure >110%) was shown in 65% of patients with alcohol-induced CP who were underweight versus 20% in patients who were of normal weight.[87]
    b) Hypermetabolism was associated with up to a 10% to 20% loss of body weight. The mechanism of hypercatabolism may include alcohol toxicity and inflammatory effects.[99–102]
15. Insulin-dependent diabetes develops on average 7 to 15 years after the diagnosis is made.
    a) 90% of the insulin-producing beta cells must be destroyed before this complication manifests.
    b) Accompanying the destruction of beta cells is the loss of glucagon-producing alpha cells.
    c) Twenty to thirty percent of these patients are insulin-dependent diabetics who are difficult to manage, with labile blood glucose levels and frequent hypoglycemic episodes.[5,103]
    d) Ketoacidosis is uncommon because of preservation of some beta cell function.[104]
    e) Wide swings in blood glucose levels and continued abnormalities in carbohydrate metabolism may contribute to delayed gastric emptying.

B. Presence of comorbid conditions. Complications seen with CP include diabetes, pseudocysts of the pancreas, biliary strictures, gastroduodenal obstruction, GI bleeding, splenic vein thrombosis, and pancreatic cancer.

IX. Focused Assessment

A. The diagnosis of CP is based on tests that assess pancreatic function and morphology.

B. An accurate nutritional assessment must be obtained in patients with CP, and evaluation of the severity of malabsorption is needed before a course of treatment can be selected.

C. Subjective global assessment, described by Detsky et al, is one measure that can be used to screen for significant nutritional risk.[105] Other data collected during the history and physical exam should include body mass index (BMI), amount of weight loss, and anthropometric measurements.

D. Laboratory data that need to be included are vitamin D and vitamin B_{12} levels.

E. The presence of steatorrhea, due to pancreatic exocrine insufficiency, can be assessed by either a quantitative or qualitative stool collection. Both methods require adherence to a strict diet of 100 g of fat per day, starting 3 days prior to the study.
   1. The quantitative method is the gold standard to estimate stool fat. Stool is collected for 72 hours; an abnormal result is the presence of >7 g of fat (or >7% of the ingested dose) per day.
   2. The qualitative method involves collecting one stool specimen, then staining for fat with Sudan III stain. Greater than 6 fat globules per high-power field is considered to be abnormal.
   3. In pediatric patients, assessment includes a 72-hour fecal fat collection while the patient is on a high-fat diet (3–4 grams of fat/kg/day) and recording all foods ingested during the stool collection period. The coefficient of fat absorption is calculated from the amount of fat ingested and excreted and normally is more than 93%.

X. Goals of Therapy

A. The goals of therapy include correction of malnutrition, improvement of nutritional status, correction of vitamin and mineral deficiencies, maintenance of glucose homeostasis, correction of malabsorption, improvement of bone mineral density, abstinence from alcohol ingestion, control of pain, and improved QOL.

B. The success of nutritional therapy is dependent upon abstinence from alcohol and control of abdominal pain. Nutritional support varies depending on disease severity.

C. Continued oral intake is preferred to the provision of artificial enteral feeds or PN.

D. Supplementation with pancreatic enzymes helps to control pain and improve digestion.

E. Specific vitamin deficiencies should be anticipated and treated appropriately.

F. Careful assessment, design of the proper nutritional regimen, and documentation of response to therapy are all required to reduce the morbidity seen in CP.

XI. Management

A. Successful intervention depends on two strategies that must be used in conjunction with nutritional therapy: absolute abstinence from alcohol and control of pain.

B. Endoscopic therapy may be needed to remove pancreatic obstructions[106] such as stones and strictures, for stent placement and drainage of pseudocysts, to block or destroy pancreatic nerves for pain control, and to place jejunal tubes for pancreatic rest.

C. Surgical therapy is indicated for patients with ongoing biliary and duodenal obstruction, pancreatic duct stenosis, and pseudocysts and consists mainly of pancreatic resection or drainage procedures for pain relief.

D. If pancreatic resection is performed, as much pancreatic tissue as possible should be conserved to decrease surgical morbidity.

E. Pain control. Controlling abdominal pain is also an important strategy for correcting malnutrition in patients with CP.
   1. Controlling abdominal pain requires putting the pancreas to rest through reduction in stimulation of pancreatic exocrine secretion.
   2. Control of pain may stimulate increased appetite and nutritional intake.

F. Oral enteral therapy
   1. Nutritional therapy may use the traditional oral route with a restrictive diet designed to reduce stimulation of the pancreas, with or without supplemental enzymes.
   2. Some patients with CP with signs of mild malnutrition may be able to consume adequate calories through an oral diet without exacerbation of abdominal pain.
      a) High-fat diets are associated with more amylase and lipase secretion than are high-carbohydrate diets.
      b) While protein may be a stronger pancreatic stimulant than carbohydrate, one study showed that varying the protein content from 10% to 40% of calories failed to produce a difference in pancreatic enzyme secretion.[107]
      c) The recommended diet for patients with CP is high in calories (35 kcal/kg/day), high in protein (1.0–1.5 g/kg/day),

high in carbohydrate percentage, and moderate in fat (0.7–1.0 g/kg/day).[108]

3. Vegetable fats are thought to be better tolerated than animal fats, because they cause less stimulation of pancreatic secretion.

G. Pancreatic enzyme replacement therapy (PERT)

1. The two goals of treatment with pancreatic enzyme supplements are control of malabsorption and relief of pain.
2. As in patients with CF, PERT is given with meals, with snacks, and sometimes at bedtime.
3. There are two types of enzyme preparations: enteric-coated (Creon, Pancrease, Ultrase) and non-enteric-coated (Viokase, pancrelipase). See Table 15-1.
4. The enteric-coated forms are designed to resist inactivation by gastric acid as the medication passes through the stomach.

TABLE 15-1. Commonly Available Pancreatic Enzyme Supplements

Brand-Name Enzymes	Manufacturer (Headquarters)	Lipase (USP Units)	Protease (USP Units)	Amylase (USP Units)
Creon Microminispheres 5	Solvay Pharmaceutical, Inc (Marietta, GA)	5000	18 750	16 600
Creon Microminispheres 10		10 000	37 500	33 200
Creon Microminispheres 20		20 000	75 000	66 400
Pancrecarb MS-4	Digestive Care, Inc (Bethlehem, PA)	4000	25 000	25 000
Pancrecarb MS-8		8000	45 000	40 000
Pancrease	Ortho-McNeil Pharmaceutical, Inc (Raritan, NJ)	4500	25 000	20 000
Pancrease MT-4		4000	12 000	12 000
Pancrease MT-10		10 000	30 000	30 000
Pancrease MT-16		16 000	48 000	48 000
Pancrease MT-20		20 000	44 000	56 000
Ultrase	Axcan Scandipharm, Inc (Birmingham, AL)	4500	25 000	20 000
Ultrase MT-12		12 000	39 000	39 000
Ultrase MT-18		18 000	58 500	58 500
Ultrase MT-20		20 000	65 000	65 000
Viokase 8 tablet	A.H. Robins Co Richmond, VA	8000	30 000	30 000
Viokase 16 tablet		16 000	60 000	60 000
Viokase each 0.7 g powder (¼ teaspoon)		16 800	70 000	70 000

USP, US Pharmacopeia

5. Once the preparation is in the proximal small bowel, the increase in pH causes dissolution of the enteric coating and the active enzymes are released.
6. Because lipase can be destroyed by gastric acid with pH <4, the non-enteric-coated forms should be given with simultaneous acid suppression (using either proton pump inhibitor or histamine-2-receptor antagonist agents).[97,109,110]
7. These two general types of enzyme preparations (enteric-coated and non-enteric-coated) are equally effective in patients with CP.[110]
8. To treat steatorrhea in adults with CP, approximately 10% of the amount of lipase normally produced by the pancreas should be delivered to the duodenum, timed to be present when the food is passing through the proximal small bowel.[111] This amount of enzyme has been shown to be equivalent to approximately 30 000 international units of lipase per meal,[112] thus requiring 4 to 8 tablets at each meal and at bedtime and 2 to 3 tablets with snacks.
9. One study showed steatorrhea to be significantly reduced from 24 to 10 g of fat/day with appropriate enzyme therapy.[113]
   a) A favorable response to treatment does not necessarily require repeat stool collection but may be determined by a clinical improvement in stool consistency, loss of visible fat in the stool, relief of diarrhea, and weight gain.[111]
   b) With correct dosing, there is usually improvement in symptoms, but steatorrhea may not be totally corrected.
   c) Tolerance of the enzyme supplements may be a problem in some patients due to nausea, bloating, cramping, constipation, or diarrhea.
   d) Failure of therapy most commonly is due to inadequate dosing, patient noncompliance, or improper use of acid-suppressive medications, as in CF.
      (1) Changing to a different preparation, decreasing daily fat intake to <60 grams, or increasing dosage to >30 000 international units of lipase per meal may improve symptomatic response.
      (2) If these measures fail to resolve symptoms, then other causes of malabsorption, such as small-bowel bacterial overgrowth, should be investigated. Intestinal bacterial overgrowth was found in approximately one third of patients with pancreatic exocrine insufficiency from CP.[114]
10. PERT can also be used to manage abdominal pain. The mechanism of pain relief from the enzyme preparations may involve suppressing the feedback mechanism of CCK-induced pancreatic secretion.
    a) Preparations high in trypsin (>50 000 international units) should be used.
    b) Surprisingly, two trials using non-enteric-coated preparations reported relief of pain, while four other trials using enteric-coated preparations did not report effective relief of pain.
    c) A recent consensus review recommended a trial of pancreatic enzymes for pain, particularly in patients with less advanced disease in whom other treatments have failed.[115]

H. PN
1. For the 10% to 15% of patients who are found to be intolerant of or unable to sustain adequate nutritional intake with a low-fat diet and pancreatic enzyme supplementation, more invasive methods for nutritional therapy may be required.[5] Either PN or enteral tube feeding can provide adequate nutritional support while minimally stimulating the pancreas, reducing abdominal pain, and decreasing the likelihood of complications associated with CP.
2. There are no reported prospective randomized trials of PN in patients with CP. Anecdotally, PN has been used to provide pancreatic rest in patients with painful symptomatic flares.
3. Disadvantages and complications from use of PN include increased cost (compared to EN), greater risk of catheter-related sepsis and thrombosis, and higher incidence of hyperglycemia and other metabolic derangements. Such PN-related complications occurred in 35% of patients in one study.[116]
4. In general, PN should be used only in patients with CP in whom signs of small-bowel dysmotility develop or enteral access to the small bowel is not available.

I. Enteral tube feeding
1. Enteral therapy (tube feeds) is helpful and has been shown to improve weight gain, improve QOL, and reduce narcotic use. The principle of reducing pancreatic stimulation by distal feeding is the same as that for acute pancreatitis.[117–121]
2. Patients with continued weight loss and poor response to oral pancreatic enzymes may gain sufficient calories from supplemental formulas containing MCT oil.
   a) MCT oil minimizes pancreatic secretion because of its direct absorption by the intestinal mucosa into the portal venous system in the absence of lipase, colipase, or bile salts.[108,122]
   b) In healthy volunteers, mean peak CCK levels were lower with the administration of formula composed of hydrolyzed peptides and MCT oil, compared to levels seen in response to an oral high-fat meal. In a 10-week pilot study of eight patients with CP and postprandial pain, daily provision of three to four cans of a small-peptide formula with MCT oil improved pain scores in 62%.[123]
3. In the few, mostly uncontrolled and retrospective studies evaluating the use of enteral feedings in patients with CP, enteral feeding has been shown to be superior to PN and in some instances to oral diet.
   a) In a group of patients with necrotizing exacerbations of CP, those on nasojejunal feedings had fewer complications, required fewer surgical interventions, and demonstrated improved healing compared to those on PN.[124]
   b) In a separate study in patients with refractory acute pancreatitis, patients sent home on jejunal feeds were less likely to be rehospitalized than patients on an oral diet.[125]
4. Enteral feedings maintain gut integrity,[126] which in turn reduces the levels of proinflammatory cytokines generated by the gut that contribute to hypermetabolism.
5. The main indication for direct enteral access is the need for prolonged (>30 days) jejunal access to manage CP and its complications.
6. Complications such as pseudocysts, ascites, and fistula are not a contraindication to jejunal feeding. For patients in whom permanent enteral access is anticipated, preliminary placement of a nasojejunal tube is recommended to see if the patient tolerates postpyloric feedings.
7. Placement of a percutaneous gastrojejunostomy, surgical jejunostomy tube, percutaneous endoscopic gastrojejunostomy, or direct percutaneous endoscopic jejunostomy depends on the patient's clinical status, the institution's expertise, and whether the patient has had previous abdominal surgery.

J. Antioxidants
1. There is some evidence supporting the use of antioxidants in patients with CP to help reduce the amount of oxidative stress created by elevated proinflammatory cytokines and the associated hypermetabolic rate.

2. Supplementation of vitamins E and C with selenium and other trace elements has shown favorable clinical outcomes, with a decrease in pain and reduced number of hospital admissions.[127,128]
3. A larger retrospective study showed that patients on antioxidant therapy had a decreased need for surgical intervention, reduced number and intensity of painful attacks, and fewer absences from work.[129]
4. Studies indicate that in pancreatic exocrine insufficiency, malabsorption of vitamin D is most likely to result in deficiency, in turn leading to osteomalacia and osteoporosis. Patients with advanced disease should be placed on vitamin D supplementation. The 25-hydroxylated form of vitamin D, calcifediol, is more readily absorbed than vitamin D_2 (calciferol). Adult dosing starts at 20 mcg per day, with maintenance dosing ranging from 20 to 100 mcg per day. Close monitoring of calcium levels is needed to avoid hypercalcemia.

XII. Background: Pancreatic Insufficiency, Including Cystic Fibrosis

A. The two most common causes of pancreatic insufficiency (PI) emerging in childhood are CF and Shwachman syndrome (PI, neutropenia, thrombocytopenia, anemia, short stature, and metaphyseal dysostosis).

B. CF is an autosomal recessive genetic disorder and is the most common inherited exocrine disease of the pancreas.
   1. It results in PI in the majority of patients with CF and is caused by mutations in the CF transmembrane conductance regulator (CFTR) gene.
   2. So far, more than 1000 CFTR gene mutations have been described.
   3. CF was once primarily a pediatric disease, since the life expectancy was low. Now, CF is fast becoming an adult disease, as patients are surviving longer.

C. EN is a mainstay of nutritional therapy for CF.

D. PN is used in critically ill patients who cannot tolerate EN or whose caloric needs cannot be met with EN.

E. It is important to sustain nutrition growth and development for improved outcome (morbidity and mortality). The many improvements in clinical care have resulted in improved survival for patients with CF.

F. It is clear that improvement in nutritional status plays an important role in maintaining pulmonary status.

XIII. Nutritional Aspects of Pancreatic Insufficiency

A. Definitions. PI refers to abnormal pancreatic exocrine function, which affects protein, fat, and carbohydrate digestion and absorption. Fat is the most significant dietary component that is malabsorbed.
   1. Pancreatic sufficiency (PS) is seen in 10% to 15% of patients with CF. These patients have sufficient (but often severely diminished) pancreatic exocrine function to achieve normal fat absorption.[130] Patients with PS have less severe mutations and disease and longer survival.
   2. Patients with CF and PS are at 900-fold increased risk for acute or recurrent episodes of acute pancreatitis[78] relative to the general population, and some of these patients go on to develop PI.[131–134] Imaging of the pancreatic and biliary trees should be done in CF patients with recurrent pancreatitis.

B. Causes
   1. Mutations in the CFTR gene result in a secretory defect in all epithelial cells. The most severe mutation is a 3-pair deletion at position delta F508 in the encoded CFTR.[130,133,134] Many other manifestations are described.
   2. Other causes of PI are rare and include Shwachman-Diamond syndrome, Alagille's syndrome, Pearson's pancreas/marrow syndrome, Jeune's thoracic dystrophy, and Johanson-Blizzard syndrome.

C. Pathophysiology
   1. Mutations in the CFTR gene result in alterations in fluid and electrolyte content of all secretions in the body due to defective CFTR anion channel transport.
      a) The damage is seen mainly in the lungs, pancreas, GI tract, liver, sweat glands, and vas deferens.
      b) These abnormalities are mainly in sodium, chloride, bicarbonate, and water content and result in changes in the viscosity of all exocrine secretions.
      c) In the pancreas, pancreatic fluid becomes viscid and obstructs smaller pancreatic ducts. This results in duct dilatation, inflammation, interstitial fibrosis, and even more obstruction and destruction of the pancreas with atrophy and fatty replacement. This process starts in utero; at birth, the majority of patients with CF have PI.
      d) In patients with PS, recurrent pancreatitis leads to ongoing damage to the pancreas.
      e) In time, PS leads to PI.[130,135,136] In older patients, endocrine function is affected, with loss of islet cells and the development of CF-related diabetes mellitus (CFRD).
   2. PI in CF manifests clinically as malabsorption, fat-soluble vitamin deficiencies, edema, hypoproteinemia, weight loss, and failure to thrive.

D. Factors causing nutritional abnormalities
   1. PI causes increased fecal losses
      a) PI leads to steatorrhea, hypoproteinemia, essential fatty acid (EFA) deficiency, and micronutrient deficiencies. Protein losses in stool are due to malabsorption.
      b) Chronic liver disease and cirrhosis associated with CF worsen maldigestion due to reduced bile salts.
      c) Patients with meconium ileus can have intestinal resections, leading to short-bowel syndrome, decreased absorptive surface area, and nutrient and bile salt losses.
      d) Older patients with CF can develop diabetes mellitus, which leads to glucosuria, further contributing to nutrient losses.
      e) Hypoproteinemia and edema are seen in infants and in patients with liver disease.
   2. Decreased intake
      a) Reduction in oral intake may occur for a variety of reasons, including post-tussive emesis, gastroesophageal reflux, esophagitis, liver disease, meconium ileus equivalent, salt depletion, micronutrient deficiency (zinc deficiency), and psychosocial causes.
      b) Patients often have a loss of appetite during acute exacerbations of pulmonary infections.
      c) Medications (eg, antibiotics) can contribute to anorexia.
      d) Some patients may have decreased intake if advised to be on a low-fat diet or prescribed unpalatable semielemental or elemental diets or supplements containing MCT.
      e) Despite a high energy intake and control of malabsorption with enteric-coated enzymes, some children remain malnourished.[137]
      f) In contrast to energy deficiency, which often exists in the malnourished child or adult with CF, protein intake is usually good.
      g) Protein deficiency is usually seen in the first year of life, when protein and energy requirements are high.

(1) Breast milk may not contain enough protein for the infant with CF, even though the protein in breast milk is more bioavailable than the protein from cow's milk–based formulas.

(2) Edema and hypoproteinemia have been described in infants with CF fed soy formulas.

3. Increased needs
   a) Children with CF have a 5% to 20% increase in resting energy expenditure, after allowing for malnutrition and lung disease.[138–140]
   b) Studies have noted greater increases in resting energy expenditures of females than males.[138–140]
   c) Chronic pulmonary infections contribute to increased energy needs.
   d) Increased energy expenditure contributes to the negative energy balance.[141] Total energy expenditure is increased, and appetite may not increase to compensate for the increased requirements and fecal energy losses.

XIV. Nutritional Alterations in Pancreatic Insufficiency

A. Growth and puberty
1. Poor growth and weight gain have been demonstrated in children and adolescents with CF.[141,142]
   a) Malnutrition can vary from mild to severe.
   b) There are critical periods in the life of a patient with CF: the first 12 months after diagnosis, birth to 12 months (for infants diagnosed prenatally), and the peripubertal period. It is critical that normal growth occur during these periods.[142]
2. Delayed puberty is seen in CF and is thought to be related to malnutrition.
   a) Swedish researchers found delayed puberty and hypogonadism in CF despite good nutritional status independent of age at menarche, growth, or nutritional or clinical parameters.[143]
   b) The CF Foundation consensus report on nutrition concluded that delayed puberty should be considered a marker for nutritional failure.[142]
3. Although growth hormone deficiency is uncommon, growth hormone therapy improves height velocity and muscle mass in patients with CF.[144–146]

B. Micronutrients
1. Deficiencies of fat-soluble vitamins (vitamins A, D, E, and K), minerals (iron, zinc), electrolytes (sodium), and EFAs can occur due to malabsorption, increased needs, and decreased intake.
2. Vitamin A deficiency is common in CF and can be seen in 15% to 40% of patients.[147–150] It may be manifested as night blindness, increased intracranial pressure, and conjunctival xerosis, or just as low levels without any clinical manifestations.
3. Vitamin D deficiency is present in 10% to 40% of patients[151] but rarely presents as rickets or osteomalacia. It is believed to contribute to the bone disease seen in CF.
4. Vitamin E deficiency is frequently seen in patients with CF and can present with hemolytic anemia, neuropathy (decreased vibration sense and proprioception), ophthalmoplegia, and ataxia.[152]
5. Vitamin K deficiency can present with coagulopathy and bone disease and is more common in infants and patients with chronic liver disease.[153]
6. Deficiencies of vitamins B_6 and B_{12} and zinc are seen in patients with CF.[142]
7. EFA deficiency is seen in patients with PI and PS.
   a) Symptoms are rare except in patients with severe deficiencies, who can have the skin changes as well as thrombocytopenia and poor wound healing.
   b) Fat malabsorption and inadequate EFA intake relative to oxidative stress or possibly from a defect in EFA metabolism are likely contributors.
8. Sodium depletion may present as hyponatremic dehydration, lethargy, weakness, and metabolic alkalosis in newly diagnosed patients and in the summer in patients who have inadequate salt intake.
9. Beta-carotene
   a) Studies have shown low levels of beta-carotene in patients with CF. These levels improved with supplementation.[154–156]
   b) There are not enough data at this time to suggest routine supplementation. The suggested intake of five servings of fruits and vegetables per day will increase the intake of beta-carotene.

C. Bone health
1. Osteoporosis and osteopenia are commonly reported complications of CF in adults. Studies have shown inconsistent results for bone mineral density in children and adolescents with CF compared to controls.[157–163]
2. Factors contributing to bone disease in CF include low body weight; gonadal dysfunction; reduced weight-bearing physical activity; poor nutritional intake; PI; malabsorption and/or decreased intake of calcium, magnesium, vitamin K, and vitamin D; corticosteroid use; pubertal delay; chronic respiratory acidosis; inflammatory cytokines; and liver disease.

XV. Focused Assessment

A. Growth and physical findings
1. According to the CF Foundation, all pediatric patients should have their weight, height/length, and head circumference (from birth to 24 months) monitored every 3 months. If growth is suboptimal, then infants should be seen every 2 to 4 weeks and older children every 4 to 6 weeks until nutritional status reaches an acceptable level.
   a) Acceptable growth is defined as % ideal body weight (IBW) 90% (all ages), weight-for-length >25th percentile (0–2 years), and BMI >25th percentile (2–20 years).
   b) Patients at risk for nutritional failure include those whose length or height has not reached genetic potential (all ages), whose %IBW is ≤90% with a history of weight loss or plateauing of weight (all ages), whose weight-for-length is between the 10th and 25th percentile (0–2 years), and whose BMI is between the 10th and 25th percentile (2–20 years).
   c) Patients with nutritional failure are those whose length/height is <5th percentile, whose %IBW is <90% (all ages), whose weight-for-length is <10th percentile (0–2 years), and whose BMI is <10th percentile (2–20 years).
2. Adult patients with CF should have their IBW determined initially. Patients should also be questioned about their usual body weight (UBW). Thereafter, at every office visit, their weight should be compared to their IBW and UBW.
   a) Malnutrition can be defined based on the %IBW as severely malnourished (<75%), moderately malnourished (75%–79%), mildly malnourished (80%–84%), underweight (85%–89%), and adequately nourished (≥90%). Improved weight gain is related to better pulmonary function.[164]
   b) BMI can also be determined at every visit and every attempt made to keep patients' BMI within a range of 20 to 25. Any

patient with a BMI of <19 is significantly malnourished and needs aggressive nutritional intervention. Arm anthropometry may also be helpful.[165]

3. Height is an effective screening tool in patients with CF.
   a) Height measurements at or below the 5th percentile for age in young children are associated with decreased life expectancy.[166]
   b) Biological parental height should be determined at diagnosis and used as a guide to determine mid-parental height and hence, growth potential.
4. The CF Foundation recommends that %IBW be used and calculated according to the Moore et al method.[167]
   a) Studies have shown that patients with mild to moderate lung disease, PI, and normal IBW had greater deficits in muscle mass than in fat stores.[137,168]
   b) Arm anthropometry should be a component of care of the patient with CF. It is recommended that arm anthropometrics be done at diagnosis and annually.
5. Pubertal status should be determined annually and may be assessed by physical examination or by the self-assessment method.[169] It is important that patients progress though puberty in a normal fashion. (See Chapter 1.)
6. Bone health is another important part of the nutritional assessment. It should include information about any history of atraumatic bone fractures, poor growth, and/or bone mineral deficits noted on previous radiographs and dual x-ray absorptiometry (DXA) studies.
   a) In the patient with growth failure and short stature, DXA results may be difficult to interpret and therefore may be more informative if obtained serially to detect a trend rather than by comparing bone densitometry values to those of age- and sex-matched controls.
   b) All children 8 years and older who have risk factors for poor bone health should have a whole-body and lumbar spine DXA done.[142]
   c) At-risk patients include those who are listed for a lung transplant and have end-stage lung disease, those who have bone fractures associated with low-impact activity, those receiving chronic corticosteroid therapy, and those with delayed puberty, nutritional failure, liver disease, or short-bowel syndrome.
   d) The CF Foundation recommends that laboratory testing (serum calcium, phosphorus, magnesium, parathormone, and 25-hydroxy vitamin D levels), as well as a detailed diet history for calcium and vitamin D intake, be obtained as part of a comprehensive assessment.
   e) Since physical activity is an important factor in bone health, an exercise history is also recommended.[159]

B. Diet history
1. A dietary history should be done by a registered dietitian at least once a year in all children with CF. It may include a 24-hour dietary recall, a 3-day written dietary record, an assessment of nutrient and supplement intake, and anticipatory dietary and feeding behavior guidance.[142]
2. Patients should be questioned about a history of enzyme use with meals and snacks.
3. More patients are trying complementary and alternative therapies,[170] so a history of the use of these therapies should be taken.
4. More frequent or detailed diet evaluations may need to be done in those patients with failure to thrive, poor weight gain, and signs/symptoms of fat malabsorption.
5. The diet history should also evaluate any abnormalities in eating behavior in the infant, toddler, child, or adolescent. Eating disorders can occur in adolescents with CF.

C. Evaluation for malabsorption
1. All patients should be evaluated for symptoms and signs of fat malabsorption at every visit. Evaluation may consist of determining whether the patient has abdominal pain, bloating, gas, floating stools, and diarrhea.
2. If patients have any of the above symptoms in conjunction with weight loss, lack of adequate weight gain, and growth failure, a more detailed assessment should be performed. It should consist of a 72-hour fecal fat determination and 3-day diet record with notes on the number of enzyme capsules used and stool description.
3. Patients with PS should have a fecal elastase level at regular intervals to monitor pancreatic function.

D. Laboratory assessment
1. It is recommended that all patients with CF have laboratory studies checked at diagnosis and at least once a year.[142] Studies include a complete blood count to screen for anemia, serum albumin, retinol, 25-hydroxy vitamin D, and alpha-tocopherol levels. EFA status should be checked in all infants and those with poor weight gain.
2. Vitamin K status should be assessed in patients at diagnosis and in those with hemoptysis, hematemesis, and liver disease. The CF Foundation recommends that a PIVKA-II level be checked.
3. The CF Foundation recognizes that there is no acceptable test currently available to check zinc status in patients with poor growth. Therefore, it is recommended that a 6-month trial of zinc supplementation be initiated, with growth status periodically reassessed to evaluate efficacy.
4. Visceral protein status should be assessed in all patients at risk of and/or diagnosed with nutritional failure by obtaining a serum albumin level.
5. Iron studies alone may not be helpful in the patient with CF, because infection will affect the reliability of the results. Soluble transferrin receptor levels are not affected by infection and inflammation and are a better reflection of iron status.

E. Presence of comorbid conditions
1. Malnourished patients should be assessed for the presence of co-existing conditions. The following conditions are known to affect nutritional status: behavioral disorders, active pulmonary disease, sinus disease, gastroesophageal reflux,[171] CFRD,[172,173] and liver disease.[174]
2. Consideration should be given to ruling out the presence of other GI disease processes, such as lactose intolerance, infections (bacterial, parasitic), bacterial overgrowth, celiac disease, inflammatory bowel disease, short-bowel syndrome, and fibrosing colonopathy. The latter should be suspected in any patient with a chronic history of ingestion of high-dose PERT, GI symptoms, and growth abnormalities.[175]

F. Determinants of disease severity
1. There is a direct association between degree of undernutrition and severity of pulmonary disease.[20] Morbidity and mortality are related to progressive lung disease.[176,177]
2. Female patients with CF appear to have a worse prognosis than males, especially during adolescence. The reasons are unknown.[178]

XVI. Goals of Therapy

A. Normal growth
1. The goals of nutritional therapy include promoting/obtaining normal growth in all patients with CF.
2. The CF team should monitor growth and nutritional status closely. This includes assessment of growth and pubertal status and early initiation of appropriate nutritional interventions.

B. Maintained or improved nutritional status
   1. All nutritional and growth abnormalities should be aggressively addressed.
   2. All abnormal vitamin and mineral and EFA levels should be corrected and periodically reassessed.

C. Promotion of optimal outcomes
   1. Optimal outcomes can be achieved by periodic assessments of adherence to PERT by the CF team, especially by the registered dietitian. In addition to a detailed history of the enzyme dose prescribed, the timing of enzyme consumption, and the storage of enzymes, a stool history and an evaluation of growth status are critical.
   2. It may be necessary to perform a 72-hour stool fat collection in addition to a 3-day diet history with documentation of PERT usage and stool pattern.
   3. Guidelines for screening and treatment of bone disease,[159] liver disease,[174] and CFRD[172] are available from the CF Foundation.
   4. DXA scans should be done in at-risk patients and at regular intervals in patients with an abnormal DXA scan.

XVII. Management

A. Energy and macronutrient needs
   1. The CF Foundation recommends a high-energy balanced diet with adequate protein and unrestricted fat appropriate for age and clinical state.
   2. The new nutrition guidelines from the CF Foundation suggest a diet that contains 35% to 40% of calories as fat.[168]
   3. There are many methods to calculate energy needs in patients with CF. In 1990, the CF consensus conference report recommended a standard method to calculate energy needs taking into account malabsorption and pulmonary status.[142] (See Table 15-2.)
   4. When weight gain is needed, energy needs are generally increased by 250 to 1000 calories.
   5. Energy needs should be periodically reassessed in conjunction with other nutritional assessment indices to ensure that energy intake is optimal.
   6. If no weight gain occurs, energy intake should be increased by 10% to 20%, with weight reassessed to determine adequacy.
   7. For adequately nourished patients with CF without associated complications (normal nutritional status, well-controlled malabsorption, and normal pulmonary function), energy requirements are generally about 105% to 115% of the recommended daily allowance (RDA).
   8. Energy needs for patients with mild to moderate lung disease, malabsorption, and nutritional failure are often in the range of 120% to 150% of the RDA.
   9. Patients with severe lung disease may require up to 200% of the RDA. However, some patients may compensate for increased energy needs by decreasing physical activity, especially when they have pulmonary exacerbations.
   10. Most patients with CF ingest a diet with adequate to high levels of protein.
   11. Patients with CF typically will require a diet with 35% to 40% of total daily energy intake contributed by fat, higher than the recommendations for the general US population (<30% of total daily energy intake as fat).
       a) Fat intake should never be restricted for patients with PI, and all patients should be prescribed a high calorie intake.
       b) Patients with recurrent pancreatitis should ingest a low-fat diet during the acute episode. These patients usually revert to their regular-fat diet once the acute episode has resolved.

TABLE 15-2. Calculations of Energy Requirements in Patients With Cystic Fibrosis

Energy needs = [REE × (AF + DC)] × 0.93/CFA
REE = resting energy expenditure or basal metabolic rate, which can be calculated using the World Health Organization energy equation for weight (*Energy and Protein Requirements.* Technical Report Series No 724. Geneva, Switzerland: World Health Organization; 1985)
AF = activity factor: 1.3 = confined to bed 1.5 = sedentary 1.7 = active
DC = disease coefficient: 0 = normal lung function or FEV1 = 80% predicted or greater 0.2 = moderate lung disease or FEV1 = 40% to 79% predicted 0.3 = severe lung disease or FEV1 = less than 40% predicted FEV = forced expiratory volume
CFA = coefficient of fat absorption; if the value is not known, use 85%

Adapted with permission from Baker RD, Borowitz D, Stallings VA. Consensus report on nutrition for pediatric patients with cystic fibrosis, 2002. *J Pediatr Gastroenterol Nutr.* 2002;35(3):246–259.

   12. Breast milk is the diet of choice for infants with CF. Some infants may need caloric supplementation using formula or molecular additives (fat and/or carbohydrate) to breast milk (eg, Polycose, vegetable oil, Microlipid, MCT, and Duocal).
       a) There is no advantage to recommending that the newly diagnosed infant with CF be given elemental or partially digested formula.
       b) If the mother chooses not to or cannot breast-feed her infant, then a cow's milk–based formula can be used.
       c) If the infant is not gaining weight appropriately, then the caloric density of formula should be increased.
   13. The timing of the introduction of solids into the infant's diet should follow the recommendation of the American Academy of Pediatrics.[179] When infants are fed cereals, breast milk or formula rather than water or juice should be used as the mixing agent to provide additional calories.
   14. Patients with short-bowel syndrome, liver disease, uncontrolled malabsorption, and/or feeding intolerances may require a partially digested or semielemental formula such as Pregestimil (Mead Johnson Nutritionals, Evansville, IN) or Alimentum (Ross Products Division, Columbus, OH) to promote optimal absorption. Butter, margarine, or vegetable oil may be added to baby food for extra calories.
   15. Toddlers, children, and adolescents benefit from a high-calorie, well-balanced diet consisting of three meals and three snacks daily, consisting of energy-dense foods and homemade or commercial shakes.
       a) Simultaneously, energy intakes typically decrease due to anorexia, fatigue, nausea, and vomiting, subsequently resulting in weight loss and deterioration in nutritional status.

b) Initiation of appropriate medical interventions (ie, IV antibiotics, increased airway clearance, etc) generally results in the return of appetite, increased energy intake, and ultimately weight gain and improved nutritional status.

16. The first step in nutritional therapy is to counsel the patient and family to increase consumption of nutritionally dense foods. It is important that any commercial supplements used do not replace the patient's usual food intake. While most practitioners use commercially available supplements for CF patients, other approaches to increasing dietary intake may be equally valid. There appears to be limited efficacy for augmenting intake orally.[180,181]
17. Patients who do not respond to the above interventions will likely need aggressive nutrition support such as tube feeds (nasogastric, gastric, and jejunal).
18. Indications for specialized nutrition support include poor weight gain for 6 to 12 months, poor nutritional status, and nutritional failure in the pre–lung transplant and pre–liver transplant patient.
19. Before the initiation of nutrition support (enteral or parenteral), patients need to be appropriately educated and the topic discussed in a positive light and proposed as supportive therapy.
    a) A trial of nasogastric tube feeds prior to gastrostomy tube placement is optimal.
    b) The patient who develops gastroesophageal reflux with nasogastric feeds that is unresponsive to medical therapy is considered a candidate for jejunal feeds after an appropriate evaluation by a gastroenterologist.
    c) Nocturnal continuous feeds are often initiated to allow for consumption of usual daytime nutrition intake and ambulation. However, this type of regimen often has a negative impact on oral intake at breakfast.
    d) Standard polymeric nutrient-dense commercially prepared enteral formulations (1–2 cal/mL) are generally well tolerated. Usually, 30% to 50% of the total daily energy intake is provided at night.
    e) Tube feeding rates need to be adjusted depending on weight gain. Infants may need 120 to 150 cal/kg/day for catch-up growth and nutritional rehabilitation. This is usually provided as a continuous nocturnal infusion for 30% to 50% of the total daily energy intake and as bolus or intermittent feeds during the day after the infant has been given an opportunity to feed orally.
    f) Signs of feeding intolerance are generally exhibited as nausea, bloating, diarrhea, and anorexia.
20. PERT is usually given at the beginning of the feed; if needed, it is also provided midway through and at the end of feeds.
21. Some patients benefit from the use of very low fat elemental formulas, which do not require PERT.
22. Feeding intolerance may be addressed through the use of a combination of enteric-coated and powdered PERT, concentrated formulas, predigested formulas containing MCT, and/or low-fat formulas.
23. Patients with CFRD may require specialized formulas as well as the use of insulin during tube feeds to avoid hyperglycemia.
    a) Patients at risk for CFRD may also develop this complication during nutritional therapy.
    b) All patients with suspected CFRD should have their blood sugars checked 2 to 3 hours after the start of the tube feeds and at the end of feeds on 2 to 3 separate nights.[114]
    c) If the serum glucose value is more than 180 mg/dL, insulin should be administered.[142]
    d) Serum glucose levels should be checked in patients at risk for developing CFRD: patients with poor weight gain, feeding intolerance, or corticosteroid use; and adolescents and young adults.
    e) If excessive bloating occurs, a prokinetic medication to improve gastric emptying and a semielemental formula can be tried.
24. PN is used infrequently in patients with CF. It is indicated in neonates with meconium ileus in the perioperative period, patients with poor nutritional status and poor oral intake who are not candidates for tube feeds or who refuse tube feeds, patients who have respiratory distress or failure while waiting for a postpyloric tube to be placed, patients who are vomiting and have significant weight loss and malabsorption, and patients with short-bowel syndrome who do not tolerate tube feeds.[182]
25. Patients with EFA deficiency (EFAD) unresponsive to enteral linoleic acid supplementation benefit from the administration of IV fat.[183]
26. Anabolic agents have been used in the management of patients with CF diagnosed with nutritional failure. Insulin has been shown to improve weight gain and fasting hyperglycemia.[184]
    a) Use of growth hormone therapy has resulted in increased growth and weight, improved pulmonary function, and fewer hospitalizations.[185]
    b) Growth hormone therapy has been shown to decrease inflammatory cytokine levels and result in less protein catabolism.[144]
    c) Growth hormone therapy is not widely used, and the decision to start therapy must be made in consultation with an endocrinologist.
    d) Trials with megestrol acetate have resulted in increased appetite and weight gain.[186]
27. Behavioral interventions are part of the management of the patient with abnormal behaviors related to feeding.[187]

B. Micronutrients

1. Standard age-appropriate doses of water-soluble vitamins should be prescribed for all patients with CF.
    a) There are age-specific recommendations for vitamins A, D, E, and K for patients with CF.[142] (See Table 15-3.)
    b) A common practice is to give patients with PI age-appropriate multivitamin doses (1–2 per day) and to give extra vitamin E.[142]
    c) It is recommended that all pediatric patients with CF receive 0.3 to 0.5 mg of vitamin K daily.
    d) Patients with liver disease and adults who have hemoptysis and are frequently on antibiotics will require significantly higher doses of vitamin K.
    e) Adult patients should ingest 2.5 to 5 mg/week of vitamin K.[164]
2. Patients consuming PERT should ingest their vitamin supplements with meals.
3. It is important to monitor fat-soluble vitamin status on a yearly basis per the CF Foundation's recommendations.
4. Adult patients consuming two tablets per day of specially formulated vitamins for CF should be ingesting sufficient vitamins.
5. Supplementation of sodium starting at diagnosis and especially during the summer months is necessary for patients with CF.
    a) This can be done by carefully adding extra salt to formula or diet in infants and by offering salty foods and sport drinks to older patients.[142]
    b) The sodium requirement for infants without CF is 2 to 4 mEq/kg/day; infants with CF have higher requirements.

TABLE 15-3. Vitamin Supplements in Patients With CF

Age	0–12 months	1–3 years	4–8 years	>8 years	Adults
Vitamin A (international units)	1500	5000	5000–10 000	10 000	10 000
Vitamin E (international units)	40–50	80–150	100–200	200–400	200–400
Vitamin D (international units)	400	400–800	400–800	400–800	400–800*

* With additional sunlight exposure.
Adapted with permission from Baker RD, Borowitz D, Stallings VA. Consensus report on nutrition for pediatric patients with cystic fibrosis, 2002. *J Pediatr Gastroenterol Nutr.* 2002;35(3):246–259.

6. All patients should consume daily reference intake (DRI) levels for calcium daily (0–6 months: 210 mg; 6–12 months: 270 mg; 1–3 years: 500 mg; 4–8 years: 800 mg; 9–18 years: 1300 mg; 19–51 years: 1000 mg; 51–70 years: 1200 mg). Note that the requirements are in milligrams of elemental calcium per day.
   a) Patients with low bone mineral content (osteopenia and osteoporosis) may need to increase their calcium intake.
   b) The upper limit for calcium is 2500 mg of elemental calcium per day.
   c) Recommended vitamin D intakes have been clearly defined by the CF Foundation.[142]
7. The CF Foundation recommends that any patient suspected of having zinc deficiency receive a trial of zinc supplements for 6 months.
   a) Growth should be monitored during this period, with improvements in growth indicative of successful treatment.
   b) Zinc supplementation is also beneficial in the patient with low vitamin A status who does not respond to vitamin A supplementation, since zinc and vitamin A deficiency are interrelated.
   c) Zinc deficiency is generally manifested as poor growth, altered taste, and skin rash (acrodermatitis enteropathica).
8. It is common practice to treat EFAD with vegetable oils that are high in linoleic/linolenic acids (eg, flaxseed oil, canola oil, walnut oil). Cold-water marine fish is another source of EFA and long-chain polyunsaturated fatty acids.
   a) All patients should meet the DRI requirements for linolenic acid.
   b) Patients with PI will need higher intakes to compensate for malabsorption.
   c) The administration of IV fat during hospitalizations using a dose of 1 g/kg/day for the duration of the hospital stay may be beneficial in patients with documented EFAD.
   d) Patients at risk for EFAD include those with nutritional failure, those with moderate to severe lung disease, and those with frequent hospital admissions for pulmonary exacerbations.
   e) There are not enough data at this time to recommend DHA supplements to all patients with CF.[139]
9. Pediatric recommendations for iron and fluoride supplementation follow the American Academy of Pediatrics guidelines.[179] Older patients and adult women with CF who are menstruating may need supplemental iron, depending on the results of blood tests of iron status.

C. Pancreatic Enzyme Replacement Therapy (PERT)

1. At diagnosis, all patients with CF should have their pancreatic function assessed. This can be done by obtaining a 72-hour collection for fecal fat, measuring fecal elastase, or measuring fecal trypsin/chymotrypsin.
2. PERT should be prescribed for all patients with CF and PI at diagnosis. (See Table 15-1.)
3. All PS patients should have their pancreatic status monitored as clinically indicated to determine if they have developed PI, especially if they have genetic mutations associated with PI.
4. PERT only partially corrects fat malabsorption.[130]
5. Excessive PERT dosing is associated with the development of fibrosing colonopathy.[175]
6. In 1995, the CF Foundation published dose recommendations for PERT. Infants should be given doses of 1500 to 2500 lipase units/kg body weight/meal, and older children and adolescents should be given doses of 500 to 2500 lipase units/kg body weight/meal. Ranges of 500 to 4000 lipase units/g of fat/day should not be exceeded. PERT should be given with all foods and milk products.[188]
7. PERT is not required with simple carbohydrates but is required when starchy foods are ingested.
   a) PERT is required with the consumption of breast milk and predigested formula, since both MCTs and long-chain triglycerides require lipase for digestion, although MCTs require less.[189]
   b) PERT should be taken before each meal and snack.
   c) If meals last longer than 30 minutes, it is recommended that the enzyme dose be split, with a half-dose given at the start of the meal and the rest of the dose given halfway through the meal.
8. Infants and children who cannot swallow the PERT capsules should be given their enzymes in applesauce immediately before eating.
   a) Parents are instructed to open the capsules and mix the beads with applesauce, which has an acidic pH.
   b) Parents and caregivers should be educated to frequently check the infant's mouth for retention of beads to prevent oral ulcerations.
   c) A skin barrier cream may be needed to prevent perianal skin irritation from the enzymes.
   d) Older children are encouraged to swallow enzyme capsules when they are able to do so.
9. Since the commonly available PERT products are porcine in origin, patients with pork allergy should not use them.
10. Significant drug interactions can occur with PERT and calcium carbonate and magnesium hydroxide. Therefore, coadministration of these products should be avoided.

11. Patients with CF have been shown to have gastric hypersecretion and pancreatic secretions that are deficient in bicarbonate. This results in an acidic duodenal pH, which does not allow for optimal function of PERT. In an effort to overcome this problem, it has been shown that concomitant use of histamine-2-receptor antagonists (eg, cimetidine) and proton pump inhibitors (eg, omeprazole) helps improve fat absorption.[190–192]
12. Data regarding the appropriate dosing of PERT with nocturnal tube feeds are limited.
    a) Erskine et al showed that tolerance of an intact formula with PERT administered before, during, and at the end of feeds was equal to tolerance of a semielemental formula without enzymes.[193]
    b) In infants, the administration of PERT with a semielemental formula resulted in better absorption.[193]
    c) Conversely, Baker et al showed that irrespective of fat content of feeds, giving the standard meal dose of PERT resulted in adequate fat absorption if PERT was given at the beginning of and midway through 8 hours of feeds.[142]
    d) Patients receiving nocturnal gastric or jejunal tube feeds appear to require PERT unless they are receiving a very low fat elemental formula.
    e) The usual premeal dose of enzymes should be taken before the feeding is started. Additional doses may need to be given midway through and at the end of the feed.[168]

D. Bone disease
1. The goals of management of pediatric bone disease in patients with CF are to optimize growth by promoting optimal intake of energy, calcium, and vitamins D and K and to ensure that the patients have regular weight-bearing physical activity.[159]
2. There are few data on the use of antiresorptive pharmacologic agents (eg, bisphosphonates) in children. These medications have been used primarily in adults with CF, especially in the peritransplant period.[5,194]
3. Patients should avoid the use of tobacco, as well as excessive alcohol and carbonated beverage intake, because these beverages have been shown to replace milk in the diet.[195]
4. Regular weight-bearing exercise is encouraged, as is optimal calcium intake of 1300 to 1500 mg/day.
5. Vitamin D intake should meet the recommendations of the CF Foundation. See Table 15-3. Serum values of 25-hydroxy vitamin D should be maintained toward the upper limit of normal.
6. Exposure to sunlight is encouraged, with the use of appropriate sunscreen measures.
7. The use of glucocorticoid therapy should be minimized, and all pulmonary infections should be treated.

E. Patient education
1. A wealth of patient educational materials is available, especially from the CF Foundation (www.cff.org).
2. Patient and family education should be part of routine care.
3. Nutritional education should include counseling regarding consumption of high-energy, high-sodium foods as well as healthy food choices.
4. The importance of adherence to the prescribed therapies (eg, vitamin and mineral supplements, PERT therapy, high-energy diet) should be reinforced.
5. All patients and their families should be included in nutritional decision making, and patients' concerns about nutritional recommendations should be addressed at every visit.

(Pancreatic disease chapters from the 1st edition were contributed by Stephen A. McClave, Harvy L. Snider, Leslie K. Sexton, Nancy Owens, Anne M. Davis, Susan S. Baker, Robert D. Baker, and Valerie Marchand)

REFERENCES

1. Bradley EL III. Acute pancreatitis: clinical classification and terminology. *Pract Gastroenterol.* 1996;20(5):8–24.
2. Bradley EL III. A clinically based classification system for acute pancreatitis. *Arch Surg.* 1993;128:586–590.
3. Corfield AP, Cooper MJ, Williamson RCN, et al. Prediction of severity in acute pancreatitis: prospective comparison of three prognostic indices. *Lancet.* 1985;ii:403–407.
4. Marulendra S, Kirby D. Nutrition support in pancreatitis. *Nutr Clin Pract.* 1995;10:45–53.
5. Holt S. Chronic pancreatitis. *South Med J.* 1993;86:201–207.
6. Koretz RL. Nutritional support in pancreatitis: feeding an organ that has eaten itself. *Semin Gastrointest Dis.* 1993;4:99–113.
7. Corcoy R, Ma Sanchez J, Domingo P, et al. Nutrition in the patient with severe acute pancreatitis. *Nutrition.* 1998;4:269–275.
8. Povoski SP, Nussbaum MS. Nutrition support in pancreatitis: fertile ground for prospective clinical investigation. *Nutr Clin Pract.* 1995;10:43–44.
9. Kelly GA, Nahrwold DL. Pancreatic secretion in response to an elemental diet and intravenous hyperalimentation. *Surg Gynecol Obstet.* 1976;143:87–97.
10. Konturek SJ, Tasler J, Cieszkowski M, et al. Comparison of intravenous amino acids in the stimulation of gastric secretion. *Gastroenterology.* 1978;75:817–824.
11. Konturek SJ, Tasler J, Cieszkowski M, et al. Intravenous amino acids and fat stimulate pancreatic secretion. *Am J Physiol.* 1979;236:E676–684.
12. Stabile BE, Debas HT. Intravenous versus intraduodenal amino acids, fats, and glucose as stimulants of pancreatic secretion. *Surg Forum.* 1981;32:224–226.
13. Saito Y, Tokutake K, Matsuno S, et al. Effects of hypertonic glucose and amino acid infusions on pancreatic exocrine function. *Tohoku J Exp Med.* 1978;124:99–115.
14. Johnson LR, Schanbachter LM, Dudrick SJ, et al. Effect of long-term parenteral feeding on pancreatic secretion and serum secretin. *Am J Physiol.* 1977;233:E524–529.
15. Hamilton RF, Davis WC, Stephanson DV, et al. Effects of parenteral hyperalimentation on upper gastrointestinal tract secretions. *Arch Surg.* 1971;102:348–352.
16. Adler M, Pieroni PL, Takeshima TT, et al. Effects of parenteral hyperalimentation on pancreatitis and biliary secretion. *Surg Forum.* 1975;26:445–446.
17. Raasch RH, Hak LJ, Benaim V, et al. Effect of intravenous fat emulsion on experimental acute pancreatitis. *J Parenter Enteral Nutr.* 1983;7:254–256.
18. Nguyen A, Barseghian G, Landel A, et al. Exocrine secretion in normal and inflamed pancreas. *J Parenter Enteral Nutr.* 1983;7:Abstr 93.
19. Klein E, Shnebaum S, Ben-Ari G, et al. Effects of total parenteral nutrition on exocrine pancreatic secretion. *Am J Gastroenterol.* 1983;78:31–33.
20. Buch A, Buch J, Carlsen A, et al. Hyperlipidemia and pancreatitis. *World J Surg.* 1980;4:307–314.
21. Silberman H, Dixon NP, Eisenberg D. The safety and efficacy of a lipid-based system of parenteral nutrition in acute pancreatitis. *Am J Gastroenterol.* 1982;77(7):494–497.
22. Grant JP, James S, Grabowski V, Trexler KM. Total parenteral nutrition in pancreatic disease. *Ann Surg.* 1984;200:627–631.
23. Grundfest S, Steiger E, Selinkoff P, et al. The effect of intravenous fat emulsions in patients with pancreatic fistula. *J Parenter Enteral Nutr.* 1980;4(1):27–31.
24. Bivins BA, Bell RM, Rapp RP, et al. Pancreatic exocrine response to parenteral nutrition. *J Parenter Enteral Nutr.* 1984;8:34–36.
25. Edelman K, Valenzuela JE. Effect of intravenous lipid on human pancreatic secretion. *Gastroenterology.* 1983;85:1063–1066.
26. Variyam EP, Fuller RK, Brown FM, et al. Effect of parenteral amino acid on human pancreatic exocrine secretion. *Dig Dis Sci.* 1980;30:541–546.

27. Noseworthy J, Colodny AH, Eraklis AJ. Pancreatitis and intravenous fat: an association in patients with inflammatory bowel disease. *J Pediatr Surg.* 1983;18(3):269–272.
28. Buckspan R, Woltering E, Waterhouse G. Pancreatitis induced by intravenous fat emulsion in an alcoholic patient. *South Med J.* 1984;77:251–252.
29. Lashner BA, Kirsner JB, Hanauer SB. Acute pancreatitis associated with high-concentration lipid emulsion during total parenteral nutrition therapy for Crohn's disease. *Gastroenterology.* 1986;90:1039–1041.
30. Havala T, Shronts E, Cerra F. Nutritional support in acute pancreatitis. *Gastroenterol Clin North Am.* 1989;18(3):525–542.
31. Niederau G, Sonnenberg A, Erkhenbrecht J. Effects of intravenous infusion of amino acids or glucose on unstimulated pancreatic secretion in healthy humans. *Dig Dis Sci.* 1995;90:446–455.
32. Stabile BE, Borzatta M, Stubbs RS, et al. Intravenous mixed amino acids and fats do not stimulate exocrine pancreatic secretion. *Am J Physiol.* 1984;246:G274–G280.
33. Leibowitz AB, O'Sullivan P, Iberti TJ. Intravenous fat emulsions and the pancreas: a review. *Mt Sinai J Med.* 1992;59:38–42.
34. Levy P, Heresbach D, Pariente EA, et al. Frequency and risk factors of recurrent pain during refeeding in patients with acute pancreatitis: a multivariate multi-centre prospective study of 116 patients. *Gut.* 1997;40:262–266.
35. Ranson JHC, Spencer FC. Prevention, diagnosis and treatment of pancreatic abscess. *Surgery.* 1977;82:99–106.
36. McClave SA, Greene LM, Snider HL, et al. Comparison of the safety of early enteral versus parenteral nutrition in mild acute pancreatitis. *J Parenter Enteral Nutr.* 1997;21(1):14–20.
37. Parekh D, Lawson HH, Segal I. The role of total enteral nutrition in pancreatic disease. *South Afr J Surg.* 1993;31:57–61.
38. Grant JP, Davey-McCrae J, Snyder PJ. Effect of enteral nutrition on human pancreatic secretions. *J Parenter Enteral Nutr.* 1987;11:302–304.
39. O'Keefe S, Broderick T, Turner M, et al. Nutrition in the management of necrotizing pancreatitis. *Clin Gastroenterol Hepatol.* 2003;1:315–321.
40. Jabbar A, Chang WK, Dryden GW, et al. Gut immunology and the differential response to feeding and starvation. *Nutr Clin Pract.* 2003;18:461–482.
41. Kudsk KA. Importance of enteral feeding in maintaining gut integrity. *Tech Gastro Endosc.* 2001;3:2–8.
42. Ammori BJ, Leeder PC, King RF, et al. Early increase in intestinal permeability in patients with severe acute pancreatitis: correlation with endotoxemia, organ failure, and mortality. *J Gastrointest Surg.* 1999;3(3):252–262.
43. Moore EE, Moore FA, Franciose RJ, et al. The postischemic gut serves as a priming bed for circulating neutrophils that provoke multiple organ failure. *J Trauma.* 1994;37:881–887.
44. Windsor ACJ, Kanwar S, Li AGK, et al. Compared with parenteral nutrition, enteral feeding attenuates the acute phase response and improves disease severity in acute pancreatitis. *Gut.* 1998;42:431–435.
45. McClave SA. Defining the new gold standard for nutrition support in acute pancreatitis. *Nutr Clin Pract.* 2004;19:1–4.
46. Abou-Assi S, Craig K, O'Keefe SJ. Hypocaloric jejunal feeding is better than total parenteral nutrition in acute pancreatitis: results of a randomized comparative study. *Am J Gastroenterol.* 2002;97(9):2255–2262.
47. Kalfarentzos F, Kehagias J, Mead N, Kokkinis K, Gogos CA. Enteral nutrition is superior to parenteral nutrition in severe acute pancreatitis: results of a randomized prospective trial. *Br J Surg.* 1997;84:1665–1669.
48. DiCarlo V, Nespoli A, Chiesa R, et al. Hemodynamic and metabolic impairment in acute pancreatitis. *World J Surg.* 1981;5:329–339.
49. Shaw JHF, Wolfe RR. Glucose, fatty acid, and urea kinetics in patients with severe pancreatitis. *Ann Surg.* 1986;204(6):666–672.
50. Dickerson RN, Vehe KL, Mullen JL, Feurer ID. Resting energy expenditure in patients with pancreatitis. *Crit Care Med.* 1991;19:484–490.
51. Sitzmann JV, Steinborn PA, Zinner MJ, et al. Total parenteral nutrition and alternate energy substrates in treatment of severe acute pancreatitis. *Surg Gynecol Obstet.* 1989;168:311–317.
52. Kohn CL, Bronzenec S, Foster PF. Nutritional support for the patient with pancreaticobiliary disease. *Crit Care Nurs Clin North Am.* 1993;5:37–45.
53. Helton WS. Intravenous nutrition in patients with acute pancreatitis. In: Rombeau JL, ed. *Clinical Nutrition: Parenteral Nutrition.* Philadelphia, PA: WB Saunders; 1990:442–461.
54. Agarwal N, Liebson C. Acute pancreatitis: systemic complications and prognostic assessment. *Pract Gastroenterol.* 1991;15:22–32.
55. Sax HC, Warner BW, Talamini MA, et al. Early total parenteral nutrition in acute pancreatitis: lack of beneficial effects. *Am J Surg.* 1987;153(1):117–124.
56. Wilson C, Heath DI, Imrie CW. Prediction of outcome in acute pancreatitis: a comparative study of APACHE II, clinical assessment and multiple factor scoring system. *Br J Surg.* 1990;77:1260–1264.
57. Larvin M, McMahon MJ. Apache-II score for assessment and monitoring of acute pancreatitis. *Lancet.* 1989;2:201–205.
58. Olah A, Pardavi G, Belagyi T, et al. Early nasojejunal feeding in acute pancreatitis is associated with a lower complication rate. *Nutrition.* 2002;18(3):259–262.
59. Louie B, Noseworthy T, Hailey D, et al. Enteral or parenteral nutrition of severe pancreatitis: a health technology assessment. *Am J Clin Nutr.* 2002;75:432S.
60. Pupelis G, Austrums E, Jansone A, et al. Randomised trial of safety and efficacy of postoperative enteral feeding in patients with severe pancreatitis: preliminary report. *Eur J Surg.* 2000;166(5):383–387.
61. Powell JJ, Murchison JT, Fearon KCH, et al. Randomized controlled trial of the effect of early enteral nutrition on markers of the inflammatory response in predicted severe acute pancreatitis. *Br J Surg.* 2000;87:1375–1381.
62. Schneider H, Boyle N, McCluckie A, Beal R, Atkinson S. Acute severe pancreatitis and multiple organ failure: total parenteral nutrition is still required in a proportion of patients. *Br J Surg.* 2000;87:362–373.
63. Cravo M, Camilo ME, Marques A, et al. Early tube feeding in acute pancreatitis: a prospective study. *Clin Nutr.* 1989;8(suppl):14.
64. Eatock FC, Chong PS, Menezes N, et al. Nasogastric feeding in severe acute pancreatitis is safe and avoids the risks associated with the nasojejunal route: a randomized controlled trial. *Gastroenterology.* 2001;120(5):A469.
65. Heyland DK, Novak F, Drover J, et al. Should immunonutrition become routine in critically ill patients? A systematic review of the evidence. *JAMA.* 2001;286:944–953.
66. Suchner U, Heyland DK, Peter K. Immune-modulatory actions of arginine in the critically ill. *Br J Nutr.* 2002;87(suppl):S121–S132.
67. Hallay J, Kovacs G, Szatmari K, et al. Early jejunal nutrition and changes in the immunological parameters of patients with acute pancreatitis. *Hepatogastroenterology.* 2001;48(41):1488–1492.
68. Olah A, Belagyi T, Issekutz A, et al. Randomized clinical trial of specific lactobacillus and fibre supplement to early enteral nutrition in patients with acute pancreatitis. *Br J Surg.* 2002;89:1103–1107.
69. Robin AP, Campbell R, Palani CK, et al. Total parenteral nutrition in severe acute pancreatitis: clinical experience with 156 patients. *World J Surg.* 1990;14:572–579.
70. Van Gossum A, Lemoyne M, Greig PD, et al. Lipid-associated total parenteral nutrition in patients with severe acute pancreatitis. *J Parenter Enteral Nutr.* 1988;12:250–255.
71. Blackburn GL, Williams LF, Bistrian BR, et al. New approaches to the management of severe acute pancreatitis. *Am J Surg.* 1976;131:114–124.
72. Kalfarentzos FE, Karavias DD, Karatzas TM, et al. Total parenteral nutrition in severe acute pancreatitis. *J Am Coll Nutr.* 1991;10:156–162.
73. Feller JH, Brown RA, MacLaren Touissant GP, et al. Changing methods in the treatment of severe pancreatitis. *Am J Surg.* 1974;127:196–201.
74. Motton G, Pistorell C, Fracastoro G, et al. Role of complete parenteral treatment nutrition in acute pancreatitis. In: Hollender LF, ed. *Controversies in Acute Pancreatitis.* Berlin, Germany: Springer-Verlag; 1982:293.
75. Goodgame JT, Fisher JE. Parenteral nutrition in the treatment of acute pancreatitis. Effect on complications and mortality. *Ann Surg.* 1977;186:651–658.
76. Ockenga J, Borchert K, Rifai K, et al. Effect of glutamine-enriched total parenteral nutrition in patients with acute pancreatitis. *Clin Nutr.* 2002;21:409–416.
77. Pederzoli P, Bassi C, Vesentini S, et al. A randomized multicenter clinical trial of antibiotic prophylaxis of septic complications in acute necrotizing pancreatitis with Imipenem. *Surg Gynecol Obstet.* 1993;176:480–483.
78. Etemad B, Whitcomb DC. Chronic pancreatitis: diagnosis, classification, and new genetic developments. *Gastroenterology.* 2001;120:682–707.

79. Lownefels AB, Maisonneuve P, Cavallini G, et al. International Pancreatitis Study Group. Prognosis of chronic pancreatitis: an international multicenter study. *Am J Gastroenterol.* 1994;89:1467–1471.
80. Ammann RW, Akovbiantz A, Largiarder F, et al. Course and outcome of chronic pancreatitis. *Gastroenterology.* 1984;86:820.
81. Copenhagen Pancreatitis Study: an interim report from a prospective multicentre study. *Scand J Gastroenterol.* 1981;16:305.
82. Everhart JE, Go VLW. Pancreatitis. In: Everhart JE, ed. *Digestive Diseases in the United States: Epidemiology and Impact.* NIH Publication No. 94-1447. Washington, DC: US Government Printing Office, US Department of Health and Human Services, Public Health Service, National Institutes of Health; 1994:691.
83. Lankisch PG, Lohr-Happe A, Otto J, et al. Natural course in chronic pancreatitis. *Digestion.* 1993;54:148.
84. Layer P, Yamamoto H, Katloff L, et al. The different courses of early- and late-onset idiopathic and alcoholic pancreatitis. *Gastroenterology.* 1994; 107:1481.
85. Worning H. Alcoholic chronic pancreatitis. In: Berger HG, Warshaw AL, Buchler MW, et al, eds. *The Pancreas.* Malden, MA: Blackwell Science; 1998:672.
86. Steer ML, Waxman I, Freedman S. Chronic pancreatitis. *N Engl J Med.* 1995;332:1482–1490.
87. DiMagno EP, Go VLW, Summerskill WHJ. Relations between pancreatic enzyme outputs and malabsorption in severe pancreatic insufficiency. *N Engl J Med.* 1973;288:813–815.
88. Scolapio JS, Malhi-Chowla N, Ukleja A. Nutrition supplementation in patients with acute and chronic pancreatitis. *Gastroenterol Clin North Am.* 1999;28:695–707.
89. Chowdhury RS, Forsmark CE, Davis RH, et al. Prevalence of gastroparesis in patients with small duct chronic pancreatitis. *Pancreas.* 2003;26: 235–238.
90. Apte MV, Keogh GW, Wilson JS. Chronic pancreatitis: complications and management. *J Clin Gastroenterol.* 1999;29:225–240.
91. Nakamura T, Tando Y, Yamada N, et al. Study on pancreatic insufficiency (chronic pancreatitis) and steatorrhea in Japanese patients with low fat intake. *Digestion.* 1999;60:93–96.
92. Twersky Y, Bank S. Nutritional deficiencies in chronic pancreatitis. *Gastroenterol Clin North Am.* 1989;18:543–565.
93. Peterson JM, Forsmark CE. Chronic pancreatitis and maldigestion. *Semin Gastrointest Dis.* 2002;13:191–199.
94. Layer P, Go VL, DiMagno EP. Fate of pancreatic enzymes during small intestinal aboral transit in humans [abstract]. *Am J Physiol.* 1986;251: G475–G480.
95. Taubin HL, Spiro HM. Nutritional aspects of chronic pancreatitis. *Am J Clin Nutr.* 1973;26:367–373.
96. Mathew P, Wyllie F, Van Lente F, et al. Antioxidants in hereditary pancreatitis. *Am J Gastroenterol.* 1996;91:1558–1562.
97. Morris-Stiff GJ, Bowrey DJ, Oleesky D, et al. The antioxidant profiles of patients with acute and chronic pancreatitis. *Am J Gastroenterol.* 1999;94: 2135–2140.
98. Haaber AB, Rosenflack AM, Hansen B, et al. Bone mineral metabolism, bone mineral density, and body composition in patients with chronic pancreatitis and pancreatic exocrine insufficiency. *Int J Pancreatol.* 2000;27:21.
99. Hebuterne X, Hastier P, Peroux JL, Zeboudj N, Delmont JP, Rampal P. Resting energy expenditure in patients with alcoholic chronic pancreatitis. *Dig Dis Sci.* 1996;41:533–539.
100. Suter PM, Schutz Y, Jequier E. The effect of ethanol on fat storage in healthy subjects. *N Engl J Med.* 1992;326:983–987.
101. Bessey PQ, Watters JM, Aoki TT, Wilmore DW. Combined hormonal infusion stimulates the metabolic response to injury. *Ann Surg.* 1984;200: 264–281.
102. Evans RD, Argiles JM, Williamson DH. Metabolic effects of tumor necrosis factor-alpha (cachectin) and interleukin 1. *Clin Sci.* 1989;37:357–364.
103. Latifi R, McIntosh JK, Dudrick SJ. Nutritional management of acute and chronic pancreatitis. *Surg Clin North Am.* 1991;71:579–595.
104. Prato SD, Tiengo A. Diabetes secondary to acquired disease of the pancreas. In: Alberti KGMM, Zimmet P, Defronzo RA, eds. *International Textbook of Diabetes Mellitus.* 2nd ed. Chichester, UK: John Wiley and Sons; 1999:189–212.
105. Detsky AS, McLaughlin JR, Baker JP, et al. What is subjective global assessment of nutritional status? *J Parenter Enteral Nutr.* 1987;11:8–13.
106. Owyang C. Negative feedback control of exocrine pancreatic secretion: role of cholecystokinin and cholinergic pathway. *J Nutr.* 1994;124:1321S.
107. Boivin M, Lanspa SJ, Zinsmeister AR, et al. Are diets associated with different rates of human interdigestive and postprandial pancreatic enzyme secretion? *Gastroenterology.* 1990;99:17763–17771.
108. Meier R. Nutrition in chronic pancreatitis. In: Buchler M, Friess H, Uhl W, eds. *Chronic Pancreatitis.* Berlin, Germany: Blackwell; 2002:421–427.
109. Heijerman HG, Lamers CB, Bakker W. Omeprazole enhances the efficacy of pancreatin (pancrease) in cystic fibrosis [abstract]. *Ann Intern Med.* 1991;114:200–201.
110. Regan PT, Malalgelada JR, DiMagno EP, et al. Comparative effects of antacids, cimetidine, and enteric coating on the therapeutic response to oral enzymes in severe pancreatic insufficiency [abstract]. *N Engl J Med.* 1977;297:854–858.
111. Forsmark CE. Chronic pancreatitis. In: Feldman M, Friedman LS, Sleisenger MH, eds. *Sleisenger and Fordtran's Gastrointestinal and Liver Disease: Pathophysiology/Diagnosis/Management.* 7th ed. Philadelphia, PA: Saunders; 2002:943–969.
112. DiMagno EP, Malagelda JR, Go VLW. Relationship between alcoholism and pancreatic insufficiency [citation]. *Ann N Y Acad Sci.* 1975;252:200–207.
113. Halgreen H, Pederson NT, Worning H. Symptomatic effect of pancreatic enzyme therapy in patients with chronic pancreatitis. *Scand J Gastroenterol.* 1986;21:104–108.
114. Trespi E, Ferveri A. Intestinal bacterial overgrowth during chronic pancreatitis. *Curr Med Res Opin.* 1999;15:47–52.
115. Warshaw AL, Banks PA, Fernandez Del Castillo C. American Gastroenterological Association technical review: treatment of pain in chronic pancreatitis. *Gastroenterology.* 1998;115:765–776.
116. Shahrudin MD, Noori SM. Pancreatic pseudocyst: the controversial value of total parenteral nutrition. *Hepatogastroenterology.* 1997;44:559–563.
117. Bodoky G, Harsanyi L, Pap L, et al. Effect of enteral nutrition on exocrine pancreatic function. *Am J Surg.* 1991;161:144–148.
118. Harsanyi L, Bodoky G, Pap A, et al. The effect of jejunal nutrition on pancreatic exocrine function. *Acta Chir Hung.* 1992;33:13–21.
119. DiMagno EP, Vay LW, Summerskill HJ. Intraluminal and postabsorptive effects of amino acids on pancreatic enzyme secretion. *J Lab Clin Med.* 1971;82:241–248.
120. Ertan A, Brooks FP, Ostrow JD, Arvan DA, Williams CN, Cerda JJ. Effect of jejunal amino acid perfusion and exogenous cholecystokinin on the exocrine pancreatic and biliary secretions in man. *Gastroenterology.* 1971; 61:686–692.
121. Vidon N, Hecketsweiler P, Butel J, et al. Effect of continuous jejunal perfusion of elemental and complex nutritional solutions on pancreatic enzyme secretion in human subjects. *Gut.* 1978;19:194.
122. Symersky T, Vu MK, Frölich M, et al. The effect of equicaloric medium-chain and long-chain triglycerides on pancreas enzyme secretion. *Clin Physiol Funct Imaging.* 2002;22:307–311.
123. Shea JC, Bishop MD, Parker EM, et al. An enteral therapy containing medium-chain triglycerides and hydrolyzed peptides reduces post-prandial pain associated with chronic pancreatitis. *Pancreatology.* 2003;3:36–40.
124. Hamvas J, Schwab R, Pap A. Jejunal feeding in chronic pancreatitis with severe necrosis. *J Pancreas.* 2001;2:112–116.
125. Gonzalez C, Silverman W. The impact of prolonged nasojejunal tube feeding in patients with refractory pancreatitis and abdominal pain: a five year retrospective review. *Gastroenterology.* 2003;124:A401.
126. DeWitt RC, Kudsk KA. The gut's role in metabolism, mucosal barrier function, and gut immunology. *Infect Dis Clin North Am.* 1999;13:465–481.
127. De Las Heras Castano G, Garcia de la Paz A, Fernandez MD, et al. Use of antioxidants to treat pain in chronic pancreatitis. *Rev Esp Enferm Dig.* 2000;92:375–385.
128. Uden S, Bilton D, Nathan L, et al. Antioxidant therapy for recurrent pancreatitis: placebo-controlled trial. *Aliment Pharmacol Ther.* 1990;4: 357–371.

129. Whiteley G, Kienle A, Lee S, et al. Micronutrient antioxidant therapy in the non-surgical management of painful chronic pancreatitis: long-term observations. *Pancreas.* 1994;9:A807.
130. Durie PR. Pancreatic aspects of cystic fibrosis and other inherited causes of pancreatic dysfunction. In: Whitcomb DC, Cohn JA, Ulrich CD, eds. *Inherited Diseases of the Pancreas.* Philadelphia, PA: WB Saunders; 2000: 609–619.
131. Sharar N, Schwarz M, Malone G, et al. Mutations of the cystic fibrosis gene in patients with chronic pancreatitis. *New Engl J Med.* 1998;339:645–652.
132. Noone PG, Zhou Z, Silverman LM, et al. Cystic fibrosis gene mutations and pancreatic risk: relation to epithelial ion transport and trypsin inhibitor gene mutations. *Gastroenterology.* 2001;121:1310–1319.
133. Cohn JA, Friedman KJ, Noone PG, et al. Relation between mutations of the cystic fibrosis gene and idiopathic pancreatitis. *N Engl J Med.* 1998; 339(10):653–658.
134. Durno C, Corey M, Zielenski J, et al. Genotype and phenotype correlations in patients with cystic fibrosis and pancreatitis. *Gastroenterology.* 2002;123:1857–1864.
135. Storman MO, Durie PR. Pathophysiologic basis of exocrine pancreatic dysfunction in childhood. *J Pediatr Gastroenterol Nutr.* 2002;35:8–21.
136. Forstner GG, Durie PR. Cystic fibrosis. In: Walker WA, Durie PR, Hamilton JR, Walker-Smith JA, Watkins JB, eds. *Pediatric Gastrointestinal Disease.* Philadelphia, PA: Mosby; 1999:1466–1485.
137. Stapleton D, Kerr D, Gurrin L, et al. Height and weight fail to detect early signs of malnutrition in children with cystic fibrosis. *J Pediatr Gastroenterol Nutr.* 2001;33(3):319–325.
138. Allen JR, McCauley JC, Selby AM, et al. Differences in resting energy expenditure between male and female children with cystic fibrosis. *J Pediatr.* 2003;142(1):15–19.
139. Shepherd RW, Greer RM, McNaughton SA, et al. Energy expenditure in the body cell mass in cystic fibrosis. *Nutrition.* 2001;17(1):22–25.
140. Zexel BS, Kawchak DA, Cnaan A, et al. Prospective evaluation of resting energy expenditure, nutritional status, pulmonary function, and genotype in children with cystic fibrosis. *Pediatr Res.* 1996;40(4):578–586.
141. Sproul A, Huang N. Growth patterns in children with cystic fibrosis. *J Pediatr.* 1964;65(5):664–675.
142. Baker RD, Borowitz D, Stallings VA. Consensus report on nutrition for pediatric patients with cystic fibrosis, 2002. *J Pediatr Gastroenterol Nutr.* 2002;35(3):246–259.
143. Johannesson M, Gottlieb C, Hjelte L. Delayed puberty in girls with cystic fibrosis despite good clinical status. *Pediatrics.* 1997;99:29–34.
144. Hardin DS, Ellis KJ, Dyson M, Rice J, McConnell R, Seilheimer DK. Growth hormone decreases protein catabolism in children with cystic fibrosis. *J Clin Endocrinol Metab.* 2001;86(9):4424–4428.
145. Hardin DS. Growth problems and growth hormone treatment in children with cystic fibrosis. *J Pediatr Endocrinol Metab.* 2002;15(2):731–735.
146. Hardin DS, Stratton R, Kramer JC, et al. Growth hormone improves weight velocity and height velocity in prepubertal children with cystic fibrosis. *Horm Metab Res.* 1998;30:636–641.
147. Palin D, Underwood BA, Denning CF. Effect of oral zinc supplementation on plasma levels of vitamin A and retinal-binding protein in cystic fibrosis. *Am J Clin Nutr.* 1979;32:1253–1259.
148. Solomon NW, Wagonfeld JB, Rieger C, et al. Some biochemical indices of nutrition in treated cystic fibrosis patients. *Am J Clin Nutr.* 1981;34:462–474.
149. Lindblad A, Diczfalusy U, Hulcrantz R, Thorell A, Strandvik B. Vitamin A concentration in the liver decreases with age in patients with cystic fibrosis. *J Pediatr Gastroenterol.* 1997;24:264–270.
150. Rayner RJ, Tyrell JC, Hiller EJ, et al. Night blindness and conjunctival xerosis in patients with cystic fibrosis. *Arch Dis Child.* 1989;64:1151–1156.
151. Feranchak AP, Sontag MK, Wagener JS, et al. Prospective, long-term study of fat-soluble vitamin status in children with cystic fibrosis identified by newborn screen. *J Pediatr.* 1999;135:601–610.
152. Winklhofer-Roob BM, van't Hof MA, Shmerling DH. Long-term oral vitamin E supplementation in cystic fibrosis patients: RRR-alpha-tocopherol compared with all-rac-alpha-tocopheryl acetate preparations. *Am J Clin Nutr.* 1996;63:722–728.
153. Strandvik B, Gronowitz E, Enlund F, et al. Essential fatty acid deficiency in relation to genotype with cystic fibrosis. *J Pediatr.* 2001;138:650–655.
154. Winklhofer-Roob BM, van't Hof MA, Shmerling DH. Response to oral beta-carotene supplementation in patients with cystic fibrosis: a 16-month follow-up study. *Acta Pediatr.* 1995;84:1132–1136.
155. Lepage G, Champagne J, Ronco N, et al. Supplementation with carotenoids corrects increased lipid peroxidation in children with cystic fibrosis. *Am J Clin Nutr.* 1996;64:87–93. Erratum in *Am J Clin Nutr.* 1997;65:578.
156. Rener S, Rath R, Rust P, et al. Effects of beta-carotene supplementation for six months on clinical and laboratory parameters in patients with cystic fibrosis. *Thorax.* 2001;56:48–52.
157. Guide to bone health and disease in cystic fibrosis consensus conference report. *CF Foundation.* 2002;10(4):1–35.
158. Gronowitz E, Garemo M, Lindblad A, et al. Decreased bone mineral density in normal-growing patients with cystic fibrosis. *Acta Paediatr.* 2003;92: 688–693.
159. Conway SP, Morton AM, Oldroyd B, et al. Osteoporosis and osteopenia in adults and adolescents with cystic fibrosis: prevalence and associated factors. *Thorax.* 2000;55:798–804.
160. Buntain HM, Greer RM, Schluter PJ, et al. Bone mineral density in Australian children, adolescents and adults with cystic fibrosis: a controlled cross sectional study. *Thorax.* 2004;59:149–155.
161. Hardin DS, Arumugam R, Seilheimer DK, et al. Normal bone mineral density in cystic fibrosis. *Arch Dis Child.* 2001;84(4):363–368.
162. Peterson ML, Jacobs DR, Milla CE. Longitudinal changes in growth parameters are correlated with changes in pulmonary function in children with cystic fibrosis. *Pediatrics.* 2003;112(3):588–592.
163. Rashid M, Durie P, Andrew M, et al. Prevalence of vitamin K deficiency in cystic fibrosis. *Am J Clin Nutr.* 1999;70(3):378–383.
164. Lloyd-Still JD, Bibus DM, Powers CA, et al. Essential fatty acid deficiency and predisposition to lung disease in cystic fibrosis. *Acta Pediatr.* 1996;85:1426–1432.
165. Yankaskas JR, Marshall BC, Sufian B, et al. Cystic fibrosis adult care: consensus report. *Chest.* 2004;125:1S–39S.
166. Beker LT, Russek-Cohen E, Fink RJ. Stature as a prognostic factor in cystic fibrosis survival. *J Am Diet Assoc.* 2001;101:438–442.
167. Moore BJ, Durie PR, Forstner GG, et al. The assessment of nutritional status in children. *Nutr Res.* 1985;57:97–99.
168. Stettler N, Kawchak DA, Boyle LL, et al. Prospective evaluation of growth, nutritional status, and body composition in children with cystic fibrosis. *Am J Clin Nutr.* 2000;72:407–413.
169. Stern RC, Canda ER, Doershuk CF. Use of nonmedical treatment by cystic fibrosis patients. *J Adolesc Health.* 1992;13:612–615.
170. Malfroot A, Dab I. New insights on gastro-esophageal reflux in cystic fibrosis by longitudinal follow-up. *Arch Dis Child.* 1991;66:1339–1345.
171. Moran A, Doherty L, Wang X, et al. Abnormal glucose metabolism in cystic fibrosis. *J Pediatr.* 1988;133:10–17.
172. Moran A, Hardin D, Rodman D, et al. Diagnosis, screening and management of cystic fibrosis–related diabetes. A consensus report. *Diabetes Res Clin Pract.* 1999;45:61–73.
173. Morris NM, Udry JR. Validation of a self-administered instrument to assess stage of adolescent development. *J Youth Adolesc.* 1980;9:271–280.
174. Sokol RJ, Durie PR, and the CF Foundation. Hepatobiliary disease consensus group recommendations for the management of liver and biliary tract disease in cystic fibrosis. *J Pediatr Gastroenterol Nutr.* 1999;28:S1–S13.
175. Fitzsimmons SC, Bukhart GA, Borowitz D, et al. High-dose pancreatic-enzyme supplements and fibrosing colonopathy in children with cystic fibrosis. *N Engl J Med.* 1997;336:1283–1289.
176. Kerem E, Reisman J, Corey M, et al. Prediction of mortality of patients with cystic fibrosis. *N Engl J Med.* 1992;32:1187–1191.
177. Konstan MW, Butler SM, Wohl ME, et al. Growth and nutritional indexes in early life predict pulmonary function in cystic fibrosis. *J Pediatr.* 2003; 142(6):624–630.
178. Kulich M, Rosenfeld M, Goss CH, et al. Improved survival among younger patients with cystic fibrosis. *J Pediatr.* 2003;142(6):631–636.
179. Kleinman RE, ed. *Pediatric Nutrition Handbook.* 5th ed. Elk Grove Village, IL: American Academy of Pediatrics; 2004.

180. Hanning RM, Blimke C, Bar-or O, et al. Relationships among nutritional status and skeletal respiratory muscle function in cystic fibrosis: does early dietary supplementation make a difference? *Am J Clin Nutr.* 1993;57:580.
181. Kalnins D, Durie PR, Corey M, et al. Are oral dietary supplements effective in the nutritional management of adolescents and adults with CF? *Pediatr Pulmonol.* 1996;(suppl 11):314–315.
182. Allen ED, Mick AB, Nicol J, et al. Prolonged parenteral nutrition for cystic fibrosis patients. *Nutr Clin Pract.* 1995;10:73–79.
183. Kusoffsky E, Strandvick B, Troell S. Prospective study of fatty acid supplementation over 3 years in patients with cystic fibrosis. *J Pediatr Gastroenterol Nutr.* 1983;2:434–438.
184. Lanng S, Thorsteinsson B, Nerup J, et al. Diabetes mellitus in cystic fibrosis: effect of insulin therapy on lung function and infection. *Acta Paediatr.* 1994:83:849–853.
185. Hardin DS, Ellis KJ, Dyson M, et al. Growth hormone improves clinical status in pre-pubertal children with cystic fibrosis: results of a randomized controlled trial. *J Pediatr.* 2001;139:636–642.
186. Marchand V, Baker SS, Stard TJ, et al. Randomized, double-blind, placebo-controlled pilot trial of megestrol acetate in malnourished children with cystic fibrosis. *J Pediatr Gastroenterol Nutr.* 2000;31:264–269.
187. Stark LJ, Jelalian E, Powers SW, et al. Parent and child mealtimes in the young child with cystic fibrosis. *J Pediatr.* 2000;136:195–200.
188. Borowitz DS, Grand RJ, Durie PR, et al. Use of pancreatic enzyme supplements with cystic fibrosis in the context of fibrosing colonopathy. *J Pediatr.* 1005;127:681–684.
189. Caliari S, Benini L, Sernbenini C, et al. Medium-chain triglycerides absorption in patients with pancreatic insufficiency. *Scand J Gastroenterol.* 1996;31:90–94.
190. Durie PR, Bell L, Linton W, et al. Effect of cimetidine and sodium bicarbonate on pancreatic replacement therapy in cystic fibrosis. *Gut.* 1980;21: 778–786.
191. Tran TM, Van den Neucker A, Hendriks JJ, et al. Effects of a proton-pump inhibitor in cystic fibrosis. *Acta Paediatr.* 1998;87(5):553–558.
192. DiMagno EP. Gastric acid suppression and treatment of severe exocrine pancreatic insufficiency. *Best Pract Res Clin Gastroenterol.* 2001;15(3): 477–486.
193. Erskine JM, Lingaard CD, Soentag MK, et al. Enteral nutrition for patients with cystic fibrosis: comparison of a semi-elemental and non-elemental formula. *J Pediatr.* 1998;132:265–269.
194. Hecker TM, Aria RM. Management of osteoporosis in adults with cystic fibrosis. *Drugs.* 2004;64(2):133–147.
195. Lytle LA, Seifert S, Greenstein J, et al. How do children's eating patterns and food choices change over time? Results from a cohort study. *Am J Health Promotion.* 2000;14(4):222–228.

William A. Faubion, Jr., MD;
Darlene G. Kelly, MD, PhD

16

Inflammatory Bowel Disease

Introduction

The inflammatory bowel diseases (IBD) primarily include Crohn's disease and ulcerative colitis. These diseases can significantly impact an individual's nutritional status, and conversely, nutritional status can alter the disease course and outcome of therapies. Nutrient deficiencies result from decreased intake, altered digestions and absorption, increased losses or requirements, and drug-nutrient interactions. This chapter will describe the disease background, therapy options, and nutritional support practices.

I. Background

A. Inflammatory bowel disease (IBD) is an incurable relapsing disorder
B. It is characterized by chronic inflammatory involvement of the small and large intestine
C. It occurs both in children and adults
D. Prevalence in U.S. only studied in Olmsted County, Minnesota[1,2]
  1. Crohn's disease (CD) for 1991 was 133 per 100,000
  2. Ulcerative colitis (UC) was 229 per 100,000 residents
  3. Similar to European data
E. Lifetime costs of care for Crohn's disease approximately $125,000 per patient[3]

II. Pathophysiology of Inflammatory Bowel Disease

A. Crohn's Disease
  1. Can involve any portion of the alimentary tract from the mouth to the anus
  2. In 80–90% of cases the small intestine is involved, particularly the terminal ileum
  3. Interspersed areas of normal mucosa are typical
  4. Inflammation of the bowel is patchy and involves the full thickness of the intestine
  5. Fistulae to other segments of involved bowel, adjacent organs (bladder, uterus), and skin occur in 20–40% of patients.
  6. Often presents with abdominal pain, fever, diarrhea, and weight loss
B. Ulcerative Colitis
  1. Mucosal disease restricted to the colon. It begins in the rectum in a continuous distribution without interspersed normal mucosa.
  2. Restricted to the left colon in 40–50% of cases (isolated rectal or rectosigmoid involvement)
  3. Remainder of cases extend proximally to involve mucosa beyond the splenic flexure. Twenty percent have pancolitis or involvement of the entire colon often with a short segment of terminal ileum involved due to "backwash ileitis."
  4. Usually presents with bloody diarrhea, urgency, and sometimes incontinence

III. Pharmacologic Therapy

A. Corticosteroid therapy most efficacious, rapidly active therapy available for moderate to severely active IBD, effective in approximately 80% of cases[4]
B. 5-ASA products (mesalamine and sulfasalazine) effective in mild to moderately active UC and CD[5–8]
  1. In UC, 5-ASA products have been shown to prolong remission.[9,10]
  2. In UC, 5-ASA products are associated with lower colon cancer rates.[11,12]
  3. The immunomodulatory agents 6-mercaptopurine (6-MP) and azathioprine are effective in the maintenance of remission in CD and are empirically believed to be effective in UC.[13–20] Azathiaprine/6-MP is also successfully used to heal fistulizing disease.[21]
C. Methotrexate useful in the induction of remission and maintenance of remission of CD in adults[22] and in children.[23]
D. Newer "biologic" therapies, such as the monoclonal antibody to TNFα, infliximab, are extremely effective in adults with moderate to severely active CD.
  1. Induction[24,25] and maintenance of remission[26,27]
  2. Perianal fistula healing[28,29]
  3. Prospective[30] and retrospective[31] studies of pediatric patients have shown similar efficacy in moderate to severely active CD, including fistulizing disease.
E. Antibiotics, particularly metronidazole and ciprofloxacin, are useful in CD
  1. Treatment of perianal disease
  2. Maintenance of post-operative remission[32,33]
  3. The high incidence of peripheral neuropathy severely limits the utility of metronidazole in CD
  4. Antibiotics have not shown a consistent effect in UC, except in the case of pouchitis post colectomy.[33]
  5. No pediatric-specific data for antibiotics

IV. Nutritional Status in Inflammatory Bowel Disease

A. Malnutrition in CD and to a somewhat lesser extent in UC is common[34]
  1. Nutritional deficiencies or inability to maintain body weight occurs in 65–78% of those with CD and in 18–62% of those with UC.[35,36]

2. Growth impairment found in 5% of children with CD.[37]
3. At some point in the course of their disease, 75% of children with CD and 10% of children with UC have growth failure.[35,38]

B. Cause of malnutrition is multi-factorial (Table 16-1).
1. Reduced oral intake caused by:
a) Pain
b) Obstructive bowel symptoms
c) Diarrhea
d) Anorexia (possibly cytokine-induced)
e) Dysgeusia (secondary to medications or zinc deficiency)[39]
f) Acutely ill children consume less than 40 to 80% of estimated needs[38]
2. Maldigestion secondary to fistulae or surgically diverted intestine
3. Malabsorption due to bacterial overgrowth, enterocyte injury, small intestinal resection, or bile acid wasting
4. Increased nutrient losses through bleeding, diarrheal losses, fistulous drainage
5. Alterations in energy expenditure
a) Total energy expenditure in quiescent and active CD is not significantly different than in normal volunteers[39,40]
b) Resting energy expenditure is increased in active CD, but activity level was decreased, making total energy expenditure identical to normals[40]
6. Drug-nutrient interactions
a) Sulfasalazine decreases absorption and alters metabolism of folic acid
b) TNFα antibody may alter protein metabolism
c) Steroids alter mineral and protein metabolism
7. Specific nutrient deficiencies
a) Vitamins: A, D, E, K, C, B_{12}, folic acid; more common in CD
b) Minerals: Copper, Calcium, Magnesium, Iron, Selenium, Zinc; more common in CD
c) Hypoalbuminemia in 25–80% of patients with CD and 26–50% of those with UC[35]
d) Anemia in about 50% of patients with CD, primarily the result of malabsorption, and in up to 80% of those with UC, largely caused by blood loss
e) Electrolytes are often depleted as a result of diarrhea in both CD and UC.

TABLE 16-1. Causes of Malnutrition in IBD

Possible causes of malnutrition	General etiology	Specific etiology
Decreased oral intake	Altered taste (Dysgeusia)	Zn deficiency or Metronidazole
	Anorexia	Cytokines (TNFa)
	Pain	Stricture, mucosal inflammation, or diarrhea
Maldigestion	Enteric fistulae	Poor exposure to digestive enzymes
Malabsorption	Carbohydrate	Enterocyte damage Bacterial overgrowth
	Fat	Enterocyte damage Bile acid deficiency (terminal ileal involvement or resection) Bacterial overgrowth Extensive surgical resection
	Protein	Inflamed tissue

V. Nutrition Support in Crohn's Disease

A. Use as primary therapy
1. Parenteral nutrition (PN) induces remission during acute attacks, but upon resuming oral diet, recurrence rates are high and do not justify the cost or risk associated with PN.[42–44]
2. No confirmed benefit for bowel rest in CD compared to enteral feedings.[45]
3. Meta-analyses comparing clinical remission with steroids was 80% versus 60% with elemental or polymeric enteral feedings[46–48]
4. No advantage for enteral elemental diets compared with semi-elemental and polymeric formula diets (61% versus 65% remission rates) in adults[47,48] and in pediatric patients[48]
5. In pediatric CD, no difference in remission rate between elemental diets and corticosteroids, each achieving remission 75–90% of the time[48–51]

B. In very extensive CD, PN may be required when the oral or tube enteral route is not possible until remission can be achieved or surgery is performed.

C. Correction of malnutrition is an important component of treatment.

D. Peri-operatively, PN in malnourished patients has shown
1. Fewer post-operative complications[52]
2. Improved clinical course[53]
3. Decreased length of bowel requiring resection, but at the expense of a longer hospitalization[54]
4. PN should be restricted to seriously malnourished patients scheduled for elective or semi-elective procedures or patients with inflammation who are not responding to pharmacologic therapy and who are not candidates for enteral nutrition support.

E. In growth failure, nocturnal enteral feeding stimulates growth[55] with significant height and weight gains compared to controls on standard therapy.[56]

F. To induce healing of enterocutaneous fistulae
1. Fistulae may result in altered nutritional status, particularly of fluid, electrolytes, and zinc.[57]
2. About 38% of fistulae initially close spontaneously with bowel rest and PN, but recurrence is common with refeeding.[58]
3. If closure of a fistula is not achieved during several weeks of PN use, infliximab can be used in an attempt to avoid surgery.

G. Dietary modification is only indicated in IBD in patients with CD where one or more non-obstructive strictures necessitates dietary fiber restriction.

VI. Nutrition Support in Ulcerative Colitis

A. No support for concept that improved nutritional status coupled with bowel rest would achieve clinical remission and avoid colectomy in UC

B. Role for specific nutrients in UC:
   1. Decreased relative risk of development of cancer or dysplasia in patients taking 0.4 and 1 mg folate daily[59]
   2. Omega-3 fatty acids as a nutritional supplement decreased disease activity and was steroid sparing[60–63]

VII. Summary

A. IBD is associated with significant nutritional risk; thus patients with these diseases require ongoing assessment and intervention to correct nutritional deficits.
B. Mechanisms for malnutrition in patients with IBD include decreased nutrient intake, maldigestion, malabsorption, increased losses, increased requirements, and drug-nutrient interactions.
C. Patients with CD do not require more energy than other patients.
D. Bowel rest with PN has no advantage over enteral nutrition in the management of patients with active CD, unless complicated by the presence of high output fistulae or high-grade small bowel obstruction, or in cases where the active disease is not responding to aggressive pharmacological therapy.
E. Elemental formulae have no advantage over polymeric diets.
F. Oral nutrition is the preferred route of feeding in patients with uncomplicated CD.
G. Peri-operative nutrition support may be indicated in patients with IBD who are severely malnourished prior to elective or semi-elective operations.
H. In children with growth failure resulting from CD, nocturnal enteral nutrition may stimulate growth.
I. In cases of fistulae associated with CD, a brief course of bowel rest and parenteral nutrition may achieve fistula healing, but relapse rates are high.
J. PN and tube enteral nutrition have no therapeutic role in uncomplicated UC.

(IBD chapter from the 1st edition was contributed by Darlene G. Kelly and Jan U. Burnes)

REFERENCES

1. Loftus EV Jr, Silverstein MD, Sandborn WJ, et al. Ulcerative colitis in Olmsted County, Minnesota, 1940–1993: incidence, prevalence, and survival. *Gut.* 2000;46:336–343.
2. Loftus EV Jr, Silverstein MD, Sandborn WJ, et al. Crohn's disease in Olmsted County, Minnesota, 1940–1993: incidence, prevalence, and survival. [erratum appears in *Gastroenterology.* 1999;116(6):1507] *Gastroenterology.* 1998;114:1161–1168.
3. Silverstein MD, Loftus EV, Sandborn WJ, et al. Clinical course and costs of care for Crohn's disease: Markov model analysis of a population-based cohort. *Gastroenterology.* 1999;117:49–57.
4. Faubion WA Jr, Loftus EV Jr, Harmsen WS, et al. The natural history of corticosteroid therapy for inflammatory bowel disease: a population-based study. *Gastroenterology.* 2001;121:255–260.
5. Sutherland L, Roth D, Beck P, et al. Azathioprine or 6-mercaptopurine for induction of remission in Crohn's disease. *Coch Data Sys Rev.* 2004.
6. Prantera C, Cottone M, Pallone F, et al. Mesalamine in the treatment of mild to moderate active Crohn's ileitis: results of a randomized, multicenter trial. *Gastroenterology.* 1999;116:521–526.
7. Thomsen OO, Cortot A, Jewell D, et al. International Budesonide-Mesalazine Study G. Budesonide and mesalazine in active Crohn's disease: a comparison of the effects on quality of life. *Am J Gastro.* 2002;97:649–653.
8. Tremaine WJ, Schroeder KW, Harrison JM, et al. A randomized, double-blind, placebo-controlled trial of the oral mesalamine (5-ASA) preparation, Asacol, in the treatment of symptomatic Crohn's colitis and ileocolitis. *J Clin Gastro.* 1994;19:278–282.
9. Anonymous. An oral preparation of mesalamine as long-term maintenance therapy for ulcerative colitis. A randomized, placebo-controlled trial. The Mesalamine Study Group. *Ann of Intern Med.* 1996;124:204–211.
10. Miner P, Hanauer S, Robinson M, et al. Safety and efficacy of controlled-release mesalamine for maintenance of remission in ulcerative colitis. Pentasa UC Maintenance Study Group. *Dig Dis & Science.* 1995;40:296–304.
11. Eaden J. Review article: the data supporting a role for aminosalicylates in the chemoprevention of colorectal cancer in patients with inflammatory bowel disease. *Aliment Pharm & Therap.* 2003;18:15–21.
12. Eaden J, Abrams K, Ekbom A, et al. Colorectal cancer prevention in ulcerative colitis: a case-control study. *Aliment Pharm Therap.* 2000;14:145–153.
13. Rhodes J, Bainton D, Beck P, et al. Controlled trial of azathioprine in Crohn's disease. *Lancet.* 1971;2:1273–1276.
14. Klein M, Binder HJ, Mitchell M, et al. Treatment of Crohn's disease with azathioprine: a controlled evaluation. *Gastroenterology.* 1974;66:916–922.
15. Present DH, Korelitz BI, Wisch N, et al. Treatment of Crohn's disease with 6-mercaptopurine. A long-term, randomized, double-blind study. *New Engl J Med.* 1980;302:981–987.
16. Ewe K, Herfarth C, Malchow H, et al. Postoperative recurrence of Crohn's disease in relation to radicality of operation and sulfasalazine prophylaxis: a multicenter trial. *Digestion.* 1989;42:224–232.
17. Willoughby JM, Beckett J, Kumar PJ, et al. Controlled trial of azathioprine in Crohn's disease. *Lancet.* 1971;2:944–947.
18. Summers RW, Switz DM, Sessions JT Jr, et al. National Cooperative Crohn's Disease Study: results of drug treatment. *Gastroenterology.* 1979;77:847–869.
19. Candy S, Wright J, Gerber M, et al. A controlled double-blind study of azathioprine in the management of Crohn's disease. *Gut.* 1995;37:674–678.
20. Oren R, Moshkowitz M, Odes S, et al. Methotrexate in chronic active Crohn's disease: a double-blind, randomized, Israeli multicenter trial. *Am J Gastro.* 1997;92:2203–2209.
21. Sandborn W, Sutherland L, Pearson D, et al. Azathioprine or 6-mercaptopurine for inducing remission in Crohn's disease. *Coch Data Sys Rev.* 2000;2:CD000545.
22. Feagan BG, Rochon J, Fedorak RN, et al. Methotrexate for the treatment of Crohn's disease. The North American Crohn's Study Group Investigators. *New Engl J Med.* 1995;332:292–297.
23. Mack DR, Young R, Kaufman SS, et al. Methotrexate in patients with Crohn's disease after 6-mercaptopurine. *J Pediatr.* 1998;132:830–835.
24. D'Haens G, Van Deventer S, Van Hogezand R, et al. Endoscopic and histological healing with infliximab anti-tumor necrosis factor antibodies in Crohn's disease: A European multicenter trial. *Gastroenterology.* 1999;116:1029–1034.
25. Targan SR, Hanauer SB, van Deventer SJ, et al. A short-term study of chimeric monoclonal antibody cA2 to tumor necrosis factor alpha for Crohn's disease. Crohn's Disease cA2 Study Group. *New Engl J Med.* 1997;337:1029–1035.
26. Hanauer SB, Feagan BG, Lichtenstein GR, et al. Maintenance infliximab for Crohn's disease: the ACCENT I randomised trial. *Lancet.* 2002;359:1541–1549.
27. Rutgeerts P, D'Haens G, Targan S, et al. Efficacy and safety of retreatment with anti-tumor necrosis factor antibody (infliximab) to maintain remission in Crohn's disease. *Gastroenterology.* 1999;117:761–769.
28. Present DH, Rutgeerts P, Targan S, et al. Infliximab for the treatment of fistulas in patients with Crohn's disease. *New Engl J Med.* 1999;340:1398–1405.
29. Ricart E, Sandborn WJ. Infliximab for the treatment of fistulas in patients with Crohn's disease. *Gastroenterology.* 1999;117:1247–1248.
30. Baldassano R, Braegger CP, Escher JC, et al. Infliximab (REMICADE) therapy in the treatment of pediatric Crohn's disease. *Am J Gastro.* 2003;98:833–838.
31. Lionetti P, Bronzini F, Salvestrini C, et al. Response to infliximab is related to disease duration in paediatric Crohn's disease. *Aliment Pharm Therap.* 2003;18:425–431.
32. Rutgeerts P, Hiele M, Geboes K, et al. Controlled trial of metronidazole treatment for prevention of Crohn's recurrence after ileal resection. *Gastroenterology.* 1995;108:1617–1621.

33. Shen B, Achkar JP, Lashner BA, et al. A randomized clinical trial of ciprofloxacin and metronidazole to treat acute pouchitis. *Inflamm Bowel Dis.* 2001;7:301–305.
34. Kelly DG, Fleming CR. Nutritional considerations in inflammatory bowel diseases. *Gastro Clin No Am.* 1995;24:597–611.
35. O'Keefe SJ. Nutrition and gastrointestinal disease. *Scand J Gastroenterology Suppl.* 1996;220:52–59.
36. Burke A, Lichtenstein GR, Rombeau JL. Nutrition and ulcerative colitis. *Baillieres Pract Res Clin Gastroenterol.* 1997;11:153–174.
37. Booth IW. The nutritional consequences of gastrointestinal disease in adolescence. *Acta Paediat Scand Suppl.* 1991;373:91–102.
38. Oliva MM, Lake AM. Nutritional considerations and management of the child with inflammatory bowel disease. *Nutrition.* 1996;12:151–158.
39. Chan AT, Fleming CR, O'Fallon WM, et al. Estimated versus measured basal energy requirements in patients with Crohn's disease. *Gastroenterology.* 1986;91:75–78.
40. Stokes MA, Hill GL. Total energy expenditure in patients with Crohn's disease: measurement by the combined body scan technique. *J Parenter Enteral Nutr.* 1993;17:3–7.
41. Geerling BJ, Badart-Smook A, Stockbrugger RW, Brummer RJ. Comprehensive nutritional status in patients with long-standing Crohn disease currently in remission. *Am J Clin Nutr.* 1998;67:919–926.
42. Shiloni E, Coronado E, Freund HR. Role of total parenteral nutrition in the treatment of Crohn's disease. *Am J Surg.* 1989;157:180–185.
43. Dickinson RJ, Ashton MG, Axon AT, Smith RC, Yeung CK, Hill GL. Controlled trial of intravenous hyperalimentation and total bowel rest as an adjunct to the routine therapy of acute colitis. *Gastroenterology.* 1980;79:1199–1204.
44. McIntyre PB, Powell-Tuck J, Wood SR, et al. Controlled trial of bowel rest in the treatment of severe acute colitis. *Gut.* 1986;27:481–485.
45. Greenberg GR, Fleming CR, Jeejeebhoy KN, et al. Controlled trial of bowel rest and nutritional support in the management of Crohn's disease. *Gut.* 1988;29:1309–1315.
46. Messori A, Trallori G, D'Albasio G, et al. Defined-formula diets versus steroids in the treatment of active Crohn's disease: a meta-analysis. *Scand J Gastro.* 1996;31:267–272.
47. Fernandez-Banares F, Cabre E, Esteve-Comas M, et al. How effective is enteral nutrition in inducing clinical remission in active Crohn's disease? A meta-analysis of the randomized clinical trials. *J Parenter Enteral Nutr.* 1995;19:356–364.
48. Griffiths AM, Ohlsson A, Sherman PM, et al. Meta-analysis of enteral nutrition as a primary treatment of active Crohn's disease. *Gastroenterology.* 1995;108:1056–1067.
49. Sanderson IR, Udeen S, Davies PS, et al. Remission induced by an elemental diet in small bowel Crohn's disease. *Arch Dis Child.* 1987;62:123–127.
50. Heuschkel RB, Menache CC, Megerian JT, et al. Enteral nutrition and corticosteroids in the treatment of acute Crohn's disease in children. *J Ped Gastro Nutr.* 2000;31:8–15.
51. Ruemmele FM, Roy CC, Levy E, et al. Nutrition as primary therapy in pediatric Crohn's disease: fact or fantasy? *J Pediatr.* 2000;136:285–291.
52. Rombeau JL, Barot LR, Williamson CE, Mullen JL. Preoperative total parenteral nutrition and surgical outcome in patients with inflammatory bowel disease. *Am J Surg.* 1982;143:139–143.
53. Eisenberg HW, Turnbull RB Jr, Weakley FL. Hyperalimentation as preparation for surgery in transmural colitis (Crohn's disease). *Dis Col Rect.* 1974;17:469–475.
54. Lashner BA, Evans AA, Hanauer SB. Preoperative total parenteral nutrition for bowel resection in Crohn's disease. *Dig Dis Science.* 1989;34:741–746.
55. Wilschanski M, Sherman P, Pencharz P, et al. Supplementary enteral nutrition maintains remission in paediatric Crohn's disease. *Gut.* 1996;38:543–548.
56. Belli DC, Seidman E, Bouthillier L, et al. Chronic intermittent elemental diet improves growth failure in children with Crohn's disease. *Gastroenterology.* 1988;94:603–610.
57. Yamazaki Y, Fukushima T, Sugita A, et al. The medical, nutritional and surgical treatment of fistulae in Crohn's disease. *Jap J Surgery.* 1990;20:376–383.
58. Afonso JJ, Rombeau JL. Nutritional care for patients with Crohn's disease. *Hepato-Gastroenterology.* 1990;37:32–41.
59. Lashner BA, Provencher KS, Seidner DL, et al. The effect of folic acid supplementation on the risk for cancer or dysplasia in ulcerative colitis. *Gastroenterology.* 1997;112:29–32.
60. Hawthorne AB, Daneshmend TK, Hawkey CJ, et al. Treatment of ulcerative colitis with fish oil supplementation: a prospective 12 month randomised controlled trial. *Gut.* 1992;33:922–928.
61. Lorenz R, Weber PC, Szimnau P, et al. Supplementation with n-3 fatty acids from fish oil in chronic inflammatory bowel disease—a randomized, placebo-controlled, double-blind cross-over trial. *J Intern Med.* 1989;225:225–232.
62. Lorenz-Meyer H, Bauer P, Nicolay C, et al. Omega-3 fatty acids and low carbohydrate diet for maintenance of remission in Crohn's disease. A randomized controlled multicenter trial. Study Group Members (German Crohn's Disease Study Group). *Scand J Gastro.* 1996;31:778–785.
63. Aslan A, Triadafilopoulos G. Fish oil fatty acid supplementation in active ulcerative colitis: a double-blind, placebo-controlled, crossover study. *Am J Gastro.* 1992;87:432–437.

Jeanette M. Hasse, PhD, RD, LD, FADA, CNSD;
Stuart S. Kaufman, MD;
Erin Fennelly, RD, CNSD

17

Liver Disease

Introduction

As a primarily metabolic organ, the liver orchestrates a complex array of physiologic and biochemical processes, one of which is the regulation of protein and energy metabolism. Consequently, it is not surprising that protein calorie malnutrition (PCM) is a common complication of advanced liver disease. The demonstration that PCM is an independent risk factor for predicting clinical outcomes in cirrhosis and the fact that nutritional intervention may improve survival, surgical outcome, liver function, and hepatic encephalopathy have made the recognition of PCM an important factor in the management of liver disease patients. The aim of the present chapter is to provide a practical approach to the nutrition management of patients with liver disease, recognizing there is insufficient information for proscriptional recommendations.

I. Overview of Liver Disease

A. Adult[1,2]
  1. Types
    a) Viral hepatitis—inflammation of the liver caused by
      (1) Hepatitis A—transmitted by the oral-fecal route
      (2) Hepatitis B and C—transmitted via body fluids
      (3) Hepatitis D—only occurs in patients infected with hepatitis B
      (4) Hepatitis E—transmitted via the oral-fecal route; hepatitis E is rare in the U.S. but is seen more often in Asia, Africa, and Mexico
    b) Alcohol—most common liver disease in the United States; progresses in 3 stages
      (1) Hepatic steatosis
      (2) Alcoholic hepatitis
      (3) Alcoholic (Laennec's) cirrhosis
    c) Cholestatic disease—involves the bile ducts
      (1) Primary biliary cirrhosis—destruction of small and intermediate-sized intrahepatic bile ducts
      (2) Sclerosing cholangitis—inflammation of segments of extrahepatic bile ducts; may involve intrahepatic ducts
    d) Toxic hepatitis—often includes:
      (1) Drug toxicity (eg, acetaminophen)
      (2) Chemical toxicity (eg, poisonous mushrooms or industrial poisons)
    e) Inherited disorders—includes metabolic diseases such as:
      (1) Hemochromatosis—iron overload
      (2) Wilson's disease—copper overload
      (3) Alpha-1-antitrypsin deficiency
    f) Other
      (1) Systemic diseases—includes rheumatoid arthritis, systemic lupus erythematosus, polymyalgia, polyarteritis nodosa, Sjögren's syndrome, autoimmune disease
      (2) Non-alcoholic steatohepatitis (NASH)
      (3) Vascular conditions—Budd Chiari syndrome, hepatic venoocclusive disease
      (4) Infectious—parasitic, bacterial, fungal, and granulomatous liver disease
  2. Duration
    a) Acute—sudden and massive destruction of liver cells[3]
      (1) Fulminant—severe liver dysfunction with hepatic encephalopathy and coagulopathy that develop within 2 weeks of illness onset; no previous history of liver dysfunction
      (2) Subfulminant—hepatic encephalopathy and coagulopathy develop in 2 to 8 weeks of onset of illness
      (3) Late-onset liver failure—hepatic encephalopathy and coagulopathy develop within 8 to 24 weeks of onset of illness
    b) Chronic—at least a 6-month course

B. Pediatric—Nutrition support is relevant primarily to chronic fibrocirrhotic disorders and acute liver failure
  1. Fulminant and subfulminant liver failure
    a) Viruses (A to G viruses)
    b) Certain inborn errors (eg, neonatal hemochromatosis)
    c) Toxins (eg, poisonous mushrooms)
  2. Chronic liver disease
    a) In infants, disorders include:
      (1) Intrahepatic and extrahepatic biliary obstructive disorders (eg, biliary atresia, familial intrahepatic cholestasis, Alagille Syndrome)
      (2) Metabolic disorders involving the hepato-biliary system such as cystic fibrosis, Niemann-Pick disease type C
    b) In older children, disorders include:
      (1) Late onset of symptomatic alpha-1-antitrypsin deficiency
      (2) Secondary hemochromatosis
      (3) Autoimmune liver disease
      (4) Chronic hepatitis C and human immunodeficiency virus (HIV; rarely)

II. Metabolic Alterations in Chronic Liver Disease

A. Accelerated starvation—The preferred fuel in cirrhotic patients is fat. This phenomenon is especially apparent after an overnight fast, as fat supplies approximately 75% of calories compared with 35% in normal subjects.[4]

B. Protein imbalance
   1. The starvation response is accelerated with increased skeletal muscle breakdown to supply substrate for gluconeogenesis and energy expenditure.[5] Protein catabolism is not as easily suppressed by feeding as in normal individuals.
   2. Hepatic encephalopathy—Neuro-psychiatric abnormalities may occur with advanced acute or chronic liver failure. These mental status alterations may range from mild behavioral changes to deep coma (Table 17-1).
      a) Sub-clinical hepatic encephalopathy is present in 70% of patients with cirrhosis and does not require any specific nutritional therapy.
      b) Hepatic encephalopathy associated with liver failure is the third most common cause of death in patients with cirrhosis and is responsible for approximately 20% of the deaths from this disease.
      c) Although the pathogenesis of hepatic encephalopathy remains poorly defined, all the proposed toxins (ammonia, mercaptans, fatty acids, γ-aminobutyric acids, altered plasma amino acid profile, and endogenous benzodiazepines) appear to be related in part to protein feeding.
      d) Overt encephalopathy is almost always associated with some precipitating event, such as gastrointestinal (GI) bleeding, infection or sepsis, fluid and electrolyte imbalances, constipation, acid-base abnormalities, or inappropriate use of sedating drugs. In 5% or less of patients with cirrhosis, hepatic encephalopathy may be precipitated by dietary protein intake (especially animal protein) without any other precipitating factor. These patients are considered protein intolerant and may benefit from a diet enriched in branched-chain amino acids (BCAA).[6–10]
      e) More than 95% of patients with cirrhosis tolerate diets of mixed proteins (up to 1.5 g/kg/d for adults, up to 4 g/kg/d for children receiving tube feeding, and up to 2.5 g/kg/d for children receiving parenteral nutrition); some studies suggest a benefit of BCAAs over standard amino acids in these patients.[6–10]

C. Metabolic alterations in alcoholic liver disease
   1. Alcohol has deleterious effects on muscle protein status independent of associated liver injury.
   2. Alcohol inhibits meal-stimulated hepatic protein synthesis.
   3. Alcohol increases intestinal permeability, which increases endotoxin uptake and cytokine-induced muscle proteolysis.
   4. Alcohol provides "empty" calories.
      a) Alcohol has a theoretic caloric density of 7 kcal/g but its calories are oxidized less efficiently than other carbohydrates and lipid.
      b) Alcohol replaces other nutrient-dense energy sources.
      c) Alcohol-induced cirrhosis generally results in decreased muscle mass but a relative sparing of fat stores compared with nonalcoholic cirrhosis.

III. Protein-Calorie Malnutrition (PCM) in Liver Disease

A. Adult
   1. Prevalence
      a) PCM is uncommon in chronic liver disease without cirrhosis. Nutritional management is based on standard recommendations that are not disease-specific.
      b) In contrast with non-cirrhotic liver disease, PCM is highly prevalent in all forms of cirrhosis.[5,11] In alcoholic cirrhosis, PCM severity correlates with liver dysfunction (as measured by serum bilirubin and international normalized ratio [INR]).
      c) Characteristics of PCM are influenced by the etiology of the cirrhosis, ie, the type of underlying liver disease (see Table 17-2).
   2. The cause of PCM is multifactorial (see Table 17-3).
      a) Anorexia is prevalent. Central appetite suppression can be caused by increased pro-inflammatory cytokine production.
      b) Diagnostic and therapeutic procedures interrupt eating and contribute to low intake. Typical intakes meet ~ 50% of needs during the first 10 days of hospitalization.[12]
      c) Early satiety can be caused by gastric compression from ascites and hepatosplenomegaly.
      d) Dysgeusia is probably related to zinc deficiency and unpalatable diets.

TABLE 17-1. Four Stages of Hepatic Encephalopathy

Stage	Symptoms
I	mild confusion, agitation, irritability, sleep disturbance, decreased attention
II	lethargy, disorientation, inappropriate behavior, drowsiness
III	somnolent but arousable, incomprehensible speech, confused, aggressive when awake
IV	Coma

Reprinted with permission from Hasse JM, Matarese LE. Nutritional care in diseases of the liver, biliary system, and exocrine pancreas. In: Mahan LK, Escott-Stump S, eds. *Krause's Food, Nutrition, and Diet Therapy.* 11th ed. Philadelphia: W.B. Saunders Company; 2004:738–767.

TABLE 17-2. Pattern of Malnutrition in Chronic Liver Disease

	Muscle Wasting	Loss of Fat Stores	Reduced Synthetic Function
Alcohol	●	■	▲
Viral	▲	▲	■
Primary biliary cirrhosis	●	●	■
Primary sclerosing cholangitis	▲	■	■

■, mild abnormalities; ▲, moderate abnormalities; ●, severe abnormalities

Reprinted from McCullough AJ. Malnutrition in liver disease. *Liver Transplant.* 2000;6(4 suppl 1):S85–S96 with permission of Wiley-Liss, Inc., a subsidiary of John Wiley & Sons, Inc.

TABLE 17-3. Etiologic Factors for Protein Calorie Malnutrition in Cirrhosis

Adults	Children
Reduced nutrient intake* • Anorexia • Increased satiety • Nausea and vomiting • Iatrogenic (protein, fluid/salt restriction)	**Reduced nutrient intake*** • Anorexia • Increased satiety • Nausea and vomiting
Malabsorption* • Pancreatic and bile salt deficiency • Enteropathy	**Malabsorption** • Pancreatic and bile salt deficiency • Portal hypertension • Small intestinal bacterial overgrowth
Altered protein and energy metabolism • Alcohol toxicity on energy and protein • Amino acid oxidation • Increased protein breakdown • Accelerated fat oxidation and gluconeogenesis	**Altered energy metabolism** • Increased resting energy expenditure • Increased active energy expenditure
Fasting status (if hospitalized) for • Diagnostic testing • Gastrointestinal bleeding • Altered neurologic status	

* Factors that can be altered or treated.

e) Fat malabsorption is usually less important than decreased intake and mainly due to reduced intestinal bile acids.
   (1) Bile acid deficiency reduces net lipid absorption from 95% to 75%.
      (a) Moderate steatorrhea (<12 g daily) is typical.
      (b) Stool fat loss may exceed 30 g daily with severe cholestasis.
   (2) Bile acid deficiency also contributes to fat-soluble vitamin deficiency (Table 17-4) and essential fatty acid deficiency, symptoms of which include dry skin and hair loss.[13]
   (3) Enteropathy may coexist with liver disease (eg, celiac sprue is associated with primary biliary cirrhosis or autoimmune disease, and inflammatory bowel disease with primary sclerosing cholangitis).
   (4) Patients with alcoholic liver disease may have exocrine pancreatic insufficiency with defective lipase secretion.
f) Increased intestinal protein losses
   (1) Prevalence—Occurs in up to 40% of patients. Enteral feeding may actually improve intestinal absorption.[14]
   (2) Bleeding due to portal hypertension contributes to intestinal protein loss. Because hemoglobin lacks the essential amino acid isoleucine, hemoglobin is a relatively low-quality protein source.
   (3) Large-volume paracentesis may also cause a loss of 10–20 g of protein.
   (4) Portal hypertension impairs GI motility and increases GI protein loss.
   (5) Small intestinal bacterial overgrowth associated with cirrhosis also increases fat and protein losses.

3. Prognosis—PCM adversely affects clinical outcomes in cirrhotic adult patients (Table 17-5). Successful nutritional intervention may improve liver function, short-term survival, and outcome following liver transplantation.

B. Pediatric considerations with PCM of chronic liver disease
1. Prevalence
   a) PCM incidence in children with liver disease is approximately 60%.[15]
   b) Metabolic and nutritional abnormalities develop and become apparent more rapidly than in adults due to higher metabolic rates associated with body growth.[5]
2. Etiology of PCM is similar to adults with chronic liver disease (Table 17-3).
   a) Reduced nutrient intake is the most important factor.
   b) Malabsorption occurs with diseases that have coincident pancreatic insufficiency (eg, Alagille syndrome and cystic fibrosis).
   c) Increased energy consumption
      (1) Resting energy expenditures (REE) are generally increased per kg of *total* body weight by about 140% to 160% or to approximately 75 kcal/kg/d.[16,17]
         (a) Increased REE results from relative increase in body cell compartment as a fraction of total body weight due to reduction in the (less metabolically active) body fat compartment.
         (b) Also, energy expenditure per unit of body cell compartment is increased, likely because of increased activity of futile metabolic pathways (eg, cyclical fatty acid synthesis and degradation) and possibly because of carnitine deficiency.
      (2) Total energy expenditures (TEE), the sum of REE and additional physical activity, are increased from the usual 160% of REE to about 200% of REE (140 to 160 kcal/kg/d).[17]
         (a) Increased energy consumption from hepatosplenomegaly and ascites contributes to increased energy expenditure.
         (b) TEE also increases intermittently as a result of infectious and inflammatory stresses.
3. Prognosis—Malnutrition predicts reduced survival after liver transplantation independent of other features of advanced liver disease.[18]
   a) Any chronic liver disease causes malnutrition; malnutrition, in turn, promotes further deterioration in liver function irrespective of the original cause.
   b) Because malnutrition reflects the severity of liver disease, correction of malnutrition does not always improve survival in the absence of transplantation.

IV. Nutrition Assessment

A. An initial comprehensive nutritional assessment includes objective and subjective parameters (see Table 17-6).

TABLE 17-4. Fat-Soluble Vitamin Supplements for Prophylaxis and Treatment for Children with Liver Disease

Vitamin	Brand	Typical Dose	Route	Deficiency	Comments
Vitamin A	ADEKs Pediatric Drops* (Axcan Pharma, Birmingham, AL) Aquaso® A Parenteral (aaiPharma, Wilmington, DE)	5,000–25,000 USP units daily 5,000–50,000 daily for 1–2 weeks	PO IM	Xerophthalmia (dry eye) Hyperkeratosis Night blindness	Normal plasma level=300–400 mcg/L Symptoms develop at 100 mcg/L Plasma levels correlate poorly with stores—aim to maintain low levels
Vitamin D (Calcitriol)	Rocaltrol (Roche Laboratories, Nutley, NJ) -Solution (1 mcg/mL) -Capsules (0.25 and 0.5 mcg/mL)	0.025 –1.0 mcg/kg daily	PO	Rickets Osteomalacia	Monitor calcium, phosphorus, intact PTH levels
Vitamin E (Tocopheryl-PEGS)	Nutr-E-Sol; 400 IU/15 mL (Advanced Nutritional Technology, Inc, Dublin, CA) ADEKs Pediatric Drops (Axcan Pharma, Birmingham, AL)	25 IU/kg/d	PO	Peripheral neuropathy Ataxia	Desired plasma level (5–15 mcg/mL) affected by serum lipids
Vitamin K (phytonadione)	Mephyton 5 mg tabs (Merck & Co., Whitehouse Station, NJ) ADEKs Pediatric Drops (Axcan Pharma, Birmingham, AL) AquaMEPHYTON (Merck & Co., Whitehouse Station, NJ)	2.5–5 mg daily 5–10 mg every 2 weeks	PO SQ	Coagulopathic hemorrhage	Monitor with prothrombin time (PT) Use SQ if PO ineffective

*ADEKs Pediatric Drops include 3,170 USP units of vitamin A, 40 IU of tocopheryl-PEGS, and 0.1 mg of phytonadione per mL.

B. If possible, REE should be measured with indirect calorimetry.
  1. REE is highly variable in cirrhosis: 30% of patients are hypometabolic and 20% hypermetabolic.[19]
  2. Prediction of energy requirements based on standard equations is unreliable.[20]
  3. If indirect calorimetry is not available, estimate energy expenditure with consideration of existing deficits and increased or decreased ongoing needs. General energy estimates are: adults ~25 to 30 kcal/kg/d, children receiving tube feeding ~130 to 160 kcal/kg/d, children receiving parenteral nutrition ~100 to 130 kcal/kg/d.
    a) Ascites increases REE by 10%.[21]
    b) If ascites or edema is present, it is controversial whether actual, ideal, or estimated "dry" weight should be used in calculation.

C. Follow-up assessment
  1. Standard monitoring can be useful in patients with chronic liver disease.[5,22] Patients with chronic liver disease must be monitored for signs of encephalopathy, fluid retention (peripheral edema and abdominal distention secondary to ascites), and gastrointestinal blood loss. Weight change can signal fluctuation in fluid retention with or without alterations in lean or fat mass.
  2. Calorie counts and/or dietary recalls are important tools to determine the adequacy of oral intake.

V. Objectives of Nutrition Therapy

A. Prevent or slow catabolism to prevent or correct PCM.

B. Attain optimal glucose control.

C. Sustain energy balance and deliver sufficient calories in children to ensure that linear growth is not limited by nutrient supply.

D. Correct or prevent vitamin deficiencies and trace element abnormalities.

E. Improve hepatic function and promote hepatocellular regeneration, benefits of which include:
  1. Reversal of existing encephalopathy and prevention of future episodes.[23]
  2. Reduction of ascites and edema and correction of electrolyte disorders (hyponatremia, hypokalemia, hypocalcemia, hypocalcemia) related to PCM and renin-angiotensin activation in chronic liver disease.

F. Preparation for transplantation (if indicated).

TABLE 17-5. Studies in Which Protein Calorie Malnutrition was Determined to be a Poor Prognostic Factor in Cirrhosis

Condition or Procedure	Clinical Outcome Measured	Study Author (year)
Cirrhosis	Survival	Caregaro (1996)[51] Merli (1996)[52]
	Immunodeficiency	Qiao (1988)[53] O'Keefe (1980)[54] Lautz (1994)[55]
Cirrhosis patients with varices	Predicting bleeding, survival	Müller (1994)[56]
Cirrhosis patients having abdominal surgery	Survival Postoperative complications	Garrison (1984)[57] Ouchi (1988)[58]
Hospitalized patients with ascites/ cirrhosis	Survival	Llach (1988)[59] Blendis (1986)[60] Franco (1987)[61]
Alcoholic hepatitis	Survival Liver function	Mendenhall (1984, 1986)[62,63]
Liver transplantation	Patient/graft survival	Shaw (1985)[64] Lautz (1992)[55] Moukarzel (1990)[18] Selberg (1997)[65] Harrison (1997)[66] Pikul (1994)[67] Hasse (1998)[68]
	Length of post-transplant hospitalization	Pikul (1994)[67] Figueirdeo (2000)[69] Stephenson (2001)[70]
Hepatectomy	Postoperative complications	Fan (1994)[71]

Adapted from McCullough AJ. Malnutrition in liver disease. *Liver Transplant.* 2000;6(4, Suppl 1):S85–S96 with permission of Wiley-Liss, Inc., a subsidiary of John Wiley & Sons, Inc.

VI. Feeding Goals

A. Background

1. Nutrition support is usually less relevant to acute liver failure secondary to drugs (eg, acetaminophen) or toxins (eg, *Amanita* mushroom) than to chronic liver disease, because recovery or death occurs quickly in the absence of liver transplantation.
2. The gastrointestinal tract functions adequately in most adult and pediatric patients with chronic liver disease, allowing correction of most deficits by oral or enteral route.
3. The fat oxidation-predominant metabolic profile of cirrhosis is similar to the fasting profile of normal individuals. Patients with cirrhosis should avoid fasting which rapidly leads to muscle catabolism.[24,25]
4. Diet composition is based on the natural history of the liver disease.
   a) In the absence of severe anorexia, patients with mildly decompensated cirrhosis, PCM, ascites, and hyponatremia, may be able to consume the desired high-calorie/protein and low-sodium/fluid diet. Carbohydrate-controlled diets are indicated for patients with diabetes mellitus.
   b) Enteral feeding improves liver function and encephalopathy in malnourished patients with cirrhosis or decompensated alcoholic liver disease.[26–29] Hirsch et al provided nutritional supplements (1000 kcal and 34 g of casein protein) for 1 year to patients with complicated alcoholic cirrhosis, reducing their need for hospitalization to treat infections[30], but positive effects on long-term survival remain difficult to demonstrate.

B. Specific nutrient guidelines (guidelines for adults with end-stage liver disease are summarized in Table 17-7)

1. Electrolytes
   a) Sodium—Dietary restriction (1500 to 2000 mg) is the cornerstone of treatment of ascites and edema, supplemented with diuretic therapy when necessary.
   b) Potassium—Potassium levels must be monitored closely, because hypokalemia can result from diarrhea or vomiting and hyperkalemia may occur in the presence of hepatorenal syndrome. Diuretics can be either potassium-wasting or potassium-sparing.
2. Fluid—Restriction to approximately 1000 mL to 1500 mL per day is indicated for hyponatremia. Conversely, patients with liver disease associated with intestinal insufficiency, for example, Crohn's disease or short bowel syndrome, may be at risk of dehydration and periodically require extra fluids.
3. Vitamins
   a) Generally, a multi-vitamin preparation is recommended.
   b) Recommendations for fat-soluble vitamin supplementation in children are listed in Table 17-2.
4. Trace elements
   a) Zinc requirements are increased[31]; children with liver disease may require up to 0.3 mg/kg/d.
   b) In patients with cholestatic liver disease receiving PN, high serum levels of copper and manganese and low levels of selenium are typical.[32] Copper and manganese should be withheld unless serum levels are low. Serum copper and manganese levels should be followed intermittently.
   c) Selenium should be given based on serum concentration (up to 5 mcg/kg/d) as should chromium (up to 0.2–0.3 mcg/kg/d).
   d) Iron—Increased losses due to chronic occult or overt gastrointestinal hemorrhage and repeated diagnostic blood testing generally indicate supplementation based on serum iron saturation. Ferritin concentration usually rises in chronic liver disease and does not reliably reflect body iron stores.

C. Additional pediatric considerations for macronutrient intake[15]

1. Protein—The usual goal is 3.5–4.0 g/kg/d in patients receiving enteral nutrition and 1.5–2.5 g/kg/d in patients receiving parenteral nutrition.
2. Energy—The usual goal for enteral intake is 130–160 kcal/kg/d, including 35% to 45% of total calories as lipid. Although medium chain triglyceride (MCT) oil in the amount of ⅓ to ½ of lipid calories is often recommended, no prospective data have confirmed a benefit compared with long-chain triglyceride (LCT)-predominant

TABLE 17-6. Nutritional Assessment in Patients with Liver Disease

Component of Assessment	Parameters	Additional considerations with children
Medical history	• Etiology, duration, and severity of liver damage • Prognosis of disease • GI function – propensity for nausea, vomiting, diarrhea, and GI bleeding • Concomitant damage to other organs (eg, chronic pancreatitis in alcoholics, diabetes and cardiomyopathy in hemochromatosis, heart and/or lung disease increasing energy expenditure, renal disease affecting fluid and electrolyte balance, glucose intolerance and hyperlipidemias)	
Nutrition history	• Diet history to assess quality and quantity of intake • Medication history to identify drug-nutrient interactions • Use of nutrition supplements including vitamin, mineral, and herbal preparations • Psychosocial and economic conditions to determine patient's or caregiver's ability to obtain/prepare food and comply with diet	• Consider route of feeding and type of formula if bottle fed
Physical examination	• Mental status • Muscle and fat stores • Edema or ascites • Skin — jaundice, bruising, excoriations (from pruritus), or xanthomas • Oral/dental health • Assessment of activity	
Anthropometric measurements	• Height • Weight history (to assess degree of fluid retention and weight loss) • Tricep skinfold and mid-arm muscle circumference measurements may be helpful if measured serially over time • Hand grip strength may be an indirect measure of muscle stores	• Height/length and percentile for age • Head circumference and percentile for age • Weight and percentile for age • Weight for length percentile • Tricep skinfold and mid-arm muscle area measurements and percentiles for age
Laboratory tests	• Tests to evaluate liver function such as bilirubin, AST, ALT, GGT, prothrombin time (or INR) • Serum electrolytes • Tests to evaluate renal function such as blood urea nitrogen and creatinine • Hepatic transport proteins are not especially helpful because concentrations are affected by fluid status, liver and kidney function, and vitamin status. • Iron studies such as serum iron, ferritin, total iron binding capacity, and iron saturation • Serum lipid levels • Fat-soluble vitamin levels (especially in patients with cholestatic liver disease)	• Urine calcium to creatinine ratio • Serum zinc and urine zinc to creatinine ratio • Fatty acid profile, including C20:3w9 • ESR, C-reactive protein
Other tests	• Subjective global assessment may be helpful as an initial assessment tool • Bioelectrical impedance is probably an inaccurate measure of PCM in cirrhosis patients with ascites or edema • Creatinine-height index is influenced by renal function • Dual-energy X-ray absorptiometry can be used to accurately measure bone density and body fat • Indirect calorimetry can accurately determine resting energy expenditure	

AST, aspartate aminotransferase; ALT, alanine aminotransferase; GGT, gamma glutamyltransferase; INR, international normalized ratio (for prothrombin time); ESR, erythrocyte sedimentation rate

TABLE 17-7. Dietary Considerations for Adult Patients with End-stage Liver Disease

Symptom	Nutrition Recommendations
Cachexia	• Provide at least 120% of estimated energy expenditure • Provide increased calories if malabsorption or malnutrition is present • Offer small, frequent meals of calorie-dense foods
Encephalopathy	• Maximize medical therapy (eg, lactulose, neomycin) • Identify and treat cause(s) of acute bouts of encephalopathy (eg, variceal bleed, infection, electrolyte imbalance, sedatives, constipation, etc.) • Restrict protein only if patient is protein sensitive (uncommon) • If patient is protein sensitive, start with 0.5 to 0.7 g protein/kg/d and increase level to tolerance, aiming for up to 1.5 g/kg/d if patient is malnourished • Consider nutritional supplements enriched with branched-chain amino acids and restricted in aromatic amino acids and methionine if intolerant to standard proteins • Supplement with zinc if deficiency is suspected • Provide adequate calories to prevent catabolism of endogenous protein stores
Ascites and edema	• Limit sodium (restriction below 2 g/d may result in inadequate calorie and protein intake) • Supplement protein if patient is undergoing frequent paracenteses
Hyponatremia	• Restrict fluid to 1000 to 1500 mL/d
Hyperglycemia	• Institute carbohydrate-controlled meal plan • Treat with insulin or oral hypoglycemic agent as needed
Hypoglycemia	• Provide frequent meals or snacks containing carbohydrate and protein • Infuse intravenous dextrose if needed
Steatorrhea	• Restrict dietary fat; if diarrhea does not resolve, discontinue fat restriction • Try medium-chain triglyceride supplementation • Supplement with fat-soluble vitamins
Osteopenia	• Maintain an appropriate weight • Encourage intake of a well-balanced diet with a wide variety of food choices • Provide enough protein to maintain muscle mass • Provide 1500 mg of calcium per day via diet and/or supplements • Provide enough vitamin D via diet and/or supplementation (may need water-miscible form) • Monitor for the development of steatorrhea and adjust the diet as needed to minimize nutrient losses • Avoid alcohol

Adapted with permission from Hasse J, Weseman B, Fuhrman MP, Loeffler M, Francisco-Ziller N, DiCecco SR. Nutrition therapy for end-stage liver disease: a practical approach. *Support Line.* 1997;19(4):8–15.

diets. When nutrition is delivered predominantly by vein, the goal is 100 to 130 kcal/kg/d with lipid providing 20% to 25% of total calories, usually up to 3 g/kg/day.[33]

VII. Methods of Nutrient Delivery

A. Oral diet

1. Dietary restrictions should be prescribed only as needed. Table 17-7 outlines guidelines for adults.
2. Oral supplements may increase total intake and preclude the need for enteral tube feeding when anorexia of chronic liver disease is mild. Supplements can be standard products or modular nutrients such as MCT oil (7.7 kcal/mL), modular protein powders, or glucose polymers (8 to 10 kcal/teaspoon).

B. Enteral feeding

1. Indication—Tube feeding is indicated when oral intake is consistently inadequate to support appropriate nutritional status.
2. Feeding routes

a) Small-caliber nasogastric or nasojejunal tubes may be used. Esophageal and gastric varices are not, in and of themselves, contraindications to feeding tube placement. However, tube feeding should be interrupted or postponed until hemorrhagic varices have been effectively treated.[34]
b) Placement of a gastrostomy or a jejunostomy tube in cirrhotic patients with ascites is usually not recommended. Potential complications include ascitic leakage, bleeding, wound dehiscence, and peritonitis.

3. Formula selection
   a) Standard polymeric (intact protein) formulas are indicated when anorexia rather than impaired digestive function is the main indication for nutrition support. Casein-based products are usually well-tolerated in patients with chronic liver disease.
   b) Hydrolyzed formulas may be tried when patients develop indications of intolerance when given polymeric formulas.
   c) Nutrient-dense formulas (greater than 1 kcal/mL) are indicated when fluid restriction is required.
   d) Renal formulas are indicated when a patient has hyperkalemia and hyperphosphatemia (usually from renal impairment).
   e) Branched-chain amino acid-enriched formulas are indicated when encephalopathy is refractory to pharmaceutical therapy and recurs with use of standard formulas.
4. Special considerations in infants and children
   a) Indications for tube feeding include subnormal weight gain for age or actual weight loss on standard diet.
   b) Route of feeding
      (1) Nasogastric tubes are easiest to use and are generally well-tolerated.
      (2) Nasojejunal tubes are indicated for infants who vomit or develop respiratory tract symptoms with gastric feedings. Unfortunately, nasojejunal tubes clog and are easily displaced making these tubes impractical for long-term use.
      (3) As in adults with chronic liver diseases and portal hypertension, gastrostomy tubes are usually contraindicated. Possible exceptions include Alagille syndrome.[35]
   c) Delivery
      (1) Intermittent daytime gavage feeding may preserve appetite but is often limited by emesis and diarrhea.
      (2) Continuous pump infusion is better tolerated with less diarrhea and emesis but often suppresses appetite.
   d) Formula selection
      (1) Formulas containing MCT oil may have 25% to 50% better lipid absorption than those containing only LCT (see Table 17-8). However, no data demonstrate superior clinical efficacy.
      (2) There is no advantage to peptide- or amino acid-based formulas in the absence of coexisting enteropathy or protein hypersensitivity.
      (3) Amino acid-based formulas are mainly indicated for hydrolysate hypersensitivity (intolerance).
      (4) Infants usually tolerate formula density up to 1 kcal/mL if mandated by need to restrict fluid, while older children usually tolerate up to 2 kcal/mL.
      (5) Appropriate tube feeding formulas for *infants* include: Alimentum (Ross Products, Abbott Laboratories, Columbus, Ohio) and Pregestimil (Mead Johnson, Evansville, IN; diluted to 0.67 to 1.0 kcal/mL).

TABLE 17-8. Proprietary Enteral Formulas Containing MCT Oil for Children with Chronic Liver Disease

Brand	Standard Density (kcal/mL)	Nitrogen (g/dL)	Lipid cals (% of total)	MCT : LCT
Elecare (Ross Products, Abbott Laboratories, Columbus, OH)	1.0	Amino acid (3.0)	43	33:67
Neocate Advance (SHS, Gaithersburg, MD)	1.0	Amino acid (2.5)	32	35:65
Alimentum (Ross Products, Abbott Laboratories, Columbus, OH)	0.67	Hydrolysate (1.8)	48	33:67
Pregestimil (Mead Johnson, Evansville, IN)	0.67	Hydrolysate (1.9)	48	55:45
Peptamen Junior (Nestle Clinical Nutrition, Glendale, CA)	1.0	Hydrolysate (3.0)	33	60:40
Deliver 2.0 (Mead Johnson, Evansville, IN)	2.0	Casein (7.4)	45	30:70
TwoCal HN (Ross Products, Abbott Laboratories, Columbus, OH)	2.0	Casein (8.4)	40	19:81

MCT, medium-chain triglyceride; LCT, long-chain triglyceride

(6) Appropriate tube feeding formulas for *children* include: Pregestimil (Mead Johnson, Evansville, IN; diluted to 1.0 kcal/mL), Peptamen Junior (Nestle Clinical Nutrition, Glendale, CA), Deliver 2.0 (Mead Johnson, Evansville, IN), and 2 Cal HN (Ross Products, Abbott Laboratories, Columbus, Ohio; diluted to 1.0 to 2.0 kcal/mL).

C. Parenteral nutrition support in liver disease
1. Indications: Severe acute and chronic liver diseases with demonstrated intolerance of enteral nutrition.
   a) Fulminant liver failure—When consciousness in impaired and aspiration risk is heightened.
   b) Chronic liver disease—Patients who develop intractable diarrhea, ileus, emesis, or fluid intolerance with EN are likely to benefit from PN. The advantage of PN is the ability to deliver a very high caloric load with easily varied macronutrient mix (based on nitrogen, lipid, and glucose tolerance) with relatively little fluid and sodium.
2. Risks of PN initiation in patients with decompensated liver disease include bleeding and infection due to placement of a central venous catheter, as coagulopathy and compromised immunity are invariably present. PN itself may also worsen liver function.
3. Route of delivery—Central PN is usually preferable to peripheral PN because of the latter's low caloric density.
4. Home parenteral nutrition—Indicated when long-term PN therapy is needed and the patient is sufficiently stable to remain at home. This situation is especially likely in the patient with both liver and intestinal failure awaiting combined liver and intestinal transplantation.
5. Amino Acids—Amino acid mixtures enriched with BCAAs (and restricted in aromatic amino acids and methionine) such as Hepatamine (B. Braun, Irvine, CA)
   a) BCAA formulas are used if standard amounts of amino acid precipitate encephalopathy.
   b) Studies demonstrating benefit are conflicting: BCAA-enriched amino acids formulas may improve encephalopathy;[36–43] and some recent studies suggest that these formulas may also improve nutritional status or survival.[7–10]
6. Special considerations in infants and children[44]
   a) Amino acids—1.5 to 2.5 g/kg/d
      (1) Taurine is conditionally essential; use TrophAmine (B. Braun, Irvine, CA).
      (2) Cysteine may be essential in chronic liver disease; add up to 1 g/L
   b) Carnitine status may be compromised, particularly with high lipid intake. If the free plasma level of carnitine is reduced, add up to 10 mg/kg/d.[45] In this patient population, serum carnitine levels should be intermittently monitored.
   c) Proprietary pediatric injectable vitamin solutions are adequate.
   d) Home parenteral nutrition—Although PN may be delivered at home, patients requiring it because of advanced liver disease usually require hospitalization.

VIII. Patient Education

Patients and/or caregivers should be given instructions regarding:

A. Diet prescription
1. Type of diet
2. Reason for diet
3. Specific food selection and preparation tips
4. Information on how to obtain foods, especially if this is a hindrance to patient compliance

B. Potential food-drug interactions

C. Vitamin/mineral supplements
1. Which type to take and which to avoid
2. Dosage

D. Food safety issues
1. General food safety guidelines (eg, avoid raw eggs; unpasteurized milk; and raw or undercooked meats, poultry, and seafood)
2. Safe handling of enteral and parenteral products

E. Complementary products (eg, milk thistle)
1. Counsel about safety and efficacy of products.
2. Milk thistle (silymarin) is most popular in the lay community.
   a) Purported anti-hepatotoxic activity and anti-inflammatory activity
   b) Scientific evidence is mixed.[46–50] A recent meta-analysis concluded that there is not adequate data to exclude benefit or harm.[50]
3. Avoid products that are potentially hepatotoxic
   a) Borage
   b) Chaparral
   c) Coltsfoot
   d) Comfrey
   e) DHEA
   f) Germander
   g) Jin bu Huan
   h) Kava Kava
   i) Liferoot
   j) Pennyroyal
   k) Periwinkle
   l) Poke root
   m) Skullcap (American)
   n) Shark cartilage

(Liver chapter from the 1st edition was contributed by Arthur J. McCullough, J. Carlos Teran, and Elizabetta Bugianesi)

REFERENCES

1. Hasse JM, Matarese LE. Medical nutritional therapy for liver, biliary system, and exocrine pancreas disorders. In: Mahan LK, Escott-Stump S, eds. *Krause's Food, Nutrition, and Diet Therapy.* 11th ed. Philadelphia: W. B. Saunders Company; 2004:738–767.
2. Liverfoundation.org [The official web site of the American Liver Foundation]. Available at: http://www.liverfoundation.org. Accessed May 4, 2004.
3. Hasse JM, Kent P. Nutritional implications of acute liver failure and emergent liver transplantation. *Support Line.* 2003;25(1):18–22.
4. Merli M, Riggio O, Romiti A, et al. Basal energy production rate and substrate use in stable cirrhotic patients. *Hepatology.* 1990:12:106–112.
5. Roggero P, Cataliotti E, Ulla L, et al. Factors influencing malnutrition in children waiting for liver transplants. *Am J Clin Nutr.* 1997;65:1852–1857.
6. Fabbri A, Mangrini N, Bianchi G, Zoli M, Marchesini G. Overview of randomized clinical trials of oral branched-chain amino acid treatment in chronic hepatic encephalopathy. *J Parenter Enteral Nutr.* 1996;20:159–164.
7. Marchesini G, Bianchi G, Merli M, et al. Nutritional supplementation with branched-chain amino acids in advanced cirrhosis: a double-blind, randomized trial. *Gastroenterol.* 2003;124:1792–1801.
8. Habu D, Nishiguchi S, Nakatani S, et al. Effect of oral supplementation with branched-chain amino acid granules on serum albumin level in the early stage of cirrhosis: a randomized pilot trial. *Hepatol Res.* 2003;25:312–318.
9. Ichida T, Shibasaki K, Muto Y, Satoh S, Watanabe A, Ichida F. Clinical study of an enteral branched-chain amino acid solution in decompensated liver cirrhosis with hepatic encephalopathy. *Nutrition.* 1995;11(2 suppl):233–244.
10. Yoshida T, Muto Y, Moriwaki H, Yamato M. Effect of long-term oral supplementation with branched-chain amino acid granules on the prognosis of liver cirrhosis. *Gastroenterol Jpn.* 1989;24:692–698.
11. McCullough AJ, Bugianesi E. Protein calorie malnutrition and the etiology of cirrhosis. *Am J Gastroenterol.* 1997;92:734–738.

12. Nielsen K, Kondrup J, Martinsen L, Stilling B, Wikman B. Nutritional assessment and adequacy of dietary intake in hospitalized patients with alcoholic liver disease. *Br J Nutr.* 1993;69:665–679.
13. Duerksen DR, Nehra V, Palombo JD, Ahmad A, Bistrian BR. Essential fatty acid deficiencies in patients with chronic liver disease are not reversed by short-term intravenous lipid supplementation. *Dig Dis Sci.* 1999;44:1342–1348.
14. Soberon S, Pauley MP, Duplantier R, Fan A, Halsted CH. Metabolic effects of enteral feeding in alcoholic hepatitis. *Hepatology.* 1987;7:1204–1209.
15. Protheroe SM. Feeding the child with chronic liver disease. *Nutrition.* 1998;14:796–800.
16. Pierro A, Koletzko B, Carnielli V, et al. Resting energy expenditure is increased in infants and children with extrahepatic biliary atresia. *J Pediatr Surg.* 1989;24:534–538.
17. Greer R, Lehnert M, Lewindon P, Cleghorn GJ, Shepherd RW. Body composition and components of energy expenditure in children with end-stage liver disease. *J Pediatr Gastroenterol Nutr.* 2003;36:358–363.
18. Mouzkarzel AA, Najm I, Vargas J, McDiarmid VS, Busuttil RW, Ament ME. Effect of nutritional status on outcome of orthotopic liver transplantation in pediatric patients. *Transplant Proc.* 1990;22:1560–1563.
19. Müller MJ, Lautz HU, Plogmann B, et al. Energy expenditure and substrate oxidation in patients with cirrhosis: the impact of cause, clinical staging and nutritional state. *Hepatology.* 1992;15:782–794.
20. Heymsfield SB, Waki M, Reinus J. Are patients with chronic liver disease hypermetabolic? *Hepatology.* 1990;11:502–503.
21. Dolz C, Ranrich JM, Ibanez J, Obrador A, Marse P, Gaya J. Ascites increases energy expenditure in liver cirrhosis. *Gastroenterology.* 1991;100:738–744.
22. Figueiredo FA, Dickson ER, Pasha TM, et al. Utility of standard nutritional parameters in detecting body cell mass depletion in patients with end-stage liver disease. *Liver Transplantation.* 2000;6:575–581.
23. Glynn MJ, Powell-Tuck J, Reaveley DA, Murray-Lyon IM. High lipid parenteral nutrition improves portasystemic encephalopathy. *J Parenter Enteral Nutr.* 1988;12:457–461.
24. Chang WK, Chao YC, Tang HS, Lang HF, Hsu CT. Effects of extra-carbohydrate supplementation in the late evening on energy expenditure and substrate oxidation in patients with liver cirrhosis. *J Parenter Enteral Nutr.* 1997;21:96–99.
25. Swart GR, Ziliikiens MC, von Vuure JK, van den Berg JWO. Effect of a late evening meal on nitrogen balance in patients with cirrhosis of the liver. *Br Med J.* 1989;299:1202–1203.
26. Kearns PJ, Young H, Garcia G, et al. Accelerated improvement of alcoholic liver disease with enteral nutrition. *Gastroenterology.* 1992;102:200–205.
27. Cabre E, Gonzalez-Huix F, Abad-LaCruz A, et al. Effect of total enteral nutrition on the short term outcome of severely malnourished cirrhotics. A randomized trial. *Gastroenterology.* 1990;98:715–720.
28. Mendenhall CL, Moritz TE, Roselle GA, et al. A study of oral nutritional support with oxandrolone in malnourished patients with alcoholic hepatitis: results of a Department of Veterans Affairs cooperative study. *Hepatology.* 1993;17:564–576.
29. Mendenhall CL, Moritz TE, Roselle GA, et al. Protein energy malnutrition in severe alcoholic hepatitis: diagnosis and response to treatment. *J Parenter Enteral Nutr.* 1995;9:590–596.
30. Hirsch S, Bunout D, De La Maza P, et al. Controlled trial on nutritional supplementation in outpatients with symptomatic alcoholic cirrhosis. *J Parenter Enteral Nutr.* 1993;17:119–124.
31. Narkowicz MR, Krebs N, Karrer F, Orban-Eller K, Sokol RJ. Correction of hypozincemia following liver transplantation in children is associated with reduced urinary zinc loss. *Hepatology.* 1999;29:830–833.
32. Navarro-Alarcon M, Lopez-Ga de la Serrana H, Perez-Valero V, Lopez Martinez MC. Selenium concentrations in serum of individuals with liver diseases (cirrhosis or hepatitis): relationship with some nutritional and biochemical markers. *Sci Total Environ.* 2002;291:135–141.
33. Handa N, Suita S, Ikeda K, Doki T, Naito K. Requirement of parenteral fat in infants with biliary atresia. *J Parenter Enteral Nutr.* 1985;9:685–690.
34. De Lédinghen V, Beau P, Mannant P-R, et al. Early feeding or enteral nutrition in patients with cirrhosis after bleeding from esophageal varices? A randomized controlled study. *Dig Dis Sci.* 1997;42:536–541.
35. Duché M, Habès D, Lababidi A, Chardot C, Wenz J, Bernard O. Percutaneous endoscopic gastrostomy for continuous feeding in children with chronic cholestasis. *J Pediatr Gastroenterol Nutr.* 1999;29:42–45.
36. Rossi-Fanelli F, Riggio O, Cascino A, et al. Branched-chain amino acids vs. lactulose in the treatment of hepatic coma. A controlled study. *Dig Dis Sci.* 1982;27:929–935.
37. Wahren J, Denis, J, Desurmont P, et al. Is intravenous administration of branched chain amino acids effective in the treatment of hepatic encephalopathy? A multicentre study. *Hepatology.* 1983;3:475–480.
38. Cerra FB, Cheung NK, Fischer JE, et al. Disease-specific amino acid infusion in hepatic encephalopathy: a prospective randomized, double-blind controlled trial. *J Parenter Enteral Nutr.* 1985;9:588–295.
39. Michel H, Bories P, Aubin JP, Pomier-layrargues G, Bauret P, Bellet-Herman H. Treatment of acute hepatic encephalopathy in cirrhotics with a branched-chain amino acids enriched versus a conventional amino acid mixture. A controlled study in 70 patients. *Liver.* 1985;5:282–289.
40. Fiaccadori F, Ginelli F, Pedretti G, et al. Branched-chain enriched amino acid solutions in the treatment of hepatic encephalopathy: a controlled trial. *Ital J Gastroenterol.* 1985;17:5–10.
41. Strauss E, Dos Santos WR, DaSilva EC, et al. Treatment of hepatic encephalopathy: a randomized clinical trial comparing a branched chain enriched amino acid solution to oral neomycin. *Nutr Supp Svcs.* 1986;6:18–21.
42. Vilstrup H, Gluud C, Hardt F, et al. Branched-chain enriched amino acid versus glucose treatment of hepatic encephalopathy. A double blind study of 65 patients with cirrhosis. *J Hepatol.* 1990;10:291–296.
43. Naylor CD, O'Rourke K, Detsky AS, Baker JP. Parenteral nutrition with branched chain amino acids in hepatic encephalopathy: a metaanalysis. *Gastroenterology.* 1989;97:1033–1042.
44. Guimber D, Michaud L, Ategbo S, Turck D, Gottrand F. Experience of parenteral nutrition for nutritional rescue in children with severe liver disease following failure of enteral nutrition. *Pediatr Transplantation.* 1999;3: 139–145.
45. Selimoğlu MA, Aydoğdu S, Yağci RV, Huseyinov A. Plasma and liver carnitine status in children with chronic liver disease and cirrhosis. *Pediatrics Int.* 2001;43:392–395.
46. Ferenci P. Critical evaluation of the role of branched chain amino acids in liver disease. In: Thomas JC, Jones ES, eds. *Recent Advances in Hepatology.* Edinburgh: Churchill Livingstone; 1986:134–154.
47. Pares A, Planas R, Torres M, et al. Effects of silymarin in alcoholic patients with cirrhosis of the liver: results of a controlled, double-blind, randomized and multicenter trial. *J Hepatol.* 1998;28(4):615–621.
48. Saller R, Meier R, Brignoli R. The use of silymarin in the treatment of liver diseases. *Drugs.* 2001;61:2035–2063.
49. Bean P. The use of alternative medicine in the treatment of hepatitis C. *Am Clin Lab.* 2002;21:19–21.
50. Jacobs BP, Dennehy C, Ramirez G, Sapp J, Lawrence VA. Milk thistle for the treatment of liver disease: a systematic review and meta-analysis. *Am J Med.* 2002;113:506–515.
51. Caregaro L, Alberino F, Amodio P, et al. Malnutrition in alcoholic and virus-related cirrhosis. *Am J Clin Nutr.* 1996;63:602–609.
52. Merli M, Riggio O, Dally L. Does malnutrition affect survival in cirrhosis? PINC (Policentrica Italiana Nutrizione Cirrosi). *Hepatology.* 1996;23: 1041–1046.
53. Qiao ZK, Halliday ML, Coates RA, Rankin JG. Relationship between liver cirrhosis death rate and nutritional factors in 38 countries. *Int J Epidemiol.* 1988;17:414–418.
54. O'Keefe SJ, El-Zayadi AR, Carraher TE, Davis M, Williams R. Malnutrition and immuno-incompetence in patients with liver disease. *Lancet.* 1980;2(8195 pt 1):615–617.
55. Lautz HU, Selberg O, Körber J, Burger M, Muller MJ. Protein-calorie malnutrition in liver cirrhosis. *Clin Invest.* 1992;70:478–486.
56. Müller MJ, Loyal S, Schwarze M, Lobers J, Selberg O, Ringe B. Resting energy expenditure and nutritional stats in patients with liver cirrhosis before and after liver transplantation. *Clin Nutr.* 1994;13:145–152.
57. Garrison RN, Cryer HM, Howard DA, Polk HC Jr. Clarification of risk factors for abdominal operations in patients with hepatic cirrhosis. *Ann Surg.* 1984;199:648–655.

58. Ouchi K, Sakai K, Sato R, Nakagawa K, Matsuno S, Sato T. Significance of perioperative nutritional support and activation of the reticuloendothelial system on the resection of the cirrhotic liver [in Japanese]. *Nippon Geka Gakkai Zasshi.* 1988;891371–1374.
59. Llach J, Gines P, Arroyo V, et al. Prognostic value of arterial pressure, endogenous vasoactive systems, and renal function in cirrhotic patients admitted to the hospital for the treatment of ascites. *Gastroenterology.* 1988;94:482–487.
60. Blendis LM, Harrison JE, Russell DM, et al. Effects of peritoneovenous shunting on body composition. *Gastroenterology.* 1986;90:127–134.
61. Franco D, Vons C, Smadja C. Results of portal shunts in the treatment of intractable ascites in cirrhosis [in Italian]. *Minerva Med.* 1987;78:689–691.
62. Mendenhall CL, Moritz TE, Roselle GA, et al. A study of oral nutritional support with oxandrolone in malnourished patients with alcoholic hepatitis: results of a Department of Veterans Affairs cooperative study. *Hepatology.* 1998;17:564–576.
63. Mendenhall CL, Tosch T, Weesner RE, et al. VA cooperative study on alcoholic hepatitis. II: Prognostic significance of protein-calorie malnutrition. *Am J Clin Nutr.* 1986;43:213–218.
64. Shaw BW Jr, Wood RP, Gordon RD, Iwatsuki S, Gillquist WP, Starzl TE. Influence of selected patient variables and operative blood loss on six-month survival following liver transplantation. *Semin Liver Dis.* 1985;5:385–393.
65. Selberg O, Böttcher J, Tusch G, Pichlmayr R, Henkel E, Muller MJ. Identification of high- and low-risk patients before liver transplantation: A prospective cohort study of nutritional and metabolic parameters in 150 patients. *Hepatology.* 1997;25:652–657.
66. Harrison J, McKiernan J, Neuberger JM. A prospective study on the effect of recipient nutritional status on outcome in liver transplantation. *Transpl Int.* 1997;10:369–374.
67. Pikul J, Sharpe MD, Lowndes R, Ghent CN. Degree of preoperative malnutrition is predictive of postoperative morbidity and mortality in liver transplant recipients. *Transplantation.* 1994;57:469–472.
68. Hasse JM, Gonwa TA, Jennings LW, et al. Malnutrition affects liver transplant outcomes [abstract]. *Transplantation.* 1998;66(8):S53.
69. Figueiredo F, Dickson ER, Pasha T, et al. Impact of nutritional status on outcomes after liver transplantation. *Transplantation.* 2000;70(9):1347–1352.
70. Stephenson GR, Moretti EW, El-Moalem H, Clavien PA, Tuttle-Newhall JE. Malnutrition in liver transplant patients. *Transplantation.* 2001;72(4): 666–670.
71. Fan ST, Lo CM, Lai ECS, Chu KM, Liu CL, Wong J. Perioperative nutritional support in patients undergoing hepatectomy for hepatocellular carcinoma. *N Engl J Med.* 1994;331:1547–1552.

ADDITIONAL SUGGESTED REFERENCES

Abbott WJ, Thomson A, Steadman C, et al. Child-Pugh class, nutritional indicators, and early liver transplant outcomes. *Hepato-Gastroenterology.* 2001;48:823–827.

Achord JL. A prospective randomized controlled study of peripheral parenteral nutrition in moderate and severe alcoholic hepatitis. *J Hepatol.* 1988;7: 200–207.

Achord JL. Malnutrition and the role of nutritional support in alcoholic liver disease. *Am J Gastroenterol.* 1987;82:1–7.

Angulo P. Nonalcoholic fatty liver disease. *N Engl J Med.* 2002;346:1221–1231.

Biel AT, Cordoba J. Hepatic encephalopathy. *Liver Transplant.* 2000;6:575–581.

Clark JM, Brancati FL, Diehl AM. Nonalcoholic fatty liver disease. *Gastroenterology.* 2002;122:1649–1657.

Donaghy A. Advances in liver disease: alcoholic hepatitis, non-cirrhotic portal fibrosis and complications of cirrhosis. Issues of malnutrition and bone disease in patients with cirrhosis. *J Gastroenterol Hepatol.* 2002; 17:462–466.

Plauth M, Egberts EH, Hamster W, et al. Long-term treatment of latent portosystemic encephalopathy with branched-chain amino acids. A double-blind placebo-controlled crossover study. *J Hepatol.* 1993;17(3):308–314.

Falck-Ytter Y, Younossi ZM, Marchesini G, McCullough AJ. Clinical features and natural history of nonalcoholic steatosis syndromes. *Semin Liv Dis.* 2001;21:17–26.

Hasse J, Strong S, Gorman MA, Liepa G. Subjective global assessment: alternative nutrition-assessment technique for liver transplant candidates. *Nutrition.* 1993;9:339–343.

Horst D, Grace ND, Conn H, et al. Comparison of dietary protein with an oral, branched chain-enriched amino acid supplement in chronic portal-systemic encephalopathy: a randomized controlled trial. *Hepatology.* 1984;4: 279–287.

Marchesini G, Bugianesi E, Forlani G, et al. Nonalcoholic fatty liver, steatohepatitis, and the metabolic syndrome. *Hepatology.* 2003;37:917–923.

Marchesini G, Dioguardi FS, Bianchi GP, et al. Long-term oral branched-chain amino acid treatment in chronic hepatic encephalopathy. *J Hepatol.* 1990;11:92–101.

McCullough AJ. Malnutrition in liver disease. *Liver Transplant.* 2000;6(4, Suppl 1):S85–S96.

Mendenhall CL, Anderson S, Weesner RE, Goldberg SJ, Crolic KA. Protein-calorie malnutrition associated with alcoholic hepatitis. Veterans Administration Cooperative Study Group on Alcoholic Hepatitis. *Am J Med.* 1984;76:211–222.

Merli M, Nicolini G, Angeloni S, et al. Incidence and natural history of small esophageal varices in cirrhotic patients. *J Hepatol.* 2003;38:266–272.

Mullen KD, Weber FL. Role of nutrition in hepatic encephalopathy. *Semin Liver Dis.* 1991;11:292–304.

Musso G, Gambino R, DeMicheli F, et al. Dietary habits and their relations to insulin resistance and postprandial lipemia in nonalcoholic steatosis. *Hepatology.* 2003;37:909–916.

Pagano G, Pacini G, Musso G, et al. Nonalcoholic steatohepatitis, insulin resistance, and metabolic syndrome: further evidence for an etiologic association. *Heptatology.* 2002;35:367–372.

Petrides AS, Matthews DE, Esser U. Effect of moderate exercise on insulin sensitivity and substrate metabolism during post-exercise recovery in cirrhosis. *Hepatology.* 1997;26(4):972–979.

Plauth M, Merli M, Kondrup J, Weimann A, Ferenci P, Müller MJ. ESPEN guidelines for nutrition in liver disease and transplantation. *Clin Nutr.* 1997;16:43–55.

Riggio O, Angeloni S, Ciuffa L, Nicolini G, Attili AF, Albanese C, Merli M. Malnutrition is not related to alterations in energy balance in patients with stable liver cirrhosis. *Clin Nutr.* 2003;22(6):553–559.

Ukleja A, Scolapio JS, McConnell JP Dickson RC, Nguyen JH, O'Brien PC. Serum and hepatic vitamin E assessment in cirrhotics before transplantation. *J Parenter Enteral Nutr.* 2003;27:71–73.

Ukleja A, Scolapio JS, McConnell JP, et al. Nutritional assessment of serum and hepatic vitamin A levels in patients with cirrhosis. *J Parenter Enteral Nutr.* 2002;26:184–188.

Elizabeth Gleghorn, MD;
Karen Amorde-Spalding, MS, RD, CSP;
Mark H. DeLegge, MD, FACG

18

Neurologic Diseases

Introduction

The spectrum of neurologic diseases is very diverse and decisions regarding nutritional intervention in cases of neurologic disease must be individualized to the patient. Neurosurgical patients requiring major spinal or intracranial interventions experience the same intense catabolism characteristic of major surgery patients. Neurologic diseases may alter the patient's ability to swallow, resulting in nutritional deterioration or death from repeated episodes of aspiration pneumonia.

The risk of nutrition problems in pediatric neurologic disease varies with the type of impairment and with its extent. Children who have cognitive and motor impairment are at higher risk for malnutrition. A team approach, with involvement of occupational and feeding therapists, social workers, psychologists, registered dietitians, as well as physicians and nurse/nurse practitioners, is required to meet the needs of these complicated patients and their families.

I. Acute Brain Injury

A. Background
1. Acute head injury (HI) accounts for approximately one fourth of all trauma deaths. These numbers have been increasing coincident with the rise in automobile-related injuries and an explosive increase in firearm-related injuries.
2. Patients with brain injury are the most recognized at-risk nutritional population of the neurological injured patient.

B. Acute medical management
1. Severely head-injured patients are usually treated in an intensive care unit (ICU), where immediate management focuses on stabilizing vital signs, reducing intracerebral pressure (ICP), and preventing further injury.
2. Cerebral edema is believed to be the key factor leading to increased ICP pressure.
   a) Vasogenic edema results from damage to capillary endothelium with resultant leakage of protein-rich material into interstitial spaces and a rise in osmolality in this tissue.[1]
   b) Free fluid flows into these highly osmotic areas and leads to the development of cerebral edema.
3. Hyperglycemia is common after brain injury.[2]
4. Assessment of neurologic function is accomplished using the Glasgow coma scale.
5. The incidence of ventilator associated pneumonia (VAP) is high. Studies have shown that VAP is multi-variable in etiology and dependent on a patient's immune function, swallowing reflex, oropharyngeal hygiene, and route of enteral feeding.
6. Mechanical ventilation is generally required. Hyperventilation can be employed to reduce intracranial pressure.
7. Dehydration and the use of osmotic diuretics, such as mannitol, are employed to reduce intravascular volume in an attempt to reduce increased cerebral pressures.
8. Impaired physical activity requires specialized attention.

C. Nutrition assessment
1. An estimate of energy needs is required to provide patient-specific nutrition support. No single test is able to predict a patient's nutritional status under all conditions.
2. The complicated physiologic response to HI makes even the simplest determination of calorie and protein needs difficult.
3. After HI, many catabolic hormones, such as cortisol and glucagon, rise significantly.[3]
4. The most commonly used formula for energy needs is the Harris-Benedict equation.
5. Resting energy expenditure (REE) can also be measured by indirect calorimetry, and is known as measured resting energy expenditure (MREE).[4] Estimated energy expenditure is calculated by multiplying the REE by an activity factor or a disease factor to arrive at a true energy expenditure.
6. Estimation of nitrogen losses plays an important role in determining a patient's protein needs. Trauma patients have both increased protein synthesis and a much larger increase in protein catabolism.[5]
7. Nitrogen losses of up to 30 g/d have been documented in acutely ill HI patients. No studies have demonstrated a direct correlation between the severity of head injury and the amount of urinary nitrogen losses.
8. Immobility may increase nitrogen losses.
9. High levels of nitrogen intake can partially reverse net nitrogen losses. However, high nitrogen excretion is not reversed by increasing caloric intake alone.[6]
10. Supplementation of branched-chain amino acids (BCAAs) may also reduce net nitrogen losses. The effect of BCAAs on patient outcome has not been studied.[2]
11. Laboratory assessment of nutritional status remains imperfect, but may provide a snapshot of the adequacy of nutrition support.
    a) Albumin production is reduced as other acute-phase reactants are produced preferentially in response to stressful stimuli.[7]
    b) Serum retinol binding protein and prealbumin may be monitored to follow the nutritional status of HI patients later in the course of their recovery.[8]
12. Global assessments of the nutritional status of critically ill patients are less accurate than for the general outpatient population.[9]

D. Nutrition goals
  1. It may be difficult to assess calorie needs accurately in the HI patient. One common approach is to provide 1.4 to 1.5 × the estimated REE.[10]
  2. In this population, setting a goal to achieve nitrogen balance may be unrealistic.
  3. Many centers aim for a protein intake between 1.5 and 2.2 g/kg/d to minimize protein losses or even achieve positive nitrogen balance for some patients.[11]
  4. In general, the peak in nitrogen losses occurs in the first few weeks following HI. It is not uncommon for nitrogen losses to lead to a loss of lean body mass of 10% in the first 7 days.

E. Nutrition therapy
  1. When the head injury is associated with other abdominal trauma, the use of the GI tract may be compromised, thus affecting the nutritional therapy options.
  2. If it is unsafe to use the gut, then parenteral nutrition (PN) may be useful until safe enteral access can be achieved.
  3. Some authors have shown no outcome difference in comparing parenteral versus enteral nutrition (EN).[12] However, many other authors have found PN to be associated with greater complications than EN in other critically ill populations.

F. Gastric function and feeding
  1. Gastric function is often abnormal in the critically ill patient. This may be secondary to cytokine influence and GI hypoxia.[13] Gastric function is also altered after severe HI.
  2. Delayed gastric emptying has been noted in the acutely HI patient population to a degree similar to patients receiving a surgical vagotomy.[14]
  3. Up to a 50% regurgitation of the volume of gastric tube feeding has been reported in some HI patients. This resulted in a marked reduction in the EN formula delivered to these patients.[15]
  4. There is a significant reduction in lower esophageal sphincter (LES) pressure in head-injured patients.[16] This lower LES pressure, in combination with gastroparesis, increases the risk of gastroesophageal reflux and aspiration associated with gastric feedings.
  5. Elevation of the head of the bed and pro-motility agents increase the tolerance of gastric feeding in HI patients.[17]
  6. A prospective trial using jejunal tube feeding in severely head-injured patients allowed full caloric delivery in approximately 4 days.[18]

G. Enteral nutrition
  1. Enteral nutrition (EN) should be used as early as possible in the hospital course of an HI patient. Although it is often easier to use parenteral nutrition due to the availability of central venous access, many potential complications are associated with parenteral nutrition.
  2. Providing energy needs to HI patients by day 7 significantly reduced mortality as compared to patients underfed for 2 weeks.[19]
  3. Patients for whom EN was initiated rapidly had fewer infectious complications, earlier hospital discharge, and better neurological outcomes at 3 months as compared to patients whose EN formula rate was slowly increased over time.[20]
  4. Head-injured patients can obtain full caloric needs in less than 5 days of jejunal feedings compared to > 10 days of gastric feeding.[21]
  5. Small bowel feedings are well tolerated during barbituate coma therapy.
  6. A potential benefit of jejunal feeding is the reduction in GI aspiration and its associated morbidity.
  7. The ultimate goal of enteral feeding is to obtain a return to oral food intake. In one study, a majority of patients with HI and a Glasgow coma scale < 8 regained sufficient cognitive function to return to oral food intake.[22]
  8. In general, the more severe the brain injury, the less likely the patient was to return to normal swallowing function. Prolonged time on the ventilator also reduced the likelihood of a return to normal swallowing.

H. Techniques for enteral access
  1. The type of enteral access a patient receives may be very dependent on the clinical expertise available at a given medical center.
  2. In the acute HI patient, a feeding jejunostomy may be the most appropriate enteral access.[23–26]
  3. Bedside placement of nasojejunal or orojejunal feeding tubes is technically difficult.
     a) Oroenteric tubes are used if trauma to the facial area prevents nasal tube passage. Oroenteric tubes are short-term feeding devices.
     b) A nasoenteric tube (NET) is one that passes through the nasal passage into or beyond the stomach, and is another short-term feeding device.
     c) An NET may cause local nasal irritation, epistaxis, and sinusitis if used long-term.
  4. Percutaneously placed gastric tubes and gastrojejunostomy tubes may be inserted either endoscopically (PEG and PEG/J) at the bedside or fluoroscopically in HI patients who may require long-term enteral access.
  5. If endoscopic or fluoroscopic attempts are contraindicated or unsuccessful, surgeons may place a gastrojejunostomy device similar to the endoscopic PEG/J tube.
  6. Comparative studies of PEG versus surgical G-tube placement have shown similar morbidity. However, the cost of PEG placement in HI patients was significantly lower than the cost of surgically placed G-tubes.[27]

I. Parenteral nutrition
  1. The absence of a functioning GI tract or the inability to obtain enteral access is an indication for the use of PN.
  2. Central venous access is required to meet calorie needs.
  3. There were early concerns about the potential for increased intracranial pressure with PN use.[28] However, a randomized study found no increases in ICP with the use of either EN and PN.[29]
  4. Hyperglycemia is most common within the first 24 hours following HI and correlates to its degree of injury.
  5. Prolonged hyperglycemia may lead to immunosuppression, placing the HI patient at greater risk for infectious complications.[30,31]

J. Nutritional outcomes
  1. Early prospective studies comparing PN to EN in HI patients demonstrated a greater delivery of calories in the parenteral group, probably secondary to ineffective enteral access techniques.
  2. Parenteral nutrition versus EN studies have not been repeated with today's better jejunal enteral access devices and feeding techniques.

K. Immune function and nutrition
  1. The incidence of infectious complications following HI is near 60%.
  2. There is a cellular immunity alteration believed to be secondary to increases in IL-1 and IL-2 with a decrease in IL-6.[2] The degree of immune alteration is directly related to the degree of head injury.
  3. EN promotes an improvement in the overall CD4 counts and lymphocyte function.

L. Specialized nutrient needs
  1. Zinc facilitates enzyme processes vital to the metabolism of fats, carbohydrates, and protein.

a) Serum zinc levels in HI patients fall and urinary zinc excretion increases.[32]
b) Zinc supplemented HI patients have shown a reduction in mortality.[33]

2. Magnesium supplementation given 1 hour post HI has been reported to decrease brain edema and improve neurologic scores 48 hours post head injury.[34]

II. Spinal Cord Injury

A. Nutritional assessment
1. Patients experiencing spinal cord injury (SCI) experience many of the same intense catabolic events as those with HI.
2. In general, directly following SCI, patients are in significant negative nitrogen balance.
3. Overall caloric needs are approximately 1.4–1.5 × BEE. The higher on the spinal cord an injury occurs, the more catabolic the patient.
4. Immobilization also leads to a rapid loss of protein muscle mass.[35] Later, these same patients may experience an increase in body fat.

B. Nutrition and immunity—A decrease in immune function and an increase in infectious episodes also occurs, similar to the HI patient.[36]

C. Nutritional therapy and outcomes
(1) The negative nitrogen balance can be reduced, but not corrected, by the provision of energy and protein.[37]
(2) The malnourished spinal cord surgery patient has a significant increase in infectious complications and an increase in hospital length of stay as compared to the well nourished spinal cord surgery patient.[38]
(3) Patients with high spinal cord transections (above T5) may experience delayed gastric emptying.[39]

III. Chronic Neurologic Diseases

A. Background
1. Depressed levels of consciousness are associated with a decreased ability to protect the upper airway from episodes of gastroesophageal reflux, vomiting, and even oropharyngeal secretions.
2. Some diseases may affect the neural or muscular coordination required for successful swallowing, while others may alter gastric or intestinal motility. This puts patients at risk for aspiration.
3. Aspiration is the entry of material below the true vocal cords.[40]

B. Dysphagia
1. A careful history is important in dividing dysphagia into 2 broad groups: esophageal dysphagia and oropharyngeal (transfer) dysphagia.
2. Esophageal dysphagia refers to difficulty with esophageal passage of a food bolus after successful passage from the pharynx to the esophagus.
3. Oropharyngeal dysphagia is difficulty swallowing due to a lesion that affects swallowing function above or proximal to the esophagus. The patient complains of difficulty moving a food bolus into the pharynx and esophagus to initiate the involuntary swallowing reflex.
4. Swallowing is a combination of integrated neural and muscular actions coordinated in the brain stem.
5. Any process that alters the fifth, seventh, ninth, or twelfth cranial nerves or the brain stem swallowing center can cause oropharyngeal dysphagia.
6. The patient may describe nasal regurgitation, dysarthria, nasal speech, or coughing during swallowing.
7. Liquids present more difficulty with oropharyngeal dysphagia than with esophageal dysphagia. In esophageal dysphagia, liquids pass easily unless the esophagus is almost totally obstructed.
8. For dysphagia evaluation, the most important test is the modified barium swallow using video fluoroscopy, which is often done by a radiologist and speech therapist.[41]

C. Gastrointestinal motility
1. Chronic HI patients may also have underlying diffuse gastrointestinal motility disorders.
2. Table 18-1 lists other neurologic diseases associated with GI motility disorders.

D. Gastroparesis
1. Delayed gastric emptying is more common in older patients and in patients with a lower Glasgow coma scale.[42]
2. Tolerance to gastric feeding is often less than 50 percent in acutely HI patients.[16,43–47] This improves in chronic HI patients.

E. Gastrointestinal motility evaluation and treatment
1. Evaluation of gastroparesis should first exclude obstruction caused by an ulcerative, inflammatory, or neoplastic process of the stomach or duodenum. This can be accomplished by upper GI endoscopy or an upper gastrointestinal barium study.
2. The gold standard for quantitative evaluation of gastric emptying is radioscintigraphic measurement (gastric emptying scan).
3. Currently available medications in the United States that can improve gastric emptying include metoclopramide, tegaserod, and erythromycin.
4. An evaluation of chronic HI patients with documented tube feeding aspiration demonstrated that the addition of a pharmacologic promotility agent allowed gastric feedings to continue without subsequent difficulties.[48,49]
5. There are no reliable pharmacologic agents for small bowel motility disorders.

F. Enteral feeding considerations for chronic neurologic patients
1. Many patients with depressed levels of consciousness tolerate intragastric feedings well.
2. Recent studies show that elevation of the head of the bed has been found to markedly decrease, but not eliminate, reflux episodes in patients on mechanical ventilation.[50,51]
3. Monitoring of patients with depressed consciousness who are fed intragastrically should include examining for abdominal distention, checking for high gastric residuals, and maintaining elevation of the head of the bed.
4. The presence of gastroesophageal reflux should be investigated in patients who experience multiple episodes of aspiration pneumonia.
5. Jejunal feeding is recommended in patients deemed to be at risk for aspiration pneumonia.[5] (Table 18-2)

TABLE 18-1. Neurologic Diseases Associated with Gastrointestinal Motility Disorders
Diabetic neuropathy and diabetic gastroparesis syndrome
Intracranial lesions
Intrinsic myopathies and neuropathies • Dystrophia myotonica • Familial gut myopathies and neuropathies • Progressive muscular dystrophy

TABLE 18-2. Patient Risk Factors for Aspiration in Adult Patients

Previous episode of aspiration
Decreased level of consciousness
Neuromuscular disorders interfering with swallowing
Endotracheal intubation
Vomiting
Persistently elevated gastric residuals
Need for prolonged supine positioning
Poor orotracheal hygiene

6. Some patients who have difficulty only with liquids may benefit from thickening agents.
7. Neurologic diseases in which the decline in swallowing function is progressive should be considered candidates for early, more permanent enteral access options, such as PEG placement.

G. Enteral access considerations for the chronic neurologic patient
1. For use less than 30 days, nasoenteric or oroenteric options are generally preferred.
2. For longer periods, gastrostomies or jejunostomies are preferred.
3. Gastric feeding is very common due to its convenience.
4. Continuous jejunostomy feeding is very effective in patients with documented tube feeding aspiration.[53,54]

H. Ethics of enteral feeding
1. Multiple criteria need to be evaluated including predicted clinical outcome, quality of patient life and attitudes and beliefs of patients and their families regarding artificial nutrition support.
2. The use of PEG in patients with cerebrovascular accident (CVA) has been shown to provide a significant improvement in survival and rehabilitation potential.[55,56]
3. In amyotrophic lateral sclerosis (ALS) patients, placement of a PEG and initiation of enteral feeding resulted in a significant stabilization of global function.[57]
4. Patients with chronic neurologic diseases, including dementia, were found to have maintained or improved their quality of life following PEG placement.[58]
5. The use of invasive enteral access in patients with dementia is very controversial. Dementia remains a progressive and ultimately fatal disease.

IV. Cerebral Palsy (CP) and Other Pediatric Conditions with Motor Disorders

A. General nutritional assessment
1. In general, nutritional assessment of these patients, most commonly children, conforms to the principles of assessment of the normal child, although it may be difficult to use and interpret anthropometric parameters.[59]
2. A greater degree of motor involvement in these children is predictive of greater feeding dysfunction and thus of increased malnutrition.[60]
3. Problems range from lack of dexterity with utensils to food spilling from the mouth to complete dysphagia.
4. Greater spasticity correlates with greater energy expenditure at rest and during feeding.[61]
5. Short stature may reflect a long-term energy deficit or relate to the underlying disorder.[62]
6. Global assessment of the child's nutritional fitness as a mechanism to avoid complications (decubiti, depletion of nutritional reserve, intertrigo, obesity-related obstructive sleep apnea) may be the most useful measurement of all.

B. Medical history
1. Certain underlying disorders may predict feeding disorders, dysphagia, or gastroesophageal reflux.
2. A large number of hospitalizations, especially recent, may predict the need for catch-up nutrition or indicate a decline in feeding skills.
3. Pulmonary complications may result from poor swallowing function, gastroesophageal reflux, or their combination.
4. Dental problems may limit intake and may increase the risk of aspiration.[63]
5. Level of activity helps predict energy needs.

C. Diet history
1. The three-day diet record gives an estimate of the amount of energy the child is using to achieve the current body habitus. However, some studies show the caretaker's reported intake estimate to be artifactually elevated by as much as 50% for orally fed, handicapped children.[64]
2. The baseline nutritional intake should be compared to published standards and also to the child's nutritional state. (Table 18-3)
3. Nutritional requirements of these children are extremely variable. If the standard recommendation does not seem to match the individual, it may be more clinically appropriate to increase or decrease energy from the reported baseline.
4. A child who needs to be bottle- or spoon-fed inappropriately for chronological age is more likely to have disorders of appetite or swallowing.
5. Reliance on one exclusive feeder stresses the role of that caretaker, limits feeding frequency, and may cause social and economic stress.
6. Respiratory symptoms such as choking, vomiting, change in voice, or difficulty breathing after feeding may predict dysphagia and/or aspiration.[63]
7. Stool output—Constipated children often vomit or refuse to eat. Diarrhea may result from infection, medication, dysmotility, or lack of fiber in the diet and may interfere with nutrient absorption
8. Urine output may be low in children who feed orally but with difficulty, reflecting low volitional free water intake. Hot weather and exercise increases fluid needs.

D. Social history
1. Family finances may be severely strained by the needs of these children. Tube-fed children incur even more costs.
2. Cultural and religious factors influence decision-making by the family.

E. Physical exam
1. Height measurement may be inaccurate because of contractures. Use of upper or lower limb measurement allows estimation of height and comparison to the measured weight.[64,65]
2. Weight should be obtained with the child sitting or standing unsupported if possible. A wheelchair scale should be used rather than having a parent hold the child and then subtracting the parental weight.
3. Measurement of skin fold thickness allows assessment of appropriate fat reserves.
4. Arm muscle area is reported to be positively associated with better subjective health of children with CP.[66]

TABLE 18-3. Recommended Energy Intake[64,73,81]

Normal children	1.5–1.89 × Resting Energy Expenditure (REE)
Spastic quadriparesis (SP), well-nourished	1.3 x REE
SP, malnourished	1.5 x REE (a)
Ambulatory developmental delay (DD) 5–12 yo	13.9 kcal/cm height
Non-ambulatory DD 5–12 yo	11.1 kcal/cm height
Very low activity Cerebral Palsy (CP)	10 kcal/cm height
Mild to moderate activity CP	15 kcal/kg height
Severe choreoathetosis	Up to 6000 kcal/d
Trisomy 21 male 5–12 yo	16.1 kcal/cm height
Trisomy 21 female 5–12 yo	14.3 kcal/cm height
Myelomeningocele	50% RDA for age, as little as 7 kcal/cm height
Prader-Willi syndrome	8–9 kcal/cm height for weight loss, 10–11 kcal/cm height for maintenance

5. Assessment of skin, hair, and other manifestations of nutrient deficit.
6. Examination of feeding device if present, including skin condition around the tube.
7. Assessment of pulmonary status can help predict the need for further investigation of swallowing and possible need for feeding intervention.
8. Assessment of development, activity level, tone, and posture will help the clinician estimate calorie needs. Higher activity and tone increases energy needs.

F. Laboratory testing
1. There is evidence that freely eating children with developmental disability may have deficiencies of Vitamin A, Vitamin C, Vitamin D, calcium, iron, thiamin, folate, and riboflavin.[64]
2. Some children with developmental disability choose very idiosyncratic diets, putting them at further risk for specific nutritional deficiencies.
3. Children who continue to grow along an appropriate curve probably should have an annual CBC and chemistry panel and indicated medication monitoring.
4. Children who continue to grow along a normal curve should not need more elaborate testing than non-handicapped children.
5. Children who are significantly underweight and then refed should be monitored for hypokalemia, hypomagnesemia, and hypophosphatemia as part of the refeeding syndrome.
6. Measured weight should be compared to the weight appropriate for the calculated height. Because these children often have low muscle mass, the tenth to thirtieth percentile weight-for-height may be suitable.

G. Swallowing dysfunction, aspiration, and gastroesophageal reflux evaluation
1. Evaluation and treatment for this problem requires a multidisciplinary team approach.
2. Certain neurological disease states are commonly associated with a risk for aspiration. (Table 18-4)

TABLE 18-4. Clinical Clues to Dysphagia and Aspiration in Neurologically Impaired Children

Conditions associated with dysphagia or aspiration	Moebius syndrome Cornelia de Lange syndrome Bulbar polio, other bulbar syndromes, stroke Familial dysautonomia Trisomies 18 and 21 Rett syndrome Guillain-Barre syndrome Arnold-Chiari malformation Muscular dystrophies and myopathies, myotonia Poliomyelitis, post-diphtheritic paralysis Cranial nerve palsy Infant botulism Brain stem glioma Long-term feeding deprivation Myelomeningocele Myasthenia gravis
Symptoms predictive of dysphagia or aspiration	Coughing, change in voice, or tachypnea after eating Recurrent respiratory infections or asthma Weak cry Nasopharyngeal regurgitation Snoring Vomiting or gagging during feeding Feeding refusal Poor trunk/neck/head tone Long time to feed
Physical exam	Tongue thrust Drooling Opisthotonus Stridor Wheezing, rales, or rhonchi

3. An upper gastrointestinal (UGI) series shows the anatomy and motor function of the esophagus and stomach.
4. A video swallow study done with the participation of a feeding therapist skilled in this evaluation.
   a) This is a good indicator of aspiration of food or fluids with swallowing.
   b) Textures varying from thin to solid are offered to the child.
   c) Techniques to increase the safety of the swallow can be identified.
5. A pH probe study counts the number of reflux events in a test period, usually overnight or up to 24 hours. This study is the most accurate test to assess for the presence of gastroesophageal reflux (GER) but also has day to day variability.[67,68] The presence of GER can predict patients who are more likely to aspirate gastric contents.
6. Gastric emptying should be measured by the use of a gastric emptying scan. Patients with delayed gastric emptying are at increased risk for reflux and aspiration of gastric contents.
7. A neurologically handicapped child shown to aspirate with feeding presents a clinical decision regarding 3 points: Should a feeding tube be used? Should oral feeding be stopped? Should an antireflux operation be performed?

H. Specialized tests
1. Bone densitometry (dual energy X-ray absorptiometry, DEXA) is likely to be abnormal in children who are mostly recumbent, because weight bearing is significantly important in building bone.
   a) Children with CP who have had fractures have less dense bone (by X-ray or densitometry) than patients who have had no fractures.[69–71]
   b) However, bone density has not been shown to predict future fractures in normal or CP children.[72]
2. Resting energy expenditure can be measured by indirect calorimetry.

I. Nutrition plan
1. Assess the child's status as overweight, appropriate weight, or undernourished based on the history, physical, and laboratory parameters. (Figure 18-1)
2. Add supplements or increase feeding volume as needed to change the child's habitus, and supplement significant micro- and macronutrient deficits caused by low energy intake and by medications that increase requirements for specific nutrients.
3. Children who are unable to meet increased oral calorie goals should be evaluated for unrecognized swallowing dysfunction and GER.
4. Behavioral modification and appetite-stimulating medicine should be used as in any child with failure to thrive.
5. A feeding therapist may be able to make the feeding process safer by altering the consistency of food and changing the feeding position.[73]
6. Antireflux surgery can decrease the risk of gastric content aspiration due to GER episode. Antireflux surgery cannot stop aspiration of saliva or food during swallowing.
7. Some families will choose to feed the aspirating child by mouth. They feel that the pleasure experienced by the child and the family in feeding is worth the potential shortening of life.
8. Orally fed children who persistently fail to improve their nutritional status should be considered for the initiation of tube feedings.
9. Antireflux surgery and tube feeding may be chosen on clinical grounds to improve management of the child with GER and aspiration.
10. Children who have GER clinically or on testing should be initially treated medically. Surgery should be reserved for medical failures, or recurrent vomiting or aspiration.
11. Often, the family is more ready for a feeding tube or antireflux surgery than the health professional initially realizes.

J. Tube feeding access and tube feeding
1. Children sometimes lose all interest in oral feeding after a gastrostomy tube is introduced. This can be very disappointing to the family.
2. Nasoenteric tubes are useful in the trial of enteral feeds. They can be used for short-term feeding in acute situations in which the child is expected to regain the ability to eat, such as after surgery.
   a) Nasogastric (NG) tubes can be placed at the bedside and placement confirmed by auscultation of insufflated air and by clinical examination of the child.
   b) NG feeding is a useful way to assess how a child will respond to gastrostomy feeding.
   c) Nasoduodenal or nasojejunal (NJ) tubes can be placed at the bedside blindly, by pH evaluation, or in the fluoroscopy or endoscopy suite under direct visualization. These tubes tend to reduce aspiration from gastroesophageal reflux.
   d) Nasally placed tubes can cause annoying problems such as increased ear and sinus infections as well as nosebleeds.
3. If the child requires permanent gastric enteral access, a percutaneous endoscopic gastrostomy (PEG) should be placed.
   a) Small bowel access is possible using a jejunal tube placed through a preexisting gastrostomy tube or gastrostomy site. Gastrojejunal tubes are more prone to mechanical complications such as tube migration and occlusion and the need for a continuous enteral formula infusion.
   b) The percutaneous enteral access techniques are usually performed by an interventional radiologist or an endoscopist.
   c) No matter who actually places the tube, a team approach (MD, nurse with feeding expertise, and registered dietitian) is needed so that complications can be resolved expeditiously.
4. Tube feedings should be given in the most physiologic manner that the child can tolerate. Bolus feeds in an amount appropriate to the child's age are usually the best way to start.
5. If the child is taking oral feeds, these should be given first. Additional formula to meet a predetermined total should be given either as a "top off" at each feed, at the end of the day, or overnight as a drip.
6. Overnight continuous drip feeds with very small boluses in the daytime may work for those intolerant of large volumes.

K. Low bone density
1. Children with CP have a high prevalence of low bone density for age.[74,75] Pathologic fractures affect up to 25% of children with CP who are in residential care.
2. Bedrest and lack of weight-bearing is an important contributor that can be treated by physical therapy.[32]
3. With their low calorie intake, children with CP may not get enough Vitamin D and calcium. They may also have insufficient sun exposure.
4. Antiepileptic drugs interfere with vitamin D metabolism.[76]
5. It is reasonable to give optimal calcium, phosphorus, and vitamin D to all children with CP.
6. Increases in vitamin D and calcium intake have been shown to increase bone density. There has been no reported toxicity of these dietary measures.

FIGURE 18-1. Nutrition Assessment and Plan for Neurologically Impaired Children

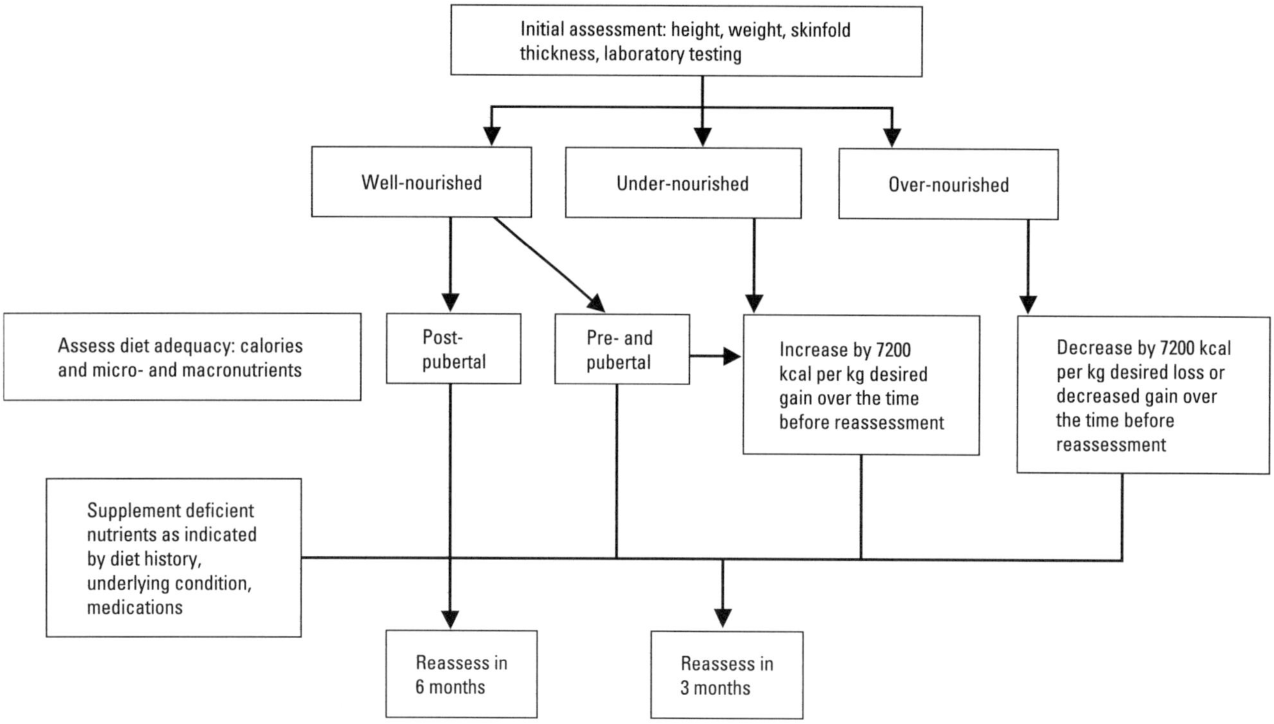

7. Intravenous and oral bisphosphonates have been successfully used to treat symptomatic low bone density in children with and without CP.[69,77,78] Pill formulations of these medications are well known to be hazardous in people with dysphagia. Therefore, IV administration, preferably in a clinic or hospital setting with close observation, would be necessary for most children with CP

V. Children with Seizures Disorders

A. Ketogenic diet
1. The ketogenic diet is an established therapy for children with intractable epilepsy.[79]
2. If conventional drug therapy fails or is accompanied by intolerable drug side effects, the ketogenic diet is an appropriate next step.
3. Ketosis can be accomplished by either fasting or consuming a high fat diet.
4. Epileptic children usually begin the ketogenic diet by fasting for a limited time (12–36 hours) to quickly establishing ketosis.
5. In order to maintain the ketosis while nourishing the growing child, a high fat diet is slowly introduced. The traditional ketogenic diet derives 80–90 % of calories from fat.
6. The long-term success of the diet requires a consistent level of ketosis which is accomplished by following a prescribed intake of energy, protein, fat, and carbohydrate.
7. A targeted ratio of total fat to protein and carbohydrate combined is routinely consumed to maintain the deep ketosis and seizure control. The most frequently used ratios are from 3:1 to 4:1.
8. This diet is designed to support near normal growth and development while maintaining seizure control.
9. This diet is effective in controlling seizures in over half of the children treated.[80]
10. Like conventional drug therapy, the ketogenic diet has the potential for both short- and long-term side effects.
    a) Side effects include acidosis, nausea, vomiting and dehydration, constipation, cholelithiasis, nephrolithiasis, pancreatitis, and cardiomyopathy.
    b) Protein-losing enteropathy has been observed in several instances.
11. Labs are monitored per a specific schedule. (Table 18-5)
12. In some cases, the need for tube feeding makes it easier to prescribe this diet, as taste and preference do not matter.
13. The ketogenic diet prescription usually limits calories and protein to less than typical allowances. This may interfere with projected normal weight gain and linear growth.
14. Once seizure control is attained, protein and calories can be titrated up to support more normal growth
    a) Overall micronutrient intake might be limited by the diet and a vitamin and mineral supplement is usually needed.
    b) A sugar-free supplement must be used.
    c) A daily calcium supplement is necessary as well.
15. The child is usually hospitalized to initiate the diet.
16. In the early weeks of the diet, the family is often overwhelmed by the dramatic change in routine.
17. Regularly scheduled follow-up appointments with the entire team are essential to assess for normal growth, metabolic complications, seizure control, and family coping.

TABLE 18-5. Ketogenic Diet Laboratory Value Assessment

	Preadmission	Admission PRN	1 month f/u	6 months f/u	Annual f/u and q 6 months
CBC	●		●	●	●
Electrolytes	●		●	●	●
Metabolic Panel	●		●	●	●
Liver Function	●		●	●	●
Uric Acid	●		●	●	●
Carnitine (Free + Total)	●		●	●	●
Urinalysis	●		●	●	●
Amylase	●		●	●	●
Lipid panel	●		●	●	●
Abdominal Ultrasound				●	●
Renal Ultrasound				●	●
EKG	●			●	●

VI. Conclusion

1. The past 3 decades have seen dramatic improvements in the nutritional care of patients with neurologic diseases.
2. Initial fears of the safety of parenteral nutrition support have been dispelled.
3. A new sense of urgency for early enteral feeding has developed because of its positive impact on patient clinical outcomes.
4. New enteral access devices have been created for this population and have been shown to allow enteral feeding early. These include PEG/J and direct percutaneous jejunostomy (DPEJ).
5. The goal of nutritional therapy in this population is to minimize loss of protein muscle mass, thereby improving clinical outcomes.
6. Patients with recurrent aspiration pneumonia should be evaluated to determine whether oropharyngeal secretions or intragastric contents are the etiology.
7. Clinical benefits of early PEG and enteral feeding in CVA and neuromuscular disorders has been proven.
8. The rationale of nutritional therapy in the demented patient needs to be clearly discussed with the patient's family and caregiver. Living wills need to be honored.
9. Children with neurologic disorders should be individually monitored for appropriate height and weight advancements.
10. The ketogenic diet plays a special role in the treatment of children with intractable seizure disorders.

(Neurologic chapter from the 1st edition was contributed by L. Glen Lewis, Shirley M. Ekvall, and Valli K. Ekvall)

REFERENCES

1. Ruelen HJ. Vasogenic brain edema. *Br J Anaesth.* 1976;48:741–752.
2. Young B, Ott L, Yingling B, et al. Nutrition and brain injury. *J Neurotrauma.* 1992;9 (suppl 1):S375–S383.
3. Ott L, Young B. Neurosurgery. In: Zaloga GP, ed. *Nutrition in Critical Care.* St. Louis, MO: CV Mosby; 1994:155–172.
4. Weir JB de V. New methods for calculating metabolic rate with special reference to protein metabolism. *J Physiol.* 1949;109:1–9.
5. Birkhahn RH, Long CL, Fitkin D, et al. Effects of major skeletal trauma on whole body protein. *Surgery.* 1980;88:294–300.
6. Ott L, Schmidt J, Young AB, et al. Comparison administration of two standard intravenous amino acid formulas to severely brain-injured patients. *Drug Intell Clin Pharm.* 1988;22:763–768.
7. Sganga G, Siegel JH, Brown G, et al. Repriorization of hepatic plasma release in trauma and sepsis. *Arch Surg* 1985;120:187–199.
8. Natolini S, Gentili P, Marini B, et al. Nutritional assessment in head injured patients through the study of rapid turnover visceral proteins. *Clin Nutr,* 1999;18:247–251.
9. Detsky AS, McLaughlin JR, Baker JP. What is the subjective global assessment of nutritional status? *J Parenter Enteral Nutr,* 1987;11:8–13.
10. Phillips R, Ott L, Young B, et al. Nutritional support and measured energy expenditure of the child and adolescent with head injury. *J Neurosurg.* 1987;67:846–851.
11. Bivins BA, Twyman DL, Young AB. Failure of nonprotein calories to mediate protein conservation in brain-injured patients. *J Trauma.* 1986;26: 980–986.

12. Borzotta AP, Pennings J, Papasadero B, et al. Enteral versus parenteral nutrition after closed head injury. *J Trauma.* 1994;37:459–468.
13. Szabo JS, Stonestreet BS, Oh W. Effects of hypoxemia on gastrointestinal blood flow and gastric emptying in the newborn piglet. *Pediatr Res.* 1985; 19:466–471.
14. Ott L, Phillips R, McClain CJ, et al. Intolerance to enteral feedings in the brain injured patient. *J Neurosurg.* 1988;68:62–66.
15. Weekes E, Elia M. Observations on the patterns of 24-hour energy expenditure changes in body composition and gastric emptying in head-injured patients receiving nasogastric tube feedings. *J Parenter Enteral Nutr.* 1996; 20:31–37.
16. Clifton GL, Robertson CS, Constant CF. Enteral hyperalimentation in head injury. *J Neurosurg* 1985;62:186–193.
17. Klodell CT, Carroll M, Carrillo EH, et al. Routine intragastric feeding following traumatic brain injury is safe and well tolerated. *Am J Surg* 2000; 179:168–171.
18. Kirby DF, Clifton GL, Turner H, et al. Early enteral nutrition after brain injury by percutaneous endoscopic gastrojejunostomy. *J Parenter Enteral Nutr.* 1991;15:298–302.
19. Rapp R, Young B, Tywman D, et al. The favorable effects of early parenteral feeding on survival in head-injured patients. *J Neurosurg.* 1991;74:43–50.
20. Harris JA, Benedict FG. *A biometric study of basal metabolism in man.* Pub. No. 279. Washington, DC: Carnegie Institution of Washington; 1919.
21. Ott L, Hatton J, McCain M, et al. Postpyloric enteral feeding costs for patients with severe head injury: blind placement, endoscopy and PEG/J vs TPN. *J Neurotrauma.* 1999;16:233–242.
22. Mackay LE, Morgan AS, Bernstein BA. Factors affecting oral feeding with severe traumatic brain injury. *J Head Trauma Rehab.* 1999;14:435–447.
23. Adams S, Delinger EP, Wertz MJ, et al. Enteral versus parenteral nutritional support following laparotomy for trauma: a randomized prospective trial. *J Trauma.* 1986;26:883–890.
24. Moore FA, Feliciano DV, Andrassy RI, et al. Early enteral feeding, compared with parenteral reduces post-operative septic complications; the results of a meta-analysis. *Ann Surg.* 1992;216:172–183.
25. Moore FA, Moore EE, Jones TN, et al. TEN versus TPN following major abdominal trauma: reduced septic morbidity. *J Trauma.* 1989;29:916–922.
26. Kudsk KA, Croce MA, Fabian TC, et al. Enteral versus parenteral feeding: effects on septic morbidity after blunt and penetrating abdominal trauma. *Ann Surg.* 1992;215:503–511.
27. Cameron BH, Blair GK, Murphy JJ, et al. Morbidity in neurologically impaired children after percutaneous endoscopic versus Stamm gastrostomy. *Gastrointest Endosc.* 1995;42:41–44.
28. Waters DC, Hoff JT, Black KL. Effect of parenteral nutrition on cold-induced vasogenic edema in cats. *J Neurosurg.* 1986;64:460–465.
29. Young B, Ott L, Haack D, et al. Effect of total parenteral nutrition upon intracranial pressure in severe head injury. *J Neurosurg.* 1987;67:76–80.
30. Fong Y, Moldawer LL, Shires T, et al. The biologic characteristics of cytokines and their implication in surgical injury. *Surg Gynecol Obstet.* 1990;170:363–378.
31. Young B, Ott L, Beard D, et al. Relationship between admission hyperglycemia and neurologic outcome of severe brain-injured patients. *Ann Surg.* 1989;210:466–473.
32. McClain CJ, Twyman D, Ott L, et al. Serum and urine zinc response in head injured patients. *J Neurosurg.* 1986;64:224–230.
33. Young B, Ott L, Kasarkis E, et al. Zinc supplementation is associated with improved neurologic recovery rate and visceral protein levels of patients with severe closed head injury. *J Neurotrauma.* 1996;13:25–34.
34. Feldman Z, Gurevitch B, Artru AA, et al. Effect of magnesium given 1 hour after head trauma on brain edema and neurological outcome. *J Neurosurg.* 1996;85:131–137.
35. Desport JC, Preux PM, Guinvarch S, et al. Total body water and percentage fat mass measurements using bioelectrical impedance analysis of anthropometry in spinal cord-injured patients. *Clin Nutr.* 2000;19:185–190.
36. Cruse JM, Lewis RE, Dilioglou S, et al. Review of immune function, healing of pressure ulcers and nutritional status in patients with spinal cord injury. *J Spinal Cord Med.* 200;23:129–135.
37. Rodriguez DJ, Benzel EC, Clevenger FW. The metabolic response to spinal cord injury. *Spinal Cord* 1997;35:569–604.
38. Klein JD, Hey LA, Yu CS, et al. Perioperative nutrition and postoperative complications in patients undergoing spinal surgery. *Spine.* 1996;21: 2676–2682.
39. Feasley RD, Szurszewski JH, Merritt JC, et al. Effects of traumatic spinal cord transection on human upper gastrointestinal motility and gastric emptying. *Gastroenterology.* 1984;87:69–75.
40. Horner J, Massey EW. Silent aspiration following stroke. *Neurology.* 1988; 38:317–319.
41. Logemann JA. *Manual for the Videofluorographic Study to Swallowing.* 2nd ed. Austin, TX: Pro-Ed; 1993.
42. Kao CH, ChangLai SP, Chieng PU, et al. Gastric emptying in head-injured patients. *Am J Gastro.* 1998;93:1108–1112.
43. Norton JA, Ott LG, McClain C, et al. Intolerance to enteral feeding in the brain-injured patient. *J Neurosurg.* 1988;68:62–66.
44. Cataldi-Betcher EL, Seltzer MH, Slocum BA, et al. Complications occurring during enteral nutrition support: a prospective study. *J Parenter Enteral Nutr.* 1983;7:546–552.
45. DeLegge MH, Duckworth PF Jr, McHenry L Jr, et al. Percutaneous endoscopic gastrojejunostomy: a dual center safety and efficacy trial. *J Parenter Enteral Nutr.* 1995;19:239–243.
46. Hunt D, Rowlands D, Allen S. The inadequacy of enteral nutritional support in head injury patients during the early post-injured period. *J Parenter Enter Nutr.* 1985;9:A121.
47. Twyman D, Young B, Ott L, et al. High protein enteral feedings: a means of achieving positive nitrogen balance in head-injured patients. *J Parenter Enter Nutr.* 1985;9:679–684.
48. Ott L, Young B, Phillips R, et al. Altered gastric emptying in the head-injured patient: relationship to feeding tolerance. *J Neurosurg.* 1991;94:738–742.
49. Altmayer T, O'Dell MW, Jones M, et al. Cisapride for the treatment of gastroparesis in traumatic brain injury. *Arch Phys Med Rehabil.* 1996;77: 1093–1094.
50. Baskin WN, Johanson JF. A novel approach to enteral nutrition in the ICU. *Gastrointest Endosc.* 1992;38:A272.
51. Torres A, Serra-Battles J, Ros E, et al. Pulmonary aspiration of gastric contents in patients receiving mechanical ventilation: the effect of body position. *Ann Intern Med.* 1992;116:540–543.
52. Ibanez J, Penafiel A, Raurich JM, et al. Gastroesophageal reflux in intubated patients receiving enteral nutrition: effect of supine and semirecumbent positions. *J Parenter Enter Nutr.* 1992;16:419–422.
53. Kirby DF, DeLegge MH, Fleming CR. AGA technical review on the use of enteral nutrition. *Gastroenterology.* 1995;108:1282–1301.
54. Welz CR, Morris JB, Mullen JL. Surgical jejunostomy in aspiration risk patients. *Ann Surg.* 1992;215:140–145.
55. Wanklyn P, Cox N, Bellfield P. Outcome in patients who require a gastrostomy tube after stroke. *Age Ageing.* 1995;24:510–514.
56. James A, Kapur K, Hawthorne AB. Long-term outcome of percutaneous endoscopic gastrostomy feeding in patients with dysphagic stroke. *Age Ageing.* 1998;27:671–676.
57. Chio A, Finnochiaro E, Meineri P, et al. Safety and factors related to survival after percutaneous endoscopic gastrostomy in ALS. *Am Acad Neurology.* 1999;53:1123–1125.
58. Weaver JP, Odell P, Nelson C. Evaluation of the benefits of gastric tube feedings in an elderly population. *Arch Family Med.* 1993;2:953–956.
59. A.S.P.E.N. Board of Directors and The Clinical Guidelines Task Force. Guidelines for the use of parenteral and enteral nutrition in adult and pediatric patients. *J Parenter Enteral Nutr.* 2002;26:1SA–138SA.
60. Dahl M, Thommessen M, Rasmussen M, Selberg T. Feeding and nutritional characteristics in children with moderate or severe cerebral palsy. *Acta Paediatr.* 1996;85:697–701.
61. Reilly S, Skuse D, Poblete X. Prevalence of feeding problems and oral motor dysfunction in children with cerebral palsy: a community survey. *J Pediatr.* 1996;129:877–882.
62. Stevenson RD, Hayes RP, Cater LV, et al. Clinical correlates of linear growth in children with cerebral palsy. *Dev Med Child Neurol.* 1994;36:135–142.
63. Toder DS. Respiratory problems in the adolescent with developmental delay. *Adolesc Med.* 2000;11:617–631.

64. Zemel BS. Energy requirements and nutritional assessment in developmental disabilities. In: Walker WA, Watkins JB, Duggan C, eds. *Nutrition in Pediatrics.* Hamilton, ON: BC Decker; 1997:170.
65. Spender QW, Cronk CE, Charney EB, et al. Assessment of linear growth of children with cerebral palsy: use of alternative measures to height or length. *Dev Med Child Neurol.* 1989;31:206–124.
66. Samson-Fang L, Fung E, Stallings VA, et al. Relationship of nutritional status to health and societal participation in children with cerebral palsy. *J Pediatr.* 2002;141:637–643.
67. Nielsen RG, Kruse-Andersen S, Husby S. Low reproducibility of 2 × 24-hour continuous esophageal pH monitoring in infants and children: a limiting factor for interventional studies. *Dig Dis Sci.* 2003;48:1495–1502.
68. Franzen T, Grahn LT. Reliability of 2-hour oesophageal pH monitoring under standardized conditions. *Scand J Gastroenterol.* 2002;37:6–8.
69. Shaw NJ, White CP, Fraser WD, Rosenbloom L. Osteopenia in cerebral palsy. *Arch Dis Child.* 1994;71:235–238.
70. Bischof F, Basu D, Pettifor JM. Pathological long-bone fractures in residents with cerebral palsy in a long-term care facility in South Africa. *Dev Med Child Neurol.* 2002;44:119–122.
71. King W, Levin R, Schmidt R, et al. Prevalence of reduced bone mass in children and adults with spastic quadriplegia. *Dev Med Child Neurol.* 2003; 45:12–16.
72. Gisel EG, Tessier MJ, Lapierre G, et al. Feeding management of children with severe cerebral palsy and eating impairment: an exploratory study. *Phys Occup Ther Pediatr.* 2003;23:19–44.
73. Trahms PP. *Nutrition in Infancy and Childhood.* WCB/McGraw-Hill; New York 1997.
74. Tasdemir HA, Buyukavci M, Akcay F, et al. Bone mineral density in children with cerebral palsy. *Pediatr Int.* 2001;43:157–160.
75. Henderson RC, Lin PP, Greene WB. Bone-mineral density in children and adolescents who have spastic cerebral palsy. *J Bone Joint Surg Am.* 1995; 77:1671–1681.
76. Lifshitz F, Maclaren NK. Vitamin D-dependent rickets in institutionalized, mentally retarded children receiving long-term anticonvulsant therapy. A survey of 288 patients. *J Pediatr.* 1973;83:612–620.
77. Henderson RC, Lark RK, Kecskemethy HH, Miller F, Harcke HT, Bachrach SJ. Bisphosphonates to treat osteopenia in children with quadriplegic cerebral palsy: a randomized, placebo-controlled clinical trial. *J Pediatr.* 2002; 141:644–651.
78. Whyte MP, Wenkert D, Clements KL, et al. Bisphosphonate-induced osteopetrosis. *N Engl J Med.* 2003;349:457–463.
79. Lefevre F, Aronson N. Ketogenic diet for treatment of refractory epilepsy in children: A systemic review of efficacy. *Pediatrics.* 2000;105:E46.
80. Freeman JM, Vining EPG, Pillas DJ, et al. The efficacy of the ketogenic diet—1998. A prospective evaluation of intervention in 150 children. *Pediatrics.* 1998;102:1358–1363.
81. Quinn HP. Cerebral palsy and developmental disabilities. In: Hendricks C, Duggan C, Walker WA. In: *Manual of Pediatric Nutrition; 3rd edition;* BC Decker and H Milton, London, UK, 2000, pg 336.

SECTION EDITOR
Juan Ochoa, MD, FACS

IV

Surgical and Critically Ill Conditions

Stephen L. Barnes, MD;
Marjorie Swintosky, MS, RD;
Andrew C. Bernard, MD;
Paul A. Kearney, MD

19

Perioperative Nutritional Support

Introduction

Malnutrition is a common problem among perioperative patients, as the primary condition may induce variable gastrointestinal obstruction, anorexia, or malabsorption. Nutrient requirements may be increased and intake diminished. This chapter will review perioperative nutrition implications, assessment, and practices.

I. Goals of Perioperative Nutritional Support.

Perioperative nutrition is an important component of perioperative care. In 1936, Studley first revealed the link in peptic ulcer patients undergoing gastrectomy,[1] demonstrating that those with preoperative weight loss of less than 20% had a 3.5% mortality rate; in contrast, those with preoperative weight loss greater than 20% had a 33% mortality rate.

A. The goals of perioperative nutritional support are as follows:
  1. Decrease surgical mortality.
  2. Decrease surgical complications and infection.
  3. Reduce the catabolic state and restore anabolism.
  4. Support the depleted patient throughout the catabolic phase of recovery.
  5. Decrease the hospital length of stay.
  6. Speed the healing/recovery process.
  7. Ensure the prompt return of gastrointestinal function to resume standard oral intake as soon as possible.

B. Perioperative nutritional support, however, is not without its own complications and cost. Risk-benefit and cost-benefit analysis must therefore be taken into account in the decision-making process regarding perioperative nutritional support.

II. Perioperative Nutritional Assessment.

Malnutrition is the result of extended periods of inadequate nutritional intake and results in changes in body composition and function, with a negative impact on all organ systems. Estimates of the prevalence of malnutrition and the incidence of associated complications vary because of the many different attempts to objectively define malnutrition.[2]

A. Individuals are generally classified as well nourished or mildly, moderately, or severely malnourished.[3]
  1. Well nourished: no significant weight change; preoperative serum albumin >3.5 g/dL
  2. Mildly malnourished: <10% weight loss; preoperative serum albumin 3.2 to 3.5 g/dL
  3. Moderately malnourished: 10% to 20% weight loss; preoperative serum albumin 2.5 to 3.2 g/dL
  4. Severely malnourished: >20% weight loss; preoperative serum albumin <2.5 g/dL

B. Perioperative nutritional assessment parameters should include a complete medical history, surgical history, social history, diet history, physical examination, anthropometric and laboratory evaluations, and indirect calorimetry when appropriate. A thorough physical assessment may also help to identify specific nutrient deficiencies and must be correlated with the patient's history and laboratory data to establish a deficiency diagnosis.[4]

C. Energy needs. Nutritional assessment also includes estimation of energy and protein requirements. While over 200 formulas exist, the most commonly employed is the Harris-Benedict equation. An adjusted body weight is used for patients who are at greater than 125% of their ideal body weight. (See Chapter 28.)

D. Visceral proteins. Visceral protein evaluation is helpful in assessing an individual's nutritional status. Visceral proteins are affected by many factors related to surgical disease, such as hydration, systemic inflammation, and metabolic state. Albumin, transferrin, prealbumin, and retinol binding protein are all indicators of nutritional status; however, albumin and prealbumin are the most clinically relevant and frequently used.

E. Stress factors. Stress factors must be incorporated into the estimation of energy needs during the perioperative period based on the operative procedure performed and the clinical condition of the patient. They help to estimate increased needs as a result of the effects of tissue repair and systemic inflammation in the perioperative period.

F. Protein requirements. An estimation of protein requirements must take into account the increased requirements postoperatively during the period of wound healing and increased metabolic activity. Protein requirements can be estimated based on the patient's age, size, physical findings, and clinical condition and the operation performed.

III. Nutritional Alterations in the Perioperative Period.

Nutrient depletion occurs in the perioperative patient due to decreased intake, increased metabolic expenditure, and altered nutrient use.

A. Metabolic response. Hormonal and inflammatory medications increase the mobilization and turnover of fatty acids, amino acids, and their precursors from skeletal muscle and adipose tissue. This redistribution of substrate ensures the functioning of essential organs, supplies building blocks for tissue repair, and supports immune response. An elective, uncomplicated operation produces a transient, modest increase in nutritional requirements that is of no clinical consequence. Greater metabolic responses occur in proportion to the severity of stressors and the degree of tissue destruction associated with the operation. Preoperative hypermetabolism may be present due to long-term inflammatory or infectious conditions (eg, inflammatory bowel disease, diverticulitis).[5]

B. Reduced preoperative intake. Preoperative reduced nutrient intake can be primary (related to the disease) or secondary to an associated or unrelated disease process resulting in the inability to maintain adequate preoperative nutrient consumption or use. Anorexia is a result of the worsening of symptoms with eating or the inability to eat secondary to obstruction. Depression, psychosocial deprivation, and physical or neurologic impairment may result in the inability to maintain adequate preoperative nutrition.

C. Preoperative malabsorption. Preoperative malabsorption may occur as a result of primary conditions or may be secondary to associated or unrelated diseases. Biliary obstruction, pancreatic insufficiency, inflammatory bowel disease, and enterocutaneous fistulas can all lead to preoperative malabsorption.

D. Reduced postoperative intake. Postoperative ileus plays an important role in the resumption of intake following surgery. All abdominal operations, including laparoscopic cholecystectomy, and major procedures outside of the peritoneal cavity are associated with impaired gastrointestinal motility in the early postoperative period.[6] The extent of ileus is directly related to the extent of dissection and degree of local and systemic inflammation. As a result, nearly all patients undergoing abdominal operations and major procedures at other sites exhibit at least transient cessation of oral intake.

E. Preoperative nutrient losses. Accelerated nutrient losses as a result of gastrointestinal fluid losses (gastric, enteric, biliary, pancreatic) that are either iatrogenic (nasogastric tubes) or due to diarrhea or fistulas can result in substantial protein loss and electrolyte disturbances as well as loss of fluid, minerals, and trace elements. Replenishment of lost fluid, electrolytes, minerals, and trace elements is mandatory in preparing a patient for surgery.

F. Postoperative nutrient losses. The postoperative patient experiences a stress-mediated increase in the requirements for sodium and water, resulting in increases in total body water and associated hemodilution. Electrolyte disturbances may be significant and can be readily identified and corrected.

G. Protein depletion. Serum albumin concentrations fall rapidly in the postoperative period in proportion to the degree of stress. This is due principally to decreased albumin synthesis and also secondary to hemodilution. Albumin thus cannot be used as the sole indicator of protein depletion postoperatively. Wound healing, tissue repair, immunologic response, and blood synthesis are all of high biologic priority in the postoperative period. Net positive protein synthesis may occur in some tissues or organs despite total body negative nitrogen balance. However, wound healing and immune responses to stress may fail in states of advanced protein depletion. The effect of intermediate degrees of protein depletion is difficult to determine clinically. Generalized protein depletion may ultimately occur, leading to an increased postoperative complication rate and other manifestations of severe protein loss.

H. Energy-store depletion. The depletion of stored carbohydrate is generally not a clinical issue because of the routine infusion of isotonic glucose solutions in the perioperative period. Depletion of stored fat is of clinical significance only in the most extreme cases, when resumption of adequate nutrient intake after recovery from the operation is significantly delayed.

I. Alterations in protein synthesis, energy stores, electrolytes, minerals, and trace elements in the perioperative period may become severe and impair recovery. Preoperative malnutrition and postoperative interruption of gastrointestinal function in the face of increases in nutrient requirements secondary to metabolic response to injury may combine to produce significant nutritional alterations and risk of complications in the perioperative patient.

IV. Perioperative Nutritional Management.

The beneficial effects of nutritional interventions are modest in well-nourished patients. In uncomplicated cases, these patients tolerate up to 10 days of starvation with no medical consequences. Moderately or severely malnourished patients may require nutritional support earlier. Severely malnourished patients are more likely to experience sepsis, pneumonia, wound infections, and other complications; they benefit from preoperative nutritional support. Perioperative nutritional support should be limited to those in whom the benefits outweigh the risks. When indicated, preoperative nutritional support can be provided only to those in whom the operation can be safely delayed, and nutrition should be continued into the postoperative period. Postoperative nutritional support comprises the majority of perioperative nutrition support and can be complicated by the site of operation, the available routes of access, and the physiologic status of the patient. As a rule, if the gut works, it should be used.

A. Indications for preoperative nutritional support. Many studies have identified the severely malnourished as benefiting from preoperative nutritional support with parenteral nutrition (PN).[3,7] Results from multiple preoperative parenteral nutrition studies of surgical patients have shown no overall reduction in perioperative mortality, but significant reductions in perioperative complications are achieved in the severely malnourished receiving more than 7 days of preoperative parenteral support. These benefits were not seen in those receiving fewer than 7 days of preoperative support. In the mildly to moderately malnourished groups, there was a trend toward increased infectious/septic-related complications.[7] Studies of preoperative enteral support are not as numerous, but available clinical evidence generally indicates a trend toward reduction in perioperative complications in the moderately and severely malnourished, as seen with preoperative PN.[3] This benefit may be amplified by the use of immune-enhancing enteral diets. (See Chapter 20 for a complete discussion of immunonutrition.)

B. Special preoperative conditions. Mental status and the ability to protect one's airway, symptoms worsened by eating, obstruction and location of the obstruction of the gastrointestinal tract, and the time frame to operation are all crucial in the preoperative nutritional support decision-making process.

C. Access. Preoperative access for preoperative nutritional support can be divided into enteral and intravenous access.

1. Nasogastric/nasoenteral tubes. In the awake, competent patient able to protect his or her airway, nasogastric or nasojejunal tube placement is the easiest form of access for preoperative enteral nutrition. The tubes can be placed by hand, with the assistance of fluoroscopy, or endoscopically with or without fluoroscopy. Bolus feeding may be used with nasogastric tubes. Continuous feeding is required with nasojejunal tubes. The major risk of nasoenteral feedings is aspiration.
2. Percutaneous endoscopic gastrostomy/jejunostomy (PEG, PEJ) tubes. Endoscopically placed gastrostomy tubes are excellent routes of access to the gastrointestinal tract. They can be placed without general anesthesia. PEG tubes allow for near-immediate gastric feedings and are useful in patients who are unable protect their airway. The traditional "pull" PEG cannot be used with carcinoma of the upper aerodigestive tract, as cancerous seeding of

the PEG tract has been reported. Newer PEG tubes can be placed percutaneously through the abdominal wall by sequential dilatation under direct endoscopic or fluoroscopic guidance. PEG tubes are not without risk during placement and can become dislodged, become infected, or migrate. For patients who do not tolerate gastric feedings or those with gastroparesis, a gastrojejunal tube can be placed. A second lumen is placed through the PEG tube and is directed past the pylorus either endoscopically or fluoroscopically. Single-piece gastrojejunal devices are available and can be placed through a mature PEG site either fluoroscopically or endoscopically. Both systems allow for simultaneous gastric drainage and jejunal feeding. In more advanced endoscopic centers, PEJ tubes can be placed. The procedure is more technically demanding than PEG tube placement but can be an effective, minimally invasive approach to long-term enteral access of the small bowel.

3. Laparoscopic gastrostomy/jejunostomy. Minimally invasive access to the abdominal cavity by way of laparoscopic surgery can allow for placement of more traditional surgical-type feeding tubes in either the stomach or the small bowel. Most procedures can be performed on an outpatient basis. Though minimal access is involved, the procedures carry risks similar to those associated with traditional open surgery.
4. Central venous access. Temporary or more permanent tunneled central venous catheters can be placed either in the operating room or at the bedside to provide central venous access for parenteral preoperative therapy. Central lines carry some risk of injury at the time of placement and ongoing risk of infection and thrombosis.

D. Indications for postoperative nutritional support. Well-nourished and mildly malnourished patients tolerate the stresses of surgery without significant difficulty, and most will not need nutritional support. Well-nourished and mildly malnourished patients who resume an appropriate oral regimen within 10 to 14 days of surgery will not benefit from postoperative nutritional support and will only incur additional cost and medical risk. Moderately malnourished and severely malnourished patients will, however, benefit from postoperative nutritional support. Early postoperative nutritional support benefits the high-risk surgical patient by decreasing septic morbidity, maintaining immunocompetence, and improving wound healing and overall recovery. Barium studies[8] have shown that small-bowel motility continues in the postoperative period, even though gastroparesis may be present for 24 to 48 hours and colonic paresis for 3 to 5 days. Given the benefits of postoperative nutritional support, early postoperative feeding is now encouraged in the high-risk surgical patient who will not resume oral intake within 10 days of surgery. Patients who are clinically and mechanically able to tolerate enteral feedings should be fed enterally. Enteral nutrition is superior to PN, with fewer postoperative infections and shorter hospital stays.[9–12] However, enteral nutrition may not be appropriate for all high-risk surgical patients. Selecting patients who will not resume oral intake within 10 days can be difficult. Preoperative nutritional status should be taken into account during surgery, as the choice of route for nutritional support can be influenced at the time of operation.

E. Special postoperative conditions. Mental status and the ability to maintain one's airway once again play a significant role in postoperative nutritional support. Location of resection, postoperative complications and the need for recurrent operations, and the return of bowel function all play significant roles in postoperative nutritional support.

F. Access. Postoperative access for nutritional support can be divided into enteral and intravenous access.

1. Nasogastric/enteral tubes. Nasogastric tubes are placed routinely during major operations. In the awake patient able to protect his or her airway, gastric feedings can proceed once the perioperative gastroparesis has resolved. Nasojejunal feeding tubes can be placed during most operations. Tube feedings can be initiated into the small bowel in the immediate postoperative period.
2. Surgical gastrostomy/jejunostomy. Traditional gastrostomy and jejunostomy tubes can be placed during surgery, allowing long-term enteral access. Selection is based on the operative procedure being performed, the preoperative nutritional state, and the presumed length of need for nutritional support. Surgical access is not without complications, and the risks must be weighed against the nutritional benefits.
3. PEG, PEJ tubes. Endoscopically placed gastrostomy tubes can be inserted intraoperatively or in the postoperative period in most cases. They can be placed without general anesthesia or during the initial procedure. PEG tubes allow for near-immediate gastric feedings and are effective in patients who are unable to protect their airway. PEG tubes are not without risk during placement and can become dislodged, become infected, or migrate. For patients who do not tolerate gastric feedings or for those with gastroparesis, a gastrojejunal tube can be placed. A second lumen is placed through the PEG tube and is directed past the pylorus either endoscopically or fluoroscopically. Single-piece gastrojejunal devices are available and can be placed through mature PEG sites either fluoroscopically or endoscopically. Both systems allow for gastric drainage and jejunal feeding. In more advanced endoscopic centers, PEJ tubes can be placed if desired, although they likely have no significant benefit over transgastric tubes.
4. Central venous access. Temporary or more permanent tunneled central venous catheters can be placed either in the operating room or at the bedside to provide central venous access for PN therapy. Central lines carry some risk of injury at the time of placement and ongoing risk of infection and thrombosis. Most high-risk surgical patients will require central venous access for other reasons during the postoperative period.

V. Practice Guidelines.

The American Society for Parenteral and Enteral Nutrition has developed evidence-based practice guidelines regarding perioperative nutrition support.[13]

1. Preoperative specialized nutrition support (SNS) should be administered for 7 to 14 days to moderately or severely malnourished patients undergoing major gastrointestinal surgery if the operation can be safely postponed.
2. PN should not be routinely given in the immediate postoperative period to patients undergoing major gastrointestinal procedures.
3. Postoperative SNS should be administered to patients who are expected to be unable to meet their nutrient needs orally for 7 to 10 days.

(Perioperative nutrition support chapter from the 1st edition was contributed by Bruce M. Wolfe)

REFERENCES

1. Studley HO. Percentage of weight loss: a basic indicator of surgical risk in patients with chronic peptic ulcer. *JAMA.* 1936;106:458–460.
2. Zaloga GP. *Nutrition in Critical Care.* St Louis, MO: Mosby; 1994.
3. Howard L, Ashley C. Nutrition in the perioperative patient. *Annu Rev Nutr.* 2003;23:263–282.
4. A.S.P.E.N. Board of Directors. Guidelines for the use of parenteral and enteral nutrition in adult and pediatric patients: nutrition assessment—adults. *J Parenter Enteral Nutr.* 2002;26(S):9SA–12SA.
5. Wilmore DW. Metabolic response to severe surgical illness: overview. *World J Surg.* 2000;24:705–711.

6. Livingston EH, Passaro EP Jr. Postoperative ileus. *Dig Dis Sci.* 1990;35: 121–132.
7. The Veterans Affairs Total Parenteral Nutrition Cooperative Study Group. Perioperative total parenteral nutrition in surgical patients. *N Engl J Med.* 1991;325:525–532.
8. Nachlas MM, Younis MT, Roda CP, Wityk JJ. Gastrointestinal motility studies as a guide to postoperative management. *Ann Surg.* 1972;175(4): 510–522.
9. Moore FA, Moore EE, Jones TN, McCroskey BL, Peterson VM. TEN vs TPN following major abdominal trauma-reduced septic morbidity. *J Trauma.* 1989;29(7):916–922.
10. Bozzetti F, Braga M, Gianotti C, Mariani L. Postoperative enteral versus parenteral nutrition in malnourished patients with gastrointestinal cancer: a randomized multicenter trial. *Lancet.* 2001;358:1487–1492.
11. Kudsk DA, Minard G, Croce MA, et al. A randomized trial of isonitrogenous enteral diets after severe trauma: an immune-enhancing diet reduces septic complications. *Ann Surg.* 1996;223(4):531–540.
12. Moore FA, Feleciano DV, Andrassy RJ, et al. Early enteral feeding, compared with parenteral, reduces postoperative septic complications: the results of a meta-analysis. *Ann Surg.* 1992;216(2):172–183.
13. A.S.P.E.N. Board of Directors. Guidelines for the use of parenteral and enteral nutrition in adult and pediatric patients: perioperative nutrition support. *J Parenter Enteral Nutr.* 2002;26(S):95SA–96SA.

SUGGESTED READINGS

Bengmark S. Aggressive perioperative and intraoperative enteral nutrition. In: Shikora S, Martindale RD, Schwaitzberg SD, eds. *Nutritional Considerations in the Intensive Care Unit.* Dubuque, IA: American Society for Parenteral and Enteral Nutrition/Kendall-Hunt; 2002:365–380.

Gottschlich MM. Early and perioperative nutrition support. In: Matarese LE, Gottschlich MM, eds. *Contemporary Nutrition Support Practice: A Clinical Guide.* 2nd ed. Philadelphia, PA: Saunders/Elsevier Science; 2003: 276–289.

Imad F. Btaiche, PharmD, BCNSP; Paul E. Marik, MD, FCCM, FCCP; Juan Ochoa, MD; Robert Martindale, MD, PhD; Jeffrey E. Salon, MD, FACP, FCCP, FCCM

20

Nutrition in Critical Illness, Including Immunonutrition

Introduction

Adequate nutrition is essential to the critically ill patient. It helps support anabolism, ameliorate uncontrolled catabolism, maintain a competent immune system, and ultimately improve patient outcome. Critically ill patients usually present with multiple medical problems that are associated with significant metabolic and nutritional alterations. Severe trauma, burns, sepsis, and head injury are associated with marked hypermetabolism and hypercatabolism, which lead to dramatic metabolic alterations, including increased glycogenolysis, gluconeogenesis, and lipolysis. Balancing nutritional needs while avoiding metabolic and iatrogenic complications is a challenge. Evidence suggests that enteral feedings should begin early to preserve gut integrity. The use of parenteral nutrition (PN) should be kept as low as possible, although concomitant use of PN may be necessary while enteral feeding tolerance is established. The pediatric intensive care patient population, with patients from birth to adolescence, encompasses a wide variety of critically ill patients, including postoperative patients and patients with trauma, congenital heart disease, severe respiratory disorders, sepsis, liver or renal failure, or multiorgan dysfunction. The prevalence of malnutrition in patients admitted to the pediatric intensive care unit (PICU) ranges between 15% and 20%, with a higher prevalence in patients with congenital heart disease. This chapter discusses the metabolic and nutritional changes that occur in adult and pediatric critically ill patients and provides guidelines for providing safe and effective nutrition support, including immunonutrition, to these patients.

I. Metabolic Response to Stress

A. Critically ill patients exhibit a characteristic metabolic response to severe illness or traumatic injury independent of cause. Both types of inciting events activate the immune system and induce a coordinated systemic inflammatory response syndrome aimed at limiting the extent of injury and restoring normal physiologic processes. The specific nature and extent of this response can vary widely based on the causative insult. See Table 20-1.

B. In critical illness, there is increased release of inflammatory mediators or cytokines (eg, interleukins 1 and 6, tumor necrosis factor) and simultaneous increased production of counterregulatory hormones (eg, catecholamines, cortisol, glucagon, growth hormone). The release of cytokines and counterregulatory hormones leads to a cascade of events that affect various body systems and have a profound impact on the patient's metabolic and nutritional status.[1] When physiologically controlled, this response can facilitate recovery. When uncontrolled, it can impair host responses to critical illness.

C. When severe infection is the etiology of the critical illness, the metabolic and physiologic responses to systemic infection are referred to collectively as "sepsis" or "sepsis syndrome." The most severe form, septic shock, is associated with the development of multiorgan dysfunction and may ultimately cause death. Sepsis leads to significant metabolic changes that result in increased energy expenditure. In nonsurgical, mechanically ventilated septic patients, energy requirements have been estimated by the Harris-Benedict (HB) equation at 20% above the basal energy expenditure (BEE).[2] Since sepsis may occur in the setting of other concomitant organ dysfunction, energy expenditure varies with the severity of illness.

D. The metabolic response to severe head injury is even more dramatic, exceeding the HB prediction of BEE by 40% to 50%. Urinary nitrogen losses exceeding 25 g/day have been reported.[3] It may take several weeks following injury to restore a neutral to positive nitrogen balance in these patients.

II. Nutritional Alterations in Critically Ill Patients.

The cascade of events following injury may affect multiple organ systems, can last from hours to days, and may be accompanied by impaired immune function and delayed wound healing. The magnitude of the response depends mainly on the severity of illness, with individual variability resulting from patient-specific illness(s) and genetic variations.

A. The rate of protein catabolism exceeds the rate of protein synthesis, resulting in negative nitrogen balance. There is loss of muscle mass and protein degradation in vital organs. The accelerated skeletal muscle proteolysis causes movement of amino acids (especially alanine and glutamine) from the periphery to the viscera for gluconeogenesis. Alanine is the major amino acid used for hepatic gluconeogenesis. Glutamine is the preferred energy source for enterocytes, cells of the immune system, and cells involved in tissue repair. It serves as a substrate for renal gluconeogenesis and for hepatic synthesis of the intracellular antioxidant glutathione. Branched-chain amino acids such as leucine, isoleucine, and valine also become important oxidative substrates during critical illness. Cytokines released from monocytes and macrophages cause the liver to reprioritize its protein synthesis, reflected by increased production of the "positive" acute-phase proteins (eg, C-reactive protein, α1-antitrypsin) and decreased synthesis of the constitutive "negative" acute-phase proteins (albumin, prealbumin, retinol-binding protein, transferrin). There are decreased blood levels of visceral proteins regardless of the patient's nutritional status.

TABLE 20-1. Metabolic Response During Starvation and Injury

Characteristic Finding	Starvation (Marasmus)	Injury (Protein-Energy Malnutrition)
Energy needs	Decreased	Increased
Primary fuel (RQ)	Lipids (0.75)	Mixed (0.85)
Insulin	Decreased	Increased (resistance)
Ketones	Present	Absent
Counterregulatory hormones	Basal	Increased
Total body water	Decreased	Increased
Proteolysis	Decreased	Accelerated
Glycogenolysis	Increased	Accelerated
Lipolysis	Increased	Increased
Body stores		
Skeletal muscle	Reduced	Reduced
Fat	Reduced	Reduced
Visceral proteins	Preserved	Increased liver/immune
Refeeding response	Net anabolism	None (unless reversed)
Weight (lean tissue loss)	Gradual	Accelerated
Typical setting	Patient with chronic diseases	Patient in hospital/ICU (cardiac, COPD, etc)

COPD, chronic obstructive pulmonary disease; ICU, intensive care unit; RQ, respiratory quotient
Adapted from Daley BJ, Bistrian BR. Nutritional assessment. In: Zaloga GP, ed. *Nutrition in Critical Care.* St Louis, MO: Mosby-Year Book; 1994:9–33 with permission from Elsevier.

B. Glucose metabolism
   1. During stress, increased endogenous glucose production is the result of increased counterregulatory hormones and cytokines that stimulate glycogenolysis and gluconeogenesis. Major substrates for gluconeogenesis are glycerol (from adipose tissues), alanine (from skeletal muscles), and lactate (from peripheral tissues and skeletal muscles). This response is believed to satisfy the glucose needs of the brain, leukocytes, and the cells involved in tissue repair.
   2. Hyperglycemia may exist even with normal or increased blood insulin level, as insulin resistance is characteristic of generalized stress. Septic patients have a significant increase in glucagon, the primary hormonal mediator of gluconeogenesis. Changes in whole-body glucose uptake and glucose oxidation in sepsis are complex. Whole-body glucose uptake and oxidation may be increased in the early stages of sepsis and endotoxemia. This is possibly the result of a cytokine-induced increase in non-insulin-mediated glucose uptake by tissues rich in mononuclear phagocytes (eg, liver, spleen, ileum, lung).

C. Lipolysis is accelerated with mobilization of glycerol and free fatty acids, and there is increased fatty acid oxidation. Overall, the patient's energy stores are reduced.

D. Critical illness is also characterized by activation of the hypothalamic-pituitary-adrenal axis with the release of cortisol from the adrenal gland. This essential response to illness and stress contributes to maintenance of cellular and organ homeostasis.

E. Significant fluid and electrolyte disturbances may occur in the critically ill patient, depending on the patient's underlying medical problems, nutritional status, and drug or resuscitative therapy. A detailed review of fluid and electrolytes disturbances can be found elsewhere.[4]

F. The physiologic response to stress and injury and its effects on the metabolic and nutritional status of pediatric critically ill patients are similar to those for adults. Due to their limited tissue reserves, pediatric patients may develop malnutrition faster than adults.

III. Nutrition Support in Critically Ill Patients

A. Assessment of nutritional status in adults
   1. The assessment of nutritional status includes a medical, surgical, and dietary history obtained from the patient or caregiver. In contrast to isolated trauma or burn patients, septic patients often have some degree of underlying malnutrition before the septic episode. This may be a predisposing factor to immune dysfunction that compromises the patient's ability to fight infection. Since no single measure can provide an accurate assessment of nutritional status, combined subjective and objective data should be used (see Chapter 1). A multitude of factors may limit the accuracy of nutritional assessment.
      a) A history of acute or chronic weight loss or gain before hospital admission is an essential indicator of the patient's nutritional status. Because body weight fluctuates with large-volume fluid resuscitation, preinjury weight in critically ill patients provides useful information on nutritional status.
      b) Anthropometric parameters including skinfold thickness and arm circumference measurements may be unreliable and are seldom used in critically ill patients because the patient's positioning and fluid status affect their accuracy.
      c) Visceral protein (eg, albumin, prealbumin) levels are affected by stress, fluid shifts, and other factors that limit their specificity and sensitivity.
      d) Delayed hypersensitivity skin testing that measures cell-mediated immunity also has limitations in the critically ill

patient. Many nonnutritional factors such as tissue disruption, acute hemorrhage, hypovolemic shock, anesthesia, surgery, and the use of steroids and immunosuppressants depress immune function, independent of nutritional status.

B. Assessment of nutritional status in pediatric patients
   1. Surgical and medical problems that may affect the patient's nutritional status should be identified. Examples in the pediatric patient include congenital defects, gastrointestinal surgeries, impaired neurological status, chronic lung disease, history of premature birth, and the presence of gastrointestinal symptoms that impair food intake or absorption, such as nausea, vomiting, constipation, or diarrhea. Among patients admitted to the PICU with a diagnosis of congenital heart disease, 15% to 20% are malnourished.[5,6]
   2. Anthropometric measurements such as length or height, weight, and head circumference should be obtained upon admission to the PICU and compared with existing standards (see Chapter 1). The measurements are compared against weight-for-age, length-for-age, and weight-for-length or BMI standard tables to determine whether the patient is adequately nourished or is experiencing moderate or severe malnutrition. Weight or length status and growth patterns are the primary parameters for nutritional assessment. Body weight should be obtained daily in the PICU patient using the same scale. Fluid shifts and imbalances are common in critically ill patients and may make weight changes an inaccurate indicator of nutritional status.

C. Energy requirements
   1. Because either overfeeding or severely restricting energy can be detrimental to the outcome of critically ill patients, sound estimates of energy requirements are necessary. Many equations have been derived to estimate energy requirements; the HB equation is the most widely used. Stress factors for various disease states have been empirically determined by the use of indirect calorimetry and are added to the estimated energy expenditure calculated using the HB equation. The stress and activity factors used to adjust for the severity of illness may be excessive and can lead to overfeeding critically ill patients. In fact, experimental studies suggest that matching nutritional intake to metabolic expenditure may exacerbate inflammation and increase mortality.[7] Although energy requirements at approximately 25 to 30 kcal/kg/day have been recommended for the critically ill patient,[8] there is increasing evidence that lower caloric intake (not exceeding 25 kcal/kg/day) may be safer in these patients. In obese patients, nutrition should be provided based on adjusted body weight (see Chapter 28).
   2. The gold standard for measuring energy expenditure in the clinical setting is indirect calorimetry (see Chapter 22). This is problematic in pediatric patients because of low gas flow rates and the use of noncuffed endotracheal tubes, which create an air leak, making gas collections incomplete.
   3. Energy requirements of the critically ill pediatric patient change with the patient's clinical status. Aside from the severity of illness and stress level, other factors that affect energy expenditure include crying, blood draws, physical therapy, and endotracheal tube suctioning.
   4. The recommended daily allowance (RDA) for age includes a 30% to 40% factor for growth in young infants and for activity in children and thus typically overestimates energy requirements for PICU patients.[9,10] Energy requirements can be estimated at 1 to 1.2 times the resting energy expenditure, depending on the nutritional status, stress level, and nutrient tolerance.

D. Protein requirements
   1. Protein requirements for critically ill adult patients are approximately 1.5 g/kg/day. Proteins are administered based on the patient's premorbid body weight or the adjusted ideal body weight in obese patients. The magnitude of nitrogen loss varies with the clinical condition (Figure 20-1) and parallels the energy expenditure and stress level. Requirements may be up to 2 g/kg/day in patients with trauma, severe burns, and head injury and as high as 2.5 g/kg/day in adult patients treated with continuous renal replacement therapy (CRRT).[11]
   2. It is the underlying paradigm that nutrition intervention is designed to sustain the body's nutritional stores until the increased energy and protein requirements subside. Since the catabolic rate exceeds the anabolic rate in critical illness, nutritional support can only limit the loss of the body's protein and calorie stores. The goal is to administer sufficient nitrogen to provide a positive or neutral nitrogen balance. This is best assessed by nitrogen balance studies, which are discussed in Section V.
   3. Protein requirements for the PICU patient vary with age and clinical status. Protein/amino acids requirements in PN support for term infants are 2.5 to 3 g/kg/day. In older children, amino acid requirements are 2 to 2.5 g/kg/day, and critically ill adolescent patients require 1.5 to 2 g/kg/day. Higher protein/amino acid amounts are required for trauma patients and those treated with CRRT to make up for the amino acid losses via the hemodiafilter.

E. Benefits of enteral feeding
   1. Enteral nutrition (EN) should be considered within the first 48 hours of injury once the patient is resuscitated and stabilized. Early initiation of EN is crucial to minimize the effects of hypercatabolism and hypermetabolism.

FIGURE 20-1. Change in nitrogen excretion in various disease states.

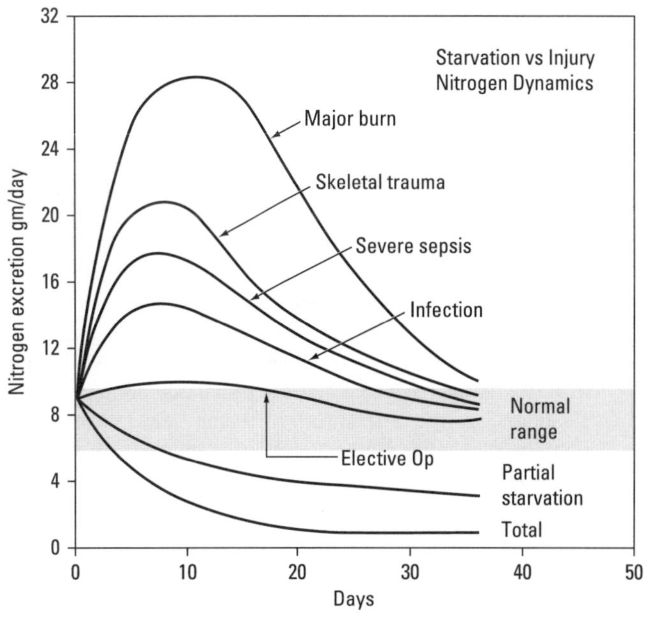

Reprinted from Long Metabolic response to injury and illness: estimation of energy and protein needs from in calorimetry and nitrogen balance. *J Parenter Enteral Nutr* 1979;3:452–56 with permission.

2. Oral nutrition is the preferred route of nutrient intake. If the patient cannot or should not be fed orally, then EN is the preferred feeding route. EN is more physiologic, cheaper, and safer than PN.
3. The gastrointestinal tract has a highly metabolically active mucosa. Lack of enteral feeding results in gastrointestinal mucosal atrophy, bacterial overgrowth, increased intestinal permeability, depletion of the liver's antioxidant enzymes, and possible translocation of bacteria and/or bacterial products. EN increases mucosal blood flow, provides a direct source of nutrients, and maintains the metabolic activity and hormonal and enzymatic balance between the gastrointestinal tract and the liver. Even low rates of enteral feeding (eg, 10 mL/hr in adults) will have protective effects on the gut mucosa and liver. Enteral feeding maintains gut integrity, prevents gut mucosal atrophy, may prevent bacterial translocation, and preserves gut-associated lymphoid tissue (GALT), which is the major source of gut mucosal immunity. EN has been shown to replete the GALT that may become depleted with PN use. While PN bypasses first-pass liver metabolism, EN allows most nutrients to go through the portal circulation. This may have a protective effect on the liver.[12]
4. Enteral feeding is also associated with lower rates of infectious complications than PN. Kudsk et al demonstrated significantly fewer cases of pneumonia, intra-abdominal abscesses, and episodes of catheter sepsis with lower septic morbidity in trauma patients who were enterally fed than in those who received PN. The most significant differences were seen in the more severely injured patients.[13]
5. EN is associated with improved wound healing, greater wound strength, and more wound hydroxyproline and collagen accumulation, which may explain the lower risk of anatomic leaks and fistulas in bowel surgery patients who receive EN instead of PN.[12]
6. Although EN has many safety and metabolic advantages over PN and is associated with fewer complications, it does not seem to affect patient mortality or the incidence of multiple organ failure.[14]

F. Enteral feeding in pediatric patients

1. Pediatric patients on an oral diet who stay longer than 5 days in the intensive care unit should have ongoing calorie count monitoring.
2. The patient's fluid requirements should be the primary consideration when the enteral formula is being selected. Then the energy and protein requirements should be considered. A 20 kcal/oz formula is equivalent to 0.67 kcal/mL, and a 24 kcal/oz formula is equivalent to 0.8 kcal/mL.
3. In infants with congenital heart disease, fluid restriction often dictates concentrating enteral formulas beyond 24 kcal/oz to meet energy and protein requirements in small volumes.
4. Enteral feeding is usually initiated at full strength since all infant and pediatric formulas are hypotonic or isotonic and there is minimal risk for hyperosmolar diarrhea with these formulas.
5. Continuous gastric or small-bowel feeding should be attempted first. Enteral feeding in infants is usually initiated at 1 mL/kg/hr and advanced to energy goal at a rate of 1 to 2 mL/kg/hr every 8 to 12 hours as tolerated. The initial volume should not exceed 50 mL/hr regardless of the patient's age or weight.

G. Immunonutrition

1. A number of specific nutritional supplements are now recognized to modulate the biologic response to injury, inflammation, and infection. Collectively referred to as immunomodulating agents, they include glutamine, omega-3 fatty acids, arginine, and antioxidants. These agents are included in various combinations in selected enteral feeding formulas.
2. Immunomodulating agents have specific favorable biological and clinical effects. Randomized clinical trials have evaluated the role of different immunomodulating enteral formulas in critically ill adult patients but not the individual components, and the results of these studies have been widely debated. A meta-analysis by Heyland et al demonstrated reductions in infectious complications, particularly in elective surgery patients, and reductions in length of stay in the intensive care unit.[15] However, the effect of these formulas on organ failure and mortality is less clear. These formulas have not yet been studied in the pediatric population.
3. Glutamine, the most abundant amino acid in skeletal muscles, is a precursor of the antioxidant glutathione and a primary nutrient for enterocytes and the GALT. Lack of glutamine may have profound effects on gut integrity and lymphoid tissue. Prophylactic administration of glutamine to critically ill patients has been attempted to improve patient outcome, but data remain inconclusive.
4. The long chain omega-3 fatty acids (eicosapentaenoic acid and docosahexaenoic acid) found in fish oil are commonly added to immunomodulating enteral formulas. Increased intake of omega-3 fatty acids instead of omega-6 fatty acids has numerous potentially positive biological effects. Eicosanoids derived from linoleic and arachidonic acids are proinflammatory. Those derived from omega-3 fatty acids are less inflammatory and less immunosuppressive than eicosanoids derived from omega-6 fatty acids.
5. Arginine, a nonessential amino acid, may become conditionally essential in the critically ill patient. Biological actions include stimulation of growth hormone, prolactin, and insulin-like growth factor. Arginine is required for the synthesis of hydroxyproline, is essential for lymphocyte function, and is the precursor of nitric oxide. Arginine levels may fall in septic patients due to decreased intake, increased metabolism to nitric oxide, and catabolism of arginine in the urea cycle as a consequence of increased arginase expression. If sepsis is potentially an arginine-deficient state, then arginine supplementation should be beneficial in septic patients. In a meta-analysis, immunomodulating enteral formulas with high arginine content resulted in a significant reduction of infectious complications[15] but had no effect on mortality. At this point, the role and safety of arginine supplementation for critically ill patients are not fully elucidated and require further studies.[16,17]

H. Parenteral nutrition

1. PN is used in patients for whom oral nutrition or EN is not feasible or is contraindicated and who are malnourished or at high risk for malnutrition (eg, critically ill patients). In adult patients who are not malnourished or at high risk for malnutrition, PN can be safely withheld for up to 5 to 7 days while the enteral route is pursued. PN should be used for the shortest duration possible.
2. PN should not be used to correct acute fluid and electrolyte deficiencies; instead, a separate intravenous solution with electrolyte supplements should be used as needed. The assessment and management of electrolyte disturbances should take into consideration electrolyte sources and losses, acid-base status, clinical conditions, and medications that affect electrolyte balance.
3. Dextrose tolerance is dependent on its rate of infusion and underlying patient conditions. Dextrose use is reduced in stressed patients, patients with diabetes, patients with acute pancreatitis, and patients treated with medications that alter glucose metabolism (eg, corticosteroids, tacrolimus, catecholamine vasopressors). Critically ill patients have a lower tolerance to dextrose

infusion compared to nonstressed subjects. In hypermetabolic burn patients, glucose oxidation reaches a plateau at a dextrose infusion rate of 5 mg/kg/min.[18] However, lower dextrose infusion rates are even better tolerated, and rates should be kept at ≤4 mg/kg/min in adult critically ill patients and should not exceed 60% of total daily energy.[19] In critically ill diabetic patients and those requiring insulin, the dextrose infusion rate should be started at no more than 2 mg/kg/min and advanced slowly over a few days to energy goal while glucose control is maintained with intensive insulin therapy. Uncontrolled hyperglycemia may cause fluid and electrolyte abnormalities, hyperglycemic hyperosmolar nonketotic syndrome, and increased susceptibility to infections. Hyperglycemia is also an early sign of sepsis, so sepsis should be ruled out in patients who are stable on PN and suddenly develop hyperglycemia or increased insulin requirements.

4. Lipid requirements
   a) Lipid clearance is reduced in stressed patients due to decreased activity of lipoprotein lipase (LPL), the main enzyme released in the bloodstream that hydrolyzes lipid particles into fatty acids. Since critically ill patients have reduced tolerance to lipid emulsion infusion, the lipid infusion rate should not exceed 0.12 g/kg/hr to avoid the development of elevated triglyceride levels.[20]
   b) A dose of intravenous lipid emulsion at 0.5 to 1 g/kg/day prevents essential fatty acid deficiency. Lipid emulsions may need to be withheld in pediatric patients when serum triglyceride concentrations exceed 275 mg/dL.
   c) Although it has been suggested that lipid emulsions may have immunosuppressive effects by helping to reduce phagocytosis and cytokine secretion, these effects have not been clinically proven.[21]
   d) There is a difference in the clearance of various lipid emulsion concentrations due to the differences in the phospholipid-to-triglyceride (PL/TG) ratio of each emulsion. The PL/TG ratios of the 10%, 20%, and 30% lipid emulsions are 0.12, 0.06, and 0.04, respectively. In critically ill patients, lower plasma triglycerides, phospholipids, and cholesterol concentrations have been seen with the use of 30% lipid emulsions compared to 10% and 20% lipid emulsions.[22–24]
   e) Structured lipids made of medium-chain triglycerides (MCT) are currently available only in Europe. These mixtures contain MCT and long-chain triglycerides (LCT) in 75/25 or 50/50 MCT/LCT ratios. The inclusion of LCT in the MCT/LCT mix provides the essential fatty acids that are not provided in MCT. MCT are oxidized faster than LCT, a possible advantage in patients with reduced lipid clearance, such as critically ill patients.[25] Although some research data showed that the MCT/LCT lipid emulsion may result in a better blood lipid profile and improved nitrogen balance, these results were not replicated in other studies.[26]
   f) In patients with acute renal failure, the clearance of both LCT and MCT was found to be equally reduced in comparison to healthy volunteers, with similar increases in serum triglyceride levels between the 2 groups.
   g) In patients with respiratory failure, variable effects have been seen in measures of respiratory function and pulmonary and arterial hemodynamics.[27–29] Hyperlipidemia during lipid emulsion infusion has been reported to affect pulmonary gas diffusion and pulmonary vascular resistance in patients with preexisting pulmonary disease.[30,31] More research is needed before routine use of the mixed MCT/LCT lipid emulsions can be recommended.
5. Multivitamin and trace element requirements
   a) Typical standard adult multivitamins and trace element formulations are added to the daily PN. However, no specific guidelines for multivitamin and trace element supplementation are available for critically ill patients. Modification of specific micronutrients is rather based on the patient's underlying diseases (eg, liver failure, wounds, burns, fistulas).[32]
   b) Blood trace element concentrations may not necessarily reflect their total body stores due to changes in tissue distribution, metabolism, or elimination. For example, during stress, blood zinc concentrations may fall due to sequestration in the liver, increased use in metabolic pathways, and increased renal elimination.
   c) Supplementation of specific micronutrients is based on the patient's underlying diseases (eg, liver failure, wounds, burns, short gut syndrome) when alterations in micronutrient metabolism and requirements are needed. The role of antioxidant supplementation (eg, supplementation of vitamins C, E, and A and selenium) in critically ill patients remains unknown.[33]
   d) Iron metabolism is also altered under stress, leading to decreased plasma iron concentrations. However, this may not necessarily indicate iron deficiency. Intravenous iron administration in the septic patient is discouraged since iron is essential for bacterial growth and may theoretically worsen sepsis.

IV. Complications of Parenteral Nutrition

A. In a meta-analysis of studies that evaluated PN use in critically ill adult patients, the benefits of PN were most noticed in malnourished patients, who also had fewer complications with PN than nonmalnourished patients given PN. Critically ill patients who received PN had almost twice the risk of mortality (relative risk 1.78; 95% confidence interval 1.11–2.85).[34] Similarly, the Veterans Affairs cooperative study showed that perioperative PN improved the outcome only of high-risk severely malnourished patients.[35]

B. The deleterious effects of PN may be most evident in critically ill patients who are at a particularly high risk for nosocomial infections. A number of studies reported an increased risk of infectious complication, longer hospital stay, and an increased risk of mortality in patients receiving PN. The Veterans Affairs study evaluated the role of perioperative PN (7–10 days before and 3 days after surgery) in patients who required noncardiac surgery. There were significantly more infectious complications in the PN group than in the control group that did not receive PN (14.1% vs 6.4%). Also, a trend toward higher 90-day mortality was observed in the PN group compared to the control group (13.4% vs 10.5%). Only those with severe malnutrition appeared to benefit from PN as administered in that study.[35]

C. PN may also be associated with a more pronounced proinflammatory response than EN. Clinical and experimental data have shown higher levels of local and systemic proinflammatory mediators with PN than EN. Higher levels of interleukins (IL-6, IL-8) were found after colorectal and major abdominal surgeries in patients receiving PN compared to patients who were fed enterally.[36,37] PN may be particularly harmful in patients with severe inflammation such as acute pancreatitis; such patients were shown to have higher infective and noninfective complications if they received PN compared to jejunal feeding.

D. A recent meta-analysis of six randomized controlled trials compared the safety and clinical outcomes of PN versus EN in patients with acute pancreatitis. Results of the meta-analysis showed that EN was associated with a significantly lower incidence of infections, shorter length of stay, and reduced surgical interventions compared to control pancreatitis patients. However, no statistically significant difference was found for mortality and noninfectious complications between the PN and EN groups.[38]

E. Complications of excess dextrose infusion include hyperglycemia, hypertriglyceridemia, hepatic steatosis, respiratory decompensation, and depression of immune function. Hyperglycemia is now thought to be a major driver of parenteral nutrition complications, which are reduced when insulin is used to maintain euglycemia.[39] (See Chapter 27.)

1. Dextrose overfeeding resulting in hyperglycemia can depress the immune system and increase infection risk. Hyperglycemia may impair cellular and humoral host defenses by reducing phagocytosis, impairing neutrophil chemotaxis and adhesion, and inhibiting complement fixation. In vitro and animal data showed a reduction in phagocytic activity of polymorphonuclear granulocytes and inhibition of immunoglobulin function with hyperglycemia. In humans, postsurgical diabetic and nondiabetic hyperglycemic patients have increased nosocomial and wound infections. Controlling hyperglycemia has resulted in improved phagocytic function as well as improved patient outcome.
2. Hyperglycemia has traditionally been defined as a random serum glucose concentration >200 mg/dL. Serum glucose concentrations of 150 to 200 mg/dL have long been considered acceptable in stressed patients because it is believed that modest hyperglycemia may promote cellular glucose uptake by glucose-dependent tissues (brain, red blood cells, wounds). However, recent data show that maintaining euglycemia between 80 and 110 mg/dL reduces complications and improves patient outcome. Van den Berghe et al, in a prospective randomized controlled study, evaluated the effects of intensive and conventional insulin therapies in 1548 adult surgical intensive care unit patients. Surgical patients were randomized to receive intensive insulin therapy to maintain serum glucose concentrations between 80 and 110 mg/dL or to receive a conventional insulin regimen to maintain serum glucose concentrations between 180 and 200 mg/dL. Study results showed that intensive insulin therapy was associated with a 34% reduction in overall in-hospital mortality and a 46% reduction in septicemia. Intensive insulin therapy significantly reduced mortality in the intensive care unit (from 8% to 4.6%) and in patients who remained more than 5 days in the intensive care unit (from 20.2% to 10.6%) compared to conventional insulin therapy. Intensive insulin therapy was also associated with reduced morbidity factors such as acute renal failure, ventilator dependency, and polyneuropathy.[39] A follow-up multivariate logistic regression analysis of the data by the same investigators showed that the benefits of intensive insulin therapy were the result of normalizing serum glucose rather than the result of the insulin dose.[40] The Van den Berghe study data are applicable to adult surgical intensive care patients; studies are under way to determine the role of tight glucose control in other intensive care and hospitalized patients.
3. In the absence of dextrose overfeeding, insulin therapy may be necessary to control hyperglycemia while meeting the patient's caloric needs, as insulin resistance is characteristic of generalized stress. Insulin stimulates glucose uptake and reduces hepatic glucose production. However, insulin does not increase glucose oxidation, and excess dextrose is largely converted to fat instead of being oxidized to carbon dioxide (CO_2). In adults, the use of a sliding scale subcutaneously administered insulin is not recommended due to variability of tissue perfusion that may lead to inadequate glycemic control between intermittent insulin dosing. The most effective way to maintain serum glucose concentrations between 80 and 110 mg/dL in hyperglycemic critically ill patients is the use of continuous insulin infusion that allows flexible titration of the insulin dose based on frequent serum glucose monitoring. A serum glucose threshold that is associated with increased morbidity and mortality has not been determined.
4. Enteral feeding is associated with fewer complications than PN and allows carbohydrate to pass through the liver with resultant hormonal/metabolic responses before reaching the systemic circulation. This reduces the hyperglycemic effect of glucose. In the Van den Berghe study,[39] patients who received exclusive PN required 26% more insulin to maintain euglycemia than those who received partial enteral feeding.[40]

F. Hypertriglyceridemia in patients receiving PN denotes excess triglyceride synthesis or reduced fat clearance. Hypertriglyceridemia during PN infusion is primarily due to dextrose overfeeding or excess lipid infusion. Stressed patients are at higher risk for hypertriglyceridemia due to increased lipolysis and hepatic fatty acid re-esterification, increased hepatic triglyceride synthesis from dextrose infusion, and decreased LPL enzyme activity that results in reduced clearance of intravenously administered lipids. Also, certain medications used in critically ill patients, such as corticosteroids and immunosuppressants (sirolimus, cyclosporine), alter fat metabolism and increase serum triglyceride levels. Patients who are especially at risk for hypertriglyceridemia include those with sepsis, multiorgan failure, diabetes, liver disease, renal failure, or pancreatitis.

G. Total energy and dextrose overfeeding may result in hypercapnia, especially in patients with borderline respiratory function and limited pulmonary reserve. Excess carbon dioxide is produced relative to oxygen (O_2) consumption during excess carbohydrate administration, resulting in an increased respiratory quotient ($RQ = VCO_2/VO_2$). The RQs for carbohydrate, protein, and fat oxidation are 1, 0.8, and 0.7, respectively. Energy-mixed substrates from fat, protein, and carbohydrates normally yield an RQ of 0.85. The RQ exceeds 1 during carbohydrate overfeeding. As a result, increased carbon dioxide generation causes increased respiratory workload and minute ventilation. Mechanically ventilated patients may have prolonged ventilator dependence. In critically ill patients, overfeeding should be ruled out when the RQ exceeds 1. When total energy intake is appropriate, reducing the carbohydrate load and substituting fat calories lowers the RQ. However, the RQ may be an insensitive indicator of overfeeding in hypermetabolic patients. Only minor changes to the RQ may occur despite major increases in minute ventilation and oxygen consumption.

H. Liver complications associated with PN include steatosis (fatty liver), cholestasis, biliary sludge, and cholelithiasis. In the critically ill intensive care unit patient, these complications are unlikely to occur, due to the short duration of PN, assuming overfeeding is avoided. Although PN-associated steatosis is more common in adults and cholestasis is more common in children, both conditions may coexist in either patient population.

1. Steatosis occurs when fat accumulation exceeds its transport from the liver. In patients receiving PN, high dextrose load is the primary cause of steatosis. However, lipid overfeeding and deficiencies of certain nutrients such choline, carnitine, and essential fatty acids may also lead to steatosis. Patients with hepatic steatosis are usually asymptomatic, and liver enzymes are poorly sensitive to the degree of fatty infiltration. Hepatic steatosis in patients receiving PN is usually reversible. The key to preventing hepatic steato-

sis is to avoid overfeeding and provide balanced PN with no more than 60% of total calories from dextrose, about 20% to 30% of total calories from fat, and the remaining calories from protein.

2. PN-associated cholestasis is more common in long-term PN patients. Factors that predispose such patients to cholestasis include PN dependence, bowel rest, overfeeding, short gut syndrome, sepsis, and premature birth in newborn babies. Elevated serum bilirubin concentrations, especially conjugated bilirubin, are the earliest clinical signs of cholestasis. Patients supported with the extracorporeal membrane oxygenation (ECMO) system may show hyperbilirubinemia because of hemolysis from the mechanical stress on red blood cells as they pass through the ECMO circuit.[41] Jaundice may or may not be present depending on the severity of cholestasis. Measures to prevent PN-associated cholestasis include initiating enteral or oral feeding, weaning off PN, avoiding overfeeding, using balanced sources of calories, and cycling PN.

V. Monitoring

A. Standard laboratory parameters are monitored in critically ill patients receiving EN and PN (see Chapters 5 and 8).

B. Nitrogen balance is a generally accepted method for evaluating the adequacy of protein intake and retention. Its validity can be limited by many factors, such as adequacy of urine collection, unrecorded nitrogen losses from large open wounds, severe burns, diarrhea, or renal failure or liver failure with nitrogen accumulating in the blood. Ideally, nitrogen balance should be measured in a "steady state," but this may be impossible in critically ill patients. Values should be interpreted in the context of the patient's clinical status. Difficulty with urine collection makes determining nitrogen balance very difficult in young pediatric patients.

(Critical care chapters in the 1st edition were contributed by Elaine B. Trujillo, Malcolm K. Robinson, Danny O. Jacobs, Theresa L. Han-Markey, and John R. Wesley)

REFERENCES

1. Martindale RG, Shikora SA, Nishikawa R, et al. The metabolic response to stress and alterations in nutrient metabolism. In: Shikora SA, Martindale RG, Schwaitzberg SD, eds. *Nutritional Consideration in the Intensive Care Unit.* Silver Spring, MD: A.S.P.E.N.; 2002:11–19.
2. Liggett SB, Renfro AD. Energy expenditures of mechanically ventilated nonsurgical patients. *Chest.* 1990;98:682–686.
3. Long CL, Schaffel N, Geiger JW, et al. Metabolic response to injury and illness: estimation of energy and protein needs from indirect calorimetry and nitrogen balance. *J Parenter Enteral Nutr.* 1979;3:452–456.
4. Vanek VW. Assessment and management of fluid and electrolyte abnormalities. In: Shikora SA, Martindale RG, Schwaitzberg SD, eds. *Nutritional Consideration in the Intensive Care Unit.* Silver Spring, MD: A.S.P.E.N.; 2002:79–100.
5. Huddleston KC, Ferraro-McDuffie A, Wolf-Small T. Nutritional support of the critically ill child. *Crit Care Nurs Clin North Am.* 1993;5:65–78.
6. Cameron JW, Rosenthal A, Olson AD. Malnutrition in hospitalized children with congenital heart disease. *Arch Pediatr Adolesc Med.* 1995;149: 1098–1102.
7. Marino PL, Finnegan MJ. Nutrition support is not beneficial and can be harmful in critically ill patients. *Crit Care Clin North Am.* 1996:12:667–676.
8. American Society for Parenteral and Enteral Nutrition Board of Directors and the Clinical Guidelines Task Force. Specific guidelines for disease—adults. Critical care: critical illness. Guidelines for the use of parenteral and enteral nutrition in adult and pediatric patients. *J Parenter Enteral Nutr.* 2002;26:90S–92S.
9. Chwals WJ. Metabolism and nutritional frontiers in pediatric surgical patients. *Surg Clin North Am.* 1992;72:1237–1266.
10. Shanbhogue RLK, Lloyd DA. Absence of hypermetabolism after operation in the newborn infant. *J Parenter Enteral Nutr.* 1992;16:333–336.
11. Scheinkestel CD, Adams F, Mahony L, et al. Impact of increasing parenteral protein loads on amino acid levels and balance in critically ill patients on continuous renal replacement therapy. *Nutrition.* 2003;19:733–740.
12. Marik PE, Zaloga GP. Early enteral nutrition in acutely ill patients: a systematic review. *Crit Care Med.* 2001;29:2264–2270.
13. Kudsk KA, Croce MA, Fabian TC, et al. Enteral vs parenteral feeding. Effects on septic morbidity after blunt and penetrating abdominal trauma. *Ann Surg.* 1992;215:503–511.
14. Cerra FB, McPherson JP, Konstantinides FN, et al. Enteral nutrition does not prevent multiple organ failure syndrome (MOFS) after sepsis. *Surgery.* 1988;104:727–733.
15. Heyland DK, Novak F, Drover JW, et al. Should immunonutrition become routine in critically ill patients? A systematic review of the evidence. *JAMA.* 2001;286:944–953.
16. Kudsk KA, Moore FA. Proceedings from summit on immune-enhancing enteral therapy. *J Parenter Enteral Nutr.* 2001;25(2 suppl):1S–63S.
17. Stechmiller JK, Childress B, Porter T. Arginine immunonutrition in critically ill patients: a clinical dilemma. *Am J Crit Care.* 2004;13:17–23.
18. Burke JF, Wolfe RR, Mullany CJ, et al. Glucose requirements following burn injury. *Ann Surg.* 1979;190:274–285.
19. Rosmarin DK, Wardlaw GM, Mirtallo J. Hyperglycemia associated with high, continuous infusion rates of total parenteral nutrition dextrose. *Nutr Clin Pract.* 1996;11:151–156.
20. Iriyama K, Miki C, Inoue T, et al. Constant infusion rates of lipid emulsions to stabilize plasma triglyceride concentrations: medium-chain triglyceride/long-chain triglyceride emulsions (MCT/LCT) versus LCT. *Surg Today.* 1998;28:289–292.
21. Waitzberg DL, Lotierzo PH, Logullo AF, et al. Parenteral lipid emulsions and phagocytic systems. *Br J Nutr.* 2002;87(suppl 1):S49–57.
22. Kalfarentzos F, Kokkinis K, Leukaditi K, Maroulis J, Onoufriou A, Alexopoulos K. Comparison between two fat emulsions: intralipid 30 percent vs intralipid 10 percent in critically ill patients. *Clin Nutr.* 1998;17:31–34.
23. Nordenstrom J, Thorne A. Comparative studies on a new concentrated fat emulsion: intralipid 30% vs. 20%. *Clin Nutr.* 1993;12:160–167.
24. Garcia-de-Lorenzo A, Lopez-Martinez J, Planas M, et al. Safety and metabolic tolerance of a concentrated long-chain triglyceride lipid emulsion in critically ill septic and trauma patients. *J Parenter Enteral Nutr.* 2003;27: 208–215.
25. Jeevanandam M, Holaday NJ, Voss T, et al. Efficacy of a mixture of medium-chain triglyceride (75%) and long-chain triglyceride (25%) fat emulsions in the nutritional management of multiple-trauma patients. *Nutrition.* 1995;11:275–284.
26. Ulrich H, Pastores SM, Katz DP, et al. Parenteral use of medium-chain triglycerides: a reappraisal. *Nutrition.* 1996;12:231–238.
27. Smirniotis V, Kostopanagiotou G, Vassiliou J, et al. Long chain versus medium chain lipids in patients with ARDS: effects on pulmonary haemodynamics and gas exchange. *Intensive Care Med.* 1998;24:1029–1033.
28. Masclans JR, Iglesia R, Bermejo B, et al. Gas exchange and pulmonary haemodynamic responses to fat emulsions in acute respiratory distress syndrome. *Intensive Care Med.* 1998;24:918–923.
29. Lekka ME, Liokatis S, Nathanail C, et al. The impact of intravenous fat emulsion administration in acute lung injury. *Am J Respir Crit Care Med.* 2004;169:638–644.
30. Periera GR, Fox WW, Stanley CA, et al. Decreased oxygenation and hyperlipemia during intravenous fat infusions in premature infants. *Pediatrics.* 1980;66:26–30.
31. Prasertsom W, Phillipos EZ, Van Aerde JE, et al. Pulmonary vascular resistance during lipid infusion in neonates. *Arch Dis Child.* 1996;74:F95–98.
32. Mason JB. Vitamins and trace elements in the critically ill patient. In: Shikora SA, Martindale RG, Schwaitzberg SD, eds. *Nutritional Consideration in the Intensive Care Unit.* Silver Spring, MD: A.S.P.E.N.; 2002:61–77.
33. Berger MM, Chiolero RL. Key vitamins and trace elements in the critically ill. In: Cynober L, Moore FA, eds. *Nutrition and Critical Care, Nestlé*

Nutrition Workshop Series, Clinical and Performance Program. Vol. 8. Vevey and Basel, Switzerland: Nestlé and S. Karger AG; 2003.

34. Heyland DK, MacDonald S, Keefe L, et al. Total parenteral nutrition in the critically ill patient. A meta-analysis. *JAMA.* 1998;280:2013–2019.
35. The Veterans Affairs Total Parenteral Nutrition Cooperative Study Group. Perioperative total parenteral nutrition in surgical patients. *N Engl J Med.* 1991;325:525–532.
36. Lin MT, Saito H, Fukushima R, et al. Preoperative total parenteral nutrition influences postoperative systemic cytokine responses after colorectal surgery. *Nutrition.* 1997;13:8–12.
37. Gianotti L, Braga M, Vignali A, et al. Effect of route of delivery and formulation of postoperative nutritional support in patients undergoing major operations for malignant neoplasms. *Arch Surg.* 1997;132:1222–1229.
38. Marik PE, Zaloga GP. Meta-analysis of parenteral nutrition versus enteral nutrition in patients with acute pancreatitis. *BMJ.* 2004;328:1407. Epu June 2, 2004.
39. Van Den Berghe G, Wouters PJ, Weekers F, et al. Intensive insulin therapy in critically ill patients. *N Engl J Med.* 2001;345:1359–1367.
40. Van Den Berghe G, Wouters PJ, Bouillon R, et al. Outcome benefit of intensive insulin therapy in the critically ill: insulin dose versus glycemic control. *Crit Care Med.* 2003;31:359–366.
41. Brown RL, Wessel J, Warner BW. Nutrition considerations in the neonatal extracorporeal life support patient. *Nutr Clin Pract.* 1994;9:22–27.

SUGGESTED READINGS

Btaiche IF, Khalidi N. Parenteral nutrition-associated liver complications in children. *Pharmacotherapy.* 2002;22:188–211.

Konstantinides FN, Konstantinides NN, Li JC, et al. Urinary urea nitrogen: too insensitive for calculating nitrogen balance studies in surgical clinical nutrition. *J Parenter Enteral Nutr.* 1991;15:189–193.

Spear ML, Stahl GE, Hamosh M, et al. Effect of heparin dose and infusion rate of lipid clearance and bilirubin binding in premature infants receiving intravenous fat emulsions. *J Pediatr.* 1988;112:94–98.

Thomson MA, Bucolo S, Quirk P, et al. Measured versus predicted resting energy expenditure in infants: a need for reappraisal. *J Pediatr.* 1995;126: 21–27.

Rosemary A. Kozar, MD, PhD;
Margaret M. McQuiggan, MS, RD, LD, CNSD;
Frederick A. Moore, MD

21

Trauma

Introduction

Nutrition support is an integral part of therapy for patients who have undergone major trauma. To determine the feasibility and need for nutrition support in trauma patients, it is necessary to understand the body's response to stress and injury. This chapter reviews the nutritional metabolic alterations associated with trauma and provides guidelines for the assessment and management of nutrition for these patients.

I. Background-Trauma

A. Trauma statistics
  1. Trauma is the leading cause of death in Americans between the ages of 1–38 years.[1]
  2. Ten percent of hospital admissions are related to trauma and range from minor abrasions and contusions to those severe cases involving multiple organs and requiring prolonged ICU stays.[2]
  3. Blunt trauma admissions are decreasing while penetrating trauma admissions are increasing, particularly in urban areas.[3]

B. Types of traumatic injuries
  1. Traumatic injuries are characterized as blunt versus penetrating, with electrical and thermal classified separately.
  2. Fifty to sixty percent of blunt trauma requiring hospital admission results from motor vehicle accidents with another 10–20 percent from falls.[3]
  3. The severity of penetrating trauma is dependent on the mechanism of injury and the organ systems involved. These types of injuries include stab and gun shot wounds.

C. Trauma presentation and outcome is also dependent on the patient's age, gender, anatomy, and pre-existing disease.[4]

(This material was borrowed from Cresci, GA and Martindale RG, Nutrition Support in Trauma. In: Gottschlich MM. *The Science and Practice of Nutrition Support: A Case-Based Core Curriculum.* Kendall/Hunt Publishing 2001 with permission from the American Society for Parenteral and Enteral Nutrition)

II. Metabolic Response to Stress

A. A variety of conditions in the trauma patient can lead to a metabolic response referred to as the "injury stress response." The systemic inflammatory response syndrome (SIRS) and its associated mediators (eg, TNFα, IL-1, IL-2, IL-6) play an important role in this response. Favorable modulation of the injury stress response is not currently feasible because the driving mechanisms are not understood. Our best options are to control the initiating insult and to provide high risk patients exogenous substrates that support the metabolic environment.

B. The injury stress response increases resting energy expenditure (REE). The increase in REE depends on both the type and severity of the insult. For example, REE can increase as much as 100% after burns, 50% with sepsis, 40% after trauma, and 30% after major surgery. To meet this increased metabolic demand, endogenous substrates are mobilized.
  1. Glucose stores (approximately 2000–3000 kcal glycogen) are quickly depleted and gluconeogenesis (principally in liver, but also in kidney) produces glucose that is shunted to glucose-dependent tissues such as brain, erythrocytes, inflammatory cells, and injured tissue.
  2. Adipose tissue is stimulated to release free fatty acids (FFA) and glycerol. The rate of lipolysis, however, exceeds lipid oxidation. As a result, plasma triglyceride levels increase and considerable re-esterification occurs in the liver. This requires energy and creates futile cycles.
  3. The increase in protein catabolism is the most dramatic effect. Skeletal muscle protein, and later constitutive proteins such as albumin, prealbumin, and transferrin are broken down. The released amino acids become substrates for acute-phase protein synthesis (clotting factors, gamma globulins, and C-reactive protein), gluconeogenesis, and energy production.
     a) Glutamine and alanine account for 70% of the amino acids released from peripheral tissues. Glutamine is the preferred oxidative fuel of enterocytes and is an important energy source for the immune system and for cells involved in tissue repair. It also may be important for hepatic synthesis of the critical intracellular antioxidant, glutathione.
     b) Alanine is the major amino acid used in hepatic gluconeogenesis.
     c) Other amino acids such as the branched-chain amino acids leucine, isoleucine, and valine become important oxidative fuels. The overall consequence of these processes is net total body protein catabolism and rapid reduction in lean body mass primarily by effects on skeletal muscle.

C. Traumatic stress also results in alterations in trace elements and minerals.
  1. Iron metabolism is altered under conditions of trauma, leading to decreased concentrations in the blood. However, it may not be advisable to administer iron under such circumstances because it is essential for the growth of many bacteria and iron supplementation in the critically ill has been reported to increase risk of systemic infection.[5,6]
  2. Plasma zinc concentrations may be decreased because zinc is sequestered in the liver during stress and is consumed in several essential metabolic pathways that are accelerated in the critically ill.

3. There are now a number of clinical trials supporting the use of antioxidants in the critically ill.[7–9] A recent study by Nathens et al demonstrated a decreased incidence of pulmonary morbidity and multiple organ failure as well as a shorter duration of mechanical ventilation and ICU stay when Vitamin E and C were administered to critically ill surgical patients at risk for organ dysfunction.[7]

D. Nutritional support needs to be tailored to the metabolic environment. The stressed trauma patient requires approximately 25–30 kcal/kg/d and 1.5–1.75 gm/kg/d of protein. As metabolic stress increases, patients become more catabolic and less tolerant to glucose.

III. Rationale for Nutrition Support

A. Prevention of acute protein malnutrition
  1. Persistent hypercatabolism results in acute protein malnutrition and is associated with cardiac, pulmonary, hepatic, gastrointestinal, and immunologic dysfunction. Delayed infections then extend hypercatabolism with the progression to full-blown multiple organ failure.
  2. A number of clinical studies have clearly demonstrated that early enteral nutrition improves outcome, as measured by improved nitrogen balance and constitutive protein levels, improved immune function, decreased infections, and decreased length of stay.[10–13]

B. Modulation of immune response
  1. Despite tremendous advances in ICU care, nosocomial infections remain a common problem. In large part, these late infections occur due to failure of local and systemic host defenses. While exact causes of late immunosuppression are not clear, it is now believed nosocomial infections occur partly as a result of dysfunctional regulation of inflammation.[14]
  2. An initial insult, whether secondary to sepsis, trauma/burns, or major operation, can precipitate early systemic hyperinflammation (ie, systemic inflammatory response syndrome, SIRS), which when intense can precipitate early multiple organ failure (MOF).
  3. Certain components of the early SIRS response are endogenously down-regulated to prevent unnecessary, potentially autodestructive inflammation. This is referred to as the compensatory anti-inflammatory response syndrome (CARS). The resulting delayed immunosuppression, however, sets the stage for secondary infection, which can either worsen early MOF or trigger late MOF.
  4. While no strategy can prevent or eliminate the dysfunctional inflammatory response, the delivery of specific immune-enhancing nutrients (generally via the gut) may prove beneficial.

C. Promotion of gut function
  1. The dysfunctional gut is believed to be a reservoir for pathogens that can then cause late MOF-associated infections.
  2. The initial insult (which could be ischemia/reperfusion, shock, or sepsis) and emergency laparotomy (via anesthesia and bowel manipulation) can cause early ileus.
  3. Disuse of the gastrointestinal tract, through the use of parenteral rather than enteral nutrition, or through commonly employed intensive care unit therapies (eg, H_2-antagonists, narcotics, or broad-spectrum antibiotics) can promote further gut dysfunction.
  4. Gut dysfunction is characterized by progressive ileus, colonization of the upper gut, increased permeability, and decreased gut-associated lymphoid tissue function. Consequently, the upper gut becomes a reservoir for pathogens. In addition, local and systemic defense mechanisms that prevent the spread of these organisms become impaired.
  5. The primary route of dissemination of pathogens that colonize the gastrointestinal tract (ie, aspiration versus translocation) is not clear. Although there is good epidemiologic evidence for this sequence of events, prospective randomized controlled trials of gut-specific therapies, such as early enteral nutrition and, more recently, immune-enhancing enteral formulas, have demonstrated a reduction in nosocomial infections.[10,15] These studies provide the most convincing evidence of the importance of the gastrointestinal tract as a source. Thus, the provision of early enteral nutrition to promote gut function is believed to prevent this cascade of events.

IV. Initiation of Nutritional Support

A. Nutritional assessment—A nutritional assessment should be performed as soon after injury as possible.
  1. Physical assessment of the patient includes evaluation of body composition, edema, wound healing, and nutrient composition of fluid losses through wounds or drains, as well as review of the laboratory and medication profile. A height and pre-admission weight are obtained and information on chronic disease, activity level, medications, previous dietary restrictions, psychosocial data, and drug and tobacco patterns is noted.
  2. A history of 10% weight loss over three months is considered significant. However, weight loss combined with physiologic impairment may be even more important, as this can be associated with increased septic complications, pneumonia, and a prolonged hospital stay.[16]
  3. Functional impairment may be assessed by crude measures such as physical assessment of triceps skinfold, decreased prehospital activity, perception of fatigue, strength of cough, and skin integrity.
  4. Body protein stores, as assessed by muscle mass and serum proteins, should be evaluated, as they correlate more closely with survival. Body composition can be assessed by a variety of techniques including caliper measurements, bioelectrical impedance analysis, and dual-energy X-ray absorptiometry for bone mineral density.
  5. Age-related loss of skeletal muscle should also be taken into consideration. The malnourished, elderly patient undergoing a catabolic illness will reach a critical cardiac or respiratory threshold much earlier than a young, previously healthy individual.

B. Estimating energy requirements
  1. The Harris Benedict Equation is a common method to estimate energy expenditure and thus determine caloric requirements. It estimates basal energy expenditure (BEE) based on age, sex, height, and weight. The BEE represents energy requirements in the fasted, resting, non-stressed state, so that in the presence of metabolic stress such as trauma, the BEE must be multiplied by an empirically derived stress factor to obtain an estimate of the caloric requirement. Typical stress multiplication factors for trauma patients range from 1.2 to 1.6.
  2. Estimates of caloric support can also be made. In general, most trauma patients should receive approximately 25–30 kcal/kg/d and 1.5–1.75 gm/kg/d of protein. Needs may decrease as patients move farther from the initial injury.

C. Monitoring response to therapy
  1. Assessment of body protein stores
    a) Serum protein status is conducted upon admission and periodically through the hospital stay. Acute phase proteins, such as C-reactive protein, rise markedly within 72–96 hours after injury, while the constitutive proteins, albumin, prealbu-

min, and transferrin, all decline. Measuring both categories of proteins concurrently helps to determine the degree of physiologic stress and the return of anabolism.

b) Once C-reactive protein falls below 10–15 mg/dl, a prompt increase in prealbumin should occur (0.5–1.0 mg/dl daily). If an appropriate increase does not occur, then the adequacy of the support should be re-assessed.

2. Nitrogen balance

a) Nitrogen balance is the difference between nitrogen intake and nitrogen output. Nitrogen intake is determined from daily dietary intake while nitrogen output is determined by measuring urinary urea nitrogen (UUN) in a 24-hour urine collection and adding 4 gm to approximate non-urea nitrogen loss in the urine and other N_2 losses.

b) The formula to calculate nitrogen balance is as follows: Nitrogen balance = (gm protein intake/6.25) – (gm nitrogen in UUN + 4)

c) UUN reflects the protein catabolic rate (degree of stress) and represents the majority of nitrogen excreted in the urine. It is therefore a rough approximation of total urinary nitrogen. As the stress level increases, the concomitant increase in protein catabolism results in an increase in urinary nitrogen. UUN may not be valid in certain patient populations, such as patients with compromised renal function (creatinine clearance < 50 mL/min) or in patients with spinal cord injury.

d) Ideally, patients should be in positive nitrogen balance (3–5 g/day).

3. Metabolic gas analysis- Also known as indirect calorimetry, metabolic gas analysis is a tool that can measure resting energy expenditure (REE). See chapter on Indirect Calorimetry for further information on this technique.

V. Enteral Nutrition

A. Benefits of early enteral nutrition

In the 1980s, three prospective randomized controlled trials demonstrated that trauma patients receiving early enteral nutrition had significantly fewer infectious complications than patients receiving parenteral nutrition, though a decrease in mortality was not demonstrated.[10–12] A meta-analysis that included eight randomized controlled trials (six published, two unpublished) verified these findings. As in the single institutional trials, this analysis concluded that fewer infectious complications developed in patients receiving enteral nutrition.[13] Even when patients with catheter-related sepsis were removed from the analysis, a significant difference in infections between groups remained. These studies provide convincing evidence that enteral nutrition is preferred to parenteral nutrition in patients sustaining major torso trauma. Data are less clear for patients with traumatic brain injury. The most recent Cochrane Review reported a trend towards better outcome (survival and disability) with the administration of early feeding.[17]

B. Role of immune enhancing agents in the trauma patient

More recent trials indicate that additional benefits can be achieved by the use of immune-enhancing agents compared to standard enteral diets. Immune-enhancing diets (IEDs) include a variety of potential immune-enhancing agents, including arginine, glutamine, omega-3-fatty acids, and nucleotides. However, the contributions of individual nutrients have not been well investigated. As a single supplement, only glutamine (added to standard enteral diets) has been shown to decrease infectious morbidity in trauma and burn patients in prospective randomized controlled trials (PRCTs).[18–20]

1. There are currently a number of commercially available formulas that contain two or more of these agents. Two formulas, Immun-Aid (McGaw, Inc., Irvine, CA) and Impact (Novartis Corp., Minneapolis, MN) have been shown in clinical studies to improve patient outcome, principally by reducing infections and improving wound healing. Other formulas have not been prospectively studied and are dissimilar enough from the tested formulas that no conclusions can be made about their use in trauma patients.

2. Five PRCTs have tested the efficacy and safety of IEDs specifically in trauma patients. The majority demonstrate improved patient outcome with the use of IEDs.[21–25] The first three studies by Brown[21], Moore[22], and Kudsk[23], all showed a reduction in infectious complications, particularly intra-abdominal abscesses. The fourth study by Mendez et al failed to demonstrate any outcome improvement and suggested that the IED may exacerbate organ failure.[24] This study had several methodologic flaws, most notably that patients receiving the immune-enhancing diets had a higher incidence of acute respiratory distress syndrome (ARDS) prior to beginning the diet (IED=31% versus SED=14%). The last study by Weimann et al demonstrated a decrease in the number of days of systemic inflammatory response syndrome and a decrease in multiple organ failure.[25] Analysis of these individual studies offers convincing evidence that IEDs provide additional benefits compared to standard enteral diets in patients sustaining major torso trauma. As with studies supporting the use of early enteral nutrition, a decrease in mortality has not been demonstrated.

(This material was borrowed from Kozar RA, McQuiggan MM, and Moore FA. Trauma, In: Cresci G , *Nutrition Support in the Critically Ill Patient.* Taylor & Francis, 2005 with permission)

C. Specialized enteral formulas in patients with ARDS

One PRCT demonstrated improved outcome in patients with ARDS who were provided an enteral diet supplemented with high omega-3 fatty acids, γ-linolenic acid, and antioxidants versus a high omega-6 formula. The control diet, a marketed high fat formula, could have worsened ARDS by increasing inflammation and the production of lipid mediators.[26]

D. Indications and contraindications of enteral nutrition

1. Patients who cannot adequately meet their nutritional goals by oral intake alone for a period of approximately seven days should be considered for enteral supplementation. Additionally, early enteral nutrition should be considered for all acutely ill patients, such as patients with major torso trauma, chronically malnourished patients, and patients with limited physiologic reserve. Early enteral nutrition is generally defined as support instituted within 48 to 72 hours of injury.

2. Contraindications to enteral nutrition can be divided into absolute and relative. Absolute contraindications include functional complications such as bowel obstruction, peritonitis, progressive ileus, massive gastrointestinal hemorrhage, and gastrointestinal ischemia associated with shock and vasopressors. Relative contraindications include intolerance to enteral nutrition. A recent bowel anastomosis is not a contraindication. Healing, in fact, may be hastened by early feeding.[27]

E. Obtaining enteral access

1. Access can be divided into gastric (and duodenal) and jejunal with push, endoscopic, radiologic, and available surgical options. Plans to obtain access should be formulated upon admission to the hospital.

2. For patients to be fed into the stomach, a soft, nonsump nasogastric tube or dobhoff can be placed. For patients anticipated to require long-term feeding access, a percutaneous endoscopic gastrostomy (PEG) is an option. Prior to instituting gastric feeds, patients should be assessed for aspiration risk including factors such as endotracheal intubation, decreased level of consciousness,

underlying neuromuscular disease, history of aspiration, recent stroke, and recent major upper abdominal surgery. If two or more risk factors are present, strong consideration for jejunal feeding should be given. Additionally, patients should be assessed for delayed gastric emptying, which may be seen with diabetes, sepsis, hyperglycemia, and traumatic brain injury. Because of a high incidence of gastroparesis in brain-injured patients, gastric feeding can be difficult.[28] Newer promotility agents may be helpful in this patient population.[29]

3. For those patients identified as candidates for jejunal feeds, access can be obtained at the time of initial laparotomy, or at subsequent laparotomy if damage control is initially performed, either as a needle catheter jejunostomy or a standard Witzel jejunostomy. Patients not undergoing laparotomy may have a "push" nasojejunal tube placed by a bedside nurse trained in this technique. If this is unsuccessful, an endoscopically-placed nasojejunal tube can be inserted. Nasojejunal feeding may be done indefinitely, but if the need for long-term access becomes apparent, a PEG with a jejunal extension limb (PEG-J) is appropriate.

F. Formula selection

1. Enteral formulas can be categorized into polymeric formulas (which contain nutrients in high molecular weight form and moderate fat loads, and require normal digestive and absorptive ability), elemental formulas (which contain one or more partially digested macronutrients or combinations of nutrients and can be absorbed in patients with compromised gastrointestinal tracts), and modular formulas (which are composed of individual nutrients but are nutritionally incomplete and intended for use as supplements or in combination with other products). Unfortunately, with the exception of the immune-enhancing formulas, very little comparative data exists to guide clinicians in selecting the most appropriate formula.
2. In general, high risk trauma patients (injury severity score ≥ 18 or abdominal trauma index ≥ 20) should be considered for an immune-enhancing diet.[30] The majority of critically ill trauma patients should receive a polymeric formula. An elemental diet should be considered for patients with proven intolerance to polymeric formulas and those high-risk patients who have received no oral or enteral nutrition for over seven days.

G. Administration of feeds—Enteral feeds should be started at 15 mL/hr of full-strength formula and advanced by 15mL/hr every 12 hours to a set goal of 60mL/hr. To assure tolerance, this rate should be maintained for 24 hours and then advanced by 15mL/hr every 12 hours to a patient-specific targeted goal.[31]

H. Identification and management of intolerance—Frequently identified indicators of intolerance include vomiting, abdominal distention or cramping/tenderness, diarrhea, and high nasogastric tube output.[32] Symptoms can be graded as mild, moderate, or severe. Mild symptoms of intolerance, such as mild abdominal distention or diarrhea, can be monitored by repeat physical exams with no change in the current rate of feeding. Moderate symptoms are managed based on the particular symptom. For distention, enteral feeds should be stopped and the patient assessed for evidence of a mechanical obstruction. If distention remains moderate, an elemental formula should be considered. Moderate diarrhea can be managed by maintaining but not increasing the current feeding rate, and repeat exams. Finally, for severe distention, enteral feeds should be stopped, intravenous hydration begun, and the possibility of nonocclusive bowel necrosis should considered. For severe diarrhea, tube feeds can be reduced and the patient should be evaluated for possible *Clostridium difficile* infection. Vomiting is managed by ensuring adequate gastric decompression and either stopping gastric feeds or decreasing the tube feed infusion rate by half for jejunal feeds. Additionally, high nasogastric output in patients fed into the small bowel can be managed by verifying postpyloric placement of the feeding tube and checking the nasogastric aspirate for glucose. Any amount of glucose is considered abnormal and enteral feeds should be withheld. Finally, enteral feeds should be discontinued if vasopressors are instituted.

I. Complications of enteral nutrition

1. Technical complications that can occur with the administration of enteral nutrition include aspiration, bowel perforation, clogged tubes, and tube malposition/dislodgement.
2. Functional complications are gastrointestinal manifestations frequently associated with intolerance and include emesis, nausea/vomiting, cramping pain or distention, and diarrhea.
3. Jejunostomy-related complications—Complication rates in trauma patients have been reported at four percent.[33] However, the majority of these complications occurred in patients with a standard, open jejunostomy rather than with a needle catheter jejunostomy. Complications included volvulus with infarction, small bowel perforation, intraperitoneal leaks, and nonocclusive small bowel necrosis.
4. Nonocclusive bowel necrosis
   a) This is a rare but devastating complication of bowel necrosis with no associated large vessel occlusion. This is similar to necrotizing enterocolitis observed in neonates. The consistent association with enteral nutrition suggests that inappropriate administration of nutrients into a dysfunctional gut plays a pathogenic role. The incidence is less than one percent but the mortality frequently exceeds 50%.[34,35]
   b) Most cases of nonocclusive bowel necrosis occur in a delayed fashion in critically injured patients with a complicated course (pneumonia, sepsis, renal failure) that requires progressively higher acuity care.
   c) Gastrointestinal signs and symptoms are nonspecific and are typically those of intolerance. Therefore, standard clinical monitoring fails to detect this entity early in its course. Though most cases will require exploratory laparotomy, less advanced presentations may be managed with cessation of feeds, broad spectrum antibiotics, and aggressive fluid resuscitation.

VI. Parenteral Nutrition

A. Indications

Whenever possible, the gastrointestinal track should be utilized for nutritional support. However, the following conditions may represent indications for parenteral nutrition: persistent or progressive ileus, bowel obstruction, massive bowel resection refractory to an enteral diet, high output fistula refractory to elemental diet, malabsorption, high risk for nonocclusive bowel necrosis if fed enterally (shock resuscitation, α-agonists, persistent severe distention or cramping), or documented intolerance to enteral nutrition. In general, parenteral nutrition should not be started in critically injured patients for at least six days post injury if the patient is well nourished at baseline. Unlike with enteral feeding, there is NO benefit to early parenteral nutrition. The only exception may be patients severely malnourished at baseline.

B. Administration

Calories are provided by a mixture of dextrose, amino acids, and fat. Although only 2–4% of total calories as linoleic and linolenic acids are required to prevent clinical essential fatty acid deficiency, most trauma patients require the use of additional fat as an alternative calorie source. The acute stress response that follows trauma is associated with glucose intolerance, which can be minimized by decreasing glucose calories and increasing fat calories, as well as by aggressive use of insulin.

C. Complications of parenteral nutrition can be divided into technical, infectious, and metabolic.
   1. Technical complications associated with the placement of a central line, required for the administration of parenteral nutrition, include injury to major veins, arteries, or nerves, and violation of the pleural space.
   2. Infectious complications include both catheter-related and -unrelated infections.
      a) Catheter-related infections most commonly stem from colonization of the patient's skin and the catheter hub. Less frequent sources of contamination include infusion of contaminated solutions or hematogenous seeding from a distal site of infection.
      b) Recent evidence suggests that glutamine-supplemented parenteral nutrition may decrease infectious complications and mortality rates in critically ill patients, with the greatest benefit with high-dose parenteral glutamine (> 0.2 g/kg/d).[36]
      c) Metabolic complications can include hyper or hypoglycemia, electrolyte abnormalities, acid/base abnormalities, liver function abnormalities, and trace mineral deficiencies.
         (1) Critical illness is frequently accompanied by hyperglycemia with resistance to insulin. Hyperglycemia can adversely affect outcome through several mechanisms, including glycosuria with inappropriate diuresis, increased risk of infection by impairment of neutrophil and immunoglobulin function, and exacerbation of cerebral edema. A recent prospective randomized clinical trial demonstrated a reduction both in infectious complications and mortality in critically ill surgical patients when glucose levels were strictly controlled between 80 and 110 mg/dL versus conventional therapy (120 to 180 mg/dL).[37,38]
         (2) The refeeding syndrome is a dramatic example of a metabolic complication that can be associated with parenteral nutrition administration. It occurs with rapid and excessive feeding of patients with severe malnutrition due to conditions commonly seen in trauma patients such as starvation, alcoholism, delayed nutritional support, or chronic malnutrition. As a result of ion fluxes into the cell, serum phosphate, magnesium, potassium, and calcium levels can drop rapidly. Additionally, severe hyperglycemia is commonly seen. Symptoms include cardiac arrhythmias, confusion, respiratory failure, and even death. The refeeding syndrome can be prevented by initiating parenteral nutrition at a rate lower than the required goal, primarily by reducing dextrose calories and adding supplemental phosphate, magnesium, potassium, and calcium in the parenteral nutrition. Exogenous insulin is also frequently required.

(Trauma material from the 1st edition was contributed by Elaine B. Trujillo, Malcolm K. Robinson, and Danny O. Jacobs)

REFERENCES

1. Cerra F. Metabolic and nutritional support. In: Feliciano D, Moore E, Mattox K (eds). *Trauma.* 3rd ed. Stamford, CT: Appleton & Lange; 1996.
2. Committee on Trauma Research. *Injury in America: A Continuing Public Health Problem.* Washington, DC: National Academy Press; 1985.
3. Shatz D, Kirton O, McKenney M, et al. *Manual of Trauma and Emergency Surgery.* Philadelphia, PA: WB Saunders; 1991.
4. Cresci GA, Martindale RG. Nutrition support in trauma. In: Gottschlich MM (ed). *The Science and Practice of Nutrition Support: A Case-Based Core Curriculum.* Dubuque, IO: A.S.P.E.N./Kendall-Hunt; 2001.
5. Bullen J, Griffiths E, Rogers H, Ward G. Sepsis: the critical role of iron. *Microbes Infect* 2000;4:409–415.
6. Robien M. Iron and microbial infection. *Support Line* 2000;22(4):23–27.
7. Nathens A, Neff M, Jurkovich G, et al. Randomized, prospective trial of antioxidant supplementation in critically ill surgical patients. *Ann Surg* 2002;236(6):814–822.
8. Bulger EM, Maier RV. An argument for Vitamin E supplementation in the management of systemic inflammatory response syndrome. *Shock* 2003; 19(2):99–103.
9. Tanaka H, Matsuda T, Miyagantani Y, Yukioka T, Matsuda H, Shimazaki S. Reduction of resuscitation fluid volumes in severely burned patients using ascorbic acid administration: a randomized, prospective study. *Arch Surg* 2000;135(3):326–331.
10. Moore EE, Jones TN. Benefits of immediate jejunal feeding after major abdominal trauma—a prospective randomized study. *J Trauma* 1986;26: 874–881.
11. Moore FA, Moore EE, Jones TN. TEN versus TPN following major abdominal trauma-reduced septic morbidity. *J Trauma* 1989;29:916–922.
12. Kudsk KA, Croce MA, Fabian TC, et al. Enteral versus parenteral feeding: effects on septic morbidity following blunt and penetrating abdominal trauma. *Ann Surg* 1992;215:503–511.
13. Moore FA, Feliciano DV, Andrassy RJ, et al. Early enteral feeding, compared with parenteral, reduces postoperative septic complications—the results of a meta-analysis. *Ann Surg* 1992;216:172–183.
14. Moore FA, Sauaia A, Moore EE, Haenel JB, Burch JM, Lezotte DC. Postinjury multiple organ failure: a bimodal phenomenon. *J Trauma.* 1996;40: 501–512.
15. Moore FA. Effects of immune-enhancing diets on infectious morbidity and multiple organ failure. *J Parenter Enteral Nutr.* 2001;25:S36–S42.
16. Windsor JA, Hill GL. Weight loss with physiologic impairment: a basic indicator of surgical risk *Ann Surg.* 1988;207(3):290–296.
17. Yanagawa T, Bunn F, Roberts I, Wentz R, Pierro A. Nutritional support for head-injured patients. *Cochrane Database Syst Rev.* 2002;(3):CD001530.
18. Houdijk APJ, Rijnsburger ER, Jansen J, et al. Randomized trial of glutamine-enriched enteral nutrition on infectious morbidity in patients with multiple trauma. *Lancet* 1998;352:772–776.
19. Wischmeyer PE, Lynch J, Liedel J, et al. Glutamine administration reduces Gram-negative bacteremia in severely burned patients: a prospective, randomized, double-blind trial versus isonitrogenous control. *Crit Care Med.* 2001;29:2075–2080.
20. Garrel D, Patenaude J, Nedelec B, et al. Decreased mortality and infectious morbidity in adult burn patients given enteral glutamine supplements: a prospective, controlled, randomized clinical trial. *Crit Care Med.* 2003;31: 2444–2449.
21. Brown RO, Hunt H, Mowatt-Larssen CA, Wojtysiak SL, Henningfield MF, Kudsk KA. Comparison of specialized and standard enteral formulas in trauma patients. *Pharmacotherapy.* 1994;14:314–320.
22. Moore FA, Moore EE, Kudsk KA, et al. Clinical benefits of an immune-enhancing diet for early postinjury enteral feeding. *J Trauma.* 1994;37: 607–615.
23. Kudsk KA, Minard G, Croce MA, et al. A randomized trial of isonitrogenous diets following severe trauma: an immune-enhancing diet reduces septic complications. *Ann Surg.*1996;224:531–540.
24. Mendez C, Jurkovich GJ, Garcia I, Davis D, Parker A, Maier RV. Effects of an immune-enhancing diet in critically injured patients. *J Trauma.* 1997;42:933–944.
25. Weimann A, Bastian L, Bischoff WE, et al. Influence of arginine, omega-3-fatty acids and nucleotide-supplemented enteral support on systemic inflammatory response syndrome and multiple organ failure in patients after severe trauma. *Nutrition.* 1998;14:165–172.
26. Gadek JE, DeMichele SJ, Karlstad MD, et al. Effect of enteral feeding with eicopentaenoic acid, gamma-linolenic acid, and antioxidants in patients

with acute respiratory distress syndrome. *Crit Care Med.* 1999;27: 1409–1420.

27. Kiyama T, Witte MB, Thorton FJ, Barbul A. The route of nutrition support affects the early phase of wound healing. *J Parenter Enteral Nutr.* 1998:22(5):276–279.
28. Ott L, Young B, Phillips R, et al. Altered gastric emptying in the head-injured patient: relationship to feeding intolerance. *J Neurosurg.* 1991; 74:738.
29. Bovin MA, Levy H. Gastric feeding with erythromycin is equivalent to transpyloric feeding in the critically ill. *Crit Care Med* 2001;29(10):1916.
30. Consensus recommendations from the US summit on immune-enhancing enteral therapy. *J Parenter Enteral Nutr.* 2001;25(2 Suppl):S61–63.
31. McQuiggan MM, Marvin RG, McKinley BA, Moore FA. Enteral feeding following major torso trauma: from theory to practice. *New Horizons.* 1999;7:131–140.
32. Kozar RA, McQuiggan MM, Moore EE, Kudsk KA, Jurkovich GJ, Moore FA. Postinjury enteral tolerance is reliably achieved by a standardized protocol. *J Surg Res* 2002;104:70–75.
33. Holmes JH, Brundage SI, Hall RA, Yuen P, Maier RV, Jurkovich GJ. Complications of surgical jejunosotomy in trauma patients. *J Trauma.* 1999;47: 1009–1012.
34. Munshi I, Steingrub JS, Wolpert L. Small bowel necrosis associated with early post operative tube feeding in a trauma patient. *J Trauma.* 2000;49(1): 163–165.
35. Marvin RG, McKinley BA, McQuiggan M, Cocanour CS, Moore FA. Nonocclusive bowel necrosis occurring in critically ill trauma patients receiving enteral nutrition manifests no reliable signs for early detection. *Am J Surg.* 2000;179:7–12.
36. Novak F, Heyland DK, Avenell A, Drover JW, Su X. Glutamine supplementation in serious illness: a systematic review of the evidence. *Crit Care Med.* 2002;30:2022–2029.
37. Van den Berghe G, Wouters P, Weekers F, et al. Intensive insulin therapy in critically ill patients. *N Engl J Med.* 2001;345:1359–1367.
38. Van den Berghe G, Wouters PJ, Boullion R, et al. Outcome benefit of intensive insulin therapy in the critically ill: insulin dose versus glycemic control. *Crit Care Med.* 2003;31:359–366.

Jennifer A. Wooley, MS, RD, CNSD

22

Use of Indirect Calorimetry in Critically Ill Patients

Introduction

A major advantage of indirect calorimetry (IC) over predictive energy expenditure equations is that it allows the clinician to measure a patient's actual energy expenditure and "match" the nutrition support regimen to the individual patient's needs. This facilitates nutrition support without the negative effects of under- or overfeeding.[1]

I. Indirect Calorimetry (IC) is Useful in Many ICU Clinical Scenarios

A. Inability to estimate accurately caloric requirements[2–5]
   1. Multiple trauma
   2. Neurological trauma
   3. Multiple Organ Dysfunction Syndrome (MODS)
   4. Sepsis
   5. Systemic Inflammatory Response Syndrome (SIRS)
   6. Respiratory distress syndrome
   7. Paralytic or barbiturate agents
   8. Large or multiple wounds
   9. Malnutrition associated with altered body composition:
      a) Underweight
      b) Overweight
      c) Paraplegia or quadriplegia
      d) Limb amputation
      e) Peripheral edema
   10. Post-operative organ transplantation

B. Inadequate response to nutrition support based on predictive equations[2–5]
   1. Malnutrition
   2. Failure to wean from mechanical ventilation
   3. Poor wound healing

C. Clinical signs of underfeeding or overfeeding[6–10]
   1. Signs of underfeeding
      a) Respiratory dysfunction
      b) Failure to wean from mechanical ventilation
      c) Low transport protein levels in the absence of infection or inflammation
      d) Poor wound healing

D. Signs of overfeeding
   1. Hyperglycemia
   2. Electrolyte imbalances
   3. Hyperlipidemia
   4. Hypermetabolism
   5. Fluid overload
   6. Organ dysfunction, such as fatty liver
   7. Failure to wean from mechanical ventilation such as elevated minute ventilation

II. Ideal Parameters for Conducting Indirect Calorimetry

A. Patients have rested in a supine position (in bed or a recliner) for more than 30 minutes before the study[2,3,5]

B. Patients receiving intermittent feedings (bolus enteral feeding, or cyclic enteral or parenteral nutrition or meals) are studied approximately 1 hour after the feeding if thermogenesis is to be included in the measured resting energy expenditure (REE), or 4 hours after the feeding if thermogenesis is to be excluded in the REE.[2,5]

C. The study is conducted in a quiet, thermoneutral environment.[2–5]

D. The rate and composition of nutrients being infused on a continuous basis are stable from at least 12 hours prior to the study until the end of the study.[2,5]

E. All sources of supplemental oxygen (nasal cannulas, masks or tracheostomy collars) are turned off during routine room air measurements, if medically feasible.[2,3,5]

F. The fraction of inspired oxygen (FiO_2) remains constant during the measurement.[2,3]

G. The study should be delayed for 90 minutes if changes are required in ventilatory settings.[2–5]

H. The patient engages in typical patterns of voluntary skeletal muscle activity (movement of the extremities) during the study.[2–5]

I. No leaks are present in the sampling system.[2–5]

J. All data used to derive REE and respiratory quotient (RQ) are taken from a period of equilibrium or steady state that has been identified according to statistically defined guidelines.[2–5]

K. The patient should not have received general anesthesia within 6–8 hours prior to the study.[2]

L. If the patient is in pain or agitated, analgesics or sedatives should be given at least 30 minutes before the study when clinically possible. Analgesics and sedatives administered should be documented and this information should be considered during the interpretation of the study.[2–4,11]

M. The study should be delayed for 3 to 4 hours after hemodialysis.[2,3,12]

N. The study should be delayed 1 hour after painful procedures have been performed.[2]
O. Routine nursing care or activities involving other health-care professionals should be avoided during the study.[2,4]

III. Technical Aspects that May Interfere with an Accurate Indirect Calorimetry Study

A. Mechanical ventilation with $FiO_2 \geq 60$[2,3]
B. Mechanical ventilation with Positive End Expiratory Pressure (PEEP) >12 cm H_2O[2,3]
C. Hyper/hypoventilation (acute changes altering body CO_2 stores)[2,3,5]
D. Leak in the sampling system[2,3,5]
E. Moisture in the system, which can affect the oxygen analyzer[2,3]
F. Continuous flow in the ventilator circuit with flow > 0 L/min during exhalation[3]
G. Inability to collect all expiratory flow[3]
H. Unstable inspiratory FiO_2 (> ±0.01%)[2,3]
I. Chest tube demonstrating the presence of an air leak (inability to collect all expired gases)[2,3]
J. Bronchopleural fistula (inability to collect all expired gases)[2,3]
K. Supplemental oxygen in spontaneously breathing patients[2,3,5]
L. Hemodialysis in progress[2,3,12]
M. Errors in calibration of indirect calorimeter[2,3]

TABLE 22-1. Situations that Can Affect VCO_2 and VO_2		
Elevated VCO_2	• Metabolic acidosis • Hypermetabolism	• Hyperventilation • Overfeeding
Decreased VCO_2	• Metabolic alkalosis • Hypometabolism • Starvation/ketosis	• Hypoventilation • Gluconeogenesis • Underfeeding
Elevated VO_2	• Sepsis • Hyperthermia • Shivering/agitation/excessive movement • Increased minute ventilation • Inotropic infusions (dopamine, dobutamine) • Hemodialysis (within 4 hours of treatment) • Overfeeding	• Hypermetabolism • Blood transfusions
Decreased VO_2	• Hypothermia • Hypothyroidism • Paralysis • Heavy sedation	• Fasting/starvation • Advanced age • General anesthesia • Coma or deep sleep

IV. Interpretation of Data Obtained from Indirect Calorimetry

A. Resting Energy Expenditure (based on the abbreviated Weir equation)

$$REE=[(3.94\times VO_2 L/min)+(1.11\times VCO_2 L/min)]1440\ min/day$$

B. Respiratory Quotient (RQ)

$$RQ = \frac{VCO_2\,(\text{carbon dioxide production})}{VO_2\,(\text{oxygen consumption})}$$

C. Measurement of urinary nitrogen excretion (UUN) is not necessary to ensure accuracy in the determination of REE.[2,3,6] Even a 100% error in the measurement of UUN will only produce an error of approximately 1–2% in the true energy expenditure.[2,6]
D. In complex patients or when steady state during an IC study is not achieved, it may be helpful to compare predicted VCO_2 and VO_2 levels using the formulas below with measured VCO_2 and VO_2 levels obtained from IC.[2] Clinical situations that can affect VCO_2 and VO_2 levels are outlined in Table 22-1.

$$\text{Normal adult } VCO_2 \text{level} = 2\text{–}3\ mL/min/kg$$

$$\text{Normal adult } VO_2 \text{level} = 3\text{–}4\ mL/min/kg$$

B. In critically ill patients, the RQ may vary significantly based on inter-patient variability, the metabolic response to stress, underlying lung disease, acid/base disturbances as well as substrate use. Low sensitivity and specificity, as a result of these variables, can limit the efficacy of using RQ as an indicator of under- or overfeeding.[13,14] However, an RQ within normal biological range (0.67–1.3) serves as a valuable marker of test reliability and validity.[2,3,13]
C. Traditional method of determining Total Energy Expenditure (TEE):

$$TEE = \text{Measured REE} \times \text{Activity Factor} \times \text{Stress Factor}$$

V. Nutrition Recommendations

A. Traditional view of RQ (Table 22-2):
1. An RQ < 0.82 suggests underfeeding. Increase caloric delivery unless contraindicated by clinical status.[5]
2. An RQ 0.85–0.95 suggests mixed substrate utilization indicating that the nutrition regimen is appropriate.[5]
3. An RQ > 1 suggests overfeeding and potential lipogenesis. Modification of the nutrition support regimen to provide less than 130% measured REE from total calories would be appropriate.[5]

TABLE 22-2. Traditional Interpretation of Respiratory Quotient

Substrate Utilization	Respiratory Quotient (physiologic range 0.67–1.3)
Ethanol	0.67
Fat oxidation	0.71
Protein oxidation	0.82
Mixed substrate oxidation	0.85
Carbohydrate oxidation	1.0
Lipogenesis	1.0–1.2

Reprinted with permission from the American Society for Parenteral and Enteral Nutrition (A.S.P.E.N) from the following: Wooley JA, Sax HC. Indirect calorimetry: applications to practice. *Nutr Clin Pract.* 2003;18:434–439.

1. Activity factor—add 5–10% to REE to account for typical physical activity of intensive care patients.[11,15–17]
2. Stress factors
   a) Thermogenesis—add 5% to REE if patient was measured in a fasting state or if feedings will be intermittent to account for thermogenesis.[4]
   b) Anabolism—If feasible from a metabolic standpoint, add up to 30% to measured REE to promote repletion.[4]
   c) TEE beyond 130% measured REE may lead to overfeeding, which often leads to metabolic and respiratory abnormalities.[6]
3. Current research has shown that feeding critically ill patients at 100% of measured REE is appropriate.[18] The addition of activity and stress factors may increase the likelihood of complications related to overfeeding.[18]
4. A specific population of critically ill patients may benefit from hypocaloric feeding,[19] (50–75% measured REE from total calories.[24] Protein provision must be aggressive (1.5–2.0 gm/kg). Some examples of appropriate candidates for hypocaloric feeding include:
   a) Class III obesity (BMI > 40)
   b) Refeeding syndrome
   c) Severe malnutrition
   d) Trauma patients following shock resuscitation
   e) Hemodynamic instability
   f) Acute respiratory distress syndrome or COPD
   g) MODS
   h) SIRS or sepsis

D. Once the caloric goal has been determined based on the measured REE, recommendations for distributing the three energy-yielding macronutrients are provided in Table 22-3.

TABLE 22-3. Designing Specialized Nutrition Support Regimens Based on Indirect Calorimetry

Carbohydrate	Stressed patients should receive approximately 50% of energy requirements as carbohydrate. Maximum glucose utilization rate is 3–5 mg/kg/min.[21]
Lipid	Stressed patients should receive ≤30% of energy requirements as lipid.[22,23] Limit total fat intake to ≤1g /kg/d via continuous infusion.[23] Monitor triglyceride levels.[23] At least 4% of total calories per day should come from linoleic acid (10% of calories as long chain fatty acids) or at least 500 mL of 10% IV lipid per week is necessary to prevent essential fatty acid deficiency.[22,23]
Protein	Stressed patients receive 15–20% of energy requirements as protein. Critically ill patients with signs of hypercatabolism require 1.5–2.0 g/kg of protein per day.[24] Trends in acute transport protein (PAB, CRP) levels and nitrogen balance studies provide insight into the patient's degree of hypercatabolism and assist with identification of the anabolic phase of recovery.[6]

VI. Frequency of IC Studies

A. There is lack of consensus in the literature on frequency of measurement.

B. IC is a "snapshot," at one point in time, of a patient's energy expenditure. Measurement of REE, at regular intervals such as weekly or whenever there is a significant change in the patient's clinical status that could affect energy expenditure, will optimize the provision of nutrition support while minimizing the likelihood of under- or overfeeding.[1,2,5,6]

VII. New Technology

Recently, a hand-held device (MedGem; Healthetech, Inc, Golden, CO) for measurement of VO2 and resting metabolic rate (RMR) in spontaneously breathing patients was introduced which may make the measurement of energy expenditure more routine in a variety of patient care settings. Validation studies comparing the performance of this handheld device to IC (open-circuit, Douglas bags, Sensormedics 2900 metabolic cart [VIASYS Healthcare, Yorba Linda, CA], Deltatrac [Datex-Ohmeda, Andover, MA] ventilator hood) have established that it is valid and reliable.[25,26]

Advantages of this device include convenience, ease of use and the reduced expense compared to a metabolic cart. Limitations are that some patients may have difficulty breathing continuously, without interruption, into the device for the entire period necessary to achieve steady state (maximum of 10 minutes) due to altered mental acuity or respiratory insufficiency, studies cannot be conducted on patients with nasal tubes or nasal cannulas and the nose clip can become uncomfortable for some patients. Furthermore, data is lacking about the most appropriate activity factors to add to the RMR in order to determine total energy expenditure.

VIII. Summary

Indirect calorimetry can make a vital contribution to the development of individualized nutrition support for critically ill patients. IC provides the most accurate method for determining energy requirements and protects the patient from extremes of under- or overfeeding. Protocols addressing the methodology required for technical accuracy and clinically useful results are necessary. The measured REE should be the energy target for nutrition support in the ICU. The addition of stress or activity factors to the measured REE is unnecessary and may increase the risk of overfeeding. Although the RQ can indicate the presence of under- and overfeeding, it should primarily be used as a marker of test validity. Optimal nutrition intervention requires continuous evaluation of all pertinent clinical data and careful monitoring of each patient's response to therapy. Therefore, the use of IC in the critically ill patient on a routine basis or in the presence of any "clinically significant" event that could affect energy expenditure would appear to be a prudent approach.

REFERENCES

1. Wooley JA, Sax HC. Indirect calorimetry: applications to practice. *Nutr Clin Pract.* 2003;18:434–438.
2. McClave S, Snider HL. Use of indirect calorimetry in clinical nutrition. *Nutr Clin Pract.* 1992;7:207–221.
3. Branson RD. The measurement of energy expenditure: instrumentation, practical considerations, and clinical application. *Respiratory Care.* 1990;35: 640–659.
4. Porter C, Cohen NH. Indirect calorimetry in critically ill patients: role of the clinical dietitian in interpreting results. *J Am Diet Assoc.* 1996;96:49–54, 57.
5. Matarese LE. Indirect calorimetry: technical aspects. *J Am Diet Assoc.* 1997;97(suppl 2):S154–S160.
6. Brandi LS, Bertolini R, Calafa M. Indirect calorimetry in critically ill patients: clinical applications and practical advice. *Nutrition.* 1997;13:349–358.
7. McClave SA, Lowen CC, Kleber MJ, et al. Are patients fed appropriately according to their caloric requirements? *J Parenter Enteral Nutr.* 1998;22: 375–381.
8. Klein CJ, Stanek GS, Wiles CE. Overfeeding macronutrients to critically ill adults: metabolic complications. *J Am Diet Assoc.* 1998;98:795–806.
9. McClave SA. The consequences of overfeeding and underfeeding. *J Resp Care Pract.* 1997;10:57–64.
10. Liposky JM, Nelson LD. Ventilatory response to high caloric loads in critically ill patients. *Crit Care Med.* 1994;22:796–802.
11. Swinamer DL, Phang PT, Jones RL, Grace M, King EG. Twenty-four hour energy expenditure in critically injured patients. *Crit Care Med.* 1987;15: 637–643.
12. Blumberg A, Keller G. Oxygen consumption during maintenance hemodialysis. *Nephron.* 1979;23:276–281.
13. McClave SA, Lowen CC, Kleber MJ, McConnell JW, Jung LY, Goldsmith LJ. Clinical use of the respiratory quotient obtained from indirect calorimetry. *J Parenter Enteral Nutr.* 2003;27:21–26.
14. McClave SA, Lowen CC, Kleber MJ, et al. Is the respiratory quotient a useful indicator of over or under feeding? *J Parenter Enteral Nutr.* 1997;21:S11.
15. Weissman C, Kemper, MS, Askanazi J, Hyman AI, Kinney JM. Day to day variation in the resting metabolic rate of mechanically ventilated critically ill patients. *Crit Care Med.* 1986;14:408.
16. White MS, Shepherd RW, McEniery JA. Energy expenditure measurements in ventilated critically ill children: within- and between-day variability. *J Parenter Enteral Nutr.* 1999;23:300–304.
17. Weissman C, Kemper M, Elwyn DH, et al. The energy expenditure of the mechanically ventilated critically ill patient: an analysis. *Chest.* 1986;89: 254–259.
18. McClave SA, Spain DA, Skolnick JL, et al. Achievement of steady state optimizes results when performing indirect calorimetry. *J Parenter Enteral Nutr.* 2003;27:16–20.
19. Zaloga GD. Permissive underfeeding. *New Horizons.* 1994;2:257–263.
20. Wolfe RR, O'Dossell TF Jr, Stone MD, et al. Investigation of factors determining the optimal glucose infusion rate in total parenteral nutrition. *Metabolism.* 1980;29:892–900.
21. Cerra FB, Benitez MR, Blackburn GL, et al. Applied nutrition in ICU patients: a consensus state of the American College of Chest Physicians. *Chest* 1997;111:769–778.
22. Fuhrman MP. Management of complications of parenteral nutrition. In: Matarese LE, Gottschlich MM, eds. *Contemporary Nutrition Support Practice A Clinical Guide.* Philadelphia, PA: WB Saunders Company;1998: 243–263.
23. Goodgame JT, Lowry SF, Brennan MF. Essential fatty acid deficiency in TPN: time course of development and suggestions for therapy. *Surgery* 1978;84:271–277.
24. Dickerson RN. Specialize nutrition support in the hospitalized obese patient. *Nutr Clin Pract.* 2004;19:245–254.
25. Nieman DC, Trone GA, Austin MD. A new handheld device for measuring resting metabolic rate and oxygen consumption. *J Am Diet Assoc.* 2003;103: 588–592.
26. Melanson EL, Coelho LB, Tran ZV, et al. Validation of the BodyGem™ handheld indirect calorimeter. *J Parenter Enteral Nutr.* 2003;27(Suppl 1):S39.

Kathleen D. Liu, MD, PhD;
Annette Stralovich-Romani, RD, CNSD;
Glenn M. Chertow, MD, MPH

23

Nutrition Support for Adult Patients With Acute Renal Failure

Introduction

Acute renal failure (ARF) is a common condition in hospitalized patients.[1–3] ARF is characterized by a decrement in the glomerular filtration rate (GFR), which leads to reduced filtration and elimination of the by-products of metabolism. Changes in serum creatinine, a product of muscle protein breakdown that is excreted by the kidney, indicate alterations in kidney function. A rise in serum creatinine usually reflects decreased filtration by the kidney. In the clinical literature, ARF is often defined as a doubling of the serum creatinine or an increase to above 0.5 mg/dL creatinine. Causes of ARF are broadly characterized as prerenal, intrarenal, or postrenal (obstructive). Hospital-acquired ARF is associated with mortality in 30% to 70% of patients.[4–6] Once the cause is identified, interventions and nourishment necessary for recovery must be prescribed. At increased risk for ARF are certain acutely ill patients, including patients with chronic kidney disease (CKD), diabetes mellitus, or liver disease; elderly patients; patients receiving certain nephritic drugs; postoperative patients; and patients with sepsis or hemorrhage. The "phase" or duration of renal injury, the volume of diuresis (oliguric vs non-oliguric), and the dialytic modality used to treat the renal failure determine the nutritional prescription.

I. Overview of ARF

A. There is no uniform definition of ARF, but it is usually characterized by an abrupt cessation or decline in renal function that may be associated with a decline in urine output. ARF may be transient or lead to permanent renal failure. In clinical practice, ARF may be defined as a doubling of serum creatinine, as a change in creatinine of 0.5 mg/dL from baseline in adults, or as a need for renal replacement therapy.

B. ARF's etiology can be broadly divided into prerenal, postrenal, or intrarenal.[3,7]
   1. Prerenal. Impaired renal perfusion from volume depletion, congestive heart failure, cirrhosis, renovascular disease, or other conditions can lead to ARF. If the underlying condition can be quickly reversed, this type of ARF may resolve rapidly. However, if the condition is long-standing or cannot be corrected, prerenal ARF may progress to ARF in the form of acute tubular necrosis (ATN).
   2. Postrenal. This type of ARF is due to obstruction of the urinary tract below the kidneys and usually resolves when the kidneys are decompressed. However, if the obstruction is long-standing, permanent kidney failure may occur.
   3. Intrarenal. Intrarenal (or intrinsic) ARF may be caused by damage to any one of the four components of the renal parenchyma: vasculature, tubules, glomeruli, or interstitium. The syndrome of a sudden and severe decline in GFR, or ATN, is common among critically ill patients. Common correlates of ATN include ischemia due to hypotension, sepsis, and nephrotoxic injury (eg, myoglobin in rhabdomyolysis, radiocontrast injury).

C. The clinical course of ARF depends on the underlying disease but typically can be divided into three clinical phases: initiation, maintenance, and recovery.[8]
   1. Initiation. During this phase, damage to the kidney starts and is reflected in a rapid reduction in GFR, which is commonly, but not always, associated with oliguria.
      a) This phase is typically recognized when the creatinine starts to rise or the urine output starts to fall. Recognition of this phase may be delayed since time is required for creatinine or other markers of kidney function to accumulate. It should be noted that small changes in serum creatinine can reflect large changes in kidney function and that serum creatinine reflects muscle mass as well as kidney function.
      b) The kidney is responsible for volume regulation. As ARF progresses, patients may become oliguric—usually defined as < 400 mL of urine output per day—and rapidly become volume overloaded, especially if they receive a large amount of intravenous colloid or crystalloid.
      c) The kidney critically regulates blood electrolytes. Serum potassium and phosphorus may rise acutely. Hyperkalemia may lead to arrhythmias and/or cardiac arrest. Hyperphosphatemia may provoke symptoms associated with hypocalcemia.
      d) The kidney regulates the excretion of organic acids. If the patient has an underlying disease that results in a large acid load (eg, rhabdomyolysis, sepsis), the patient may become profoundly acidemic.
      e) Patients with ARF may manifest systemic signs of uremia, including nausea, vomiting, and altered mental status (including confusion and seizures).
   2. Maintenance. During this phase, ARF is established and recovery has not occurred. In cases due to reversible causes of ARF, such as pre- and postrenal ARF, patients may start to recover rapidly. During the maintenance phase of intrinsic ARF, there are fewer dynamic changes. The patient may require dialysis or hemodiafiltration to control acidosis, electrolytes, and/or volume status. These therapies have important implications for the provision of selected nutrients, including amino acids and water-soluble vitamins. Dialysis removes amino acids, typically in the range of 8 to 10 g per intermittent hemodialysis (IHD) session—and potentially

more with high-efficiency continuous renal replacement therapy (CRRT).[9–10]

3. Recovery. As the name implies, this phase is characterized by improving kidney function. During this phase, patients frequently "auto-diurese," leading to a large and inappropriate loss of fluid and electrolytes, while tubular function remains impaired. Fluid and nutrition prescriptions may need significant modification during this phase, particularly if dialysis or hemodiafiltration is reduced or discontinued.

D. The methods of estimating renal function are described below.

1. Creatinine clearance rate and GFR are measures of kidney function. The normal GFR of a young, healthy adult is approximately 130 mL/min. GFR declines by about 1 mL/min per year after the age of 40.[11] It is not usually feasible to measure GFR (determined by injection of inulin or iothalamate and measuring clearance over time) in a critically ill patient. In ARF, the GFR can be estimated by calculating a creatinine clearance only if (1) the patient is not receiving dialytic support and (2) the serum creatinine concentration is stable on a day-to-day basis.
2. Kidney function may be estimated using the Cockcroft-Gault estimated creatinine clearance[12] or the modification of diet in renal disease (MDRD) estimated GFR equations,[13] if the above two conditions are met. The Cockcroft-Gault equation is as follows: ([140 – age] × weight [in kg])/(serum creatinine [in mg/dL]) × 72) × 0.85 for women. The simplified MDRD equation is GFR = $186 \times (\text{plasma creatinine})^{-1.154} \times (\text{age})^{-0.203} \times 0.742$ if female × 1.210 if African American.
3. Alternatively, a timed urine collection can be obtained and creatinine clearance may be calculated using the following equation: Creatinine clearance = (urine volume × urine creatinine)/(plasma creatinine × number of minutes of timed collection). Again, to obtain an accurate measurement, the serum creatinine needs to be stable and the patient cannot be receiving dialysis. Typically, timed urine collections are clinically useful only in the recovery phase of ARF.

E. Dialytic support may be provided as IHD or as CRRT.

1. Peritoneal dialysis is not commonly used to treat ARF due to issues with access and solute clearance and the inability to use after abdominal surgery.[3]
2. IHD compares with CRRT as follows:
   a) Both IHD and CRRT require vascular access, in the form of either an arteriovenous fistula or graft or a double-lumen catheter placed in a large vessel. Few patients with ARF have preexisting angioaccess; therefore, the majority require placement of a dialysis catheter.
   b) IHD is generally performed at least 3 times a week for 3 to 4 hours per session. A recent study demonstrated that patients with ARF may benefit from more frequent IHD.[14]
   c) CRRT generally causes less hemodynamic stress than IHD and over time can provide for greater clearance and tighter control of electrolytes and acidosis. However, it is labor-intensive and requires the patient to be connected continuously to the dialysis machine.
   d) The decision to use IHD or CRRT is based on many factors, including the hemodynamic stability of the patient, physician preference, and nursing/staff resources. Data regarding the relative benefits of these two modalities to patient outcome are limited.[15–17]
   e) A hybrid dialysis modality has been used more frequently of late: slow, low-efficiency dialysis (SLED).[18] SLED is intended to combine the benefits of CRRT and IHD and is typically performed over 6 to 12 hours, 6 or 7 days per week.

II. Nutritional Aspects of ARF

A. General effect on nutrition. The wide range of nutritional requirements of patients with ARF reflects the broad spectrum of disease severity. Metabolic derangements may be attributable to uremia as well as to underlying disease processes. Critical illness typically precipitates a hypercatabolic and hypermetabolic response and is frequently associated with ARF.[19] Patients with multiorgan dysfunction from sepsis, pancreatitis, trauma, burns, neurological injury, or other causes may be profoundly catabolic and have very high protein and energy requirements. In contrast, some patients, such as those with isolated ARF due to nephrotoxic injury such as aminoglycoside or radiocontrast-associated injury, may have energy requirements that do not differ significantly from those associated with other diseases of modest severity. Moreover, nutritional requirements are affected by whether the patient is on dialysis.

B. Energy. While ARF alone does not lead to a significant rise in energy expenditure, it is frequently associated with an underlying disease state that leads to a large increase in energy expenditure (eg, sepsis, neurological injury, burns, trauma).[20,21] Thus, assessment of the underlying medical condition must be part of the initial nutritional evaluation.

C. Carbohydrate. ARF is frequently associated with disease states characterized by high levels of counterregulatory hormones that lead to hyperglycemia. ARF is usually associated with insulin resistance, reduced renal gluconeogenesis, and accelerated hepatic gluconeogenesis, which in sum typically result in increased serum glucose levels. However, the kidney is also a major site of insulin degradation, so serum insulin levels tend to be higher in patients with ARF.[22] Hyperglycemia is common among patients with ARF. There is growing evidence that aggressive glycemic control reduces intensive care unit (ICU) mortality and complication rates in hospitalized patients.[23] In adults, this possibility must be balanced against the risk of hypoglycemia in ARF.

D. Lipid

ARF leads to an impairment of lipolysis that may be further exacerbated by metabolic acidosis, a frequent complication of ARF.

E. Protein

1. ARF leads to an increase in protein catabolism. Increased protein catabolism is due to both accelerated breakdown of muscle protein and abnormal use of amino acids by skeletal muscle.[24,25]
2. Accelerated protein breakdown is due to several factors. These factors include stimulation of hepatic gluconeogenesis, which cannot be fully suppressed even when an exogenous substrate (eg, glucose) is added, and insulin resistance and acidosis, both of which promote muscle protein breakdown.[26] Levels of endogenous counterregulatory hormones (cortisol, glucagon, epinephrine, and norepinephrine) are frequently elevated in states associated with ARF; these elevated levels increase protein catabolism. Cytokine release also contributes to the acceleration in muscle proteolysis seen with critical illness.
3. Metabolism of certain amino acids is affected by a lack of kidney function. Thus, amino acid pools are often altered.[27] Several amino acids that are usually considered nonessential (eg, glutamine) may become required in ARF. Lack of supplementation with these amino acids can lead to hyperammonemia, metabolic acidosis, and coma.

F. Fluid administration and volume status. Patients with ARF are often given large quantities of intravenous fluid in an attempt to augment urine output. In addition, many patients have reduced urine output. These factors conspire to create volume overload. In particular, volume overload complicates the management of patients with ARF who are not yet receiving dialysis. Volume overload may also influence the recognition of ARF, since large increases in total body water can dilute the concentrations of creatinine and urea nitrogen, the usual markers of renal failure early in the course of ARF. Clinicians commonly use diuretics to try to reduce volume overload; often, dialysis is required to control volume overload.

G. Electrolytes
   1. Serum electrolytes will vary considerably depending on the underlying disease state and on whether the patient is receiving dialysis. Electrolyte abnormalities present at the recognition of ARF are corrected with dialysis in most patients. Meticulous electrolyte and mineral management is critical to the successful management of ARF.
   2. Hyperkalemia is frequent. Hyperkalemia may be due to impaired renal potassium excretion, as well as to changes in the extracellular and intracellular distribution of potassium due to the metabolic acidosis associated with ARF. Endogenous or iatrogenic hyperglycemia can also contribute to hyperkalemia.
   3. Over the course of therapy, some patients develop hypokalemia (and hypophosphatemia).

H. Minerals
   1. Hyperphosphatemia is frequently observed as a result of impaired renal phosphate excretion as well as increased release from cells.
   2. Patients with ARF frequently present with hypocalcemia. Hypocalcemia is a multifactorial process, due at least in part to hyperphosphatemia as well as reduced formation of $1,25(OH)_2$ vitamin D_3, leading to reduced calcium absorption from the gastrointestinal tract. Hypercalcemia is rare in critically ill patients with ARF, except those with particular underlying disorders otherwise associated with hypercalcemia (eg, fungal or mycobacterial infection, lymphoma, milk alkali syndrome). Immobilization can contribute to hypercalcemia, particularly in adolescent and young adult patients.
   3. As noted for potassium, over the course of therapy some patients develop hypophosphatemia. Hypophosphatemia may need to be corrected to prevent weakness and rhabdomyolysis. Hypophosphatemia may be a particular problem during the diuretic or recovery phase of ARF, as well as during "refeeding."

III. Nutritional Assessment in Patients with ARF

A. The usual procedures for nutritional assessment are followed (see Chapter 1).

B. The clinical assessment must include evaluation of the current whole body fluid status. Patients with ARF are often fluid overloaded. The usual, or ideal, weight of the patient is used to determine nutritional status and nutrient requirements, and to monitor response to nutritional therapy.

C. Ongoing assessment of volume status can be made by following daily weights and maintaining accurate records of intake and output, along with physical examination findings (eg, jugular venous pressure). Sometimes, invasive monitoring such as monitoring of central venous pressure is needed.

D. Caliper skinfold measurements are of limited utility in patients with ARF because of edema. There are limited data on bioelectrical impedance in patients with ARF.[28]

E. Biochemical measurements include the following:
   1. Serum sodium, potassium, chloride, bicarbonate, urea nitrogen, creatinine, calcium, magnesium, and phosphorus should be obtained at the initial assessment and up to several times a week, depending on the clinical stability of the patient.
   2. If a serious acid-base disorder is suspected, arterial blood gas should be obtained with the initial assessment.
   3. For patients undergoing IHD, laboratory values should be obtained at the start of or before the dialysis session.
   4. Various serum proteins have been used in the assessment of nutritional status. Albumin and thyroxine-binding prealbumin are most commonly used clinically.[9] The advantages of serum albumin include wide availability and low cost of measurement. However, due to the multiple factors that can reduce serum albumin, little credence should be given to albumin as a marker of nutritional status or response to nutritional therapy during periods of metabolic stress, which are common in conditions associated with ARF.
   5. Like that of albumin, the synthesis of prealbumin decreases independent of nutritional status during metabolic stress. In addition, prealbumin may be falsely elevated in ARF due to reduced renal clearance.
   6. Hypertriglyceridemia is more common in patients with ARF than in patients without ARF. As is done for all patients on total parenteral nutrition (PN), baseline and serial triglyceride concentrations should be obtained for ARF patients.
   7. Nitrogen balance can be calculated for patients with ARF, but the usual technique must be modified (Table 23-1). Studies of nitrogen balance in patients with CKD suggest that nonurinary losses can be estimated based on body weight.[29,30]

TABLE 23-1. Calculation of Nitrogen Balance in Adult Patients Receiving Dialytic Support

Nitrogen balance in g/day = (protein intake in g/day/6.25) – nitrogen loss/day

A. Patients receiving intermittent hemodialysis

Nitrogen loss in g/day = 0.97 × UNA + insensible losses (2–4 g of nitrogen/day) + dialysis amino acid losses (approximately 1 g of nitrogen/dialysis session)

UNA = UUN + [(BUN2 – BUN1) × (0.6 × BW1)] + (BW2 – BW1) × BUN2

Where UNA = urinary nitrogen appearance in g/day; UUN = urine urea nitrogen in g/day; BUN1 = initial blood urea nitrogen in g/L (eg, postdialysis); BUN2 = final BUN in g/L (eg, predialysis); BW1 = initial body weight in kg; BW2 = final body weight in kg; 0.6 = estimated fraction of BW that is water.

B. Patients receiving continuous renal replacement therapy

Nitrogen loss in g/day = dialysate urea nitrogen losses in g/day + amino acid losses across continuous renal replacement therapy membrane in g/day + UUN in g/day + insensible losses (2–4 g/day)

Dialysate urea nitrogen losses in g/day = total dialysate ultrafiltrate volume in L × average ultrafiltrate urea nitrogen in g/L

Amino acid losses can be approximated as follows: 1.5 g nitrogen/day for 1 L/hour flow rate and 2.0 g nitrogen/day for 2 L/hour flow rate

Adapted with permission from Dr. Thomas Baumgartner

IV. Nutritional Requirements and Goals of Therapy in ARF

A. Overall goals of therapy
  1. Maintain appropriate hydration.
  2. Establish and maintain acid-base equilibrium.
  3. Establish and maintain electrolyte balance.
  4. Control uremia.
  5. Maintain normal body composition during ARF and critical illness, which should improve immune function, wound healing, and host resistance.

B. Nutritional support for patients with ARF
  1. General requirements. Nutritional requirements for patients with ARF will vary based on underlying nutritional status, degree of hypermetabolism and hypercatabolism, residual renal function, and clinical condition. In addition, plans for dialysis or ultrafiltration may strongly influence the prescription for enteral nutrition or parenteral nutrition (PN). Patients with ARF may differ from patients with CKD (discussed in Chapter 31) with regard to protein and energy requirements and, therefore, nutritional goals.
  2. Energy requirements. Among patients with ARF, energy requirements can be estimated in several ways, including by the Harris-Benedict equation with adjustment for illness severity or by indirect calorimetry using a metabolic chart (see Chapter 22).[31,32] The resting energy expenditure should not be measured during intermittent hemodialysis treatments, because of changes in organ perfusion and other factors that may influence energy use.
  3. Protein requirements. Protein requirements will vary depending on the underlying clinical state and on whether or not the patient is receiving IHD or CRRT. Table 23-2 outlines recommendations regarding protein intake in ARF, with or without dialysis.
     a) Some have advocated that a limited subset of patients with ARF who have little to no protein depletion, who have no clinical evidence of uremia, and who are likely to recover rapidly from ARF can be treated with a restricted, essential amino acid regimen,[24] but this is rarely done. In fact, at present it is virtually impossible to predict the time course of recovery from ARF.
     b) Most patients with ARF are catabolic. Therefore, protein intake should generally not be limited to forestall dialysis. Rather, adequate nutrition should be provided early in the course of illness, and dialytic support should be used to allow provision of adequate nutrition. Indeed, when ARF accompanies sepsis or multiorgan dysfunction or failure, the combination of underlying disease and the provision of nutrition nearly always makes initiation of dialysis necessary.
     c) Patients receiving CRRT or "daily" dialysis in the form of IHD or SLED may require higher doses of protein or amino acids. Patients receiving continuous hemodiafiltration should receive at least 1.0 g/kg/day of protein, and many patients will require at least 1.5 to 1.8 g/kg/day of protein or amino acids. A number of groups have recently used up to 2.5 g/kg/day of amino acids in these patients and demonstrated no apparent complications,[33,34] assuming that adequate solute clearance can be achieved. Nutritional goals need to be serially reevaluated based on net nitrogen balance on an ongoing basis.
  4. Vitamin and trace mineral requirements. These are not well defined for ARF.[24,35]
     a) Vitamin and mineral status is affected by dialysis. Patients undergoing IHD lose water-soluble vitamins into the dialysate. Vitamin supplementation is needed to compensate for the losses. Excessive doses of vitamin C (>1 g/day) should be avoided, given the impaired excretion of oxalate, a vitamin C by-product, in ARF. Vitamin B_{12} losses may be less than losses of other water-soluble vitamins, as this vitamin is protein bound.
     b) Vitamin A supplementation should be avoided, at least initially, in light of observations that patients with CKD have elevated serum concentrations of vitamin A. Usual doses of vitamin A have been reported to cause toxicity.

V. Enteral Nutrition in ARF

A. Choice of enteral nutrition
  1. Enteral nutrition provides significant benefits to the patient with ARF,[19] as it does for most other patients. PN requires a larger fluid load than enteral nutrition, which can make it less appealing for use in ARF patients.
  2. Special enteral formulas (with reduced concentrations of sodium, potassium, and phosphorus, and often with reduced protein content) have been developed for patients with CKD and are often used in patients with ARF. These formulas are more concentrated than standard formulas, usually supplying 1.5 to 2.0 kcal/mL. Since the patient may undergo dialysis regularly, providing adequate energy and protein, rather than providing a particular volume of the formula, should be the primary focus, and it may be possible to use a standard formula. Once dialysis is stopped, one of the low-electrolyte "renal" formulas may be preferable.
  3. Essential amino acid enteral formulas are no longer commonly used in ARF.
  4. The use of immune-enhancing formulas is discussed in Chapter 20.

B. Access. Most enteral formulas can be taken orally. In patients who are unable to meet their nutritional goals or who are intubated and unable to eat, a feeding tube may be placed.

C. Complications. Three major types of complications—mechanical, gastrointestinal, and metabolic—are associated with enteral nutrition in patients with ARF.
  1. A recent study compared the rate of complications of enteral feeding in patients with ARF and those without ARF.[36] The only complication that was more frequent in ARF was delayed gastric emptying. However, this complication did not result in additional episodes of aspiration or aspiration pneumonia.
  2. For patients on tube feeds, phosphate binders (calcium carbonate, calcium acetate, sevelamer hydrochloride) may be required to reduce the amount of absorbable phosphorus in the feeding.
  3. Phosphate binders, particularly sevelamer hydrochloride, a hydrogel that expands upon contact with liquid, may clog feeding tubes. Sevelamer hydrochloride should not be administered via this route without extensive postadministration tube flushing.
  4. Sodium polystyrene sulfonate (eg, Kayexalate, Sanofi Winthrop Pharmaceuticals) and aluminum hydroxide (eg, Amphojel, Wyeth-Ayerst Laboratories) should not be co-administered, as these medications polymerize to form an insoluble compound.
  5. Electrolyte disturbances are common, in particular hyper- and hypokalemia, hyper- and hyponatremia, and hyper- and hypophosphatemia.
     a) Some medications may cause potassium loss, in particular amphotericin, semisynthetic penicillins such as piperacillin, and potassium-wasting diuretics.
     b) Some of the penicillins are formulated as either potassium or sodium salts and may lead to hyperkalemia or volume overload, respectively.
     c) If patients are receiving concentrated enteral formulas, they may require free water (which can be given enterally or intra-

venously) to prevent or correct hypernatremia. Hypernatremia may be particularly common in the early recovery phase of ARF (perhaps in response to high concentrations of retained osmotically active, noncharged, and nonmeasured solutes).

D. Monitoring. The major goals of monitoring are to minimize the complications of enteral therapy and to maintain the patency of the small-bore feeding tube. Basic monitoring in ARF patients on enteral tube feeds is similar to that of other patients on enteral tube feeds. The patient's intake and output, as well as serum electrolytes, should be strictly monitored (see Section II for commonly found biochemical abnormalities).

VI. Parenteral Nutrition in ARF

A. The fluid tolerance of a patient with ARF depends on many factors, including the phase of ARF, whether the patient is receiving dialytic support, and whether the dialysis is continuous or intermittent. Attention must be paid to the volume of solution infused on a daily basis.

B. Standard amino acid solutions should be used for patients with ARF. There is no clear advantage to administering essential amino acids alone.[35]

C. The "dose" of protein in the form of amino acids that is appropriate to the patient's age and stress level, plus an additional component for losses from dialysis or hemodiafiltration (see Table 23-2), should be prescribed. The A.S.P.E.N. guidelines state that patients with ARF should receive both essential and nonessential amino acids. In addition, the guidelines recommend that patients undergoing CRRT should receive at least 1 g/kg/day of protein and that patients with ARF who are severely malnourished or hypercatabolic should receive 1.5 to 1.8 g/kg/day of protein. However, whenever possible these decisions should be guided by nitrogen balance calculations.

D. Patients with ARF receiving PN should receive fat emulsions. Intravenous fat emulsions are not cleared with dialysis.[37] The optimal dose or frequency of fat administration is unknown. While some clinicians favor a high fat-to-carbohydrate formula and severe fluid restriction to delay dialysis, it is generally preferable to base nutrition therapy on needs and side effect profiles, rather than pursuing the usually futile course of trying to delay or avoid initiation of dialysis.

E. The PN's electrolyte composition should be assessed and adjusted daily according to changes in the patient's clinical condition and serum chemistries. Special attention should be paid to serum potassium and phosphorus levels, which will usually rise with ARF. However, as dialytic support is initiated and anabolism returns, serum concentrations may fall abruptly, and appropriate amounts need to be provided.

F. The balance of acetate and chloride needs to be adjusted in the PN solution based on the patient's acid-base status. While typically complicated by acidosis, ARF can be accompanied by a wide variety of metabolic disturbances. The PN prescription will depend on whether the patient's underlying disease is characterized by high levels of organic acid production and whether the patient is receiving dialysis.

G. Means of access must be considered carefully.
   1. Because of its high osmolality, PN needs to be administered through a central line or peripherally inserted central catheter (PICC). Patients with ARF typically have a large-bore hemodialysis catheter in a large central vessel (eg, internal jugular or femoral). Recently, new triple-lumen dialysis catheters, which contain a third lumen for medication administration, have been developed. While it is generally accepted that PN should not be administered through the large ports of a double-lumen dialysis catheter, there are insufficient safety data regarding using the third lumen for nutrition infusion.
   2. PICC lines have been shown to have lower risks of infection than other central lines and thus may be preferable for administering PN.[38] A potential disadvantage to PICC lines in patients with ARF is scarring of the basilic and cephalic veins that might later be used for permanent vascular access (in the form of either an arteriovenous fistula or a synthetic graft) if ARF does not resolve but the patient survives. In ARF, the obvious focus of care should be on recovery from the acute illness rather than long-term dialysis access. However, if the latter can be preserved while the necessary goals within the ICU are accomplished, there is additional potential for long-term patient benefit.

H. Monitoring patients with ARF on PN is similar to monitoring other patients on PN, although the PN prescription and fluid balance need to be frequently reassessed.

I. A number of potential complications must be considered.
   1. Patients with ARF are prone to the mechanical, metabolic, and infectious complications of TPN to which other PN patients are prone.
   2. Hyperglycemia is common among patients with ARF. In hospitalized patients, there is growing evidence that aggressive glycemic control reduces ICU mortality and complication rates.[23] However, patients with kidney disease are at increased risk for hypoglycemia (see above).

TABLE 23-2. Approximate Protein Requirements for Adults

Normal renal function	
Maintenance	0.8–1.2 g of protein/kg/day
Moderate stress	1.3–1.5 g of protein/kg/day
Severe stress	1.5–2.0 g of protein/kg/day
Renal failure	
Nondialyzed	0.8–1.2 g of protein/kg/day
Hemodialyzed	1.0–1.4 g of protein/kg/day (may need to be adjusted based on frequency of dialysis)
Continuous renal replacement therapy	1.5–2.5 g of protein/kg/day

REFERENCES

1. Nolan CR, Anderson RJ. Hospital-acquired acute renal failure. *J Am Soc Nephrol.* 1998;9:710–8.
2. Thadhani R, Pascual A, Bonventre J. Acute renal failure. *N Engl J Med.* 1996;334:1448–60.
3. Brady H, Clarkson M, Lieberthal W. Acute renal failure. In: Brenner BM, ed. *Brenner and Rector's The Kidney.* 7th ed. St Louis, MO: WB Saunders; 2003.
4. Brivet FG, Kleinknecht DJ, Loirat P, et al. Acute renal failure in intensive care units: causes, outcome and prognostic factors of hospital mortality: a prospective, multicenter study. *Crit Care Med.* 1996;24:192–8.
5. Liano F, Pascual J, The Madrid Acute Renal Failure Study Group. Epidemiology of acute renal failure: a prospective, multicenter, community-based study. *Kidney Int.* 1996;50:811–8.
6. Metnitz P, Krenn C, Steltzer H, et al. Effect of acute renal failure requiring renal replacement therapy on outcome in critically ill patients. *Crit Care Med.* 2002;30:2051–8.
7. Holley J. Clinical approach to the diagnosis of renal failure. In: Greenberg A, ed. *Primer on Kidney Diseases.* 3rd ed. San Diego, CA: Academic Press; 2001.

8. Brady H, Singer G. Acute renal failure. *Lancet.* 1996;346:1533–40.
9. Davies S, Reaveley D, Brown E, et al. Amino acid clearances and daily losses in patients with acute renal failure treated by continuous arteriovenous hemodialysis. *Crit Care Med.* 1991;19:1510–15.
10. Frankenfield D, Badellino M, Reynolds H, et al. Amino acid loss and plasma concentration during continuous diafiltration. *J Parenter Enteral Nutr.* 1993;17:551–61.
11. Choudhury D, Raj D, Levi M. Effect of aging on renal function and disease. In: Brenner B, ed. *Brenner and Rector's The Kidney.* 7th ed. St Louis, MO: WB Saunders; 2003.
12. Cockcroft D, Gault M. Prediction of creatinine clearance from serum creatinine. *Nephron.* 1976;16:31–41.
13. Levey A, Bosch J, Lewis J, et al. A more accurate method to estimate glomerular filtration rate from serum creatinine: a new prediction equation. Modification of Diet in Renal Disease Study Group. *Ann Intern Med.* 1999;130:461–70.
14. Schiffl H, Lang, S, Fischer R. Daily hemodialysis and the outcome of acute renal failure. *N Engl J Med.* 2002;346:305–310.
15. Kellum J, Angus D, Johnson J, et al. Continuous versus intermittent renal replacement therapy: a meta-analysis. *Intensive Care Med.* 2002;28:29–37.
16. Mehta R, McDonald B, Gabbai F, et al. A randomized clinical trial of continuous versus intermittent dialysis for acute renal failure. *Kidney Int.* 2001;60:1154–63.
17. Tonelli M, Manns B, Feller-Kopman D. Acute renal failure in the intensive care unit: a systematic review of the impact of dialytic modality on mortality and renal recovery. *Am J Kidney Dis.* 2002;40:875–85.
18. Marshall M, Golper T, Shaver M, et al. Sustained low-efficiency dialysis for critically ill patients requiring renal replacement therapy. *Kidney Int.* 2001;60:777–85.
19. Stralovich-Romani A, Mahutte C, Matthay M, et al. Administrative, nutritional, and ethical principles for the management of critically ill patients. In: George R, Light RW, Matthay MA, Matthay RW, eds. *Chest Medicine.* 5th ed. Philadelphia, PA: Lippincott Williams & Wilkins. In press.
20. Goldstein S, Elwyn DH. The effects of injury and sepsis on fuel utilization. *Ann Rev Nutr.* 1989;9:445–73.
21. Schneeweiss B, Graninger W, Stockenhuber F, et al. Energy metabolism in acute and chronic renal failure. *Am J Clin Nutr.* 1990;52:596–601.
22. Druml W. Nutritional support in patients with acute renal failure. In: Molitoris B, Finn W, eds. *Acute Renal Failure: A Companion to Brenner and Rector's The Kidney.* Philadelphia, PA: WB Saunders; 2001.
23. Van den Berghe G, Wouters P, Weekers F, et al. Intensive insulin therapy in the critically ill patient. *N Engl J Med.* 2001;345:1359–67.
24. Kopple J. Nutritional management of acute renal failure. In: Kopple J, Massry S, eds. *Nutritional Management of Renal Disease.* 2nd ed. Philadelphia, PA: Lippincott Williams & Wilkins; 2004.
25. Druml W. Protein metabolism in acute renal failure. *Miner Electrolyte Metab.* 1998;24:47–54.
26. Clark AS, Mitch WE. Muscle protein turnover and glucose uptake in acutely uremic rats. Effects of insulin and the duration of renal insufficiency. *J Clin Invest.* 1983;72:836–45.
27. Druml W, Burger U, Kleinberger G, et al. Elimination of amino acids in acute renal failure. *Nephron.* 1986;42:62–67.
28. Bioelectrical impedance analysis in body composition measurement: National Institutes of Health technology assessment conference statement. *Am J Clin Nutr.* 1996;64:524S–532S.
29. Maroni B, Steinman T, Mitch W. A method for estimating nitrogen intake of patients with chronic kidney failure. *Kidney Int.* 1985;27:58–65.
30. Kopple J, Gao X, Qing D. Dietary protein, urea nitrogen appearance and total nitrogen appearance in chronic renal failure. *Kidney Int.* 1997;52:486–94.
31. McClave S, Snider H. Use of indirect calorimetry in clinical nutrition. *Nutr Clin Pract.* 1992;7:207–21.
32. Ireton-Jones C, Borman K, Turner W. Nutritional considerations in the management of ventilator-dependent patients. *Nutr Clin Pract.* 1993;8:60–64.
33. Bellomo R, Seacombe J, Daskalakis M, et al. A prospective comparative study of moderate versus high protein intake for critically ill patients with acute renal failure. *Ren Fail.* 1997;19:111–20.
34. Scheinkestel C, Adams F, Mahony L, et al. Impact of increasing parenteral protein loads on amino acid levels and balance in critically ill anuric patients on continuous renal replacement therapy. *Nutrition.* 2003;19:733–40.
35. Bellomo R. Nutritional management of patients treated with continuous renal replacement therapy. In: Kopple J, Massry S, eds. *Nutritional Management of Renal Disease.* 2nd ed. Philadelphia, PA: Lippincott Williams & Wilkins; 2004.
36. Fiaccadori E, Maggiore U, Giacosa R, et al. Enteral nutrition in patients with acute renal failure. *Kidney Int.* 2004;64:999–1008.
37. Bellomo R, Martin H, Parkin G, et al. Continuous arteriovenous haemodiafiltration in the critically ill: influence on major nutrient balances. *Intensive Care Med.* 1991;17:399–402.
38. O'Grady N, Alexander M, Dellinger E, et al. Guidelines for the prevention of intravascular catheter infections. *Am J Infect Control.* 2002;30:476–89.

Carolyn L. Abitbol, MD;
Marie Rossique, PharmD;
Mirta Rios, RD

24

Nutritional Support of the Pediatric Patient with Acute Renal Failure

Introduction

Children present a unique challenge in nutritional and metabolic support during periods of acute renal failure (ARF). The challenge is to make an appropriate assessment and prescribe interventions that provide necessary replacement and sustenance for recovery. As in adults, causes of ARF in infants and children are broadly characterized, as pre-renal, intra-renal and post-renal (or obstructive). The "phase" or duration of renal injury, the volume of diuresis (oliguric versus non-oliguric) and the effects of any needed form of renal replacement therapy determine the nutritional prescription.

I. Overview of Pediatric Acute Renal Failure

A. The pathophysiology and principles of management of ARF are described in Chapter 23. This chapter presents information specifically related to managing pediatric patients with ARF.

B. Estimation of kidney function in the pediatric population is based on the serum creatinine (Scr) and the child's height using the formula of Schwartz, et al.[1] Estimation of the severity of deterioration in renal function in normovolemic pediatric patients, including preterm neonates with small muscle mass, is a doubling of the baseline Scr, especially when associated with a fall in urine flow to < 0.5 to 1 ml/kg/hr.[2,3] This applies equally to preterm neonates prone to vasomotor nephropathy.[3]

II. Nutritional Aspects of Pediatric ARF

A. Nutritional requirements for macronutrients should be estimated based on the patient's needs and current intakes. Enteral and parenteral nutrition must be determined in coordination with the plans for fluid allowance and required dialysis modalities including continuous renal replacement therapies (CRRT).

B. Infants and children are metabolically and hormonally primed for maintaining growth and positive nitrogen balance. Although their energy requirements are inversely proportional to their age and size, their metabolic vulnerability to stress may be less than in adults who begin in a state of nitrogen equilibrium.

C. Response to bodily injury in a child is extremely variable and is primarily dependent on age, degree of organ maturity, underlying nutritional status and the severity of the traumatic insult.

D. The acute metabolic response to injury or stress is catabolism. It involves the mobilization and utilization of endogenous substrates (protein, fat, and carbohydrates) rather than tissue deposition and growth.[4]

E. Respiratory quotients indicate that the proportion of macronutrient utilization/expenditure during childhood stress is approximately 33% from carbohydrate, 53% from fat and 14% from protein oxidation[5], in contrast to normal substrate utilization of approximately 55% carbohydrate and 30% fat.

F. Early "overnutrition" or "overfeeding," particularly with excessive concentrations of carbohydrate, may jeopardize the subsequent hospital course.[4] Studies using indirect calorimetry in critically ill pediatric patients indicate that the percent of energy from carbohydrate is lower than previously predicted.[5,6]

G. Over-feeding with carbohydrate in the face of insulin resistance and compensatory gluconeogenesis may lead to hyperglycemia, hypertriglyceridemia and hyperosmolality.[4] Recent reports indicate that critically ill infants and children who demonstrated early and sustained hyperglycemia > 126 mg/dL (7 mM/L) had a 3 fold risk of mortality over those with well controlled glycemia.[7]

III. Nutritional Assessment in Pediatric Patients with ARF

A. Nutritional assessment in ARF patients uses standard approaches described in Chapter 1.

B. Of particular importance is itemization of fluid intake and output with a relative "balance" estimate. This is used in conjunction with the clinical assessment of current whole body fluid status.

C. Laboratory data at initial assessment should include the BUN, Scr, electrolytes, calcium and phosphorus, total protein and serum albumin, lactic acid and magnesium.

D. See Table 24-1 for the Pediatric Intensive Care Global Nutritional Assessment

IV. Nutritional Goals and Requirements

A. Maintain adequate hydration and avoid "over-hydration" or dehydration
B. Establish and maintain acid-base equilibrium
C. Establish and maintain electrolyte and bone-mineral balance
D. Assess and reverse the catabolic stress (negative nitrogen balance)
E. Provide "co-factors" of metabolism
F. Avoid "toxic" overload of macro and/or micro-nutrients
G. Meet energy needs.

TABLE 24-1. Pediatric Intensive Care Global Nutritional Assessment Used in ARF

Age	Parameter	Notations	
Primary Diagnosis			
Time in ICU		**Yes**	**No**
Co-Morbid Profile	ARF		
	Anemia		
	Sepsis		
	Edema		
	Surgery/Trauma		
Output	Urine		
	Stool		
	Emesis/NG		
	Ostomy		
	Dialysis		
Fluid Intake	Enteral		
	Intravenous (PN+IV)		
	Crystalloid		
	Colloid		
Fluid Balance			
Nutritional Assessment	General Physical Exam		
	Estimated Wt/Ht SDS		
	Albumin;Pre-Albumin		
	Na+, K+, Cl-, Ca++, P, Mg++		
	BUN, Scr		
	Serum Bicarbonate		
	Lactate:Pyruvate		
	mNB (Urea Kinetics)		
Nutritional Intake	Enteral		
	CHO		
	Protein		
	Fat		
	Parenteral		
	CHO		
	Protein		
	Fat		

(*Continued*)

TABLE 24-1. Pediatric Intensive Care Global Nutritional Assessment Used in ARF (*Continued*)

Assessment Summary
Dialysis Plans
Enteral Feedings
Parenteral Nutrition
______________________ Signature

1. Formulas commonly used to predict resting energy expenditure (REE) with modifications for stress factors in critically ill pediatric patients have been shown to be unreliable.[4] Indirect calorimetry, when available, gives valuable insight into individual patient requirements.
2. Carbohydrate-The utilization of carbohydrate (CHO) is unpredictable in critically ill infants and children, making glucose monitoring extremely important. Although hypoglycemia may occur, the pediatric patient more often exhibits intolerance to rapid glucose infusions resulting in potentially lethal hyperglycemia and hyperosmolality.[7] Insulin infusions may be required to maintain normoglycemia.

H. Protein

1. A dietary protein prescription at the higher end of the recommendation for infants and toddlers is appropriate (Table 24-2) with a goal of maintaining the serum albumin > 3 g/L and BUN > 50 and < 60 mg/dL.
2. Nitrogen Balance-Adjusted Protein Catabolic Rate. In renal failure, protein nitrogen requirements are typically estimated from urea nitrogen appearance.[6] The recently published Kidney Disease Outcomes Quality Initiative (K/DOQI)[2,8] now term this *normalized Protein Nitrogen Appearance* (nPNA).
3. During ARF without dialysis, endogenous catabolic nitrogen is estimated by urea kinetics (change in total body urea nitrogen plus total urinary urea nitrogen). This must be added to any urinary protein or total nitrogen losses, which may be extreme if the nephrotic syndrome, proteinuria (>1 $g/m^2/day$) is present.
4. Impact of dialytic modality on nutrition
   a) All dialytic modalities, including peritoneal (PD), hemodialysis (HD), and continuous renal replacement therapy (CRRT) or continuous veno-venous hemofiltration (CVVH), result in increased nitrogen and micronutrient losses.[9–13]
   b) Peritoneal Dialysis.
      (1) Advantages of PD include slower osmolar fluid shifts and avoidance of the dialysis disequilibrium syndrome.[11] While PD imposes a greater loss of proteins through the dialysate than HD, it is often the only feasible modality for small infants with ARF. Protein loss is inversely related to body size. A general estimate is 10 grams per liter of ultrafiltrate per treatment.[13] In infants and children, 1 to 4 grams/kg/day of protein losses must be added to the total daily protein intake.
      (2) The energy from dialysate glucose should be included in the total carbohydrate intake in patients treated with PD.

TABLE 24-2. Recommended Protein Intake(s) and Estimated Losses During Dialysis Treatments

Age (Weight Range)	RDI	Est'd PD Losses	Est'd HD Losses	Est'd CRRT Losses	Daily PI Goal
Infant Size Age <2 Yrs (≤10 kg)	1.6–2.2	2.0-4.0	0.5–1.0	2.0–3.0	2.0–6.0
Small Child Age 1–6 Yrs (>10 ≤ 25 kg)	1.0–1.2	2.0-3.0	0.5–1.0	2.0–3.0	1.0–3.0
Older Child Age 7-14 Yrs (>25 ≤ 40 Kg)	0.8–1.2	1.0-2.0	0.5–1.0	2.0–3.0	1.0–2.0
Adolescent Age 15-21 Yrs (>40 ≤ 70 kg)	0.8–1.0	1.0-2.0	0.5–1.0	2.0–3.0	1.0–2.0

Values are expressed as grams of Protein / kilogram / day. RDI = Recommended dietary intake for normal children.[20] Estimated losses by peritoneal dialysis (PD) vary widely and are inversely related to size. Estimated losses by hemodialysis are per treatment and are relatively stable according to size. There are no definitive data regarding protein requirements for children on dialysis, especially small children. Individualized recommendations for protein intakes of children with renal failure are best determined by estimated losses and modified nitrogen balance (mNB) studies. The broad "goal" is to maintain the blood urea nitrogen (BUN) >40 mg/dl < 80 mg/dl.

Peritoneal dialysate glucose absorption increases total energy intake by 7 to 10 kcal/kg/day. Too often, infants on chronic PD accumulate excessive fat mass due to supplementation with non-protein calories and inadequate protein intake relative to losses through the PD.

c) Hemodialysis and CRRT
   (1) When dialytic or ultrafiltration treatment is required, dialysate nitrogen losses must be estimated for dialysis modality and added to the nitrogen requirements. Nitrogen loss during HD is primarily free amino acids during the 2 to 3 hours of treatment and accounts for 3 to 12% of the patient's daily protein requirement.[10,11] This is equivalent to as much as 0.1 to 0.3 g/kg/treatment of protein as amino acids.[13]
   (2) Continuous veno-venous hemofiltration and/or dialysis (CVVHD) entails continuous loss of plasma free amino acids, as well as all unbound nutritional cofactors in plasma water. Because of the associated nitrogen losses, when CVVHD is maintained for greater than 24 hours, it should be accompanied by continuous parenteral nutrition via a separate central venous or through a port beyond the replacement port to maintain a positive nutritional status.[12]

5. Urea kinetics
   a) Following urea kinetics allows assessment of protein nitrogen balance as well as dialysis efficiency (Table 24-3). Adjustment of pediatric dialysis prescriptions, particularly in ARF, requires careful attention to avoiding the acute disequilibrium syndrome which is acute brain swelling following too rapid lowering of plasma osmolality by rapid hemodialysis solute removal. Urea kinetics are used to estimate nitrogen balance (NB) from the following equation:

$$NB = NI - \left[\Delta V_{urea} + (U + PD)_{urea} + (U + PD)_{protein}/6.25\right]$$

   where NI is nitrogen intake from parenteral or dietary intake, ΔV is change in total body urea in 24 hours. The V is calculated as 60 to 70% of total body weight. U is 24 hour urine. If the patient is being treated with PD, the 24 hour peritoneal dialysate is assayed for total urea and protein nitrogen. Estimates of proteinuria are made from 24 hour urine protein determinations or spot urine protein to creatinine ratios (Up/c). The Up/c estimates daily proteinuria in $g/m^2/day$.[14] This number, in turn, is adjusted to "nitrogen" by dividing by the factor 6.25. For the NB assessment, results are reported in grams per kilogram per day. These calculations are provided in Table 24-3.
   b) In summary, the calculation involves an estimate of nitrogen intake from dietary / nutritional intake minus the total nitrogen output which includes the urea nitrogen generation (urine urea nitrogen, total body urea nitrogen appearance, dialysate urea nitrogen clearances) plus total protein losses from urine and/or dialysate corrected for nitrogen content (i.e., total protein/ 6.25 g/gram nitrogen).

6. Protein:energy ratio. Few studies are available that allow estimation of optimal protein:energy ratio in critically ill children. Standard maintenance diets provide a total energy (calories)-to-nitrogen (g) ratio of 250. In metabolic studies, the mean ratio achieving nitrogen balance is lower, averaging 193 ± 96 or approximately 13% of calories from protein.[4]
7. Adjustment of protein dose based on Blood Urea Nitrogen
   a) A rapid assessment of protein catabolic rate, especially in children, can be made from blood urea nitrogen (BUN), *not* the BUN to creatinine ratio. Infants and children with unusual physical stress, such as those undergoing visceral transplants, trauma or infection, for example with the Human Immuno-

TABLE 24-3. Formulae for Calculating Nitrogen Parameters in Pediatric Patients With ARF

	Formula	Normal Values
Creatinine Clearance[1] (Ccr)	Ccr = Ht(cm)*k ÷ Scr k = 0.35 (infant); 0.55 (child); 0.75 (adolescent male)	95–110 mL/min/1.73m²
Oliguria (Inadequate or low urine output)	<0.5 to 1 mL/kg/hr	10kg > 500 mL/d (>2 mL/kg/hr) 20kg > 750 mL/d (>1.5 mL/kg/hr) 30kg > 875 mL/d (>1.2 mL/kg/hr) 50kg > 1000 mL/d (>1 mL/kg/hr)
Modified Nitrogen Balance (mNB) Pre-Dialysis or HD	mNB = NI – [Δ Vurea + Uurea] + Uprotein/6.25	Zero to 0.3 gram N/kg/d (2 grams Protein/kg/d) ; Never negative
Modified Nitrogen Balance (mNB) for PD	mNB = NI – [Δ Vurea + (U + PD)urea + (U + PD)protein/6.25]	
V = Est'd Total Body Water	60 to 70% of Body Weight (kg = liters)	Higher estimate recommended in ill patients.
Kt/Vurea		
Hemodialysis (HD)	Kt/V = 1.2 [–Ln R] Ln = Natural log R = Post/Pre plasma BUN ratio	Goal Kt/V > 1.3
Peritoneal Dialysis (PD)	K = PD urea × Dialysate Volume [Initial Drain + (Infusion Volume × Cycles) + Ultrafiltrate Volume] ÷ Plasma urea t = time (days) V = Body Weight (kg) × 0.7	Wide Variation: CAPD: Kt/V = 1.75 to 2.0 CPPD: Kt/V = 2.0 to 2.5 per week

deficiency Virus (HIV), may be chronically malnourished with wasted muscle mass and will have a low serum creatinine. These patients often have subclinical renal disease and are sensitive to the effects of endogenous catabolism, as well as excessive nitrogen administered either enterally or parenterally. A safe target is to limit the protein to energy ratio to that which will maintain the BUN > 50 and < 60 mg/dL. This is usually of 10–15% of total energy as protein. If the BUN jumps quickly to > 100 mg/dL, the protein content of the PN can be cut in half for a brief period, then increased as possible to maintain $S_{Alb} > 3.0$ g/dL.

b) It is well established that a *low* pre-dialysis BUN (< 50 mg/dL) reflects an increased risk of mortality associated with poor or inadequate protein intake, regardless of dialysis modality. This same premise seems applicable in children with ARF who are not on dialysis, even in those who seem to have a relatively large fat mass (as in infants or obese adolescents).

I. Fluid and Solute Requirements-Ongoing losses from naso-gastric drainage or from diuresis that frequently occur in the *recovery phase* should be replaced with solutions matching the concentrations of sodium (Na^+) to the total from chloride (Cl^-), bicarbonate (HCO_3^-), or acetate. Anuric (no urine flow) or oliguric (< 0.5–1 mL/kg/hr) patients are likely to require restriction of fluids. If parenteral fluids are required for resuscitation or as vehicles for medications, they should contain at least 60 to 140 mEq/L of Na+ to prevent dilutional hyponatremia. As with adults, limiting fluids or nutritional support in an effort to delay the need for dialysis is usually unsuccessful and is not recommended.

V. Enteral Nutritional Support

A. Enteral supplements and food feedings used in ARF are included in the Table 24-4.

B. Carbohydrate supplements, polymerized glucose, have traditionally been added to oral and enteral feedings. They contribute to carbohydrate "overfeeding," particularly in patients on PD who absorb the glucose from the dialysate solutions. These supplements are discouraged, particularly if dialysis therapy is to continue for longer than 2 weeks.

C. Fat supplementation to provide energy and essential fatty acids may include long-chain fats and medium chain triglycerides (MCT). These preparations can contribute significantly to the overall energy content of the diet. Eicosapentanoic acid (EPA) and fish oils are potentially therapeutic entities for renal injury and repair.[15]

D. Protein supplementation should be closely monitored and adjusted on a daily basis until the patient demonstrates some degree of stability. As nitrogen balance becomes positive, requirements for minerals increase, such as potassium and phosphate, which are used in protein and lean tissue synthesis. Protein supplements are usually required in infants and children on PD.

TABLE 24-4. Commercial Enteral Preparations Used in ARF[21–24]

Indication(s)	Description	Examples
Infant Formulas		
Decreased Renal Function	Whey: Casein (approximately 60 : 40) Ca:P (2 : 1)	Similac PM 60:40 Premature Formula
Pediatric Enteral Formulas (1–10 Years)		
Decreased Kidney Function	2 Kcal/cc, lactose free, 7.5 g/dL Protein	Magnacal Renal
	2 Kcal/cc, lactose free, 7 g/dL Protein	Nepro; Nutrirenal
	2 Kcal/cc, lactose free, low Vit A,D, Phos, 3 g/dL Protein	Suplena
	2 Kcal/cc, semi-elemental, lactose free, low electrolytes, 3.4 g/dL Protein	Renalcal

E. Phosphate binders (calcium carbonate, calcium acetate, sevelamer) may be added to the feedings to help maintain normal phosphate levels.[16]

VI. Parenteral Nutritional Support in Pediatric ARF

A. Hemofiltration (CVVH) offers an exceptional, effective modality for treatment of prolonged ARF with anuria/oliguria, intractable lactic acidosis, and/or hepato- renal syndrome. Once the patient becomes metabolically stable, continuous parenteral nutrition can be administered at physiologic rates of glucose administration through the post-filter port of the CVVH circuit. Although this avoids the need for a second central venous catheter, the risk of sudden loss of dextrose infusion due to catheter clotting should be considered.

B. Micronutrient Requirements

1. Electrolytes, Minerals and Trace elements.

a) Sodium, chloride, and bicarbonate. These three electrolytes are the main components of plasma electroneutrality and tonicity. Narrow limits (within 5 mEq/L) should be maintained for each of these according to the following ratios ($Na:Cl:HCO_3::135:105:25$) with no more than 5 mEq/L of unmeasured anion. When preparing the prescription for PN or CVVH replacement fluids, these ratios should always be maintained. Infants and stressed children *do not* metabolize lactate to bicarbonate in a predictable fashion. For this reason, we do not recommend the use of Lactated Ringer's solution for fluid resuscitation or any parenteral solutions containing lactate as the primary buffer. This includes CVVH replacement solutions and/or dialysate solutions. Only acetate and bicarbonate are used in such solutions.

b) Potassium. Potassium intake is essential for cell anabolism but can become lethal during periods of ARF and catabolic stress. For this reason, potassium supplementation is withheld during ARF until a stable anabolic process is confirmed. This is usually simultaneous with a concurrent fall in serum phosphorus. Transient falls in serum potassium to < 3.0 mEq/L are common following dialysis (with 0 to 2 mEq/L dialysate bath) and are routinely followed by a "rebound" phenomenon. If these levels are treated aggressively with "bolus" potassium, the consequences may be lethal. Therefore, we recommend *not* to treat any potassium level ≥ 2.0 mEq/L, unless it is sustained and/or associated with electrocardiographic (EKG) evidence of arrhythmia. Hyperkalemia (≥ 6.0 mEq/L) should be treated with kayexalate resin as a retention enema or mixed with enteral feedings if possible. The dose is 0.5 to 1 gram/kg as necessary 1 to 3 times daily. When mixed with sorbitol, it causes diarrhea and has been associated with bowel necrosis. The powdered form of kayexalate may thicken in the intestine and, in the presence of other products, cause constipation and bezoars. This can be avoided by mixing the resin with the liquid formula, allowing it to settle, then decanting the formula from the residue.[17]

c) Calcium and phosphorus. The serum Ca × P product in ARF is extremely labile, particularly in infants and during parenteral alimentation. Too often, only the serum Ca is measured and both Ca and P are added to the PN solution. With small amounts of intravenous P, the serum P will rise and cause the serum Ca to fall precipitously causing seizures or tetany. The rapid correction of the serum Ca with IV calcium chloride ($CaCl_2$) may cause acute intravascular and intrapulmonary calcifications when the serum P is ≥ 7 mg/dL. It is imperative to always monitor the Ca × P product in ARF in children. *Do not add phosphorus to the PN solution until the serum P is ≤ 4 mg/dL. Never infuse $CaCl_2$* solution with a serum P ≥ 7 mg/dL.

d) Iron deficiency is a common complication of patients undergoing treatment for ARF and is multifactorial. Intravenous supplementation is *not* recommended due to frequent hypersensitivity reactions and its association with septicemia.

e) Magnesium (Mg). Although Mg is essential for intermediary metabolism, it accumulates rapidly with ARF. Supplementation should be cautious and monitored by serum levels. Infants are especially prone to toxicity.

f) Trace Elements—These micronutrients are key elements in immune and antioxidant defenses and are rapidly depleted in critically ill patients, especially those undergoing dialysis or CRRT.[18] Please see Table 24-5 for age and size adjusted recommendations for parenteral nutritions solutions.

2. Vitamins

a) Water soluble

(1) Folate and B_{12} are frequently low and require supplementation. Oral supplementation 400 µg to 1 mg/day of folate in pediatric patients with ARF is recommended. B_{12} is poorly absorbed in patients with ARF due to achlorhydria. Supplementation is recommended. (See Tables 24-5 and 24-6).

(2) Vitamin B_6 (pyridoxine) is lost during dialysis treatment and is an important co-factor in protein metabolism. Its deficiency has been associated with seizures in infants and children. Supplementation is recommended. (See Tables 24-5 and 25-6).

(3) Thiamine (B_1) and riboflavin (B_2) are also lost in dialysis and are important co-factors in carbohydrate and protein metabolism.

TABLE 24-5 Components of Pediatric Parenteral Nutrition Formulations[18–22]

	Weight		
Components	**≤10 Kg**	**10–20 Kg**	**>20 Kg**
Fluid Maintenance	100–150 ml/kg	1000 ml + 50 ml/kg >10 Kg	1500 ml + 25 ml/Kg >20 Kg
Dextrose (3.4 kcal/gram) Grams/Kg/day	10–25	8–20	5–20
Amino Acid (+Losses) 1 gram=0.16 gram nitrogen	1.6–2.2	1–1.2	0.8–1.2
Fat (Lipids) (grams/Kg/day)	0.5–4	1–3	1–3
Total Calories (Kcal/kg/day)	75–110	50–80	30–70
Sodium (mEq/Kg/day) Not to exceed 152 mEq/L	2–4	2–3	2–3
Potassium (mEq/Kg/day) Not to exceed 40 mEq/L	0–3	0–3	0–2
Bicarbonate or acetate mEq/Kg/day	1–3	1–2	1–2
Vitamins and Trace Minerals			
Pediatric MVI (See Table 24-6)	2 ml/day	2-5 ml/day	5 ml/day
Zinc	0.2 mg/kg/day		Adult Dose 5 mg
Copper	20 μg/kg/day		Adult Dose 2 mg
Manganese	5 μg/kg/day		Adult Dose 500 μg
Chromium	0.2 μg/kg/day		Adult Dose 20 μg
Selenium	2 μg/kg	2 μg/kg/day (Maximum 30 μg/day)	

(4) Vitamin C, a water soluble vitamin, is metabolized to oxalate which accumulates in tissues of patients with chronic kidney disease (CKD) but this is not documented in ARF patients. Dialysis patients may become deficient without minimal supplementation. Supplement at no more than the recommended dietary intake (RDI) of 60 mg/day. (See Tables 24-5 and 24-6).

b) Fat soluble vitamins are potentially toxic since they are not dialyzed and may accumulate in CKD. If ARF is not prolonged (i.e., > 2 weeks), supplementation is usually recommended. (See Tables 24-5 and 24-6).

(1) Vitamin A is decreased in ARF and requires supplementation.

(2) Vitamin E in ARF is decreased and may require supplementation. It may improve leg cramping but may also increase blood clotting. Supplementation is recommended.

(3) Vitamin D. $25(OH)D_2$ and $1,25(OH)_2D_2$ are the hydroxylated derivatives of calciferol. The vitamin is actually a hormone that requires hydroxylation in the liver after sterol isomerization in the skin by the sun. The most active form is $1,25(OH)_2D$, calcitriol, which has been hydroxylated in the kidney. Any renal injury, acidosis, or fluctuation(s) in the Ca × P product with parathyroid hormone (PTH) can markedly alter the production of calcitriol. Supplementation is not within the nutritional prescription. Dosing and administration must be a component of the medical management of Ca × P and intact PTH (iPTH) levels.

(4) Vitamin K, synthesized by intestinal bacteria, may be compromised in children with renal failure, especially during antibiotic therapy. Supplementation is recommended.

3. Other Micronutrients and supplements. Carnitine deficiency occurs in all dialyzed patients. It is easily supplemented either

TABLE 24-6 Oral Vitamin & Mineral Supplements for Pediatric Patients With ARF

Supplement	Recommendation	Dose & Formulation[20-24]	Parenteral Pediatric MVI/ 5 ml
Vitamin A	Caution	Not to Exceed RDA*	0.7 mg (2300 IU)
Vitamin E	Caution	Not to Exceed RDA*	7 mg (7 IU)
Vitamin D	Cholecalciferol	400 µg /day; calcitriol separate from nutritional prescription	10 µg (400 IU)
Vitamin C	Caution	≤60 mg/ day	80 mg
Thiamine (B1)	Recommended	0.2 to 1.0 mg/day	1.2 mg
Riboflavin (B2)	Recommended	0.3 to 1.0 mg/day	1.4 mg
Pyridoxine (B6)	Recommended	6.25 to 50 mg/day	1 mg
Folate	Recommended	0.4 to 1.0 mg/day	140 µg
Vitamin K	Caution	5 to 60 µg/day	200 µg
Vitamin B12	Recommended	0.5 to 2.5 µg/day	1 µg
Carnitine	50–300 mg/kg/day	Levocarnitine (Carnitor) 330 mg/cap (or 1 gram/10 mL PO/IV)	Separate Additive

RDA* Recommended Dietary Allowances for Age

orally or parenterally and is well tolerated.[18] Supplementation is recommended.

WEB RESOURCE

National Kidney Foundation's Kidney Disease Outcomes Quality Initiative http://www.kidney.org/professionals/kdoqi/guidelines_updates/doqi_nut..html

(Pediatric renal chapter from the 1st edition was contributed by Robert Wolk, Rowena Stokowski, and Peter Yorgin)

REFERENCES

1. Schwartz GJ, Brion LP, Spitzer A. The use of plasma creatinine concentration for estimating glomerular filtration rate in infants, children, and adolescents. *Pediatr. Clin. North Am.* 1987;34:571–590.
2. Hogg RJ, Furth S, Lemley KV, et al. National Kidney Foundation's Kidney Disease Outcomes Quality Initiative. Clinical practice guidelines for chronic kidney disease in children and adolescents: evaluation, classification, and stratification. *Pediatrics.* 2003;111(6 Pt 1):1416–1421.
3. Drukker A, Guignard JP. Renal aspects of the term and preterm infant: a selective update. *Curr Opin Pediatr.* 2002,14(2):175–182.
4. Chwals WJ. Overfeeding the critically ill child: fact or fantasy? *New Horizons.* 2:147–155, 1994.
5. Coss-Bu JA, Jefferson LS, Walding D, David Y, Smith O, Klish W. Resting energy expenditure in children in a pediatric intensive care unit: Comparison of Harris-Benedict and Talbot predictions with indirect calorimetry values. *Am J Clin Nutr.* 1998;67:74–80.
6. Coss-Bu J, Jefferson L, Walding D, David Y, Smith O, Klish W. Resting energy expenditure and nitrogen balance in critically ill pediatric patients on mechanical ventilation. *Nutrition* 1998;14:649–652.
7. Srinivasan V, Spinella PC, Drott HR, Roth CL, Helfaer MA, Nadkarni V. Association of timing, duration, and intensity of hyperglycemia with intensive care unit mortality in critically ill children. *Pediatr Crit Care Med.* 2004;5(4): 1–17.
8. K/DOQI Clinical Practice Guidelines for Nutrition in Chronic Renal Failure. *Am J Kidney Dis.* 2000;35(S2):S17–S104.
9. Wassner SJ, Sanders R, Orloff S, Sheldon GF, Holliday MA. A comparison of essential and general amino acid infusions in protein-depleted patients receiving parenteral alimentation. *Am J Clin Nutr.* 1979;32: 1497–1504.
10. Abitbol CL, Mrozinska K, Mandel S, McVicar M, Wapnir RA. Effects of amino acid additives during hemodialysis of children. *J Parenter Enteral Nutr.* 1984;8(1):25–26.
11. Ikizler TA, Flakoll PJ, Parker RA, et al. Amino acid and albumin losses during hemodialysis. *Kidney Int.* 1994;46: 830–837.
12. Maxvold N, Smoyer W, Custer J, Bunchman T. Amino acid loss and nitrogen balance in critically ill children with acute renal failure: A prospective comparison between classic hemofiltration and hemofiltration with dialysis. *Crit Care Med.* 2000;28:1161–1165.
13. Quan A, Baum M. Protein losses in children on continuous cycler peritoneal dialysis. *Pediatr Nephrol.* 1996;10:728–731.
14. Abitbol C, Zilleruelo G, Freundlich M, Strauss J. Quantitation of proteinuria with urinary protein/creatinine ratios and random testing with dipsticks in nephrotic children. *J Pediatr.* 1990;116:243–247.

15. Kielar ML, Jeyarajah DR, Zhou XJ, Lu CY. Docosahexaenoic acid ameliorates murine ischemic acute renal failure and prevents increases in mRNA abundance for both TNF-alpha and inducible nitric oxide synthase. *J Am Soc Nephrol.* 2003;14:389–96.
16. Mahdavi H, Kuizon BD, Gales B, Wang HJ, Elashoff RM, Salusky IB. Sevelamer hydrochloride: an effective phosphate binder in dialyzed children. *Pediatr Nephrol.* 2003;18:1260–1264.
17. Fassinger N, Dabbagh S, Mukhopadhyay S, Lee DY. Mineral content of infant formula after treatment with sodium polystyrene sulfonate or calcium polystyrene sulfonate. *Adv Perit Dial.* 1998;14:274–7.
18. Druml W. Nutritional management of acute renal failure. *Am J Kid Dis.* 2001;37(1): S89–S94.
19. Evangeliou A, Vlassopoulos D. Carnitine metabolism and deficit—when supplementation is necessary? *Curr Pharm Biotechnol.* 2003;4(3):211–219.
20. Yates AA, Schlicker SA, Suitor CW. Dietary Reference Intakes: The new basis for recommendations for calcium and related nutrients, B vitamins, and choline. *J Am Diet Assoc.* 1999;98:699–706.
21. Committee on Nutrition, American Academy of Pediatrics. *Pediatric Nutrition Handbook (ed 5).* pp 391–403, 643–652, 921–929, 1032–1057, 1140–1142, 2004.
22. Makoff R, Micronutrient requirements in dialysis patients. Parts 1 & 2. HDCN. ASN 2002 Renal Week_Philadelphia, PA_Congress of Nephrology.htm
23. Makoff R. Water-soluble vitamin status in patients with renal disease treated with hemodialysis or peritoneal dialysis. *J Renal Nutr.* 1991;1: 56–73.
24. Malone A. The clinical benefits and efficacy of using specialized enteral feeding formulas. *Support Line.* 2002;24:3–11. 2002.

Michele M. Gottschlich, PhD, RD;
Theresa Mayes, RD

25

Burns

Introduction

Nutrition support following burns represents a unique challenge because of the complex interactions of injury, organ function, wound healing, and immunocompetence. Nutrition is an important effector of each of these events, and in burn patients, inefficient diet therapy will exacerbate pathophysiologic abnormalities and catabolic sequelae, such as erosion of lean body mass, bone, and blood proteins. The clinician is therefore faced with important decisions regarding what and how to feed burn patients. This chapter outlines the impact of acute thermal injury on metabolism and nutritional needs. Options for nutrient delivery as well as guidelines for nutrition assessment and monitoring are presented.

I. Pathophysiology of Burns

A. Physical destruction of the skin
   1. The severity of a burn is measured by evaluating the surface area involved and the depth of the tissue destroyed. These two parameters successfully predict outcome and determine metabolic arrangements and therapeutic interventions. The size of a burn injury is expressed as a percentage of the total body surface area (TBSA). Burn size is classified using the rule of nines or, more accurately in children, using the Lund and Browder chart.[1]
   2. Burns are also classified by the depth of skin injury (Figure 25-1). First degree burns affect the epidermal layers of the skin. Second degree burns involve the epidermis and some of the dermis. Third degree (full thickness) burns destroy all layers of the skin.

B. Metabolic response[2–5]
   1. The early phase of burn injury is characterized by a decrease in cardiac output, oxygen consumption, and resting energy expenditure. This is similar to the response observed following other traumatic injuries. After resuscitation, a hypermetabolic response is observed and includes increased oxygen consumption, cardiac output, and metabolic rate.
   2. Large thermal injuries cause the greatest degree of hypermetabolism of all stress states. This metabolic response is proportional to the extent of the burn injury. Other factors that contribute to hypermetabolism include fever, sepsis, surgery, environmental temperature, physical activity, and medications. Metabolic rate increases and peaks approximately 5–12 days postburn. Catecholamines may be an important stimulus for increased oxygen consumption and increased energy needs.
   3. Hypermetabolic responses continue throughout the course of burn recovery. Patients are in a net whole-body protein catabolic state with protein anabolism increased approximately one-third above normal and protein catabolism increased two-thirds above normal. Extensive nitrogen losses occur from burn wound exudate as well as in the urine, both of which can result in massive daily nitrogen losses. In the first week postburn, protein losses are particularly high, and then slowly decrease over the course of convalescence. Abnormal protein loss is not observed once wounds and donor sites have healed.
   4. The metabolic response to thermal injury results is increased glucose production from gluconeogenesis in response to the altered hormonal and inflammatory mediator environment. The burn wound itself metabolizes large quantities of glucose via anaerobic glycolytic pathways, producing large amounts of lactic acid as an end product. Support of gluconeogenesis requires accelerated net protein catabolism and movement of amino acids from the periphery to the viscera.

II. Energy and Nutrient Requirements of Burn Patients

A. Energy requirements are heightened postburn; therefore, adequate (but not excessive) calories should be provided. Nutrition intervention is designed to provide adequate amounts of protein and calories to burn patients. Inadequate interventions result in over- or under-feeding, both of which can harm the patient. Metabolic needs are difficult to predict; therefore, numerous formulas are used to estimate energy needs in burn patients.[6–10] Most take into account weight and percentage of total body surface area burned; formulas may also include factors such as patient age and activity. Mathematical equations for estimating the energy requirements of pediatric and adult burn patients are listed in Table 25-1. Whenever possible, indirect calorimetry should be used to better assess caloric needs.[2] A factor of 20–30% above the measured energy expenditure is commonly added to account for increased energy demands from physical therapy along with the stresses of wound care.[5]

B. Immediately after thermal injury, fluid, electrolytes and protein escape from the vascular compartment to the interstitial area surrounding the burn wound. As a consequence, prompt provision of intravenous fluid resuscitation is required to restore tissue blood flow and to prevent shock. The most popular fluid replacement formula is the Parkland formula,[11] which must be modified for children, who require more fluid per square meter of body surface area than adults with burns.[12]

C. As protein is essential for wound healing, close attention should be paid to protein status.[2] Protein losses may be massive in burned patients secondary to both increases in net whole body catabolism

FIGURE 25-1. Interpretation of burn classification based on damage to the integument.

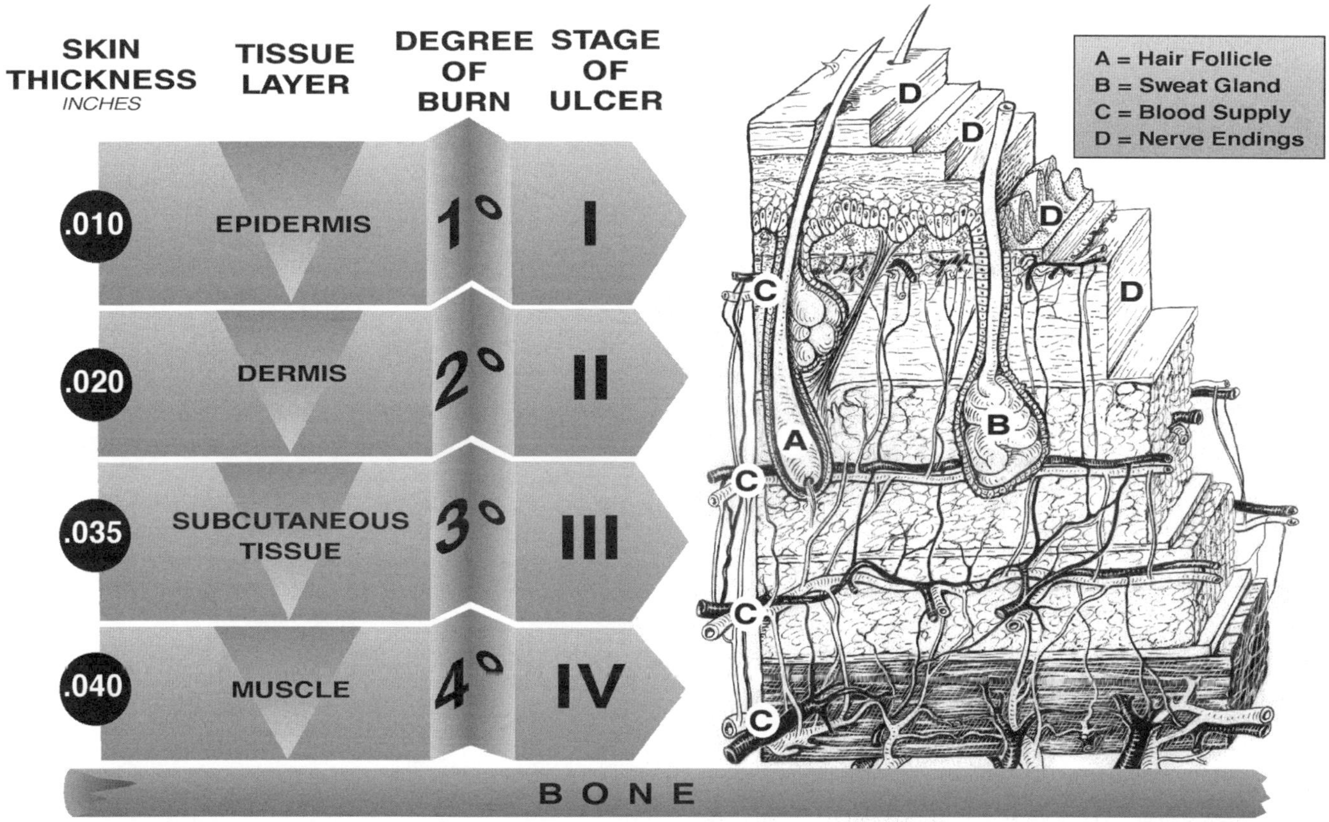

Reprinted from Mayes T, Gottschlich MM. Burns. In: *Contemporary Nutrition Support Practice.* Matarese L, Gottschlich MM, eds. Philadelphia, PA: WB Saunders Co; 2003:595–615, with permission from Elsevier.

and protein loss from the burn wound itself. Protein needs are higher in burn patients than in other stress states and should compose approximately 20 to 25% of total calorie needs.[5,9,13] Most burn patients require protein intake of 1.5 to 2 g/kg/d depending on the size of the burn. Some practitioners use 1.5 g/kg/d for burn wounds that cover <20% of body surface area and 2.0 g/kg/d for wounds that cover >20% body surface area.

D. Carbohydrates have a protein-sparing effect in the postburn patient and therefore should comprise approximately 60% of the energy provided. Over-feeding of carbohydrates, however, can lead to hepatic steatosis and increased carbon dioxide production. Therefore, in the adult burn patient, it is recommended that glucose administration not exceed 5 mg/kg/min.

E. Although lipid is calorically dense, its administration in excessive amounts can lead to side effects including immunosuppression. Modest use of fat is recommended in burn patients, and diets containing 15 to 20% of calories as fat may be optimal.

F. Burned individuals also have increased vitamin and mineral needs. Current knowledge supports administration of daily multivitamins until wound healing has been achieved.[5] Vitamin A, which is important for maintaining the immunologic response and for epithelialization of wounds, should approximate 5000 IU per 1000 kcal of enteral nutrition. Vitamin C is a coenzyme that is important for collagen synthesis and immune function and should be provided at a dose of 500 mg twice daily. Zinc is a cofactor in energy and protein metabolism and should be supplemented at a dose of 220 mg of zinc sulfate per day. In addition, burn patients may benefit from further supplementation with vitamins D, K and folic acid; however, specific intake guidelines do not yet exist.[14–17]

III. Nutritional Therapy for Burn Patients

A. Nutritional intervention should be initiated as soon as the patient is stabilized from the initial burn and other associated injuries.

B. Nutrition support of the burn patient has changed substantially over the past 30 years. It was routine in the 1970s to use parenteral nutrition (PN) as a means of providing the large calorie and protein loads that are required by burn patients. It is now clear that PN offers no advantage. In addition, the high incidence of septic complications, mucosal atrophy, and expense associated with PN,[2,18] has led many clinicians to restrict its use to supporting those burn patients with severe diarrhea, gastrointestinal dysfunction, or intra-abdominal pathology.

C. Nutrient delivery is best accomplished enterally.[2] A high calorie, high protein oral diet may be sufficient to meet needs in patients with burns <20% surface area. However, patients with larger burns and those presenting with facial injury, inhalation injury, psychological difficulties, or preburn malnutrition generally require a feeding tube to ensure adequacy of intake. Gastric ileus, which limits use of the stomach for enteral nutrition, is common and often resurfaces with surgery, sepsis, major dressing changes, or other complications. As such, transpyloric feedings are commonly used in an effort to avoid the necessity for tube feeding interruptions.[19]

TABLE 25-1. Formulae for Calculating Energy Requirements of Pediatric and Adult Burn Patients

Reference	Age (yr)	% BSAB	Calories per day
Curreri[6]	0–1 yr	<50	Basal + (15 × % BSAB)
	1–3 yr	<50	Basal + (25 × % BSAB)
	4–15 yr	<50	Basal + (25 × % BSAB)
	16–59 yr	Any	(25 × W) + (40 × % BSAB)
	>60 yr	Any	Basal + (65 × % BSAB)
	Adult	Any	20/kg + 70% BSAB
Davies and Liljdahl[21]	>60 yr	Any	Basal + (65 × % BSAB)
	Adult	Any	20/kg + 35% BSAB
	Child	Any	60/kg + 35% BSAB
Long modification of the Harris-Benedict equation[20]	Male	Any	(66.47 + 13.7W + 5H – 6.76A) × (activity factor) × (injury factor)
	Female	Any	(655.1 + 9.56W + 1.85 – 6.68A) × (activity factor) × (injury factor)
Hildreth[7]	<15 yr	>30	(1800/m² BSA) + (2200/m² burn)
Hildreth[7]	<12 yr		(1800/m² BSA) + (1300/m² burn)
Mayes[8]	<3 yr	10–50	108 + 68W + 3.9 × % BSAB
	5–10 yr	10–50	818 + 37.4W + 9.3 × % BSAB

BMR, basal metabolic rate; BSA, body surface area; BSAB, body surface area burned; W, weight in kg; A, age in years; H, height in cm.

Activity factor:
(a) confined to bed, use 1.2
(b) out of bed, use 1.3

Injury factor:
(a) severe burn, use 2.0

D. Provision of adequate nutrition can attenuate whole-body catabolism but rarely prevents or reverses loss of lean body mass by conventional management principles. This has led to the adjunctive use of anabolic agents such as growth hormone and oxandrolone in critically ill burn patients.[20] Clinical benefits reportedly include increased healing rate and decreased length of hospital stay and mortality. Clinical risks include hyperglycemia and increased mortality (growth hormone) and nausea and virilism (oxandralone).

IV. Nutrition Assessment and Management of Burn Patients[5,21]

A. Regular assessment of the appropriateness of nutrition intervention should continue until achievement of 95% wound closure at a minimum.

B. Tables 25-2 and 25-3 summarize guidelines for initial, daily, weekly, and discharge evaluation of nutrition status. The initial nutrition assessment (Table 25-2) determines the appropriate route of feeding, formula selection, and nutrition goals. The purpose of nutrition reassessment (Table 25-3) is to track restoration and maintenance of nutrition stores due to their importance for wound healing and immunity.

C. Energy and protein from enteral and parenteral sources should be calculated daily. Cumulative caloric balance ([current 24-hour caloric intake – measured energy expenditure × 1.3] + cumulative caloric balance from the previous day) should be evaluated daily. A cumulative balance within +/– 7000 calories over a patient's hospital course is desirable.

D. Gastrointestinal tolerance of enteral feedings is monitored daily. Periodic, non-infectious diarrhea is often successfully managed by the use of scheduled constipating medications (consider a combination of an anti-motility and bulking agent) without compromising the patient's infusion rate or concentration of tube feeding.

E. The clinical dynamics of the burn patient fluctuate daily. These alterations influence nutrition status and thus the appropriateness of the care plan. Daily monitoring of changes in medications, infectious episodes, surgical needs, and respiratory status dictate adjustments in nutrition goals and methods of therapy.

F. Burn patients commonly experience hypophosphatemia, hypomagnesemia, and hypocalcemia. Serum electrolytes and minerals should be routinely monitored in patients with burns in excess of 25% TBSA. Intravenous supplementation via maintenance fluid adjustment is most effective in stabilizing levels.

G. Adequacy of protein intake in burn patients can be determined by serial measurements of nitrogen balance using the following formula:

$$\text{Nitrogen balance} = \text{nitrogen intake} - (\text{total urinary nitrogen} + \text{fecal nitrogen loss} + \text{burn wound nitrogen loss})$$

where all of the above parameters are measured in grams per 24 hours. The collection of wound exudate, however, is not routinely practiced and, therefore, many clinicians estimate wound nitrogen losses as follows:

$\leq$10% open wound = 0.02 g of nitrogen per kg of body weight per day

TABLE 25-2. Acute Burns—Guidelines for Initial Nutrition Assessment

Collect objective data	Obtain appropriate histories	Determine preburn nutritional status	Calculate	Determine appropriate route of feeding	Initiate assessment tools
Age Total percent body surface area burn Body areas burned Inhalation injury Ventilatory status Gastric decompression initiated Anthropometrics: • Weight • Height/length • Head circumference (≤3 yrs)	Past medical history Social history Concomitant injuries Routine medications Diet history Referring hospital course, as applicable	Usual food intake protein needs Food preferences Food restrictions/ allergies Dentition Appetite Vitamin/mineral supplementation	Calorie and protein needs Vitamin/mineral supplementation recommendations Weight percentage: • Percent ideal body weight • NCHS* percentile (≤18 years)	Oral Nasoenteral Parenteral	Obtain indirect calorimetry measurement within 24 hours of admission Begin 24-hour urinary urea collection for nitrogen balance determination Obtain nutrition labs (transferrin and prealbumin) Begin monitoring calorie and protein intake

*NCHS, National Center for Health Statistics

Reprinted with permission from Mayes T, Gottschlich MM. Burns and Wound Healing. In: Gottschlich MM. *The Science and Practice of Nutrition Support A Case-Based Core Curriculum.* Silver Spring, MD: A.S.P.E.N.; 2001:391–419 with permission from the American Society for Parenteral and Enteral Nutrition (A.S.P.E.N.).

TABLE 25-3. Acute Burns—Recommendations for Nutrition Reassessment

Daily	Weekly	Upon discharge
Calorie and protein intake Labs: • Albumin • BUN/creatinine • Glucose • Electrolytes • Nitrogen balance Tolerance (nausea, vomiting, distention, diarrhea, constipation) Clinical course (sepsis, infection, surgeries, fluid status, medications, respiratory status) Appropriateness of diet, enteral or parenteral alimentation order	Weight (once edema resolved) Transferrin Prealbumin Nitrogen balance trend Wound healing (% open wound) Indirect calorimetry: • Resting energy expenditure • Respiratory quotient	Percent preburn weight at discharge Adequacy of oral intake Nutrition supplementation requirements Need for nutrition follow-up in the outpatient setting

BUN, blood urea nitrogen

Reprinted with permission from Mayes T, Gottschlich MM. Burns and Wound Healing. In: Gottschlich MM. *The Science and Practice of Nutrition Support A Case-Based Core Curriculum.* Silver Spring, MD: A.S.P.E.N.; 2001:391–419 with permission from the American Society for Parenteral and Enteral Nutrition (A.S.P.E.N.).

11% to 30% open wound = 0.05 g of nitrogen per kg of body weight per day

≥31% open wound = 0.12 g of nitrogen per kg of body weight per day

Fecal nitrogen losses can be estimated to be approximately 2–4 g/d. It should be noted that serial nitrogen balance measurements are more reliable, as individual 24-hour urine nitrogen contents may vary significantly. In the first 3 days postburn, nitrogen loss is very high and then decreases 4 to 16 days postburn. It should be realized that it is difficult, if not impossible, to achieve nitrogen equilibrium or a positive nitrogen balance in burn victims initially despite aggressive nutrition support.

H. Burn patients usually exhibit some degree of fluid retention. This normal postburn response interferes with the use of weight to assess nutritional or fluid status in the acute postburn phase. An admission weight, before the onset of edema, or reliable statement of preburn weight from the patient or family member, provides important baseline weight data. Resolution of edema may take weeks. Once this occurs, however, biweekly weight measurement and comparison to dry/preburn weight is essential. Achievement of 90% to 110% of preburn weight indicates optimal energy provision.

I. Assessment of visceral protein status should consist of weekly evaluation of either transferrin or prealbumin. Weekly trends of these biochemical indices provide insight as to the adequacy of protein provision.

J. Wound healing should be assessed weekly. This includes monitoring the healing status of partial thickness wounds and donor sites, as well as graft adherence.

K. Assessment of energy needs is guided by indirect calorimetry a minimum of once per week. Respiratory quotient (RQ) is a component of this test that further assists in determining the adequacy of nutrient provision. An RQ between 0.80 and 0.95 is indicative of appropriate substrate utilization.

L. Recent evidence suggests loss of bone mass postburn.[15,17] Dual energy X-ray densitometry (DEXA) can be used to monitor changes in bone mineral content as well as lean body and fat mass.

(Burns material from the 1st edition was contributed by Elaine B. Trujillo, Malcolm K. Robinson, and Danny O. Jacobs)

REFERENCES

1. Lund CC, Browder NC. The estimate of area of burns. *Surg Gynecol Obstet.* 1960;79:352–358.
2. ASPEN Board of Directors. Burns. In: August D, ed. Guidelines for the Use of Parenteral and Enteral Nutrition in Adult and Pediatric Patients. *J Parenteral Enteral Nutr.* 2002;26:88SA–90SA.
3. Mayes T, Gottschlich MM. Burns and wound healing. In: Gottschlich MM, ed. *The Science and Practice of Nutrition Support: A Case-based Core Curriculum.* Dubuque, IA: Kendall/Hunt Publishing Co; 2001:391–419.
4. Gottschlich MM, Mayes T. Nutrition support in the burned pediatric patient. In: Samour P, King K, Lang C, eds. *Handbook of Pediatric Nutrition.* 3rd ed. Boston: Jones & Bartlet; *in press.*
5. Mayes T, Gottschlich MM. Burns. In: *Contemporary Nutrition Support Practice.* L. Matarese L, Gottschlich MM, eds. Philadelphia, PA: WB Saunders Co; 2003:276–289.
6. Gottschlich MM, Ireton-Jones CS. The Curreri Formula: A landmark process for estimating the caloric needs of burn patients. *Nutr Clin Prac.* 2001;16:172–173.
7. Hildreth MA, Herndon DN, Desai MH, Duke MA. Caloric needs of adolescent patient with burns. *J Burn Care Rehabil.* 1989;10:523–526.
8. Mayes T, Gottschlich MM, Khoury J, Warden GD. An evaluation of predicted and measured energy requirements in burned children. *J Am Diet Assoc.* 1996;96:24–29.
9. Long CL, Schaffel N, Geiger JW. Metabolic response to injury and illness: Estimations of energy and protein needs from indirect calorimetry and nitrogen balance. *J Parenter Enteral Nutr.* 1979;3:452–456.
10. Davies JWL, Liljedahl SL. Metabolic consequences of an extensive burn. In: Polk HC, Stone HH, eds. *Contemporary Burn Management.* Boston: L Little, Brown & Co; 1971:151–169.
11. Baxter CR, Shires T. Physiologic response to crystalloid resuscitation in thermally injured children. *Ann NY Acad Sci.* 1968;150:874–894.
12. Merrell SW, Saffle JR, Sullivan JJ, Navar PD, Kravitz M, Warden GD. Fluid resuscitation in thermally injured children. *Am J Surg.* 1986;152:664–669.
13. Alexander JW, MacMillan BG, Stinnett JD, et al. Beneficial effects of aggressive protein feeding in severely burned children. *Ann Surg.* 1980;192: 505–517.
14. Gottschlich MM. Fat soluble vitamins in wound healing. In: Molnar JA, ed. *Nutrition in Wound Healing.* CRC Press; *in press.*
15. Gottschlich MM, Mayes T, Khoury J, Warden GD. Hypovitaminosis D in pediatric burn patients. *J Am Diet Assoc.* 2004;104:931–941.
16. Jenkins ME, Gottschlich MM, Kopcha R, Khoury J, Warden GD. A prospective analysis of serum vitamin K and dietary intake in severely burned pediatric patients. *J Burn Care Rehabil.* 1998;19:75–81.
17. Klein GL, Herndon DN, Rutan TC, et al. Bone disease in burn patients. *J Bone Miner Res.* 1993;8:337–345.
18. Herndon DN, Stein MD, Rutan TC, Abston S, Linares H. Failure of TPN supplementation to improve liver function, immunity and mortality in thermally injured patients. *J Trauma.* 1987;27:195–204.
19. Gottschlich MM, Jenkins ME, Mayes T, Khoury J, Warden GD. An evaluation of the safety of early versus delayed enteral support and effects on clinical, nutritional, and endocrine outcomes after severe burns. *J Burn Care Rehabil.* 2002;23:401–415.
20. Demling RH. Comparison of the anabolic effects and complications of human growth hormone and the testosterone analog, oxandrolone, after severe burn injury. *Burns.* 1999;25:215–221.
21. Mayes T, Gottschlich MM, Warden GD. Clinical nutrition protocols for continuous quality improvements in the outcomes of patients with burns. *J Burn Care Rehabil.* 1997;18:365–368.

Winston W. K. Koo, MB, BS, FRACP;
Kathleen McLaughlin, MS, RNC, NNP; and
May Saba, PharmD, BCNSP

26

Neonatal Intensive Care

Introduction

Nutrition support by the parenteral and/or enteral route is freely available in any neonatal intensive care unit (NICU) and plays an important role in the management of sick neonates and infants. It can reduce metabolic complications and minimize the interruption to normal growth. However, nutrition support is frequently applied inappropriately—that is, "too little too late" or "too much too quickly." The former often occurs when the infant is considered "too sick" or "too immature," and the latter often occurs when there is an unreasonable expectation that the effects of prior prolonged periods of inadequate nutritional support can be dramatically reversed. This overview, therefore, aims to provide a practical basis upon which optimal nutrition support can be provided to patients in the NICU, taking into account the unique challenges posed by the sick infant.

I. Special Considerations.

Nutrition support of sick infants, especially preterm infants, in the NICU must take into consideration the following issues:

A. Tissue stores of nutrients are rapidly depleted if exogenous nutrient intake is not begun immediately. The critical role of early complete nutrition support in minimizing potential problems is shown in Table 26-1.
B. The capacity of enzyme and organ systems is limited.
   1. Gastric capacity and intestinal motility may be limiting factors for the delivery, digestion, and absorption of nutrients.
   2. The limited capacity of enzyme systems can result in diminished tolerance of nutrients such as glucose and lipids.
   3. Limited organ function, for example, decreased renal capacity is associated with lower renal tubular glucose absorption and contributes to glucose intolerance.
   4. Neurobehavioral and neuromotor immaturity can impede normal nipple feeding.
   5. There is an increased risk for disease conditions associated with premature birth (e.g., respiratory distress syndrome, necrotizing enterocolitis).
C. Different problems are associated with underlying illnesses.
   1. Nutrient delivery needs to be tailored to the clinical situation and biochemical parameters. For example, if nipple feeding is unsuccessful, a different route of delivery for enteral nutrients or the use of parenteral nutrition (PN) may be needed. Different amounts or combinations of nutrients may be needed in renal or hepatic failure.
   2. Therapies for the illness may interfere with nutritional status.
      a) Long-term diuretic therapy results in increased loss of minerals and trace metals, nephrocalcinosis, and metabolic bone disease.
      b) Corticosteroid therapy to shorten the duration of mechanical ventilator support can result in negative nitrogen balance, delayed growth, glucose intolerance, and possibly bone demineralization and neurodevelopment impairment.
      c) Bowel resection decreases the mucosal area for digestion and absorption of nutrients and fluid.
   3. After resolution of the acute illness, catch-up growth needs to occur.
D. Nutrition support has several phases (Table 26-2). Metabolic response in the critically ill infant is proportional to the degree of stress and involves an increase in the turnover of proteins, fats, and carbohydrates. The resting energy expenditure is high, with protein degradation rates elevated out of proportion to synthetic rates, and resultant negative protein balance. Appropriately designed nutritional support that has a mixed fuel system and is replete in protein does not quell this metabolic response. However, it can minimize the morbidity and mortality associated with depletion of the limited body stores of nutrients and may result in anabolism and continued growth at a rate appropriate to the gender and gestational and postnatal age. Therefore, no infant is too sick to receive nutrition support. It is a matter of whether the nutrients are delivered parenterally or enterally and the composition of the formulation.

II. Parenteral Nutrition

A. Indications. PN can be used as the sole source of complete nutrition support for infants who cannot be fed enterally or as an adjunct to enteral feeding. In sick infants, PN allows prompt resumption of growth and expedites the transition to full-volume enteral feeding by providing supplemental nutrition while enteral tolerance is reduced. Any infant unable to tolerate adequate enteral feeding for more than 2 or 3 days should receive PN support. However, to optimize nutritional support and minimize complications, PN and/or enteral nutrition (EN) should begin within 24 hours after birth.[1–4]
B. Preparation. Because of stability and sterility issues[5] and the need for adjustments to various nutrient components during the initial phase of nutrition support, PN solutions are usually prepared daily for infants in the NICU. See Table 26-3 for PN macronutrient recommendations for neonates. Major groups of nutrients include the following:
   1. Protein
      a) During the immediate newborn period, sick infants, especially preterm infants, may not tolerate standard amounts of nutrients normally delivered to clinically stable infants and may not tolerate adequate energy intakes for optimal utilization of amino

TABLE 26-1. Nutritional Issues in the NICU*

Problem**	Potential solutions
Low tissue energy store	Multiple sources of energy (carbohydrate, fat, protein) from PN or EN
Obligatory tissue (protein) catabolism ≥ 0.5 g/kg/d	Adequate protein and energy intake from PN or EN
Essential fatty acid deficiency	Essential fatty acids and adequate energy intake from PN or EN
Disturbance to circulating concentrations of electrolytes (sodium, potassium, chloride) and minerals (calcium, magnesium, phosphorus) and hydrogen ion	PN or EN with some modifications as necessary
Hyperbilirubinemia	EN to decrease enterohepatic circulation of bilirubin
Glucose intolerance	Complete nutrition support, including nutrients such as thiamine and chromium from PN or EN
Delayed tolerance to full enteral feeding	PN plus trophic feeding
Incomplete catch-up growth and development	Early complete nutrition support

EN, enteral nutrition; NICU, neonatal intensive care unit; PN, parenteral nutrition
* For neonates unable to receive adequate enteral feeding, the use of parenteral dextrose (+/– electrolytes) and water should be limited to the brief period pending the routine availability of PN.
** Pathogenesis begins at birth.

acids. The administration of glucose alone may result in hyperglycemia and cannot fully prevent tissue catabolism. Early administration of protein as amino acids may decrease the risk for hyperglycemia and promote nitrogen retention. The usual starting dose for amino acids is 1 to 2 g/kg/day. The dose is increased by similar amounts each day to the desired goal, depending on the weight of the infant. Generally, the extremely low birth weight (ELBW, birth weight up to 1 kg) infant may require up to 3.5 to 4 g/kg/day, the very low birth weight (VLBW, birth weight up to 1.5 kg) infant may require up to 3 to 3.5 g/kg/day, and the term infant may require up to 2–3 g/kg/day.[1–4,6] Once EN is started, the volume (and therefore the amount) of nutrients from PN is correspondingly decreased.

b) Commercial amino acid solutions used for infants are formulated to result in plasma amino acid profiles comparable to those of breast-fed infants. Like human milk, these "pediatric" amino acid formulations contain taurine, tyrosine, histidine, aspartic acid, and glutamic acid. They contain lower concentrations of glycine, methionine, and phenylalanine than the amino acid preparations intended for older patients. Preparations with other sources of nitrogen, including dipeptides, are under study.

c) Cysteine (a conditional essential amino acid for infants that also enhances calcium and phosphorus solubility), glutamine (a primary fuel for enterocytes, lymphocytes, and macrophages as well as a precursor for nucleotides and glutathione), and carnitine (required for optimal metabolism of fatty acids) are not currently included in commercial pediatric amino acid formulations because of problems with short shelf life and uncertain efficacy. Cysteine hydrochloride can be added to PN infusate at a dose of 40 mg/g of amino acids.

d) Carnitine can be added to PN infusate in varying amounts depending on institutional practice (see Section II.B.2.b).

e) Glutamine supplement to PN is not recommended. Glutamine at a dose of 20% of total amino acids of PN had no effect on decreasing mortality, late-onset sepsis or necrotizing enterocolitis, or improving tolerance of enteral feeds or growth in ELBW infants.[7]

2. Energy. Carbohydrate and lipid emulsion are the major sources of energy used in PN. Provision of adequate energy is essential for optimal use of other nutrients for tissue synthesis and growth. Energy requirements are influenced by many factors. Factors that increase energy requirements include prematurity (increased absorptive loss and heat loss), preexisting nutritional status (small for gestational age versus appropriately grown infants), physiologic stress (fever, sepsis, respiratory failure, etc), type (enteral (versus parenteral) nutrients have absorptive loss) and method of feeding (nipple versus gavage feeding), and rate of growth (tissue synthesis).[8] Preterm infants receiving an energy intake as low as 70 kcal/kg/d can achieve positive nitrogen balance[9] because there is no absorptive or digestive loss of energy with PN. In the presence of adequate protein intake, adequate weight gain occurs at a parenteral energy intake of 80 to 130 kcal/kg/day. Excessive energy intake is associated with increased fat deposition and greater carbon dioxide production, which further complicates any underlying respiratory illness.[10,11]

a) Carbohydrate

(1) Dextrose, hydrated glucose solution, is the standard source of carbohydrate used in PN. It may be initiated at a rate of about 4 to 8 mg/kg/min. This is comparable to the range of endogenous glucose production rate in clinically stable infants.[12,13] Normally, dextrose can be started at 10% concentration, which delivers a glucose load of ~7 mg/kg/min at 100 mL/kg/d. However, immediately after birth or during acute stress events such as sepsis or corticosteroid therapy, the sick or preterm infant may tolerate <5% dextrose solution, which provides a much lower glucose infusion rate. Dextrose concentration can be increased gradually at about 2.5g/100 mL per day to deliver a load of 12 to 14 mg/kg/min. For infants who need PN after a period of adequate enteral feeding, a PN infusate containing 10% or 12.5% dextrose can be used from the onset, provided the blood glucose is normal.

(2) A trace amount of glucosuria is not uncommon in critically ill infants, although glucosuria of >1% is of concern and the rate of glucose infusion may need to be decreased. The use

TABLE 26-2. Phases of Nutrition Support for Critically Ill Infants

Phase	Duration*	Primary Source of Nutrient	Goal
Immediate newborn period and during acute illness	Days to weeks	Parenteral nutrition**	Minimize catabolism. Begin nutrition support within 24 hours after birth. Aim to maintain normal biochemical status and some somatic growth, if possible.
Later neonatal period and during hospitalization	Weeks to months	Enteral nutrition***	"Catch-up" growth. Aim to reach normal centile channel for gestation and postnatal age.
Post–hospital discharge	Months to years	Enteral nutrition****	Slower growth rate than phase 2 but still may require additional nutrients. Aim to achieve growth rate comparable to postmenstrual age–matched infants born at term.

* May vary somewhat depending on the extent of functional immaturity and the course of underlying illness.
** Most critically ill infants require a period of PN during the transition to full enteral feeding.
*** Term infants require human (own mother's) milk or standard infant formula. Preterm infants require human milk with fortifier or specifically designed preterm formulas.
**** Ad libitum breast-feeding or standard formula. Preterm infants may require additional supplementation or use of specific postdischarge infant formula.

TABLE 26-3. Recommendations for Parenteral Nutrition Macronutrients for Neonates

Source	Initiation	Advancement	Goal	Neonate	Blood or plasma monitoring
Amino acids	1.5–2 g/kg/d	0.5–1 g/kg/d	2–3 g/kg/d	Term	BUN, ammonia, arterial pH
	1.5–2 g/kg/d	0.5–1 g/kg/d	3.5–4 g/kg/d	ELBW	
	1 g/kg/d	0.25–0.5 g/kg/d	3–4 g/kg/d	Septic, hypoxic	Lactate concentration
Dextrose	8 mg/kg/min	1–3 mg/kg/min	12–14 mg/kg/min*	≥1 kg	Glucose <150 mg/dL
	6 mg/kg/min	1–3 mg/kg/min	12–14 mg/kg/min	<1 kg	Glucose <125 mg/dL
Fat	1–2 g/kg/d	0.5–1 g/kg/d	3 g/kg/d**	Term	Triglycerides <200 mg/dL*** and ****
	0.5–1 g/kg/d	0.25–1 g/kg/d	3 g/kg/d	Preterm	Bilirubin, glucose
	0.5 g/kg/d*****	0–0.5 g/kg/d	1–2 g/kg/d	Hyperbilirubinemic****** Sepsis Severe respiratory distress	Bilirubin*******
Energy			90–108 kcal/kg/d	Term	
			100–120 kcal/kg/d	Preterm	
Fluid			130–150 mL/kg/d	Term	
			130–180 mL/kg/d	Preterm	

BUN, blood urea nitrogen; ELBW, extremely low birth weight; FFA, free fatty acids
* Maximum recommended upper limit for glucose intake.
** May consider slightly higher dose in growth failure.
*** Heparin 1 unit per milliliter parenteral nutrition solution improves lipid clearance.
**** IV fat emulsion infusion over 24 hours maximizes clearance.
***** Minimum fat needed to prevent essential fatty acid deficiency.
****** Bilirubin approaching exchange transfusion levels.
******* IV lipid dose can be increased to normal range when bilirubin is below 50% of exchange level and when sepsis and respiratory distress is under adequate control
Adapted from: A.S.P.E.N. Board of Directors and the Clinical Guidelines Task Force. Guidelines for the use of parenteral and enteral nutrition in adult and pediatric patients. *J Parenter Enteral Nutr.* 2002;26(1 suppl):1SA–138SA with permission.
Nash MA. The management of fluid and electrolyte disorders in the neonate. *Clin Perinatol.* 1981;8:251–262 with permission.
Table 26-3 adapted from work contributed by Gordon Sacks, Susan Mayhew, and Debbie Johnson.

of insulin to treat hyperglycemia and promote growth in infants is not well established. Insulin infusion at 0.05 unit/kg/hr[14] has been associated with the development of lactic acidosis. However, bolus doses of crystalline insulin may be useful to treat persistent hyperglycemia (blood glucose >200 mg/dL) after lowering the dextrose concentration. In our experience, 0.05 to 0.1 unit/kg of crystalline insulin as an intravenous bolus may be effective as an initial dose. Repeated monitoring of blood glucose and acid-base status at 1- to 4-hour intervals is needed to determine whether there is a further need for insulin. Insulin administration should be discontinued when the blood glucose is <100 mg/dL. It is important to monitor for and manage other conditions (e.g., sepsis) that could contribute to hyperglycemia.

b) Fat emulsions. Available commercial fat emulsions provide a source of concentrated calories and prevent essential fatty acid deficiency (EFAD). Fat emulsions are isotonic. When fat and amino acid–dextrose solutions are infused simultaneously into the same vessel, the patient receives a higher energy and lower osmolar solution (which helps spare peripheral veins from thrombophlebitis) than with amino acid–dextrose alone. Commercial fat emulsion is available as 10% (1.1 kcal/mL) and 20% (2 kcal/mL) soy or soy-safflower oil. These preparations contain >40% by weight linoleic acid and >4% by weight linolenic acid. The use of 20% emulsion is preferred since it is more energy-dense and contains the same amount of phospholipid (1.2% by weight) and same osmolarity as the 10% emulsion. Phospholipid is believed to inhibit lipoprotein lipase, the main enzyme for intravenous lipid clearance. Newer lipid preparations not available in North America include those containing structured triglycerides (mixture of long- and medium-chain fatty acids on a glycerol backbone) and water-soluble short-chain triglycerides, which may have some metabolic advantages compared with the available lipid emulsions with long-chain triglycerides. However, none of the fat preparations appear to be able to support the normal rate of intrauterine accumulation of very long chain polyunsaturated fatty acids of the n-3 and n-6 families in developing infant tissues.

Administration of fat emulsion in an energy-deficient state may not adequately prevent development of EFAD because EFAs can be oxidized to meet energy needs. However, in the presence of adequate energy intake, a minimum of 0.5 to 1 g/kg/d of commercial fat emulsion containing the C18 fatty acids, linoleic acid, and linolenic acid is needed to prevent clinical EFA deficiency. Fat emulsion can be started on the first day of PN at 0.5 to 1 g/kg/d and increased by a similar amount daily up to 3 g/kg/d. To maximize lipid clearance, the daily amount of fat emulsion is generally infused over 18 to 24 hours. Smaller increments and lower total dose may be prudent for acutely ill or ELBW infants.

Jaundice and sepsis are not absolute contraindications to the use of fat emulsions. The dose probably should be in the range of 1 to 2 g/kg/d if serum bilirubin is near the exchange level[15] and during the acute phase of sepsis. Parenteral fat can be increased to the normal dose once the serum bilirubin or sepsis is controlled.

Carnitine plays an essential role in the metabolism of long-chain fatty acids. However, no convincing evidence of clinical benefit has been demonstrated in infants receiving carnitine-supplemented PN; specifically, there was no evidence of effect on weight gain, lipid utilization, or ketogenesis.[16] Nevertheless, since both breast milk and infant formulas contain carnitine, infants who received PN without carnitine have very low tissue levels of carnitine. Since fatty acid oxidation is impaired when the tissue carnitine levels fall below 10% of normal, it seems reasonable to provide L-carnitine at 2 to 10 mg/kg/d. This approximates the amount provided in human milk and the in utero rates of tissue carnitine accretion. There is no evidence that pharmacological concentrations of carnitine provide greater benefit in infants in the absence of (rare) metabolic defects of carnitine metabolism.

3. Electrolytes and minerals
   a) Sodium and potassium are available as chloride, acetate, and phosphate salts. During the first one to two days after birth, parenteral nutrition for small preterm infants need not contain potassium until regular urine output is assured; and sodium phosphate can be used as the only source of sodium. The latter practice allows the flexibility to use small amounts of sodium bicarbonate as needed and minimizes the risk of hypernatremia if there is high insensible loss of water. The normal range of maintenance intake for sodium and potassium is 2 to 4 mEq/kg/d.
   b) Calcium is usually delivered as 10% calcium gluconate. Phosphorus is added as either a sodium or a potassium salt. During the first one to two days after birth, the parenteral nutrition for small preterm infants may contain about half the maintenance phosphorus content to minimize the risk for hyperphosphatemia. Sodium phosphate is preferred unless there is a risk for hypernatremia. Potassium phosphate can be used in the presence of adequate urine output. Maintenance calcium and phosphorus are usually added at 500 to 600 mg of elemental calcium per L and 350 to 500 mg of elemental phosphorus per L of PN at a weight ratio of ~1.3 to 1.7:1 (or 1 to 1.3:1 by molar ratio). The ability to maintain calcium and phosphorus solubility in PN solution depends on a number of factors, particularly the type and amount of amino acid and the presence of cysteine. The amount of calcium and phosphorus delivered in PN is several times greater than that absorbed from human milk.
   c) Magnesium is usually added to PN at 25 to 50 mg/L of elemental magnesium. The amount of magnesium may need to be decreased in sick infants with impaired renal function or transiently withheld or provided in a lower amount for infants whose mothers received intrapartum magnesium sulfate infusion.
   d) Chloride and other anions are normally provided in sufficient quantities if the minerals or cations are given in the recommended amounts. Current commercial amino acid preparations for infants contained minimal amount of chloride at 0.46 to 0.97 mEq per gram of amino acid. Some clinicians also use small amounts of acetate (10–20 mEq/L PN solution) as part of anion intake and as a source of base to lower the risk of metabolic acidosis.
   e) Supplemental iron usually is not provided with PN for patients in the NICU. However, if PN is provided exclusively for >2 months after birth or if iron deficiency develops, parenteral iron can be administered at 0.1 to 0.2 mg/kg/d, up to as high as 10 mg/kg/d.[17] Three parenteral products are currently available in the United States: iron dextran, sodium ferric gluconate complex in sucrose, and iron sucrose. Except for iron dextran, the experience with use of iron products in children is extremely limited.
4. Trace minerals. Trace mineral preparations are commercially available as single agents or as combinations of various trace min-

erals. There is no compelling reason to avoid providing trace minerals for infants requiring short- term PN, and they probably should be provided from initiation of PN. Recommended normal daily trace mineral intakes are the same for preterm and term infants, except for zinc. Recommended intakes are as follows: chromium 0.2 mcg/kg; copper 20 mcg/kg; iodide 1 mcg/kg; manganese 1 mcg/kg; molybdenum 0.25 mcg/kg; and selenium 2 mcg/kg.[4] Zinc dosing for preterm infants is 400 mcg/kg; for term infants <3 months, 250 mcg/kg; and at >3 months, 100 mcg/kg. The use of both single and combination trace mineral preparations is usually needed to provide the recommended doses. Most institutions provide PN solutions containing chromium, copper, manganese, selenium, and zinc.

5. Multivitamins. Two commercial multivitamin products are available for use in infants. Both products have the same contents in the same concentration. Neither provides the exact range of estimated needs for all vitamins,[4] and none of the several recommended dosages has been demonstrated to be superior for sick infants. The manufacturers recommended that for infants weighing <1 kg, 1 to 3 kg, and >3 kg, the intake should be 30%, 65%, and 100% of a 5-mL vial. The American Academy of Pediatrics[4] recommends 2 mL/kg/day up to one vial (5 mL) of multivitamins. The American Society of Clinical Nutrition[18] recommends 40% of a 5-mL vial (2 mL) to patients less than 2.5 kg, and one vial (5 mL) to patients >2.5 kg up to 11 years.

C. Delivery
1. Peripheral or central catheters
   a) Peripheral catheter. To minimize thrombophlebitis, only PN solutions with amino acids and a <12.5% concentration of dextrose are delivered via a peripheral intravenous catheter.[4] Coinfusion of fat emulsions reduces the degree of venous irritation.
   b) Central catheter. Higher dextrose concentrations (>12.5%) can be delivered through the central catheter to a large vessel with high blood flow. Insertion of the catheter into the central venous system by cutdown, percutaneously, or through the umbilical artery or vein is widely used in neonates. Central catheter placement must be confirmed by x-ray before infusion of PN solution.
2. Volume. The delivery of adequate amounts of nutrients parenterally often is limited by the amount of fluid that the sick infant needs or can tolerate. In situations of severe fluid restriction, the concentration of all nutrients must be increased, resulting in extremely high osmolarity and possibly exceeding the limits of solubility of calcium and phosphorus salts. In contrast, in situations of high fluid requirements (>200 mL/kg/d) in preterm infants with low renal thresholds for many nutrients, a diluted infusate must be provided to prevent delivery of excessive nutrients, particularly dextrose. Normally, adequate amounts of parenteral nutrients can be delivered in a total volume of 120 to 160 mL/kg/d. Some flexibility in the tolerance to the volume infused can be achieved by manipulating environmental factors. For example, caring for the neonate under a radiant warmer results in greater insensible fluid loss, thus allowing delivery of a larger volume of PN (Table 26-4).
3. Infusion rate. In the NICU, amino acid–dextrose solution is infused continuously over 24 hours to improve tolerance, particularly if higher concentrations of dextrose are used. Fat emulsion is also better tolerated if infused over 18 to 24 hours each day. Infusing fat emulsion over about 18 hours allows the measurement of plasma triglyceride level immediately prior to the next day's infusion, which makes it possible to determine tolerance to fat emulsion without concern about interference from the triglyceride content of the lipid emulsion.

TABLE 26-4. Factors Affecting Water Requirements[19]

Environmental Factors	Infant Factors
Factors increasing water requirements	
Radiant warmers	Physiologic
Conventional single-walled isolette	Increased permeability of the skin
	Larger body surface area relative to body weight
Phototherapy	Increased blood flow to the skin
Ambient temperature above the neutral thermal range	Pathologic
	Increased respiratory distress
	Elevated body temperature
	Glycosuria with osmotic diuresis
	Gastric or intestinal losses
Factors decreasing water requirements	
Thermal blankets	Physiologic
Double-walled isolette	Increasing gestation and postmenstrual age
Above-ambient humidity	Pathologic
	Renal oliguria

Adapted from Doyle LW, Sinclair JC. Insensible water loss in newborn infants. *Clin Perinatol.* 1982;9:453–482, with permission from Elsevier.

4. A 2-in-1 versus a 3-in-1 solution. The amino acid–dextrose solution and lipid emulsion can be provided separately as a 2-in-1 solution and delivered together through a Y connector to the peripheral or central venous catheter or through umbilical venous or arterial catheters. In some institutions, PN is delivered as a total nutrient admixture (TNA) or 3-in-1 solution (i.e., mixing all nutrient components in the same container). The disadvantages of TNA in the NICU are that the stability of each component of TNA is not completely defined, it is impossible to determine whether there is a precipitation of nutrients in the admixture, and a 1.2 micron filter must be used instead of the standard 0.22 micron bacterial filter. TNA also may be a better bacteria growth medium than amino acid–dextrose solution.[4]
5. Light exposure. Amino acid–dextrose solution containing vitamins and other additives and lipid emulsion should be protected from direct exposure to phototherapy light to avoid photodegradation. Some NICUs routinely protect PN infusate from exposure to ambient light.

D. Monitoring (see Tables 26-3 and 26-5).

E. Complications. The potential complications of PN are all seen in the NICU patient.
1. Mechanical
   a) Kinking, compression, or tearing of the catheter can occur with all central catheters, but the thin-walled percutaneously inserted Silastic catheters used in neonates appear to be more prone to kinking and compression. Pneumothorax and brachial plexus injury may complicate the percutaneous insertion of a subclavian catheter.
   b) Catheter occlusions presumed to be associated with thromboses are treated with 0.25 to 2 mg (0.25–2 mL) of tissue plasminogen activator (tPA) or 5000 units (1 mL) of urokinase instilled

TABLE 26-5. Guidelines for Metabolic Monitoring During Parenteral Nutrition

Variable to Be Monitored	Initial Period*	Later Period**
Growth***		
• Weight	Daily	Daily
• Head circumference	Baseline	Twice weekly
• Length	Baseline	Weekly
Intake and output	Every shift	Daily
Glucose reagent strips	1 to 3 times/day	As indicated
Serum electrolytes, urea nitrogen, creatinine	Baseline and every 1 to 3 days	Every 1 to 2 weeks
Serum calcium, magnesium, phosphorus	Baseline and every 2 to 3 days	Every 1 to 2 weeks
Serum triglycerides****	Daily during dose increase	Every 1 to 2 weeks
Serum glucose	As needed	As needed
Total and direct bilirubin	Baseline, as needed clinically	Every 1 to 2 weeks
Total protein and albumin	Baseline	Every 2 to 3 weeks
Alanine aminotransferase, aspartate amino-transferase, and alkaline phosphatase	Baseline	Every 2 to 3 weeks
Complete blood cell count	Baseline	Every 2 to 3 weeks
Vitamin and trace mineral status and other specific tests	As indicated	As indicated

*The period before reaching maximum doses of glucose, amino acids, and lipid emulsion, or during any period of metabolic instability. This period normally lasts 3 to 4 days.

**The period during which the patient is in a metabolic steady state. For clinically stable infants receiving the desired intake of nutrients, the interval between laboratory measurements may be increased beyond the above recommendations.

***All measurements should be plotted on growth charts appropriate for sex, gestation[62] and postnatal[63] age. Growth charts based on postnatal growth of preterm infants are biased for nutritional management regimens and should not be used.

****Target level <200 mg/dL.

in the catheter for 30 to 60 minutes; then the blood and tPA or urokinase is aspirated from the catheter. This may be repeated once. For chemical (e.g., calcium phosphate) or medication precipitate, 0.1N hydrochloric acid (HCl) (1 mL) or 0.1N sodium hydroxide (NaOH) (1 mL) may be used with the same technique. For lipid-related occlusion in TNA, 70% ethanol (1 mL) may be used with the same technique. Some clinicians flush tPA or urokinase through the catheter to gain patency of the catheter. In infants, experience with the use of these agents as therapy for catheter occlusion, particularly for the percutaneous Silastic catheter, is limited.

c) Extravasation of nutrient infusate into interstitial space resulting in skin slough is a frequent complication associated with the use of peripheral intravenous catheters in infants. This complication can be reduced by meticulous observation of the catheter insertion site and removal of the catheter at the first sign of swelling or thrombophlebitis. Extravasation of nutrient infusate into the pleural or pericardial space occurs rarely but may be associated with acute metabolic (decreased plasma glucose), circulatory, or respiratory compromise requiring symptomatic support, including drainage of the fluid.

2. Sepsis
   a) Source identification. Sources of infection can be catheter related, involving the catheter insertion site, the subcutaneous tunnel, or line sepsis (see Chapter 8). Non-catheter-related sources of sepsis should also be considered.
   b) Diagnosis. Cultures of blood drawn from the catheter, a non-catheterized blood vessel, and obvious sites of septic foci are needed.
   c) Therapy. Empiric antibiotic therapy should be started whenever sepsis is suspected (e.g., sudden, unexpected glucose intolerance or temperature instability). Initial therapy should be based on the clinical status of the neonate and the antibiotic sensitivities of microbial organisms prevalent in the NICU. Antibiotics should be adjusted on the basis of culture results. Catheter removal is indicated if sepsis is not promptly resolved. Some clinicians recommend immediate catheter removal if there is evidence of a fungal infection or some gram- negative rods such as Klebsiella. Antibiotic lock and antimicrobial- impregnated central venous catheters are not routinely used in NICU patients.
3. Metabolic. Most metabolic complications are related to excessive, imbalanced, or inadequate intake.[1] A recent shortage of multivitamin preparations resulted in more than 30 cases of vitamin deficiency.[20]
   a) Glucose disturbances. Hyperglycemia from excessive glucose load or during short-term stress such as sepsis may result in glucosuria, osmotic diuresis, and dehydration. Treatment of the underlying cause, a decrease in glucose load, and even the use of insulin for brief periods may be needed to correct hyperglycemia. Hypoglycemia may occur with abrupt discontinuation of lipid-free PN containing >12.5% dextrose.
   b) Hypertriglyceridemia. Plasma triglyceride >200 mg/dL may occur during lipid infusion. The infusion of lipids over 18 to 24 hours and the use of heparin in a dose of 1 unit/mL may increase lipid clearance. The latter increases lipoprotein lipase activity. The use of carnitine may be beneficial in clearing triglycerides.
   c) Mineral (calcium, phosphorus, magnesium), blood urea nitrogen (BUN), and acid-base disturbances. Hyper- or hypocalcemia and hyper- or hypophosphatemia can result from

excessive or inadequate infusion of these minerals. In addition, phosphate deficiency with hypophosphatemia and secondary parathyroid hormone resistance can cause hypercalcemia even in the presence of low calcium intake.[21] Phosphorus must be added to the PN if serum phosphorus is <4 mg/dL during infancy. Hyperphosphatemia (and secondary hypocalcemia) may occur in preterm infants receiving high phosphorus intake because of limited renal excretory capacity. Adjustments may be needed for one or both minerals. Hyper- or hypomagnesemia can result from excessive intake or inadequate renal excretory capacity, or inadequate intake or replacement of gastrointestinal losses.[22]

d) The potential for metabolic acidosis is higher during the immediate newborn period and during acute stress. Abnormal serum chloride levels from inappropriate intake or inadequate replacement of losses can be associated with metabolic acidosis or alkalosis.

e) Increased BUN or plasma ammonia has been reported only in infants who received >4 g protein/kg/d and from the use of earlier amino acid preparations.[4] Starvation and tissue catabolism is a more likely cause of raised BUN in the absence of documented renal failure. Underlying disease processes also may result in disturbances of acid-base status. Occasionally, symptomatic treatment of metabolic acidosis with sodium or potassium acetate and treatment of metabolic alkalosis with sodium or potassium chloride may be appropriate.

f) Decreased nutrient availability. Decreased nutrient availability may result from adsorption to delivery systems (e.g., insulin, vitamin A), light (especially phototherapy) degradation (e.g., tryptophan, methionine, histidine, riboflavin, vitamin A), and increased nutrient loss (e.g., electrolyte, mineral, or trace metal loss from loop diuretics and to a lesser extent from thiazide diuretics; potassium and magnesium loss with amphotericin B).

g) Toxic products. Toxic products in PN can be found as contaminants of nutrients or from exposure to the environment during preparation, storage, or delivery to the patient.
   (1) Aluminum is the best-studied contaminant of parenteral nutrients. Aluminum has no known physiologic role, and preterm infants and infants with severe renal impairment are at risk for aluminum toxicity. Many nutrient components of PN are contaminated with aluminum, and the same nutrients from different manufacturers can have different degrees of aluminum contamination.[23] Calcium salts alone accounted for >80% of the total aluminum load from PN.[23] The Food and Drug Administration has labeling requirements concerning aluminum contents on all PN components, and efforts should be made to use products with the lowest aluminum contamination.
   (2) Formation of toxic lipid peroxidation products is also of potential concern. Ambient and especially phototherapy light increase peroxidation of fatty acids lipid emulsion to form lipid hydroperoxides[24] and also increase hydrogen peroxide generation from multivitamins, in particular the riboflavin in amino acid–dextrose solutions.[25]

f) PN flush solutions and drug-nutrient interactions. All medications not compatible with PN infusate should be administered as close to the catheter entry site as possible or via a separate catheter. Most, but not all, medications can be flushed with normal saline before and after infusion of medication to minimize any risk of drug-nutrient interaction. Normal saline flush solutions can result in significant sodium intake. Generally, this is well tolerated by many VLBW infants because of the greater sodium needs secondary to decreased renal tubular absorption of sodium or concurrent diuretic therapy. Glucose in the flushing solution can cause swings of blood sugar in VLBW infants. Only preservative-free flush solutions should be used.

g) PN-associated cholestasis[26–28]
   (1) Risk factors. The incidence varies inversely with the degree of prematurity, the duration of PN (>2 weeks), excessive intake of calories and nutrients (e.g., glucose, lipids, amount and type of amino acids, copper, manganese), sepsis, and impaired intestinal function, including dysmotility, bowel rest, and lack of enteral feedings.
   (2) Management. Enteral feedings should be initiated and continued if feasible. However, PN should not be discontinued if the infant is unable to tolerate enteral feeding. Excessive intake of nutrients, particularly the nutrients that require normal metabolic or excretory function of the liver, should be avoided. For example, protein intake should be the minimum that allows adequate growth and good nutritional status, and copper and manganese supplements may need to be held or reduced and their status monitored. Use of pediatric amino acids solutions and change from continuous infusion to cyclic PN may improve the cholestasis. Medications such as cholecystokinin, ursodeoxycholic acid, and phenobarbital have been used with varying success to stimulate bile flow and lower the bilirubin level.

h) Metabolic bone disease[21,29–31]
   (1) Risk factors. Metabolic bone disease incidence varies directly with degree of prematurity, duration of PN (>4 weeks), prolonged volume restriction, PN solutions with low mineral (calcium and phosphorus) content, secondary vitamin D deficiency from calcium and/or phosphorus deficiency,[29,31] aluminum contamination of nutrients, delayed initiation and delay in achieving the full volume of appropriate enteral feeding, and prolonged excessive pharmacotherapy, in particular, with loop diuretics and corticosteroids. Excessive force (e.g., physical restraint during surgery) or during physical therapy has occasionally caused fractures in osteopenic patients.
   (2) Management. Enteral feedings should be initiated and continued if feasible. However, PN should not be discontinued if the patient is unable to tolerate enteral feeding. The recommended minerals, vitamin D, and other nutrients should be maintained in the PN solution. Pharmacotherapy and physical therapy should be reassessed and modified if necessary. Supplementation with calcium and/or phosphorus alone is not recommended since a balanced intake of all nutrients is necessary for normal bone growth.

i) Oral aversion. Oral aversion may occur in chronically ill infants who have not been fed for many months. Difficulty in achieving adequate nipple feeding is particularly notable in ELBW infants and those who have experienced hypoxic insults. Nonnutritive sucking during the course of illness does not appear to improve the ability to nipple-feed; actual oral feeding is necessary for the development of sucking behavior.[32]

III. Enteral Nutrition

A. Assessing readiness for enteral feeding. For the healthy neonate born at term, transition from the placental source of nutrients to enteral feeding usually occurs within a few hours after birth once physiologic adaptation to the extrauterine environment is achieved. For the sick and/or premature neonate, indicators of readiness for enteral feeding include the following:

1. Absence of gastrointestinal anomalies that interfere with adequate delivery, digestion, or absorption of enteral nutrients
2. Cardiorespiratory stability as indicated by the absence of respiratory distress and consistently normal vital signs. The prone or side-lying position with the head of the bed elevated generally improves respiratory gas exchange and decreases gastroesophageal reflux and aspiration.
3. Controversial issues. There are generally no contraindications to enteral feeding under the following conditions, provided the infant is clinically stable:
   a) Mechanical ventilation or continuous positive airway pressure
   b) Indwelling umbilical vein or arterial catheters
   c) Perinatal asphyxia
   d) Inotropic, sedative, or indomethacin therapy

B. Enteral preparations

1. Human milk. The advantages to the use of human milk include psychosocial benefits to the mother and easy digestibility, low formula and renal solute load, and potential benefits from immunologic and trophic factors for the infant.[33] Human milk contains long-chain polyunsaturated fatty acids (LCPUFA) of the n-3 and n-6 fatty acid families, and some data show possible neurological or visual developmental advantages in preterm infants fed human milk compared to those fed formulas without LCPUFA supplementation.[34] There are very few contradictions to feeding human milk.[33] These include the presence of certain maternal systemic infections such as tuberculosis and human immunodeficiency virus, and certain metabolic disorders affecting the infants, including galactosemia. A number of drugs may be secreted into human milk, but not all are thought to be of concern to the infant.[35] The mother should be encouraged to discuss any use of prescription drugs, over-the-counter drugs, or herbal medications with the physician. Presence of jaundice (if determined to be breast milk–associated jaundice) does not preclude continuation of breast-feeding, although a 24- to 48-hour substitution with infant formula may be useful as a diagnostic test and for management.
   a) Human milk can be the exclusive source of nutrition for all term infants for 4 to 6 months after birth.[33] For small preterm infants, breast milk has insufficient amounts of protein, energy, sodium, calcium, phosphorus, vitamin D, zinc, and probably folic acid to for adequate growth. Commercial powder or liquid human milk fortifier containing multiple nutrients should be used to supplement all small preterm infants fed human milk, at least until ad libitum breast-feeding begins.
   b) Critically ill infants are usually unable to nipple-feed and may not tolerate enteral feeding, and mother's milk is collected for delivery via gavage feeding or stored for later use. A lactation specialist may be helpful in teaching and assisting in breast-pumping techniques and for support in maintaining lactation for the mother. Manual expression of breasts or mechanical aids can be used depending on the mother's preference. An electric breast pump that allows simultaneous emptying of both breasts shortens the duration of milk expression and tends to encourage the most milk production. Breast pumping should begin within 24 hours after delivery and should be done every 3 to 4 hours during the day and once or twice at night. A sterile bottle or plastic bag should be used for each collection. Maternal stress and fatigue can decrease milk production. Encouragement and support of the mother may be needed to maintain the milk supply. Routine use of oxytocin nasal spray to promote a let-down response or metoclopramide to stimulate prolactin secretion, and the use of herbal products to stimulate milk production, are not recommended.
   c) Plastic containers are preferred to glass containers for storage of breast milk.[36] Fresh breast milk can be refrigerated for 48 hours without significant microbial growth. During transport from the home to the hospital, fresh milk should be cooled or frozen by packing tightly in a cooler with freezer gel packs. Frozen milk can be stored for about 3 months in a home freezer at −20 degrees Celsius (−4 degrees Fahrenheit).[37] Frozen milk should be thawed in the storage container in a refrigerator or under cool running water. Boiling or microwave heating can affect the nutritional and immunologic properties of human milk. Thawed or refrigerated milk is often warmed under hot water and several drops of milk should be dripped onto the dorsum of the hand to confirm that it is not too hot prior to feeding the baby.
   d) The use of donated human milk is controversial, and the practice remains regional.
2. Commercial preparations
   a) Infant formulas are designed to substitute for human milk in the event that the mother decides not to breast-feed or in the presence of contraindications to breast-feeding. For infants born at term or small preterm infants beyond 6 to 12 months of postnatal age, standard cow milk–based infant formulas should be used. There are limited indications for soy formula[38] or partially hydrolyzed protein formulas.[39] Highly modified infant formulas based on extensive protein hydrolysates or amino acids are used in certain allergic or intestinal disorders (see Section IV).

      For small preterm infants, only formulas designed specifically to meet the nutrient requirements of VLBW infants should be used.[40] The two commercially available iron-fortified preterm infant formulas contain whole protein with a whey-casein weight ratio of 60:40, long-chain and medium-chain triglycerides in an approximate weight ratio of 1:1, and lactose and glucose polymers in an approximate weight ratio of 1:1. All other nutrients, including LCPUFA, are added in amounts designed to meet the nutrient requirements of preterm infants when fed at about 150 mL/kg/d. Both commercial preterm infant formulas are available in 20 or 24 kcal/oz preparations and all are isotonic. The higher nutrient density preparation can be used as the initial feeding and there is no advantage in the use of the lower density preparation.

      Soy protein–based formula should not be used because of uncertain mineral absorption and higher concentrations of some trace elements such as manganese and aluminum. Protein hydrolysate formulas with other highly modified macronutrients, including a high proportion of medium-chain triglycerides with glucose polymers as the sole source of carbohydrate, theoretically can improve absorption of these nutrients. However, VLBW infants who receive these formulas may have distortions of the plasma aminogram, lower total nitrogen absorption and retention, and lower phosphorus absorption compared with those fed formulas designed specifically for VLBW infants. Elemental formulas containing free amino acids are rarely needed and should be used only under the supervision of physicians with special knowledge of nutrition support in infants. It is important to note that commercial milk powder preparations are not sterile and are not recommended for in-hospital use for small preterm infants unless there is no suitable alternative.[41]

Careful preparation and handling of all infant formulas, particularly those prepared from powder, is warranted. All formulas should be fed immediately or refrigerated and fed within 24 hours of preparation. For infants requiring continuous infusion of milk feeding, the "hang time" of each feed type depends on institution practice. In any case, hang time of >4 hours is not recommended for enteral feeding.[42,43] For human milk containing human milk fortifier, the maximum suggested hang time is 4 hours.

b) Commercial human milk fortifiers are available from two manufacturers in North America. They provide additional energy and multiple nutrients when added to human milk. The contents of the two commercial fortifiers differ, and when the fortifiers are added to human milk in the recommended amounts, the final nutrient compositions tend to resemble the commercial preterm infant formulas from the respective manufacturers. The optimal level of iron content in human milk fortifier is controversial. In vitro studies indicated that a higher iron content may adversely affect the bacteriostatic properties of human milk against Escherichia coli, Staphylococcus, Enterobacter sakazakii, and group B streptococcus,[44] and results in greater generation of free radicals and lipid peroxidation products.[45] Thus, use of a low iron–containing human fortifier may be preferable. However, one report of short term (up to 28 days) use of human milk fortifier with 1.44 mg of iron added to 100 mL of human milk showed there was no increase in the incidence of sepsis or necrotizing enterocolitis.[46] The low-iron, insoluble calcium salt-containing human milk fortifier also resulted in better growth than the one with soluble calcium salts.[47] In terms of product sterility, there is no alternative to powdered human milk fortifier for in-hospital use. When mixed with human milk, the fortified milk should be used within 4 hours of preparation. A sterile liquid human milk fortifier is available, but when used according to the manufacturer's directions, it reduces human milk intake by 50%.

c) Vitamin D supplementation is recommended for all infants receiving human milk as an exclusive source of nutrition.[48] It is often part of commercial infant multivitamin preparations. Preterm infants, especially ELBW infants, are often given additional multivitamin supplementation containing 400 international units of vitamin D early in their course, whether they are receiving fortified human milk or preterm infant formula. Anecdotal reports exist for hypercalcemia with or without hypervitaminosis D in VLBW infants receiving preterm formula or fortified human milk with additional vitamin D or multivitamin supplementation. In any case, vitamin supplementation is unnecessary when these infants reach about 2 kg and are receiving adequate feedings of fortified human milk or preterm infant formula.

d) For term infants, adequate intake of iron during the first 6 months is <0.3 mg/d and can be met by breast-feeding alone. For the small preterm infant, the recommended daily iron intake is 1.7 to 2.5 mg elemental iron/100 kcal (2–4 mg/kg) during early infancy. Iron supplementation can be started once the infant achieves full enteral feeding and continues for the first year up to a maximum of 11 mg of elemental iron per day.[49] For infants receiving erythropoietin therapy, the iron requirement is substantially higher, and 10 mg/kg/d has been used.[17] Prolonged contact of human milk with iron may impede bacteriostatic activities and increase generation of free radicals and peroxidation products.[44,45] Medicinal iron given as once or twice daily supplementation is a proven effective therapy and may be preferably to the continuous contact of human milk to the high iron containing fortifier. No fluoride supplementation is recommended for infants in the first 6 months of life. Thereafter, daily supplementation of 0.25 mg of fluoride until 3 years of age is recommended if the drinking water contains <0.3 ppm of fluoride.[50]

e) Commercial modular nutrient components are available to meet the increased or altered dietary needs of infants in the NICU. These components include carbohydrate, fat, and protein modules. Modular protein products may be used to increase protein density (but are only available in powder), and emulsified fat products, medium-chain triglyceride, or glucose polymer may be used to increase caloric density. The use of modular nutrients may result in imbalanced intake of various nutrients. For example, increased protein density may result in an abnormal plasma aminogram, and increased caloric density may result in excessive fat deposition as adipose tissue and in various organs (including the liver), with adverse consequences. Thus, sick infants without significant gastrointestinal problems can have the infant formula concentrated. For those without the need for severe fluid restriction, the use of a greater volume of mother's milk or infant formula is preferred since the intake of all nutrients is proportionally increased. The experimental use of recombinant human lactoferrin, oligosaccharides, prebiotics, and probiotics in the diet holds promise to improve the gastrointestinal function and growth of sick and healthy infants.

C. Feeding methods. Enteral feeding methods should be individualized on the basis of gestational age, clinical status, and expected tolerance to feeding. Before about 32 weeks postmenstrual age (PMA), most preterm infants require gavage feeding because the integration of sucking, swallowing, gastrointestinal motility, and breathing necessary for successful oral feeding is generally inadequate. Between 32 and 36 weeks PMA, the preterm infant may need a combination of gavage and bottle (or breast) feedings. Once a coordinated suck and swallow are present, the change to full oral feedings usually can be established within 1 to 2 weeks.[51] Avoidance of hypoxemia is critical to successful enteral feeding. Use of a pulse oximeter should be part of the management during the transition from gavage to oral feedings. Parameters that should be evaluated include heart rate, respiration, and oxygenation relative to baseline through sucking and the postfeed period. Illnesses, particularly those affecting the central nervous system—whether congenital or secondary to severe asphyxia insult—can affect the normal maturation of the physiologic actions needed for successful nipple feeding.

1. Gastric gavage

a) Indications include infants with a poor suck-and-swallow reflex, such as extremely premature infants and infants with congenital or acquired neuromuscular disorders. Gavage feeding may be used during the transition from PN to EN or during the establishment of nipple feedings. Some infants with high respiratory rates may require gavage feeding, although enteral feeding probably should be withheld if the respiratory rate exceeds 80 breaths per minute to minimize the risk of aspiration.

b) The appropriate size gavage tube, which ranges from a 5F to an 8F catheter for intermittent gavage feeding, or an anchored indwelling naso- or orogastric catheter, should be selected. For ELBW infants, the smaller catheter is preferred to minimize occlusion of the nares, although an anchored orogastric tube may result in less airway resistance and less impairment of minute ventilation than a nasogastric tube.

c) Clinical verification of correct tube placement must be done immediately after insertion, at regular intervals during each nursing shift, and prior to each bolus feeding.

d) Polyvinyl chloride catheters should be changed every 24 to 48 hours to prevent stiffening of the plastic and potential gut perforation. Silastic or polyurethane catheters are preferable if a feeding tube is to be left indwelling for more than 72 hours.

e) For continuous gavage feedings, the amount of breast milk or formula placed on the constant-rate infusion pump should be only the amount that is to be delivered for a 3- to 4-hour period. Possible advantages compared with bolus feeding include less abdominal distention, improved intestinal absorption, better tolerance to feeding, and faster growth rates. Possible disadvantages may include increased risk of aspiration from the potential for increased gastroesophageal reflux (common in this population) or dislodgment of the feeding tube from the stomach to above the gastroesophageal junction. In addition, when breast milk is continuously infused, large amounts of fat may be lost with separation and layering of fat in the delivery system. This loss can be minimized by tilting the infusion pump so the fat is delivered before the water-soluble portion.

f) For bolus gavage feeding, most infants weighing >1500 g will tolerate feedings every 3 hours. Each feeding can be delivered by gravity or infused over 15 to 20 minutes. Smaller infants may require delivery over 1 to 2 hours to improve tolerance to intermittent bolus feeding. Possible advantages compared with continuous gavage feedings include more complete delivery of nutrients. For example, there is less risk of mineral sedimentation from high-mineral preterm infant formula or separation of human milk fat during delivery. In addition, bolus gavage feeding is simple to administer and requires minimal equipment. Possible disadvantages may include an increased risk of gastric residuals, abdominal distention, and gastroesophageal reflux.

g) Potential complications of gavage feedings
   (1) Misplacement of the tube into the trachea
   (2) Irritation or perforation of the pharynx, esophagus, or stomach
   (3) Vagal stimulation resulting in apnea and bradycardia
   (4) Gastroesophageal reflux and aspiration with subsequent pneumonia

h) Infants showed variable responses to non-nutritive sucking. Some studies reported benefits in weight gain, energy intake, heart rate, oxygen saturation, and intestinal transit time, and decreased time to full oral feeds.[52] A pacifier may be offered to infants during gavage feedings, although actual oral feeding is necessary for the development of sucking behavior.[32]

2. Transpyloric feeding. The transpyloric feeding route is rarely used because of multiple potential complications, including abdominal distention, diarrhea, fat malabsorption, bacterial overgrowth, necrotizing enterocolitis, malposition or dislodgment of the tube, and perforation of the intestine.

3. Gastrostomy tube

   a) Indications. Infants who have a functional stomach and intestine but a major impairment in swallowing or an esophageal obstruction are candidates for gastrostomy feeding. For example, a gastrostomy tube can be used as a long-term route for feeding infants with severe neurological deficits or as a temporary measure in infants with congenital esophageal atresia.

   b) Placement method. Gastrostomy tubes are percutaneously placed by radiologists with skill in invasive procedures or by surgeons as a specific surgical procedure. Tubes can be easily replaced 2 to 3 weeks after the initial operative procedure.

   c) Potential complications
      (1) Risk of surgical and anesthesia procedures
      (2) Local skin breakdown
      (3) Leakage of gastric contents around the gastrostomy tube insertion site
      (4) Accidental removal of tube or tube migration
      (5) Gastroesophageal reflux worsening with gastrostomy without fundoplication

4. Nipple feeding

   a) Breast-feeding. General hygienic practice is essential. This includes hand washing and making sure the breast/nipple area is clean before feeding. A lactation consultant or clinician can teach and support the mother to help ensure effective breast-feeding. Postsurgical infants may need additional positioning supports to minimize stress on the surgical incision. The infant should be assessed for respiratory and gastrointestinal tolerance, sucking strength, and coordination. The feeding duration on each breast should start at 3 to 5 minutes, thereafter increasing daily by 1 to 2 minutes, up to a total of 10 to 12 minutes per breast per feeding. For some infants, supplemental gavage feedings after breast-feeding attempts may be needed during the transition to complete breast-feeding. Continued support and education helps promote a let-down reflex and a positive breast-feeding experience for both the mother and the infant. Test weighing after breast-feeding to determine the volume of milk ingested is unnecessary. Observing the infant during breast-feeding, monitoring urine and stool patterns, and following daily and preferably weekly weight gains are better indicators of successful breast-feeding. If there is a local breast infection, milk should be expressed from the breast and discarded.

   b) Bottle feeding. Appropriate flow from the nipple is important. Too slow a flow requires excessive effort and may not allow adequate intake; excessive flow may result in choking or aspiration. Typically, more time is required to complete a feeding in the preterm or sick infant compared to the healthy term infant. The infant should be allowed to set the pace of bottle feeding so less energy is expended for feeding. Force-feeding or overstimulation of the infant may result in hypoxia or vomiting. It is important that the infant be held comfortably and securely during the feeding. The infant's head should be higher than the rest of the body to minimize the risk of gastroesophageal reflux. The bottle should be held so the infant sucks in only milk and not air through the nipple. The bottle should never be propped in the bed for feeding.

D. Transition from PN and initial feeding

1. Achieving adequate enteral intake may require considerable time depending on the infant's gestational age and clinical status. PN should be continued until about 70% of intended intake is provided through the enteral route. However, in extremely small preterm infants weighing <1 kg, PN should be continued even at 1 mL/hr since this is equivalent to as much as 50 mL/kg/d for infants with birth weight of <500g, a substantial source of nutrition support.

2. Full-strength feedings can be attempted whenever the infant is clinically stable. There is no advantage to the use of diluted milk for initial feedings. Human milk should never be diluted. Some clinicians prefer that infants first tolerate some enteral feeding,

~30 mL/kg/d, before adding human milk fortifier. Formula-fed preterm infants should start with 81 kcal/dL formulations since they are isotonic and there is no advantage in the use of 67 kcal/dL formulations. Some clinicians use protein hydrolysate formula with the aim of maximizing macronutrient absorption. However, this type of formulation was not designed to meet the nutrient needs of the preterm infant, and specific indications for the term infant are limited. Their use in small preterm infants has been associated with altered plasma amino acid patterns.

E. Feeding volume and energy. In contrast to PN, in which the content of multiple nutrients and fluid volume can be adjusted, EN support is limited to the type of milk and the volume provided to the infant. For the vast majority of infants in the NICU, the type of milk would be mother's milk or standard infant formula for those born at term, and mother's milk with fortifier or preterm infant formulas for those born prematurely. The fortified human milk and the preterm infant formula provide a caloric density of 24 kcal/oz, with fixed content of specific nutrients in the range to meet the estimated requirement.[40] The practice in most NICUs is to start with small volumes and advance slowly to allow for adaptation of the gastrointestinal tract (GIT) to avoid distention, emesis, and diarrhea.
   1. A typical starting volume is 10 to 30 mL/kg/d, advanced daily in increments of similar amounts as tolerated until the fluid goal is reached. Smaller, sicker infants generally tolerate the smaller initial volume of feeds and a slower rate of increase.
   2. The volume of feedings needs to be adjusted daily or on alternate days with increasing body weight to maintain the fluid and nutrient goals for growth. Consistent weight gain usually occurs with an intake between 150 and 200 mL/kg/d.
   3. Sick infants, particularly preterm infants, even if they are not expected to tolerate much milk feeding, may benefit from minimal enteral feeding (<10 mL/kg/d) soon after birth once clinically stable. This minimal enteral feeding is intended as trophic stimulus for gut growth and function. Trophic feeding alters gastrointestinal disaccharidase activity, hormone release, blood flow, motility, and microbial flora. The clinical benefits appear to include improved milk tolerance, greater postnatal growth, reduced systemic sepsis, and shorter hospital stay.[53] There is no evidence of any adverse effects from trophic feeding.
   4. Energy requirements for enterally fed infants are generally 10% to 20% higher than for parenterally fed infants because of individual variability in digestion and absorption. Generally, an enteral intake of 110 to 130 kcal/kg/d (~136 to 160 mL/kg/d of 24 kcal/oz milk) should allow adequate growth in most sick infants, even those born prematurely.

F. Complementary feeding. Additional foods or fluids are rarely needed. For patients in the NICU, the priority is to achieve adequate intake of mother's milk (with or without fortification, depending on the infant's weight, as discussed in Section III.B) or nutritionally complete infant formulas. There is no nutritional indication to add complementary foods before 4 to 6 months. Infants who are ready to receive complementary feeding for the purpose of adding variety in texture and taste to the diet normally would have been discharged from the NICU. In a few infants being prepared for home ventilator support, the use of complementary feeding should be similar to that for healthy infants, with one "single-ingredient" new food introduced at a time and at the consistency or texture appropriate for oral motor development.[54]

G. In-hospital monitoring
   1. Daily body weight in addition to intake and output, twice-weekly head circumference, and weekly body length should be measured. All measurements should be plotted on appropriate growth charts. See Chapter 1.
   2. The type and frequency of laboratory monitoring should be based on the individual needs of the infant and his or her tolerance of enteral feedings. Laboratory studies may be similar to those needed for PN but are oriented toward determining hematologic and biochemical homeostasis and improving nutritional status.
   3. If an infant has signs or symptoms such as lethargy, abdominal distention, increased gastric residuals, vomiting, bilious aspirate, diarrhea, or bloody stools, feedings should be stopped to allow for assessment of the cause and appropriate management instituted.
   4. Apnea, bradycardia, and desaturation may result in or be caused by feeding intolerance. Care should be taken to define the origin of these signs so the infant can be treated appropriately. Head up with prone or right lateral positions are best during gavage feeding to maximize gastric emptying and minimize respiratory impairment. After hospital discharge, the head-up feeding position can be maintained, but a supine sleep position is strongly recommended.[55] Caution should be exercised with the prolonged use of antireflux medication.
   5. Gastric residual is normally used as an indicator of feeding tolerance. There is no specific cutoff for the amount of residual as a predictor of additional complications such as necrotizing enterocolitis.[56]
      a) With gavage feedings, check for aspirates before each feeding.
      b) The aspirate volume should be less than the volume infused over the previous hour if fed by continuous infusion, or 10% to 20% of the bolus volume. Refeed the aspirate, give the intended volume for the next feed, and continue with the same feeding schedule.
      c) If the aspirate is >20% of the volume fed, assess the infant for other signs of intolerance such as abdominal distension. If no other signs are noted, reduce the feeding volume to the previously tolerated volume and adjust the PN intake accordingly. Continue to assess the infant for signs of intolerance.
      d) If feeding intolerance continues or other signs of intolerance develop, stop feedings immediately and assess the infant for complications.

IV. Nutrition Support for Sick Infants With Specific Disorders

The key to maintaining optimal nutritional status in the critically ill infant is to begin appropriate nutrition support via the enteral or parenteral route within 24 hours of admission. Nutrition support should include taking into account the influence of the underlying pathophysiology of the disease process and minimizing the use of therapeutic measures that might interfere with nutrient utilization and tolerance. Nutrition support of all infants depends on a number of factors. See Table 26-6.

A. Functional capacity of the GIT and cardiorespiratory stability. If the GIT function is intact and the cardiorespiratory status is stable, then the use of enteral feeding with standard enteral preparations (see Section III.B) is appropriate, except in patients with inborn errors of metabolism. The route (see Section III.C) of feeding will vary depending on the neurodevelopmental maturity of the patient.

   GIT function is significantly impaired in primary or secondary short-bowel syndrome or severe intractable diarrhea. The presence of enterostomy (especially at the upper small bowel), motility disorder, or bacterial overgrowth also may complicate the nutritional management. To improve digestion and absorption of nutrients, protein

TABLE 26-6. Nutrition Support for Critically Ill Infants

Nutrition concerns	Nutritional management
Impaired function of gastrointestinal tract from • Primary or secondary shortening • Motility or mucosal dysfunction	• Modify protein (hydrolysate or amino acids), carbohydrate (glucose polymer), and fat (medium-chain triglyceride) components of milk. • Supplement other nutrients (eg, electrolytes, vitamins) as needed. • Give continuous infusion rather than bolus feeding. • Use total or supplementary parenteral nutrition.
Impaired function of other organ function	• Modify fluid goal and components of milk as needed. • Limit nutrients that require the metabolic or excretory capacity of the organ (eg, fluid and electrolyte restriction in renal impairment, copper and manganese restriction in hepatic impairment).
Underlying disease	• Modify route of delivery (eg, nasogastric or gastrostomy feeding in patients with impairment of sucking and swallowing). • Increase nutrient density of standard milk preparations (eg, small preterm infants, infants with poorly controlled cardiac failure). • Adjust nutrient (glucose and/or lipid) load in septic subjects. • Replace abnormal losses (eg, gastric, enterostomy, or diarrhea losses). • Provide specific formulation for cow milk protein or soy protein allergy, and inborn errors of metabolism.
Therapy for underlying illness	• Adjust glucose load in patients receiving systemic steroid therapy. • Minimize therapy that might increase nutrient losses or adversely affect nutrient digestion, absorption, metabolism, or excretion (eg, proton pump inhibitor, corticosteroids, phenobarbital, chronic diuretics). • Use appropriate analgesia and anesthesia to minimize tissue catabolism.

hydrolysate formula with modified fat and carbohydrate delivered by continuous infusion is usually used as the initial feeding. The amount can be increased slowly, depending on the volume of gastric residual and the quality and quantity of stool. Gastric residuals may be reduced by continuous gavage feeding, and the short-term use of a prokinetic agent may be helpful. There is no agreement on the amount of stool or enterostomy output that is acceptable. A decrease in enteral intake and supplemental PN is generally indicated if the volume of output is >20% to 30% of enteral intake and the infant fails to gain weight, head circumference, and length.

There are some differences in the contents of the two commercial protein hydrolysate formulations. The most convenient and important indicator of its adequacy would be clinical tolerance and adequate growth. An amino acid–based elemental formula containing modified fat and carbohydrate source can be used[57] if a protein hydrolysate formula is not tolerated. Supplementation of fluid and multiple nutrients such as electrolytes, minerals, trace minerals, and vitamins such as B_{12} and fat-soluble vitamins are frequently needed. Pharmacotherapy to modulate intestinal motility, intestinal fluid loss, gastric acid production, and the use of growth hormone and other intestinal growth–enhancing agents in short-bowel syndrome (see Chapter 14) may be needed. Early provision of a central venous catheter is necessary in these infants to allow easy access for supplemental or total PN, including home PN, as necessary.

To optimize nutrition support, it is better to provide the infant a small volume of full-strength milk formula and employ supplemental PN rather than providing a high volume (but nutritionally insufficient) of diluted milk formula alone. Maintaining even a minimal amount of enteral feeding, if tolerated, may be helpful to intestinal growth and adaptation. The rate of intestinal adaptation to EN varies with the gestation of the infant (preterm infants may have better potential than term infants for compensatory intestinal growth), the site and length of residual bowel (upper or lower small bowel with or without the presence of ileocecal valve, or colon), the response to other medical and surgical therapy, and the ability to maintain or improve the nutritional status throughout the course of illness. In any case, meticulous attention to details of fluids and electrolytes, and all aspects of macro- and micronutrient status, is essential. If a small preterm infant with impaired GIT function has tolerated protein hydrolysate formula, cautious introduction of preterm formula with more appropriate nutrient composition for the infant's needs should be attempted. Ultimately, functional adaptation of the intestine may allow gradual transition to a normal diet. Management of these infants by a small group of multidisciplinary professionals is strongly recommended.

B. Functional capacity of organs other than the GIT system. This also is important to the tolerance and type of nutrients delivered. For example, with renal disorders, most infants can be fed human milk or "humanized" infant formulas, depending on the extent of renal impairment and the treatment for it. Close monitoring of serum electrolytes, minerals, urea nitrogen, and albumin status is needed. Infants with biliary atresia often have reduced intake and impaired digestion and absorption of nutrients, particularly long-chain fats and fat-soluble vitamins. The use of protein hydrolysate formula rich in medium-chain triglycerides, supplementation of multivitamins, and continuous enteral feedings may be needed to maximize digestion and absorption of nutrients to promote growth until definitive treatment for the underlying disease can take place.

C. Constraints imposed by the underlying disease state. Fluid restriction may limit the amount of nutrient that can be delivered in infants with acute renal failure or the syndrome of inappropriate antidiuretic hormone secretion. However, an increase in fluid intake may be feasible with manipulation of environmental factors (Table 26-4). In other situations such as infants with poorly controlled cardiac failure, can be fed with standard infant formula concentrated to 80 to 100 kcal/dL as necessary. Infants receiving the highly concentrated formulas should be observed for gastrointestinal tolerance, and use of the concentrated formula should be terminated if the infant is having other problems such as gastroenteritis.

With surgical operation and sepsis, the increased metabolic demands return to normal upon resolution of the primary conditions. After most elective operations in otherwise normal infants, the increase in metabolic demand often lasts only 4 to 6 hours[58] and no change to standard nutrition support is needed. Septic infants frequently do not tolerate the increased amount of nutrients needed to compensate for their greater metabolic demands, and complications such as hyperglycemia may develop while they are receiving the previously tolerated PN infusate. Replacement of losses such as enterostomy losses of electrolytes is needed. The clinician also must be cognizant of the loss of minerals and trace minerals in addition to electrolytes, since the content of minerals such as magnesium[22] or trace minerals such as zinc[59] and many other nutrients in the fecal or enterostomy fluid is rarely measured. Zinc status may be the limiting factor in immunologic and numerous other functions and growth.

Infants with demonstrated allergy to cow milk or soy protein may require protein hydrolysate formula. The use of elemental amino acid infant formula and even PN also may be needed. Infants with inborn errors of metabolism such as phenylketonuria have specific needs and therapy regardless of gestational age or birth weight. These groups of patients should be comanaged by a physician and a dietitian familiar with the management of these disorders.

D. Alteration in the form of nutrients and adjunctive support. Changes in the form of nutrients are not necessary for many complications commonly found in patients in the NICU. For example, some conditions such as feeding difficulties associated with central nervous system complications require a change in the route of delivery rather than a change in the form of nutrients. Even gastrointestinal complications normally do not require modification of standard PN infusate or enteral feeding unless there is a significantly shortened intestinal tract or dysmotility problems. Infants requiring extracorporeal membrane oxygenation (ECMO) therapy generally have severe respiratory failure. Protein catabolism in these infants is markedly elevated, consistent with their severe illness. A surplus of dietary caloric intake does not improve protein catabolism and merely increases carbon dioxide production in the highly stressed neonates.[60] Thus, excess nutrient intake, especially during the acute phase of illness, including the period on ECMO, is not warranted and may be detrimental. Some infants on ECMO show intolerance to nutrients such as carbohydrate load, as other sick infants do, and some develop hypercalcemia if they are receiving PN solutions high in calcium. Hyperglycemia and hypercalcemia are transient and resolved with temporary lowering of dextrose and calcium in PN. Occasionally, calcium may need to be withheld from PN for 2 or 3 days. Many infants who received ECMO therapy suffer from variable periods of hypoxia and are at risk for increased intestinal permeability with the potential for bacterial translocation and sepsis. However, neonates on ECMO have tolerated some enteral feeding without further clinical deterioration.[61] The major complication with feeding is the poor nipple-feeding effort of many infants after discontinuation of ECMO therapy, and almost all infants require a period of gavage feeding. There are no data to indicate that the nutrient requirement for infants needing ECMO would differ from that of other sick infants with non-GIT problems, and there is no indication to use milks other than human milk or standard infant formula.

Infants with chronic disease states such as Bronchopulmonary Dysplasia (BPD) may require relative fluid restriction but possibly have increased energy needs because of increased respiratory effort. Increased energy intake in this situation should be managed with the understanding that excessive carbohydrate load also may increase the work of respiration and that balanced macronutrient content is needed.

All pharmacotherapy including but not limited to diuretics, corticosteroids, proton pump inhibitors, and phenobarbital must be regularly reassessed to determine its continuing need. This could minimize the adversely effect on nutrient digestion, absorption, metabolism and excretion. Adequate analgesia and anesthesia are proven means of reducing the catabolism associated with sick and stressed infants and are useful adjuncts to optimize the nutritional management.

REFERENCES

1. Koo WWK, Cepeda E. Parenteral nutrition in neonates. In: Rombeau JL, Rolandelli RH, eds. *Clinical Nutrition: Parenteral Nutrition.* 3rd ed. Philadelphia, PA: WB Saunders; 2000:463–475.
2. Ziegler EE, Thureen PJ, Carlson SJ. Aggressive nutrition of the very low birthweight infant. *Clin Perinatol.* 2002;29:225–244.
3. A.S.P.E.N. Board of Directors and the Clinical Guidelines Task Force. Guidelines for the use of parenteral and enteral nutrition in adult and pediatric patients. *J Parenter Enteral Nutr.* 2002;26(1 suppl):1SA–138SA.
4. Committee on Nutrition. Parenteral nutrition. In: Kleinman RE, ed. *Pediatric Nutrition Handbook.* 5th ed. Elk Grove Village, IL: American Academy of Pediatrics; 2004:369–389.
5. Ockerman AV. Compounded sterile preparations. An overview of the new standards in USP <797>. *U.S. Pharmacist.* 2004;29:46–62.
6. Thureen PJ, Melara D, Fennessey PV, Hay WW Jr. Effect of low versus high intravenous amino acid intake on very low birth weight infants in the early neonatal period. *Pediatr Res.* 2003;53:24–32.
7. Poindexter BB, Ehrenkranz RA, Stoll BJ, et al. Parenteral glutamine supplementation does not reduce the risk of mortality or late-onset sepsis in extremely low birth weight infants. *Pediatrics.* 2004;113:1209–1215.
8. O'Leary MJ. Nourishing the preterm and low birthweight infant. In: Pipes PL, ed. *Nutrition in Infancy and Childhood.* St. Louis, MO: McGraw-Hill; 1985:145.
9. Zlotkin SH, Bryan MH, Anderson GH. Intravenous nitrogen and energy intakes required to duplicate in utero nitrogen accretion in prematurely born human infants. *J Pediatr.* 1981;99:115–120.
10. Jones MO, Pierro A, Hammond P, Nunn A, Lloyd DA. Glucose utilization in the surgical newborn infant receiving total parenteral nutrition. *J Pediatr Surg.* 1993;28:1121–1125.
11. Chwals WJ. Overfeeding the critically ill child: fact or fantasy? *New Horiz.* 1994;2:147–155.
12. Lafeber HN, Sulkers EJ, Chapman TE, Sauer PJ. Glucose production and oxidation in preterm infants during total parenteral nutrition. *Pediatr Res.* 1990;28:153–157.
13. Sunehag A, Gustafsson J, Ewald U. Glycerol carbon contributes to hepatic glucose production during the first eight hours in healthy term infants. *Acta Paediatr.* 1996;85:1339–1343.
14. Poindexter BB, Karn CA, Denne SC. Exogenous insulin reduces proteolysis and protein synthesis in extremely low birth weight infants. *J Pediatr.* 1998;132:948–953.
15. American Academy of Pediatrics, Subcommittee on Hyperbilirubinemia. Management of hyperbilirubinemia in the newborn infant 35 or more weeks of gestation. *Pediatrics.* 2004;114:297–316.
16. Cairns PA, Stalker DJ. Carnitine supplementation of parenterally fed neonates [Cochrane Review]. *The Cochrane Library.* 2004;issue 2.
17. Ohls RK, Ehrenkranz RA, Wright LL, et al. Effects of early erythropoietin therapy on the transfusion requirements of preterm infants below 1250 grams birth weight: a multicenter, randomized, controlled trial. *Pediatrics.* 2001;108:934–942.

18. Greene HL, Hambidge KM, Schanler R, Tsang RC. Guidelines for the use of vitamins, trace elements, calcium, magnesium, and phosphorus in infants and children receiving total parenteral nutrition. *Am J Clin Nutr.* 1988;48: 1324–1342.
19. Doyle LW, Sinclair JC. Insensible water loss in newborn infants. *Clin Perinatol.* 1982;9:453–482.
20. Nelson RE, Biberdorf RI. Nationwide drug shortage: it's time to take the lead. *Nutr Clin Pract.* 1998;13:295–297.
21. Koo WWK. Neonatal calcium and phosphorus disorders. In: Lifshitz F, ed. *Pediatric Endocrinology: A Clinical Guide.* 4th ed. New York, NY: Marcel Dekker; 2003:481–515.
22. Thoren L. Magnesium deficiency in gastrointestinal fluid loss. *Acta Chir Scand.* 1963;306(suppl):1–65.
23. Koo WWK, Kaplan LA, Horn J, Tsang RC, Steichen JJ. Aluminum in parenteral nutrition solution—sources and possible alternatives. *J Parenter Enteral Nutr.* 1986;10:591–595.
24. Neuzil J, Darlow BA, Inder TE, et al. Oxidation of parenteral lipid emulsion by ambient and phototherapy lights: potential toxicity of routine parenteral feeding. *J Pediatr.* 1995;126:785–790.
25. Chessex P, Lavoie JC, Rouleau T, et al. Photooxidation of parenteral multivitamins induces hepatic steatosis in a neonatal guinea pig model of intravenous nutrition. *Pediatr Res.* 2002;52:958–963.
26. Kaufman SS. Prevention of parenteral nutrition-associated liver disease in children. *Pediatr Transplant.* 2002;6:37–42.
27. Btaiche IF, Khalidi N. Parenteral nutrition-associated liver complications in children. *Pharmacotherapy.* 2002;22:188–211.
28. Forchielli ML, Walker WA. Nutritional factors contributing to the development of cholestasis during total parenteral nutrition. *Adv Pediatr.* 2003;50: 245–267.
29. Koo WWK, Steichen JJ. Osteopenia and rickets of prematurity. In: Polin R, Fox W, eds. *Fetal and Neonatal Physiology.* 2nd ed. Philadelphia, PA: W. B. Saunders; 1998:2335–2349.
30. Koo WWK. Preterm infants with fractures. In: Kleerekoper M, Siris E, McClung M, eds. *The Bone and Mineral Manual. A Practical Guide.* 2nd ed. San Diego, CA: Academic Press. In press.
31. Koo WWK, Warren L. Calcium and bone health in infants. *Neonatal Netw.* 2003;22:23–37.
32. Mizuno K, Ueda A. Development of sucking behavior in infants who have not been fed for 2 months after birth. *Pediatr Int.* 2001;43:251–255.
33. American Academy of Pediatrics, Committee on Nutrition. Breastfeeding and the use of human milk. *Pediatrics.* 2005;115:496–506.
34. Koo WWK. Efficacy and safety of docosahexaenoic acid and arachidonic acid addition to infant formulas: can one buy better vision and intelligence? *J Amer Coll Nutr.* 2003;22:101–107.
35. American Academy of Pediatrics, Committee on Drugs. The transfer of drugs and other chemicals into human milk. *Pediatrics.* 2001;108:776–789.
36. Committee on Nutrition. Breastfeeding. In: Kleinman RE, ed. *Pediatric Nutrition Handbook.* 5th ed. Elk Grove Village, IL: American Academy of Pediatrics; 2004:55–85.
37. Robbins ST and Baker LT. Infant Feedings: Guidelines for Preparation of Formula and Breastmilk in Health Care Facilities. Chicago, IL: American Dietetic Association; 2004:71–75.
38. American Academy of Pediatrics, Committee on Nutrition. Soy protein-based formulas: recommendations for use in infant feeding. *Pediatrics.* 1998;101:148–153.
39. American Academy of Pediatrics, Committee on Nutrition. Hypoallergenic infant formulas. *Pediatrics.* 2000;106:346–349.
40. Klein CJ, ed. Nutrient requirements for preterm infant formulas: a report from the American Society for Nutritional Sciences, Life Sciences Research Office. *J Nutr.* 2002;132:1395S–1577S.
41. U.S. Food and Drug Administration. Recalls and safety alerts. FDA warns about possible *Enterobacter Sakazakii* infection in hospitalized newborns fed powdered infant formula. *MMWR.* 2002;51:298–300.
42. American Dietetic Association. *Preparation of Formula for Infants: Guidelines for Healthcare Facilities.* Chicago, IL: American Dietetic Association; 2002:64.
43. Food and Drug Administration, USA. Letter to health-care professionals. October 2002. Available at: http://www.cfsan.fda.gov. Accessed August 15, 2004.
44. Chan GM. Effects of powdered human milk fortifiers on the antibacterial actions of human milk. *J Perinatol.* 2003;23:620–623.
45. Raghuveer TS, McGuire EM, Martin SM, et al. Lactoferrin in the preterm infant's diet attenuates iron-induced oxidation products. *Pediatr Res.* 2002; 52:964–972.
46. Berseth CL, Van Aerde JE, Gross S et al. Growth, efficacy, and safety of feeding an iron-fortified human milk fortifier. *Pediatrics* 2004;114: 699–706.
47. Reis BB, Hall RT, Schanler RJ, et al. Enhanced growth of preterm infants fed a new powdered human milk fortifier: a randomized, controlled trial. *Pediatrics.* 2000;106:581–588.
48. Gartner LM, Greer FR on behalf of Section on Breastfeeding and Committee on Nutrition, American Academy of Pediatrics. Prevention of rickets and vitamin D deficiency: new guidelines for vitamin D intake. *Pediatrics.* 2003;111:908–910.
49. Food and Nutrition Board, Institute of Medicine. *Dietary Reference Intake for Iron.* Washington, DC: National Academy Press; 2001:290–393.
50. Committee on Nutrition. Nutrition and oral health. In: Kleinman RE, ed. *Pediatric Nutrition Handbook.* 5th ed. Elk Grove Village, IL: American Academy of Pediatrics; 2004:789–800.
51. Lemons PK, Lemons JA. Transition to breast/bottle feedings: the premature infant. *J Am Coll Nutr.* 1996;15:126–135.
52. Pinelli J, Symington A. Non-nutritive sucking for promoting physiologic stability and nutrition in preterm infants. *Cochrane Database Syst Rev.* 2001; 3:CD001071.
53. McClure RJ. Trophic feeding of the preterm infant. *Acta Paediatr.* 2001; 90(suppl):19–21.
54. Committee on Nutrition. Complementary feeding. In: Kleinman RE, ed. *Pediatric Nutrition Handbook.* 5th ed. Elk Grove Village, IL: American Academy of Pediatrics; 2004:103–118.
55. American Academy of Pediatrics, Task Force on Infant Sleep Position and Sudden Infant Death Syndrome. Changing concepts of sudden infant death syndrome: implications for infant sleeping environment and sleep position. *Pediatrics.* 2000;105:650–656.
56. Kenton AB, Fernandes CJ, Berseth CL. Gastric residuals in prediction of necrotizing enterocolitis in very low birth weight infants. *Pediatrics.* 2004; 113:1848–1849.
57. Bines J, Francis D, Hill D. Reducing parenteral requirement in children with short bowel syndrome: impact of an amino acid–based complete infant formula. *J Pediatr Gastroenterol Nutr.* 1998;26:123–128.
58. Pierro A. Metabolism and nutritional support in the surgical neonate. *J Pediatr Surg.* 2002;37:811–822.
59. Wolman SL, Anderson GH, Marliss EB, Jeejeebhoy KN. Zinc in total parenteral nutrition. Requirement and metabolic effects. *Gastroenterology.* 1979;76:458–467.
60. Shew SB, Keshen TH, Jahoor F, Jaksic T. The determinants of protein catabolism in neonates on extracorporeal membrane oxygenation. *J Pediatr Surg.* 1999;34:1086–1090.
61. Piena M, Albers MJ, Van Haard PM, et al. Introduction of enteral feeding in neonates on extracorporeal membrane oxygenation after evaluation of intestinal permeability changes. *J Pediatr Surg.* 1998;33:30–34.
62. Alexander GR, Himes JH, Kaufman RB, Mor J, Kogan M. A United States national reference for fetal growth. *Obstet Gynecol* 1996;87: 163–168.
63. Kuczmarski RJ, Ogden CL, Grummer-Strawn LM, et al. 2000 CDC growth charts: United States. Advance data from vital and health statistics; no 314. Hyattsville, Marylands: *National Center for Health Statistics.*

SECTION EDITOR
W. Frederick Schwenk, MD

V

Metabolic Conditions

M. Molly McMahon, MD

27

Diabetes Mellitus

Introduction

In practice, most nutrition clinicians will manage the care of hospitalized patients with diabetes mellitus who require parenteral nutrition or enteral tube feeding. An important management goal in the care of the hospitalized patient with diabetes is to avoid the extremes of hypoglycemia and hyperglycemia. This chapter provides an approach to achieving glucose control in stressed hospitalized patients with diabetes who are receiving nutrition support.

I. Background Information

A. Diabetes mellitus is a metabolic disorder caused by an absolute (Type 1; previously called insulin-dependent diabetes mellitus) or a relative (Type 2; previously called non-insulin-dependent diabetes mellitus or stress-induced hyperglycemia) lack of insulin.[1]
   1. Type 1 diabetes is associated with onset at an earlier age, a tendency toward ketosis, and an absolute dependency on insulin.
   2. Type 2 diabetes, by far the more common type, is associated with adult onset, obesity, and need for larger doses of insulin.

B. Because of the increasing prevalence of diabetes, the co-morbidity of the disease, and the number of patients with stress-induced hyperglycemia, many hospital clinicians will manage patients with hyperglycemia receiving nutrition support. A third of all patients admitted to an urban general hospital had fasting glucose levels exceeding 126 mg/dL or two or more random glucose levels exceeding 200 mg/dL, and a third of these patients did not have known diabetes.[2]

C. Carbohydrate metabolism is closely regulated in both the postabsorptive (overnight fasted state) and postprandial periods in healthy, nondiabetic subjects.
   1. In the postabsorptive period, euglycemia is maintained because the rate of hepatic glucose production approximates the rate of glucose uptake by the liver, brain, and peripheral tissues. These rates average 2 mg/kg/min or approximately 200 g/d in a 70-kg person.
   2. After a meal, the increase in plasma glucose and insulin decreases hepatic glucose release and increases peripheral glucose uptake, thereby decreasing the amount of glucose that must be used by extrahepatic tissues.

      As the plasma glucose and insulin concentrations decrease after a meal, the rates of hepatic glucose production and peripheral glucose uptake are restored to basal levels, allowing glucose production to increase and glucose uptake to decrease.

      The postprandial glucose concentration rarely exceeds 150 mg/dL.

D. The homeostatic mechanisms that maintain euglycemia in the postabsorptive state and blunt the postprandial glycemic response in nondiabetic subjects are impaired in patients with diabetes. These patients have both preprandial and postprandial hyperglycemia because of excessive hepatic glucose production, impaired glucose uptake, and decreased insulin secretion or action.

E. Under conditions of severe stress, patients without an antecedent diagnosis of diabetes mellitus may develop hyperglycemia.[3]
   1. Severe stress is accompanied by marked increases in the plasma concentration of counterregulatory hormones (ie, glucagon, epinephrine, cortisol, and growth hormone) and cytokines.
      a) Hyperglycemia results from increased hepatic glucose production and decreased peripheral glucose uptake.
      b) Stress causes a greater derangement in glucose metabolism in diabetic patients because they cannot increase insulin secretion as a compensatory response and this is one mechanism for the deterioration in glucose control often observed in sick diabetic patients.[4]

II. Unique Nutritional Issues Associated with Diabetes Mellitus

A. Although the nutrition assessment, indications for nutrition support, and estimate of nutritional needs for critically ill diabetic patients are similar to those of nondiabetic patients, special attention should be focused on caloric requirements. Overfeeding should be avoided because excessive calories can cause hyperglycemia.
   1. Studies using the Harris-Benedict equation have shown that the measured energy expenditure of most hospitalized patients is between 100% and 120% of predicted resting energy expenditure.[5]
   2. Many patients with diabetes are overweight, yet data are limited and there is no consensus about the nutritional requirements of obese patients.
   3. Certain groups recommend that, in obese patients, the weight used to estimate caloric requirements should be the weight halfway between ideal and current weight. Others recommend feeding ~75% of the Harris-Benedict estimate of energy requirements based on the current weight. Outcome studies are needed.

B. Although the nutrition assessment, indications for nutrition support, and estimate of nutritional needs for critically ill diabetic patients are similar to those of nondiabetic patients, special attention should be focused on diabetes-related gastrointestinal complications.
   1. Diabetic gastroparesis denotes gastric atony and delayed gastric emptying; however, symptoms are related to dysmotility not only of the stomach but also of the small bowel.[6]

      Common manifestations of diabetic enteropathy include heartburn, dysphagia, early satiety, postprandial vomiting (especially partially digested food retained from earlier meals), and epigastric pain.

Although demonstration of delayed gastric emptying establishes the diagnosis of gastroparesis, the diagnosis should be strongly suspected from the history.

Peripheral neuropathy, retinopathy, and nephropathy are frequently found in patients with symptomatic diabetic gastroparesis.

Delayed gastric emptying makes regulation of glucose control difficult. Hyperglycemia may further delay gastric emptying, whereas hypoglycemia may develop in patients treated with insulin or with oral diabetic agents who do not absorb ingested food normally because of a delay in gastric emptying.

Glucose levels should be carefully monitored and appropriately managed because gastric emptying can be slowed by hyperglycemia.

Accurate diagnosis of gastroparesis is important to avoid attributing the gastrointestinal symptoms to tube feeding alone or to other factors capable of slowing gut motility.

The patient's medication profile should be reviewed for medications with potential to slow gastric emptying, such as anticholinergics, antidepressants, α_2-adrenergic agonists, calcium channel blockers, and opiates.

Knowledge of the fat content of the tube feeding formula is important because enteral fat can decrease gut motility.

If tube feeding is required, most patients tolerate jejunal tube feeding, provided that iso-osmolar feedings are started at a low rate and are advanced slowly. Certain patients require a decompression (venting) gastrostomy tube.

Parenteral nutrition (PN) should be reserved for patients who have severe small bowel dysmotility and who have failed a reasonable trial of nasojejunal tube feeding.

C. Constipation, diarrhea, or fecal incontinence may also develop with long-standing diabetes.

III. Glucose Goals and Rationale of Therapy

A. There are limited data establishing "ideal" glucose goals in hospitalized patients.

1. In an effort to balance potential benefits derived by prevention of hyperglycemia and risks due to hypoglycemia, aiming for a glucose goal range of 80 to 120 mg/dL is recommended for critically ill patients in intensive care unit settings.
2. Aiming for a range of 100 to 150 mg/dL is recommended for non-critically ill patients in ward settings. Safe achievement of tighter glucose goal ranges is difficult, as nurse to patient staffing ratios are different in ward and intensive care unit settings and many patients are managed with subcutaneously administered insulin regimens. Finally, studies showing an outcome advantage with tight glucose control did not include non-critically ill patients on ward settings. Additional studies are required to establish risks, benefits, and goals for differing subsets of hospitalized patients. In addition, to date studies have not included pediatric patients.
3. Aggressive treatment of hyperglycemia is indicated regardless of whether a previous diagnosis of diabetes has been established.

B. Avoidance or minimization of hypoglycemia is important as hypoglycemia can cause adrenergic or neuroglycopenic symptoms.

1. Adrenergic symptoms include sweating, palpitations, anxiety, tachycardia, and hunger; neuroglycopenic symptoms include headache, visual changes, and alterations in behavior.
2. Identification of the neuroglycopenic or adrenergic symptoms of hypoglycemia is difficult in severely ill patients who are sedated or ventilator-dependent.
3. In addition, patients with long-standing diabetes may develop hypoglycemic unawareness, a loss of the ability to recognize warning symptoms of hypoglycemia.
4. To minimize subsequent hypoglycemia, clinicians should attempt to identify the factor(s) responsible for hypoglycemia.
5. Potential causes include excess insulin dose, unanticipated discontinuation of nutrition support in patients receiving insulin, resolution of severe stress, discontinuation or decreased doses of corticosteroids or sympathomimetic agents, renal dysfunction, severe hepatitis, sepsis, or diabetic gastroparesis.

C. Avoidance or minimization of hyperglycemia is important during short-term hospitalization to avoid adverse effects on fluid balance.

1. As the filtered load of glucose increases, it eventually exceeds tubular reabsorptive capacity.
2. As a result, glucose remains in the tubular lumen and acts as an osmotic diuretic, increasing the urinary loss of electrolytes and water.

D. Avoidance or minimization of hyperglycemia is also important to enhance immune function.

1. Hyperglycemia is associated with abnormalities in granulocyte adhesion, chemotaxis, phagocytosis, respiratory burst function, and intracellular killing; significant improvement occurs with control of blood glucose.[7–12]
2. Hyperglycemia can impair complement function.[9] Glucose can attach to complement, preventing its attachment to a microbe and impairing opsonization.
3. The association between hyperglycemia and infections with the yeast *Candida albicans* is well known and a potential mechanism has been identified.[7–8]
   a) The yeast expresses a surface protein that is homologous with the alpha chain of the neutrophil receptor for complement and its expression is increased with hyperglycemia.
   b) This surface protein can impair phagocytosis by binding to complement and mediate adhesion of the yeast to endothelial surfaces.
4. Clinical evidence has linked hyperglycemia to nosocomial infection in stressed hospitalized patients.
   a) Hyperglycemia (plasma glucose concentration > 200 mg/dL) within 3 days before the diagnosis was the most common risk factor for candida infection.[7]
   b) A meta-analysis summarizing results from prospective randomized trials comparing parenteral with enteral nutrition in critically ill patients reported that significantly fewer enterally fed patients experienced septic complication (16% versus 35%, respectively). Hyperglycemia may have been one variable responsible for the increased infection rate, as the mean glucose concentration at the conclusion of the study was 230 mg/dL in the parenterally fed patients compared with 130 mg/dL in the enterally fed group.[13]
   c) Hyperglycemia itself may be an independent risk factor for development of infection.[14] Investigators who monitored perioperative glucose control in 100 previously uninfected patients with diabetes and followed the subsequent development of postoperative infection found that hyperglycemia (glucose level in excess of 220 mg/dL) on postoperative day 1 was associated with a higher rate of infection.
5. Observational studies indicate that hyperglycemia in patients without known diabetes is a risk factor for adverse outcome in patients experiencing acute illnesses.
   a) A meta-analysis of observational studies quantified the impact of hyperglycemia on the prognosis of patients without known

diagnoses of diabetes following myocardial infarction. In patients immediately following myocardial infarction, glucose values in excess of 110 to 144 mg/dL were associated with a 3-fold increase in mortality and a higher risk of heart failure.[15]

b) In patients suffering ischemic strokes, glucose values in excess of 108 to 144 mg/dL (range) were associated with a 3-fold increase in mortality and appear related to the degree of permanent disability after stroke.[16]

6. Randomized trials of interventions in critically ill patients have documented association between hyperglycemia and adverse outcomes.
   a) The Veteran Administration Cooperative Study was designed to test the hypothesis that perioperative parenteral nutrition would prevent serious complications following major surgery.[17] While patients receiving parenteral nutrition had fewer noninfectious complications, infections were twice as common as in control patients. This higher infection rate was associated with severe hyperglycemia and provision of excess calories. A serum glucose concentration greater then 300 mg/dL occurred in 20% of patients receiving parenteral nutrition and in 1% of the control group.
7. Control of hyperglycemia during acute illness has been associated with improved outcomes.
   a) In an observational study, implementation of an insulin infusion to maintain glucose levels between 150 and 200 mg/dL decreased by 58% the risk of sternal wound infections following coronary artery bypass grafting.[18]
   b) This same group of investigators compared insulin infusion with subcutaneous insulin management in diabetic patients undergoing coronary artery bypass grafting procedures. Insulin infusion resulted in improved glucose control, and decreased mortality by 57%.[19]
   c) Malmberg et al conducted a randomized trial of intensive insulin therapy (from admission to 3 months after discharge) in patients with diabetes after myocardial infection.[20] In this study known as the DIGAMI Trial, the 1-year mortality was 29% lower in patients receiving insulin therapy compared with the standard treatment group.
   d) Van den Berghe et al conducted a randomized trial of intensive glycemic control (glycemic goal of 80 to 110 mg/dL) compared with usual care in a surgical intensive care unit.[21] Patients received intravenous dextrose day one and then either parenteral nutrition, enteral nutrition, or combined parenteral and enteral nutrition. The mean caloric intake was ~19 nonprotein calories per kilogram body weight. At the end of the study period, patients with average blood glucose levels of 103 mg/dL (study group) experienced 44% lower mortality than patients with average blood glucose of 153 mg/dL. Intensive insulin treatment also reduced bloodstream infections, acute renal failure requiring dialysis or hemofiltration, median number of red cell transfusions, and critical illness polyneuropathy. However, there was a 60% increase in the risk of hypoglycemia (defined as glucose concentration below 40 mg/dL).
8. Benefits may be due to insulin, correction of hyperglycemia, or a combination.
9. The cause or causes of hyperglycemia must be identified.
   a) Potential causes include illness or infection, overfeeding (nutrition support, dextrose-containing crystalloid, dextrose absorption during peritoneal dialysis, and medications formulated in lipid emulsion, such as propofol), medications (eg, corticosteroids, sympathomimetic infusion, or immunosuppressants), insufficient insulin, and volume depletion
   b) Unexplained hyperglycemia may be a harbinger of infection so potential sources should be evaluated.

IV. Management

A. Special aspects of diet and nutritional supplements
   1. The American Diabetes Association position statement on nutrition states that although selected soluble fibers are capable of delaying glucose absorption from the small intestine, the effect of dietary fiber on glycemic control is probably insignificant.[22] Therefore, the fiber intake recommendations for diabetics are probably the same as for the general hospitalized population.
   2. The availability of enteral formulas lower in carbohydrate and higher in fat content than standard formulas has prompted studies examining their effects on glycemic control.
   3. Evidence from single meal and short-term studies report better glycemic control. However, no prospective randomized trials have compared continuous or gravity feeding of these formulas compared with standard formulas in hospitalized patients. Thus, whether these products are helpful in these patients has yet to be established.[23] See Chapter 4 for further detail on formulas.

B. Special aspects of enteral and parenteral nutrition[24]
   1. Although many approaches can be used to achieve glucose control, the following approach works effectively in an institution where many clinicians prescribe nutrition.[25]
   2. Although it is not recommended to initiate long-acting (eg, Ultralente or Glargine) insulin programs in hospitalized patients, it is recommended to continue basal doses of these insulins for patients admitted to the hospital on established multiple daily insulin programs (Table 27-1).

C. Enteral nutrition
   1. Although subcutaneous (SQ) insulin administration aims to prevent hyperglycemia in patients receiving enteral calories, glycemic control can be difficult to achieve.

TABLE 27-1. Insulin Preparation Pharmacokinetics

Insulin	Route	Onset	Peak	Effective duration
Rapid-acting	SQ			
• Lispro		5–15 min	30–90 min	5 hr
• Aspart		5–15 min	30–90 min	5 hr
Short-acting				
• Regular	SQ	30–60 min	2–3 hr	5–8 hr
	IV		0.5 hr	3.5 hr
Intermediate-acting	SQ			
NPH	2–4 hr	4–10 hr	10–16 hr	
Lente	2–4 hr	4–10 hr	10–16 hr	
Long-acting	SQ			
Ultralente		6–10 hr	10–16 hr	18–24 hr
Glargine		2–4 hr	No peak	20–24 hr

a) Measurement of glucose by reflectance meter is recommended because the results are rapidly obtained and the need for venipuncture is avoided. However, a control program including meter calibration, personnel training, comparison measurements, and monitoring of results must be established to ensure accuracy of results.
b) Oral diabetic agents may be administered by feeding tube in medically stable patients with well-controlled type 2 diabetes mellitus and normal renal and hepatic function.
c) Use of metformin in hospitalized patients is not recommended because a major (although very uncommon) risk of metformin use is lactic acidosis, which can occur in patients with hepatic or renal disease or in those with tissue ischemia.
d) When initiating tube feeding, use of short-acting insulin is recommended to minimize the risk of hypoglycemia which could result from continued absorption of insulin from NPH (insulin suspension, isophane) or Lente (insulin zinc suspension) preparations after unexpected discontinuation of tube feeding.
e) Once the tube feeding infusion rate has reached 30 to 40 mL/h, the use of NPH or Lente insulin preparation (intermediate-acting insulin) generally is safe.
f) If tube feedings are administered during the day, begin by providing one-half of the patient's preadmission morning insulin dose as intermediate-acting insulin, while adhering to the SQ regular insulin algorithm (Table 27-2), and then appropriately adjust the following day's doses of intermediate-acting insulin.
g) For some patients with type 2 diabetes receiving nocturnal tube feeding, administration of intermediate-acting insulin prior to the initiation of nocturnal feeds is adequate.
h) Twice daily administration of intermediate-acting insulin may be required if tube feedings are administered continuously over 24 hours.
i) If feedings are infused by gravity administration, the glucose concentration should be checked immediately before the feeding is initiated and no sooner than 4 hours after the end of the prior feeding.
j) Although some patients receiving gravity feeding can be managed with intermediate-acting insulin alone, others need combined treatment with intermediate-acting and short-acting insulin.

TABLE 27-2. Guidelines for SQ Regular Insulin Supplementation

Adjustment of algorithm may be required for differences in patient weight, response to insulin, and treatment goals. Insulin should not be administered more often than every four to six hours. Initiate supplementation if two consecutive glucose values exceed 150 mg/dL.

Glucose, mg/dL	SQ Regular Insulin Dose, Units
150–200	1–2
201–250	2–4
251–300	3–6
301–350	4–8
>350	5–10

k) Increases in the tube feeding infusion rate should be avoided until adequate glucose control has been achieved. Insulin doses should be appropriately adjusted.

Although gastroparesis may make tube-feeding tolerance more difficult, most patients tolerate jejunal feedings when iso-osmolar formulas are started at a low rate (eg, 20 mL/h) and advanced slowly (eg, increased at increments of 10 to 20 mL/h every 12 hours) to the goal infusion rate. Avoidance of higher fat formulas is needed because enteral fat may decrease gastric emptying. In addition, review of the patient's medication profile is important. Certain medications (eg, anticholinergics, antidepressants, α_2-adrenergic agonists, calcium channel blockers, and opiates) may decrease gut motility and, if not needed, should be discontinued. Prokinetic agents remain the treatment of choice. Selected patients require use of a venting decompression tube.

Unexpected discontinuation of tube feeding may cause hypoglycemia in patients treated with subcutaneous injections of insulin. A protocol to treat hypoglycemia is shown in Table 27-3.

TABLE 27-3. Treatment of Hypoglycemia in Hospitalized Adult Patients with Hyperglycemia on Insulin or Oral Diabetic Agents

I. Presumed symptomatic hypoglycemia should be treated without waiting to check plasma or blood glucose level.
   A. If patient able to swallow safely, administer ~15 grams carbohydrate in one of the following forms:
      1. 5 sugar packets dissolved in 4 ounces (½ cup) of water
      2. 4 ounces (½ cup) of fruit juice
      3. Glucose Oral Gel 15 grams orally must be used for those on Acarbose or Miglitol
   B. If the patient has a functioning feeding tube, administer one of the following by feeding tube:
      1. 4 ounces (½ cup) of fruit juice (not orange juice or other pulp-containing juice)
      2. 5 sugar packets dissolved in 4 ounces (1/2 cup) of water
   C. If patient not able to take oral feeding safely or NPO:
      1. If IV access available, administer $D_{50}W$ 25 mL (12.5 grams) intravenously
      2. If no IV access present, administer Glucagon 1 mg by SQ injection. Following Glucagon treatment, for patients not NPO, provide snack to prevent subsequent hypoglycemia.
   D. Contact the service responsible for the patient's diabetes management
II. For treatment of asymptomatic hypoglycemia (glucose less than or equal to 60 mg/dL) follow steps A through C above
III. Glycemic monitoring following treatment
   A. Measure reflectance meter glucose level in 15 minutes. If glucose not greater than 80 mg/dL, repeat treatment outlined above. Recheck glucose value in 15 minutes. Repeat further treatment (and glucose checks at 15 minutes intervals) until glucose level greater than 80 mg/dL.

An IV insulin infusion should be initiated (Tables 27-4 and 27-5) for severe hyperglycemia or if glucose goals cannot be achieved with subcutaneous insulin. We use different infusion algorithms in intensive care unit settings compared with ward settings. As discussed earlier, outcome studies testing degrees of glucose control have not included patients on ward settings. In addition, nursing staff to patient ratios are typically different in intensive care unit and ward settings, and safe achievement of tighter glucose goals is a challenge. Appropriate adjustment of the insulin infusion is required for effective use of infusions. Studies testing which insulin infusion achieves desired goals are limited.

D. Special aspects of parenteral nutrition[25]

1. A glucose level should be measured before initiation of PN. Avoid overfeeding and limit PN dextrose to ~ 150–200 g on the first day of nutrition.
2. Measuring glucose levels on the first and second morning following implementation of PN is recommended in all patients. The frequency of subsequent monitoring should be individualized. For patients with diabetes or significant hyperglycemia we initially measure glucose levels two to four times per day until glucose values are stable. Subsequently, glucose levels are checked twice daily.
3. The majority of diabetic patients require supplemental insulin when glucose is infused.
   a) For patients previously treated with insulin or oral diabetic agents or for patients with two more glucose values > 120 or 150 mg/dL (120 mg/dL for intensive care unit settings and 150 mg/dL for ward settings), adding a basal amount of insulin to PN solutions is recommended.
   b) A common starting point is 0.1 units of insulin per g of dextrose (eg, 10 units/L of 10% dextrose [100 g/L], 20 units/L of 20% dextrose [200 g/L]).
   c) This ratio of insulin to dextrose is unlikely to cause hypoglycemia and thus minimizes the need to discard a bag of PN because it contains too much insulin.
   d) If needed, supplemental SQ regular insulin is administered according to an algorithm (Table 27-2) to supplement the PN insulin.

TABLE 27-4. Intravenous Insulin Infusion Algorithm for ICU Use

Column 1		Column 2		Column 3		Column 4	
Dedside glucose (mg/dL)	Insulin infusion rate (units/hr)	Dedside glucose (mg/dL)	Insulin infusion rate (units/hr)	Dedside glucose (mg/dL)	Insulin infusion rate (units/hr)	Dedside glucose (mg/dL)	Insulin infusion rate (units/hr)
>400	8	≥360	12	≥360	16	≥270	20
351–400	6	330–359	8	330–359	14	240–269	16
301–350	4	300–329	7	300–329	12	210–239	12
251–300	3	270–299	6	270–299	10	180–209	8
200–250	2.5	240–269	5	240–269	8	150–179	4
150–199	2	210–239	4	210–239	6	120–149	2
120–149	1.5	180–209	3	180–209	4	100–119	1
100–119	1	150–179	2	150–179	3	<100	Off
<100	Off	120–149	1.5	120–149	2		
		100–119	1	100–119	1		
		<100	Off	<100	Off		

1. Glucose goals should be determined for each patient. In critically ill patients, a glucose goal range of 80 to120 mg/dL is appropriate. This infusion algorithm is designed for the average 70-kg patient and may require modification for smaller or larger patients. This infusion is not appropriate for the treatment of diabetic ketoacidosis or hyperosmolar states.
2. Choose appropriate columns for insulin infusion. Follow a column for two hours and if reflectance meter glucose (RMG) is still greater than 120 mg/dL or is not decreasing, proceed to next column. If patient treated by column 3 or 4 has RMG less than 120 mg/dL for 4 hours, then go to the next lowest column.
3. Instructions for use of columns: Use if any of the following criteria listed for each column are met. Column 1: RMG 120 to 200 mg/dL; not on corticosteroids or sympathomimetic infusion.
   Column 2: Initial RMG greater than 200 mg/dL; receiving oral or IV corticosteroids (excludes inhaled or ophthalmic); on sympathomimetic infusion; has not reached RMG range of 80 to 120 mg/dL within two hours of using Column 1.
   Column 3: Patient who has not reached RMG of 80 to 120 mg/dL within two hours using Column 2.
   Column 4: Patient who has not reached RMG range of 80 to 120 mg/dL within two hours using Column 3.
4. Glucose level should be measured hourly until glucose concentration has stabilized in the desired goal range for four hours. Testing frequency may then be decreased to every two hours. Return to hourly monitoring with any of the following: change in nutritional status, RMG is above goal for two consecutive readings or below 100 mg/dL, or change in clinical status or column use.

TABLE 27-5. IV Insulin Infusion for Use in Non-ICU Settings

Glucose mg/dL	IV infusion rate mL/hr	Insulin infusion rate units/hr
>400	8	8
351–400	6	6
301–350	4	4
250–300	3	3
200–249	2.5	2.5
150–199	2	2
120–149	1.5	1.5
100–119	1	1
70–99	0	0
<70	0	0

1. Guidelines are for the average 70-kg patient and modifications may be necessary for smaller or larger patients. Guidelines not appropriate for treatment of patients with diabetic ketoacidosis or hyperosmolar states.
2. Glucose should be measured hourly until glucose concentrations have stabilized in the patient's goal glucose range for 4 hours. Frequency of testing may then be decreased to every 2 hours, and once glucose control remains stable, frequency of testing may be reduced to every 4 hours.
3. If glucose value is >200 mg/dL and does not decrease by at least 50 mg/dL by 2 hours, increase insulin infusion by 50% increment for each glucose range >150 mg/dL. Make the same adjustment if glucose <200 mg/dL (but >150 mg/dL) and does not decrease by at least 25 mg/dL by 2 hours. Risk of hypoglycemia may be greater if infusions are increased for glucose ranges <150 mg/dL.
4. When converting from an IV to SQ insulin program, continue infusion for 1 to 3 hours after administration of first SQ insulin dose.

If over a 24-hour period glucose values consistently exceed the desired goal, the PN insulin is increased by 0.05 units of insulin injection per g of dextrose each day to 0.2.

Order forms to standardize use of insulin infusions are presented in Tables 27-4 and 27-5.

If two consecutive glucose values exceed 120 mg/dL in patients in intensive care units, it is reasonable to initiate an insulin infusion. On wards, guidelines for when to initiate infusions are less clear as data is limited. It is recommended to continue providing PN insulin for patients treated with an insulin infusion. However the SQ insulin algorithm should be discontinued.

In general, the dextrose content of the PN should not be increased until the glucose concentrations during the previous 24-hour period are in goal range.

Insulin in the PN should be proportionally increased or decreased when the PN dextrose content is increased or decreased.

If the patient develops hypoglycemia, parenteral dextrose should be administered (Table 27-3) and the PN insulin content should be reduced by approximately 50% to minimize recurrent hypoglycemia.

Similar reductions in the PN insulin should also be made if there is a significant decrease in the mean glucose concentration over a 24-hour period to values below the goal range.

Symptomatic hypoglycemia after sudden discontinuation of PN is uncommon provided that the patient has not received excess calories.

If PN is discontinued it is important to remember that the PN insulin also will be stopped.

Subcutaneous insulin should be administered several hours before discontinuation of intravenous insulin infusion to avoid rebound hyperglycemia. For example, in patients treated with combined intermediate and short-acting insulin programs, administration of small amounts (eg, 4 to 5 units) of short-acting insulin combined with a 'basal' insulin (eg, glargine or ultralente insulin or small doses of NPH insulin) is recommended.

While the technology to deliver tight glucose control in the intensive care unit is widely available, implementing a safe and effective program may present logistical challenges.[26] One safety concern of tight glucose control is the potential increase in the risk of hypoglycemia.

E. Focused monitoring/goals assessment—In addition to the usual careful monitoring required after initiation of nutrition support in a malnourished patient, special attention should be focused on glucose control (discussed above), fluid balance, sodium, potassium, magnesium, phosphorus, and triglyceride values.
  1. A baseline glycated hemoglobin value is useful to establish recent glucose control and to determine the appropriate diabetic treatment after dismissal from the hospital.
  2. The presence of high urine output, negative fluid balance, weight loss, or hypernatremia should prompt a review of recent glucose trends to be certain hyperglycemia is not causing an osmotic diuresis.
  3. Hyperglycemia may cause a pseudohyponatremia. In general, each incremental increase in plasma glucose of ~60 mg/dL reduces the plasma sodium concentration by 1 mEq/L.
  4. Hyperkalemia, if accompanied by hyperglycemia, if often effectively treated by an increase in insulin supplementation.
  5. Hyperinsulinemia due to refeeding or insulin administration may lead to a decrease in plasma levels of potassium, magnesium, and phosphorus.[27]
  6. Hyperinsulinemia shifts potassium and magnesium into skeletal muscle and hepatic cells.
  7. Glucose and insulin-stimulated glycolysis increases cellular uptake and utilization of phosphorus for phosphorylation of glucose and fructose and for synthesis of adenosine triphosphate.
  8. Serum potassium and phosphorus concentrations should be monitored daily (and appropriately managed) until values are in the normal range.
  9. For patients with known hypertriglyceridemia receiving PN, triglycerides should be checked before initiation and during fat emulsion administration. Measuring a triglyceride level before initiation of PN is also recommended in patients with pancreatitis or poorly controlled diabetes and in those receiving medications formulated in fat emulsion.
  10. Although there are limited data regarding infusion of fat emulsion in patients with hypertriglyceridemia, if the plasma triglyceride concentration exceeds 350 to 400 mg/dL reducing the amount of fat or discontinuing fat altogether is recommended, as lipoprotein lipase-mediated triglyceride uptake may be saturated above this level.[28] Triglyceride-rich lipoproteins are removed from the circulation by zero- and first-order kinetics and therefore, when sat-

urated, plasma triglyceride concentrations will increase exponentially with incremental changes in the rate of infusion of intravenous fat emulsion.

F. System of care
  1. Implementation of a safe and effective program for glucose control is required.
  2. One safety concern relates to the potential increase in the occurrence of hypoglycemia in patients with a goal of tight glucose control.
  3. Well-defined algorithms to manage high and low glucose levels are required as well as education of managing staff.

(Diabetes chapter from the 1st edition was contributed by Susan A. Romanski and M. Molly McMahon)

REFERENCES

1. The Expert Committee on the Diagnosis and Classification of Diabetes Mellitus. Report of the expert committee on the diagnosis and classification of diabetes mellitus. *Diabetes Care.* 1997; 20:1183–1197.
2. Umpierrez GE, Isaacs SD, Bazargan N, et al. Hyperglycemia: an independent marker of in-hospital mortality in patients with undiagnosed diabetes. *J Clin Endocrinol Metab.* 2002;87:978–982.
3. Shamoon M, Hendler R, Sherwin R. Synergistic interactions among anti-insulin hormones in the pathogenesis of stress hyperglycemia in humans. *J Clin Endocrinol Metab.* 1981;52:1235–1241.
4. Shamoon M. Hendler R, Sherwin R. Altered responsiveness to cortisol, epinephrine, and glucagon in insulin-infused juvenile-onset diabetes. *Diabetes.* 1980;29:284–301.
5. McMahon MM, Farnell MB, Murray MJ. Nutritional support of critically ill patients. *Mayo Clin Proc.* 1993;68:911–920.
6. Camilleri M. Advances in diabetic gastroparesis. *Rev Gastroenterol Disord.* 2002;2:47–56.
7. Hostetter M. Perspectives in diabetes: Handicaps to host defense: effects of hyperglycemia on C3 and Candida albicans. *Diabetes.* 1990;39:271–275.
8. Gustafson KS, Vercellotti GM, Bendel CM, et al. Molecular mimicry in Candida albicans: role of an integrin analogue in adhesion of the yeast to human endothelium. *J Clin Invest.* 1991;87:1896–1902.
9. Hostetter M. The third component of complement: new functions for an old friend. *J Lab Clin Med.* 1993;122:491–496.
10. McCowen KC, Malhotra A, Bistrian BR. Stress-induced hyperglycemia. *Crit Care Clin.* 2001;17:107–124.
11. McMahon M, Bistrian BR. Host defenses and susceptibility to infection in patients with diabetes mellitus. *Infect Dis Clin N Am.* 1995;9:1–9.
12. Bistrian BR. Hyperglycemia and infection. Which is the chicken and which the egg? *J Parenter Enter Nutr.* 2001;25:180–181.
13. Moore FA, Feliciano DV, Andrassy RJ, et al. Early enteral feeding, compared with parenteral, reduces postoperative septic complications. The results of a meta-analysis. *Ann Surg.* 1992;216(2):172–83.
14. Pomposelli JJ, Baxter JK, Babineau TJ, et al. Early postoperative glucose control predicts nosocomial infection rate in diabetic patients. *J Parenter Enter Nutr.* 1998;22:77–81.
15. Capes SE, Hunt D, Malmberg K, Gerstein HC. Stress hyperglycemia and increased risk of death after myocardial infarction in patient with and without diabetes. A systematic overview. *Lancet.* 2000;355:773–778.
16. Capes SE, Hunt D, Malmberg K, et al. Stress hyperglycemia and prognosis of stroke in nondiabetic and diabetic patients: A systematic overview. *Stroke.* 2001;32:2426–2432.
17. The Veterans Affairs Total Parenteral Nutrition Cooperative Study Group. Perioperative total parenteral nutrition in surgical patients. *N Engl J Med.* 1993;325:525–532.
18. Furnary AP, Zerr KJ, Grunkemeier GL, et al. Continuous intravenous insulin infusion reduces the incidence of deep sternal wound infection in diabetic patients after cardiac surgical procedures. *Ann Thorac Surg.* 1999;67:352–362.
19. Furnary AP, Guangqiang G, Grunkemeier GL, et al. Continuous insulin infusion reduces mortality in patients with diabetes undergoing coronary artery bypass grafting. *J Thorac Cardiovasc Surg.* 2003;1125:1007–1021.
20. Malmberg K, for the DIGAMI Study Group. Prospective randomized study of intensive insulin treatment on long-term survival after acute myocardial infarction in patients with diabetes mellitus. *Br Med J.* 1997;314:1512–1515.
21. Van den Berghe G, Wouters P, Weekers F, et al. Intensive insulin therapy in critically ill patients. *N Engl J Med.* 2001;345:1359–1367.
22. American Diabetes Association. Nutrition recommendations and principles for people with diabetes mellitus. *Diabetes Care.* 1995;18:16–19.
23. Nutrition Subcommittee of the Diabetes Care Advisory Committee of Diabetes UK. The implementation of nutritional advice for people with diabetes. *Diabet Med.* 2003;20:786–807.
24. A.S.P.E.N. Board of Directors. Clinical pathways and algorithms for delivery of parenteral and enteral nutrition support in adults. Silver Spring, MD: American Society for Parenteral and Enteral Nutrition; 1998:4–11.
25. McMahon M. Management of parenteral nutrition in acutely ill patients with hyperglycemia. *Nutr Clin Practice.* 2004;19:120–128.
26. Montori VM, Bistrian BR, McMahon M. Hyperglycemia in acutely ill patients. *J Am Med Ass.* 2002;288:2167–2169.
27. Knochel JP. Complications of total parenteral nutrition. *Kidney Int.* 1985;27:489–496.
28. Carpentier YA. Intravascular metabolism of fat emulsions. *Clin Nutr.* 1989;8:115–1.

Julie L. Roth, MD; Robert F. Kushner, MD; Eden Bateman, MS, RD, LD

28

Obesity

Introduction

One third of Americans and over 50% of minority women are considered obese, while 15% of US children and adolescents are overweight. Obesity, defined as a body mass index (BMI) of greater than or equal to 30 kg/m^2, is associated with several chronic degenerative diseases that often require medical and surgical attention. Nutritional care of obese individuals requires expertise in management of the associated comorbidities, assessment of energy and protein requirements, special techniques of access, and delivery and monitoring of nutrition support.

I. Background

A. Prevalence. The 1999 National Health and Nutrition Examination Survey (NHANES 1999) found that 34% of the adults in the United States aged 20 and over are overweight, and 27% are obese.[1] This represents a 100% increase in obesity prevalence from the 15% reported during NHANES II (1976–1980).[2] For these population surveys, adults were classified as overweight when their BMI (defined as the weight in kilograms divided by the height in meters squared [kg/m^2]) was 25 to 29.9 kg/m^2 and obese when their BMI was greater than or equal to 30 kg/m^2.

B. Etiology. Obesity is a heterogeneous disease involving genetic, environmental, psychological, and other factors. The current view holds that genetics determines vulnerability (penetrance) while environment determines the presence in vulnerable individuals and the extent of disease. Regardless of the etiology, however, obesity occurs when energy intake exceeds the amount of energy expended over time.

1. Obesity is considered a disorder of energy balance. Persons become overweight when a positive energy balance is produced whenever (1) energy intake is increased, (2) energy output is lowered, or (3) both occur. In contrast, maintenance of the obese state is sustained when the individual is once again in energy balance, produced when either (1) energy intake and output are both low or (2) energy intake and output are both high.
2. The role of genetics in human obesity may involve appetite regulation, metabolic partitioning of nutrients, and thermogenesis.
3. Although genetics influences the tendency to become obese, the development and severity of obesity depend on the environment. Improving on the unhealthy eating and physical activity habits of Americans forms the basis for several initiatives of the Public Health Service's Healthy People 2010 campaign.[3]

II. Nutritional Alterations

A. The nutritional alterations of obesity primarily include changes in body composition and energy expenditure. These variables are interrelated, since body weight (kg) is a function of energy balance (calories).

1. Body composition. A positive energy balance produced and sustained over time must result in the storage of excess calories and a gain in body weight. These excess calories are stored in adipose tissue (fat mass) and used to synthesize adipose tissue-free mass (lean body mass [LBM]). Forbes et al found the increase in LBM accounts for 29% (range 20%–40%) of the excess weight.[4] This LBM/body weight relationship is not linear, however; the fatter the individual, the less will be the relative contribution of LBM to the total weight.
2. Total energy expenditure (TEE). TEE increases with increasing body weight in both men and women. Interpersonal variability in this relationship is due to genetic determinants, body composition, and level of physical activity. TEE is composed of three distinct factors: basal metabolic rate (BMR), thermogenic effect of food, and physical activity. The increased energy expenditure observed in obesity is primarily attributed to an elevated BMR that results from increased LBM. Differences in energy requirements within and between individuals are primarily due to differences in physical activity. Since the energy cost of a given activity (workload) is proportional to body weight, total absolute energy expended in physical activity is higher in healthy obese individuals than in their lean counterparts. However, when energy expenditure or physical activity is normalized for BMR (physical activity level index = TEE/BMR), the influence of body weight disappears. An average physical activity level index (light to moderate activities) can be assumed to be 1.55 to 1.65, whereas sedentary individuals (chair-bound or bed-bound) exhibit a physical activity level index of 1.2 (an index that is commonly seen among hospitalized patients).[5]
3. Substrate metabolism. Studies by Jeevanandam et al[6,7] suggest that the sources of endogenous metabolic fuels differ significantly in obese and nonobese patients in response to injury. Whereas nonobese patients displayed an increase in net fat oxidation, obese patients derived a significantly lower percentage of their energy requirements from mobilization of fat. Energy was produced instead from oxidation of carbohydrates and protein. Thus, there is concern that obese patients have both a reduced ability to mobilize fat stores after acute injury and a limited capacity to oxidize fat.

B. Health alterations

1. Endocrine system
   a) Glucose intolerance. Increasing severity of obesity is associated with the development of reduced insulin sensitivity, increased insulin secretion, glucose intolerance, and type 2 diabetes

mellitus. Thus, the occurrence of acute illness, administration of anti-insulin medications (eg, corticosteroids), or infusion of intravenous dextrose often results in glucose intolerance and uncontrolled hyperglycemia.

b) Dyslipidemia. Obesity is associated with a higher prevalence of hypertriglyceridemia, low levels of high-density lipoprotein (HDL) cholesterol, and elevated total cholesterol. The administration of intravenous fat may cause hypertriglyceridemia and requires close monitoring.

2. Metabolic syndrome

a) The metabolic syndrome is a constellation of cardiovascular disease (CVD) risk factors that is present in approximately 24% of US adults.[8] According to the Adult Treatment Panel definition of the metabolic syndrome,[9] three of the following five criteria must be present for diagnosis: increased abdominal girth (>35 inches for women or >40 inches for men), increased triglyceride levels (≥150 mg/dL), decreased HDL cholesterol levels (<50 mg/dL for women or <40 mg/dL for men), increased blood pressure (≥130/85 mm Hg), and increased fasting glucose (≥110 mg/dL).

b) Lemieux et al[10] have suggested that simultaneous measurement of waist circumference and fasting triglyceride levels could be used to identify individuals who meet the metabolic syndrome criteria. Presence of the metabolic syndrome increases risk for development of type 2 diabetes and CVD.[11]

c) The syndrome is also associated with insulin resistance; small, dense low-density lipoprotein particles; increased biomarkers of chronic inflammation (eg, C-reactive protein, tumor necrosis factor-α); a prothrombotic state; endothelial dysfunction; and hemodynamic changes (increased sympathetic nervous system activity and renal sodium retention)—although these are not routinely measured.[12] Recent studies have linked the metabolic and inflammatory abnormalities seen in obesity to the secretion of adipocyte and adipose connective tissue products, or adipokines. Peptides secreted by the adipocyte include leptin, plasminogen activator inhibitor-1 (PAI-1), interleukin-6, adiponectin, angiotensinogen, and tumor necrosis factor-α.[13]

3. Respiratory system

a) Pulmonary function. The most frequently described alterations in pulmonary function of the obese patient are restrictive defects: a decreased functional residual capacity (FRC) and a decreased expiratory reserve volume (ERV). These changes result from reduced compliance of the chest wall and lung tissue, primarily due to the cephalad displacement of the diaphragm and increased weight of fat tissue on the chest wall during tidal breathing. The loss of FRC and ERV results in airway closure, alveolar dysfunction, and ventilation/perfusion abnormalities. Increased metabolic requirements for oxygen consumption and carbon dioxide excretion may exceed pulmonary capacity.

b) Obesity hypoventilation syndrome (OHS) and obstructive sleep apnea (OSA). More severe degrees of obesity may result in further impairment of pulmonary function and development of hypoventilation, hypoxia, hypercarbia, and obstructive sleep apnea. Patients with OHS and/or OSA should be closely monitored with pulse oximetry and capnography during nutrition support. Use of continuous positive airway pressure in both hospitalized and ambulatory patients should be instituted if obstructive sleep apnea is detected.

4. Cardiovascular system

a) The increased metabolic demands of obesity with increased V_{O_2}, V_{CO_2}, and blood volume require an increased cardiac output. This is accomplished by increasing stroke volume; heart rate usually remains normal. Over time, an increased cardiac preload results in increased left ventricular end-diastolic volume, wall stress, and development of eccentric left ventricular hypertrophy. Development of hypertension and increased cardiac afterload results in concentric left ventricular hypertrophy. The consequences of increasing severity and duration of obesity include coronary artery disease and congestive heart failure. Hypoventilation and obstructive sleep apnea result in increased pulmonary artery pressure, right-sided hypertension, and cor pulmonale. The fluid-overloaded status and congestive changes of the severely obese patient require that fluid administration be carefully monitored.

b) Obesity is often associated with peripheral venous stasis and risk for thromboembolism. This increased risk may be due to a deficiency in antithrombin III, a serum protein that inhibits thrombin activity, and other prothrombotic factors, including increased plasma PAI-1, fibrinogen, and factor VIII. The thrombotic tendency is of particular concern when an indwelling venous catheter is placed for intravenous fluids and nutritional support. Thus, obese patients require primary prevention that often includes pneumatic compression of the lower extremities combined with subcutaneous or intravenous unfractionated heparin or low-molecular weight heparin.

5. Gastrointestinal system. Obese patients' increased risk for developing gallbladder disease is proportional to their higher BMI, with a significant increase above 30 kg/m^2.[14] Obese patients are also at increased risk for developing nonalcoholic fatty liver disease, gastroesophageal reflux disease, and colon cancer.

6. Psychiatric issues. Obese patients often suffer from depression that may or may not be diagnosed. One study found higher depression scores in women, younger subjects, and those with body image issues at baseline; these scores significantly decreased with surgically induced weight loss at 4-year follow-up.[15]

7. Nursing care issues. The heavy body weight and immobility of the obese patient increases the risk for skin breakdown, development of decubitus ulcers, and infection. Necrosis and infection may quickly spread through the subcutaneous tissue with little warning. Intertriginous areas, such as under the breasts, on inguinal folds, beneath the abdominal pannus, and on inner thighs, are often sites for skin maceration and fungal infections. Care is needed to prevent skin breakdown by frequently rolling the bedridden patient, closely examining all skin areas, and using beds specially designed to facilitate care of the severely obese patient.

III. Focused Assessment

A. History

1. Obesity is associated with the coexistence of multiple diseases. Therefore, a detailed history of the obese patient should include a collection of medical information related to any comorbid conditions, use of medications that may influence body weight (including a history of medications specifically related to the treatment of obesity), a family history of obesity and related diseases, and a history of surgeries specifically related to the treatment of obesity. A thorough medication history should be obtained, looking for possible drug-induced weight gain. Medications associated with weight gain are listed in Table 28-1.[16]

2. Dietary assessment is an important tool to identify premorbid nutritional risk factors, to provide information about previous attempts at weight reduction, and to document current intake.

TABLE 28-1. Medications Associated With Body Fat Weight Gain

Psychiatric/neurological
- Antipsychotic agents: phenothiazines, olanzapine, clozapine, risperidone
- Mood stabilizers: lithium
- Antidepressants: tricyclics, MAOIs, SSRIs (paroxetine), mirtazapine
- Antiepileptic drugs: gabapentin, valproate, carbamazepine

Steroid hormones
- Corticosteroids
- Progestational steroids

Antidiabetes agents
- Insulin, sulfonylureas, thiazolidinediones

Antihypertensive agents
- Beta- and alpha-1 adrenergic receptor blockers

Antihistamines
- Cyproheptadine

HIV protease inhibitors: lipodystrophy

HIV, human immunodeficiency virus
Reprinted from Kushner RF, Roth JL. Assessment of the obese patient. *Endocrinol Metab Clin N Am.* 2003;32:915–933 with permission from Elsevier.

3. For long-term planning it is important to know which member of the household is primarily responsible for shopping and meal preparation. This person should be involved in discharge planning and education.
4. Weight history is essential to gain an understanding of the patient's weight patterns and potential for successful, long-term weight management. Patients who have made recent attempts to lose weight and have suffered nutritional deficiencies may need a period of refeeding or nutritional replenishment prior to a surgical procedure.
5. Habitual physical activity level and limitations should be assessed. Information regarding actual activities as well as the duration and frequency of the activities prior to admission should be documented.

B. Physical examination
  1. Anthropometric measurements
     a) Measurement of an obese patient's body weight is useful for nutrition calculations and medical management. The admission weight is used for the calculation of nutrient requirements and medication dosing. However, several disease states can cause physically undetectable increases in fluid retention or total body water in the severely obese patient. Any calculations that include excess fluid weight will introduce error into the final estimate. Daily weights obtained with the same scale will assist the clinician with monitoring alterations in fluid, as opposed to indicating changes in nutritional status.
     b) BMI (weight divided by height squared [kg/m^2]) is the most useful and practical measure for assessing body fatness.[17] The calculation can also be easily performed by dividing the weight by height twice, for example, kg/m/m. The BMI uses a ratio of height to weight, thus eliminating the need to compare weight to a reference value. Several classifications of obesity have been proposed based on health outcomes. The Expert Panel on the Identification, Evaluation, and Treatment of Overweight and Obesity in Adults recommends the classification shown in Table 28-2.[18] BMI measurements should be used as a screening tool in all hospitalized patients.
  2. Assessment of body composition/fat distribution
     a) Waist measurements are commonly used to evaluate the distribution of body fat, especially in persons with a BMI less than 35 kg/m^2. A waist circumference ≥35 inches (85 cm) in women or ≥40 inches (100 cm) in men leads to an increased risk of developing obesity-related comorbidities regardless of the BMI classification. The presence of excess fat stores in the abdominal visceral depot has significant prognostic importance. Patients with greater upper body fat tend to have greater visceral fat stores and increased risk for developing hyperinsulinemia, glucose intolerance, hypertriglyceridemia, hypertension, diabetes mellitus, and coronary artery disease than individuals with lower body obesity.[19] According to the Practical Guide,[20] "To measure waist circumference, locate the upper hip bone and the top of the right iliac crest. Place a measuring tape in a horizontal plane around the abdomen at the level of the iliac crest. Before reading the tape measure, ensure that the tape is snug, but does not compress the skin, and is parallel to the floor. The measurement is made at the end of a normal expiration."
     b) Skinfold measurements are used to estimate the quantity of subcutaneous fat. Measurements can be taken from various body sites and then compared with standard reference values. These estimates are most useful when serial measurements are taken over time to assess changes in body composition. For this reason, skinfold measurements are rarely used to assess nutritional status in the acute care setting. The reliability of skinfold measurements decreases as body fat increases because there are large fat folds that the caliper cannot accurately measure.[21] In the

TABLE 28-2. Classification of Overweight and Obesity by BMI

	Obesity Class	BMI (kg/m^2)
Underweight		<18.5
Normal		18.5–24.9
Overweight		25.0–29.9
Obesity	I	30–34.9
Obesity	II	35–39.9
Extreme obesity	III	≥40.0

BMI, body mass index
Reprinted from National Heart, Lung, and Blood Institute. Clinical Guidelines on the Identification, Evaluation, and Treatment of Overweight and Obesity in Adults. The evidence report. *Obes Res.* 1998;6(suppl 2):51S–210S with permission from the North American Association for the Study of Obesity.

acute care setting, skinfold measurements can be taken if the patient intends to follow up for long-term weight management.

C. Laboratory data
   1. Abnormalities seen in obese patients may include hyperglycemia, hyperinsulinemia, dyslipidemia, elevated uric acid levels, and abnormal liver function tests. Patients with OHS may present with hypoxemia and hypercarbia.
   2. Laboratory abnormalities seen in patients who have previously undergone malabsorptive procedures for obesity include iron deficiency anemia, vitamin B_{12} and folate deficiency, and calcium deficiency. Laboratory evaluation may demonstrate elevated parathyroid hormone levels with depressed 25-hydroxyvitamin D and normal calcium levels.[22]

IV. Approach to the Patient

A. Objectives/goals of therapy. Traditional practice is to provide adequate energy for weight maintenance or to provide enough calories to support anabolism. More recently, though, practitioners have started to implement nutrition care plans for obese patients that promote gradual loss of body fat while maintaining or replenishing LBM. This therapy is often referred to as a protein-sparing modified fast (PSMF). The PSMF is designed to promote use of endogenous fat stores for energy while maintaining nitrogen balance, maintaining LBM, and promoting anabolism. The PSMF has been used for years to treat nonstressed obese people. More recently, the PSMF theory has been applied to metabolically stressed obese patients who require enteral nutrition or parenteral nutrition (PN) support. Dickerson et al[23] found that obese patients given hypocaloric PN achieved a beneficial clinical outcome with complete wound healing, weight loss, and improved plasma proteins. Using a randomized, prospective, double-blind, controlled trial design, Choban et al[24] demonstrated that obese patients receiving hypoenergetic feedings achieved a nitrogen balance comparable to that of patients given conventional PN regimens.

B. Clinical considerations
   1. Severity of obesity. Patients with mild obesity may benefit from a weight maintenance feeding regimen until they are medically stable. This is especially true if the patients are not motivated to continue with weight loss after discharge from the hospital. Moderately and severely obese patients may develop comorbidities related to their excess weight. For these patients, hypocaloric feedings for gradual weight loss may be beneficial.
   2. Comorbid considerations. Hypocaloric, protein-sparing therapy can be useful for patients with poor respiratory status, hyperglycemia, and positive fluid balance. A reduction of total calorie input reduces carbon dioxide production and enhances diuresis, which can improve ventilation and facilitate liberation from the ventilator. The low glucose load from the hypocaloric feeding reduces the risk of carbohydrate intolerance and can decrease insulin requirements.
   3. Premorbid nutritional status. Patients assessed as having malnutrition may need a maintenance nutrition care plan during the critical phase of their illness or until nutritional replenishment/refeeding has occurred. Hypocaloric feeding is most appropriate for obese patients who are not malnourished upon admission.

C. Assessment of energy requirements
   1. Calculated
      a) The Harris-Benedict equation was developed with the use of healthy subjects and, therefore, requires the addition of stress factors that involve subjective judgment of the patient's stress level (Table 28-3). This introduces bias and error to the final estimate of energy requirements. The Ireton-Jones equation was developed specifically for hospitalized patients and takes into account mechanical ventilation and obesity (Table 28-3). Amato et al[25] compared these formula estimates, as well as their own estimate of 21 kcal/kg of actual weight/day for obese patients, to actual measured energy expenditure (MEE) by indirect calorimetry. With a total of 188 measurements on 113 obese mechanically ventilated patients, they found an overall precision of ± 400 kcal between the calculated requirements and MEE, thus suggesting that the use of predictive equations should be limited to situations in which actual measurement of resting metabolic rate by indirect calorimetry is not available. One of the most controversial aspects of using predictive equations to estimate energy requirements for obese patients is choosing which weight to use in the calculation: actual, ideal, or adjusted. It is thought that if the actual weight of an obese patient is used, then the estimate will be significantly above the actual energy requirement, since adipose tissue is less metabolically active than LBM. Obese people are known to have higher LBM than nonobese people of equal stature.[26] If ideal body weight (IBW) is used to calculate energy requirements, the final estimate will fail to account for the increased metabolic activity of the extra LBM and underestimate the total energy requirement. The adjustment of body weight for an obese patient is based on an average increase in LBM of approximately 25% (as discussed in Section II.A.1) to account for metabolically active tissue (Table 28-3).

TABLE 28-3. Predictive Equations to Estimate Energy Expenditure

Harris-Benedict

Men: $66.47 + 13.75(W) + 5.0(H) - 6.75(A)$

Women: $655.1 + 9.56(W) + 1.85(H) - 4.68(A)$

W, weight (kg); H, height (cm); A, age (yr)

Ireton-Jones

$EEE(V) = 1925 - 10(A) + 5(W) + 281(S) + 292(T) + 851(B)$

$EEE(S) = 629 - 11(A) + 25(W) - 609(O)$

V, ventilator; S, spontaneous breather; A, age (yr); W, weight (kg); S, sex (male = 1, female = 0); T, trauma (present = 1, absent = 0); B, burns (present = 1, absent = 0); O, obesity (present = 1, absent = 0)

Amato

EE = 21 kcal/kg (kg in actual weight)

Adjustment of body weight for obesity

Adjusted body weight = [(actual weight − ideal weight) × 0.25) + ideal weight]

EE, energy expenditure; EEE, estimated energy expenditure

Reprinted from Amato P, Keating K, Quercia R, et al. Formulaic methods of estimating calorie requirements in mechanically ventilated obese patients: a reappraisal. *Nutr Clin Pract.* 1995;10:229–232, with permission from the American Society for Parenteral and Enteral Nutrition (A.S.P.E.N.).

      b) A recent study evaluated four different equations (Harris-Benedict, Harris-Benedict using adjusted body weight in obese individuals, Owen, and Mifflin) in nonhospitalized obese and nonobese subjects. The Mifflin calculation (men: kcal/day = 879 + 10.2 [weight in kg]; women: kcal/day = 795 + 7.2 [weight in kg]) provided a more accurate estimate of actual resting metabolic rate in the largest percentage of obese and nonobese subjects, with a low rate of overestimation.[27] This study confirmed the tendency to underestimate resting metabolic rate with the Harris-Benedict equation when using an adjusted body weight.

c) Another study assessed the use of bioelectrical impedance analysis to develop predictive equations for resting energy expenditure (REE).[28] This method provided an REE estimate that was significantly more accurate than the Harris-Benedict equation in 75% of patients. In male subjects, the mean error of the estimate using the Harris-Benedict equation was 372 kcal/d, whereas it was 242 kcal/d with the predictive equation. In female subjects, the mean error of the estimate with the Harris-Benedict equation was 343 kcal/d, whereas it was 158 kcal/d using the predictive equation

$$\text{Men: EE} = [858 - 4.6 \text{ age} + 12.1 \text{ FFM} + 15.0] \text{ (stress factor)}$$

$$\text{Women: EE} = [812 - 5.57 \text{ age} + 15.2 \text{ FFM} + 5.61\text{FM}] \text{ (stress factor)}$$

where EE is energy expenditure, FFM is fat-free mass (in kg), and FM is fat mass.

2. MEE with use of indirect calorimetry is the most accurate, reliable, and practical method of assessing energy requirements in critically ill patients. Continuous indirect calorimetry is ideal for measuring REE as well as the metabolic and mechanically induced rises in energy expenditure. Unfortunately, few hospitals have the resources to routinely conduct continuous indirectly calorimetry. Commonly, intermittent indirect calorimetry is conducted over 30 to 60 minutes at various times during the hospitalization to periodically determine average energy expenditures. Indirect calorimetry is the ideal method for determining energy requirements in the obese patient population, since the measurement eliminates the need to use judgment with regard to body weight, alterations in body composition, and stress factors.
3. If weight loss is desired during an acute illness, the preferred mode is to institute hypocaloric nutrition support. This type of regimen will induce weight loss while minimizing loss of LBM. The basic approach is to provide 50% to 60% of MEE or calculated energy requirements,[23,28] with adequate protein to preserve LBM, and minimal or no fat. Shikora and Muskat[29] favor the use of adjusted body weight, which accounts for the larger LBM, when calculating the energy requirements for a patient receiving hypocaloric feedings. Choban et al[24] base their caloric requirements on a fixed total energy-to-nitrogen ratio (kcal/g of nitrogen) of 75:1, where all patients receive 2 g of protein/kg of IBW. This form of nutrition support has been used for patients with weights 130% or greater than ideal. The nutrients for hypocaloric nutrition support can be delivered enterally or parenterally. A more recent study[30] cautions against the use of hypocaloric high-protein nutritional support in hospitalized stressed obese patients over the age of 60. In this study, 5 of 12 patients over the age of 60 had negative nitrogen balance.

D. Protein requirements can be calculated after an assessment is made of serum protein status, renal function, and metabolic stress level. A review of the literature indicates a general practice of using IBW when protein requirements are calculated.[31] Based on this practice, the following guidelines should be used for calculating protein requirements:
   1. Maintenance[32]: 1.0 g/kg IBW
   2. Stress[32,33]: 1.5 to 2.0 g/kg IBW

E. Vitamin and mineral requirements for obese patients are based on dietary reference intakes. Any deficiencies should be corrected with supplements. Close attention must be paid to the vitamins and minerals provided by hypocaloric feedings. It is likely that patients who receive hypocaloric feedings in an oral diet or via enteral nutrition support will need daily vitamin and mineral supplements.

F. Periodic reassessment of the patient's nutritional status and goals should be conducted every 2 weeks, or earlier if there is a change in the patient's medical condition. Calorie and protein requirements should be more frequently assessed for patients being treated with hypocaloric feedings, as weight loss may alter energy expenditure.

V. Management

A. Special aspects of diet and nutritional supplements
   1. Dietary modifications
      a) A balanced-calorie weight maintenance diet is appropriate for obese patients who do not desire weight loss or for whom it is not indicated. A macronutrient distribution of 45% to 65% carbohydrate, 10% to 35% protein, and 20% to 35% fat is recommended by the Institute of Medicine,[34] although guidelines should be consistent with those for any comorbidities, for example, 2 g of sodium for renal dysfunction or 20% of calories from protein for wound healing. These patients should have an adequate serum protein status and should be hemodynamically stable. The total daily calorie deficit should not exceed 500 kcal/d for very gradual weight loss.
      b) In very low calorie diets (VLCD), usual food intake is replaced by specific liquid or food formulations containing 800 kcal/d or less.[35] Patients are considered appropriate for VLCD when they have failed at more conventional approaches to weight loss, are well motivated, and have a BMI of greater than 30 kg/m^2. Patients should undergo a thorough history and physical examination before beginning VLCD. Initial laboratory testing should include complete blood cell count, serum electrolytes, liver function tests, serum urea nitrogen and creatinine, a fasting or postprandial blood glucose, and uric acid. Patients on VLCD must be closely monitored in clinic and generally lose 1.5 to 2.5 kg/week, with total weight loss of 20 kg at 12 to 16 weeks. The risk for gallstone formation increases exponentially at rates of weight loss above 1.5 kg/week.[36] Prophylaxis against gallstone formation with ursodeoxycholic acid, 600 mg/day, is effective in reducing this risk.[37] Usually within 1 week, diabetic patients' glycemic control improves, with blood pressure improving at a slower rate.
      c) Progression of diet in a hospitalized critically ill obese patient is similar to that of a nonobese patient. Ideal dietary intake consists of food taken orally. If patients are unable to take food orally or if they are unable to meet their caloric needs in this manner, then enteral nutrition is the next-best option. If patients are unable to tolerate oral food or enteral nutrition (eg, owing to bowel obstruction, bowel ischemia, or severe pancreatitis), then PN should be employed.
   2. Dietary considerations after surgical treatment of obesity, which depend upon the procedure performed
      a) Patients who have undergone a Roux-en-Y gastric bypass (RYGB) procedure are at risk of developing dumping syndrome

because of alterations of the intestinal anatomy that involve bypassing the pyloric valve. These patients should restrict their intake of simple sugars to reduce the risk of dumping hypertonic gastric contents into the small bowel, which can cause abdominal cramping, osmotic diarrhea, and vasomotor changes.

b) The RYGB and laparoscopic adjustable silicone gastric banding procedures reduce the capacity of the stomach, so small, frequent meals are required. Often the diet is initiated with clear liquids and advanced slowly to pureed or soft foods. The ideal dietary composition of the liquids is high protein (usually 60–100 g protein/d), moderate carbohydrate, and very low fat. Intake of carbonated beverages should be limited to avoid excess pressure on the remnant pouch and the gastric outlet port. Beverages consumed by patients should be no calorie or low calorie.

c) Post-bariatric surgery patients should consume a clear liquid diet for the first 1 to 2 days, progressing to a full liquid diet. At the time of discharge, patients are generally eating a pureed/soft diet. At 4 to 6 weeks, patients should gradually transition to a regular-consistency low-fat, controlled-energy diet. Patients should be instructed to avoid consuming fluids for at least 30 minutes before and after meals. Minimum daily protein intake should be 60 to 75 grams divided into four to six small meals daily. Patients should also keep food logs, including foods not tolerated, for discussion with the dietitian at follow-up.[38]

3. Supplements

a) Dietary supplements for obese patients can be used for calorie and protein supplementation. The supplements that are fat-free or low fat can help to meet the dietary goals without providing excess fat. Hospitalized obese patients who are eating food and taking supplements should be monitored with daily weights and calorie counts to help prevent overfeeding and weight gain.

b) Vitamin and mineral supplements should be prescribed for all patients who are on a calorie-restricted, carbohydrate-restricted, or specific nutrient-restricted diet. Specialized vitamin preparations may be required for patients who have had surgical treatment of their obesity. Gastric bypass patients need calcium, iron, folate, and vitamin B_{12} supplements. A typical supplement regimen includes a prenatal vitamin daily, 500 to 1000 mcg vitamin B_{12} daily (or monthly injections), and 1000 mg calcium citrate with vitamin D daily in divided doses (the dosage may be decreased if there is significant calcium intake in the diet).

B. Special aspects of enteral nutrition

1. Obtaining enteral access. As with nonobese patients, in obese patients, access to the gastrointestinal tract can be achieved nasoenterically, surgically, endoscopically, or laparoscopically. These procedures can often be technically challenging when performed in the severely obese.[39] Often they cannot be performed because of difficulty with patient cooperation or lack of special instrumentation. In the case of endoscopic placement or nasoenteric placement, which often require fluoroscopy, patients whose weight exceeds 300 lb (136 kg) will be unable to undergo this procedure in certain institutions where damage to the operating, movable roentgenogram table is likely. When patients undergo techniques that require light sedation without airway security or general endotracheal intubation, extreme caution should be used, and continuous arterial saturation monitoring with or without capnography is recommended. Patients who are severely obese frequently have either congestive heart failure or sleep apnea syndrome, and very light sedation with simple draping of the face and neck can significantly increase the P_{CO_2}. Therefore, with any approach to enteral access in the severely obese, maintenance of an adequate airway and assurance of normal oxygenation and ventilation are mandatory. An increase in morbidity and mortality is associated with pickwickian syndrome (sleep apnea syndrome and obstructive hypoventilation syndrome), benzodiazepine use, epidural use, and morphine administration.

a) Surgical gastrostomy. Surgical gastrostomy or gastrojejunostomy can be performed primarily for enteral access in severely obese patients. A midline incision is preferred. The severely obese can develop significant debilitating and serious wound infections from a simple gastrostomy. These techniques can also be performed laparoscopically with excellent results and avoid the complications of a midline incision. The rate of incisional hernia following midline incisions in severely obese patients approaches 30%, so laparoscopic techniques may be advantageous.

b) Surgical jejunostomy. Jejunostomy in the severely obese is often associated with many complications: subcutaneous abscess formation, small-bowel obstruction, feeding into the subcutaneous space, and peritonitis. This option is best reserved for cases in which gastrostomy or gastrojejunostomy cannot be performed.

c) Percutaneous endoscopic gastrostomy (PEG) or gastrojejunostomy. PEG or gastrojejunostomy is useful for the severely obese patient requiring enteral access. In patients greater than 300 lb, the technique can be difficult to perform if the endoscope is unable to transilluminate the abdominal wall.

2. Selecting an enteral formula

a) The nutrient composition of an enteral formula should be based on the assessed calorie, protein, and volume requirements or restrictions. If hypocaloric feedings are instituted, then a very high protein, low-fat formula should be used. This may require the addition of a modular protein supplement to the enteral formula to ensure adequate protein input to spare LBM.

b) The vitamin and mineral composition of the enteral formula used for the hypocaloric feeding should be compared with the recommended daily allowances (RDAs). Daily vitamin and mineral supplementation may be required.

C. Special aspects of PN

1. Obtaining venous access. Securing central venous access for monitoring or PN administration is a formidable task in the severely obese.[40] Central venous access is defined as catheter placement in the superior vena cava–right atrial junction. Monitoring and positioning are key elements in the successful and safe placement of temporary and permanent central venous access. In the severely obese patient with congestive heart failure or sleep apnea syndrome, central venous access should be obtained only with an anesthesiologist or nurse anesthetist monitoring the airway and with the administration of intravenous sedation. Studies have demonstrated that Trendelenburg's position or the head-down position can result in a 35% to 50% decrease in the functional residual capacity of the lung, significantly impairing gas exchange. Therefore, cardiac monitoring and pulse oximetry are recommended. Because the placement of central venous catheters can require extended operating time and because the airway is often draped, capnography is also strongly recommended. It is very helpful in patients without well-defined landmarks to define the anatomy of the jugular and subclavian venous system with duplex imaging preoperatively. Indelible markings can be made and followed during placement.

a) Internal jugular vein. The internal jugular vein is the most accessible site for central line placement in the severely obese. If an assistant pulls the skin overlying the pectoralis muscle and the anesthetist provides countertraction, the anterior triangle of the neck will be defined and internal jugular cannulation allowed without difficulty. The central venous catheter can then be placed with use of fluoroscopic guidance. The internal jugular vein is often the first choice for patients who weigh greater than 300 lb.

b) External jugular vein cutdown. An alternate site for central venous catheterization in the severely obese is the external jugular vein. This can often be identified and marked preoperatively by duplex imaging. Cutdown avoids the complications of pneumothorax or local hematoma, which can contribute to airway compromise. The severely obese may not clinically manifest a neck hematoma; the first sign may be stridor. This approach is both safe and practical for many patients.

c) Subclavian vein catheterization. While considered by many the preferred site for venous cannulation, the subclavian vein can be extremely difficult and dangerous to access in the severely obese. Landmarks are ill-defined, which can make this approach a formidable undertaking. Furthermore, even when cannulation is successful, passage of the dilators and indwelling catheters is often impossible because of the circuitous route of entry into the vein from the skin puncture. If a pneumothorax develops or bleeding occurs within the chest, both tube thoracoscopy and thoracotomy are fraught with technical difficulty and high morbidity in this group of patients. However, if this approach is necessary, in experienced hands it can be successfully accomplished and safe. For patients who are superobese (greater than 400 lb [182 kg]), the posterior approach (supraclavicular and posterior to the subclavian vein) can be useful. Venous access with a peripherally inserted central catheter obviates many of these problems.

2. Selecting a formula

a) The nutrient composition of PN support for obese patients depends on the overall nutrition care plan. If weight maintenance is desired, then a mixed-nutrient formula that provides 100% of the required nutrients is appropriate. To avoid essential fatty acid deficiencies, approximately 4% of total daily energy should be provided as linoleic acid. This can be accomplished by using 500 cc of 10% intralipid solution twice weekly.[41]

b) The infusion regimen depends on the patient's hemodynamic and metabolic stability, the anticipated length of support, and the desired outcome. Continuous infusions of PN are usually required when a patient is hemodynamically unstable (requiring constant infusion rates) or when serum glucose control is difficult to optimize. Cyclical PN should be considered for patients who are hemodynamically and metabolically stable, have increasing activity and mobility, need long-term support (months to years), or need mobilization of lipid stores. In a review article by Matuchansky et al,[42] the benefits of cyclic PN were cited as producing higher rates of lipid oxidation, lower rates of lipid storage, gains in visceral protein, and less fluid imbalance compared with continuous infusion of PN. These benefits are especially important for patients who already have excess fat stores and for patients on hypocaloric support who need to maintain LBM and liberate lipids from stores for essential fatty acids. Optimally, PN should be cycled over 12 hours a day; however, some acutely ill patients may not tolerate the high infusion rates needed to feed the total volume required. The length of PN infusion should be gradually decreased by 1 to 3 hours each day, as the patient can tolerate, to the goal of 12 hours per day.

D. Focused monitoring/goals assessment

1. Complications and postoperative considerations. While meticulous attention to aseptic technique and intraoperative monitoring are key to reducing postoperative morbidity, being aware of the self-care limitations of some severely obese patients is important. Some patients are unable to provide care and hygiene to feeding access sites and cannot recognize serious problems. Follow-up care is important. Soft-tissue infection can be insidious and virulent because of the depth of the subcutaneous fat and the number of microbes that establish a niche in moist and excoriated skin folds. Patients may fail to recognize and seek attention for these problems. Patients with diabetes may harbor particularly hostile microbes. Since severely obese patients do not tolerate surgical complications well, the best strategy is to avoid them.
2. Special needs. An area of growing concern is the need for facilities equipped to care for the morbidly obese patient. Hospitals and physicians' offices are often not equipped with larger beds, gowns, and blood pressure cuffs. Many radiology tables cannot accommodate patients weighing greater than 300 or 350 pounds, leading to difficulty in obtaining tests in these patients.

E. Patient/caregiver education

1. Obese patients and their family members should receive education about the long-term effects of carrying excess body weight (as discussed in Section II), the high rate of comorbid diseases related to obesity, and the options for treatment. Information related to the health benefits of reducing weight and maintaining a lower body weight should be provided during the education phase.
2. Many weight management programs are available. If a patient is motivated to lose weight, the various options should be discussed prior to discharge from the hospital. To date, most people who attempt weight loss are unable to maintain a significant weight loss for more than 5 years. However, this fact should not prevent an obese patient from attempting to lose weight, since as little as a 5% to 10% decrease in weight can have health benefits. The ideal weight management program uses a multidisciplinary approach to modify behavior and eating habits, provide emotional support, incorporate physical activity, and monitor the patient's physical well-being. Participation of obese family members or cohabitants can be motivational and supportive to the patient as well as provide health benefits to the other participants.
3. Patients who choose to undertake weight management after recovery from an acute illness should modify their home environment before attempting to lose weight. Modification of the types of foods procured, food preparation methods, and general eating habits of all cohabitants may be necessary to allow for successful weight management of the obese patient.

(Obesity chapter from the 1st edition was contributed by Robert F. Kushner, Elizabeth Wall-Alonso, and John Alverdy)

REFERENCES

1. Flegal KM, Carroll MD, Ogden CL, Johnson CL. Prevalence and trends in obesity among US adults, 1999–2000. *JAMA*. 2002;288:1723–1727.
2. Kuczmarski RJ, Flegal KM, Campbell SM, et al. Increasing prevalence of overweight among US adults. The National Health and Nutrition Examination Surveys, 1960 to 1991. *JAMA*. 1994;22:205–211.
3. *Healthy People 2010. National Health Promotion and Disease Prevention Objectives*. Washington, DC: US Government Printing Office, US Department of Health and Human Services, Public Health Service; 2000.

4. Forbes GB, Welle SL. Lean body mass in obesity. *Int J Obes.* 1983;7:99–107.
5. Prentice AM, Black AE, Cole TF. Energy expenditure in overweight and obese adults in affluent societies: an analysis of 319 doubly-labelled water measurements. *Eur J Clin Nutr.* 1996;50:93–97.
6. Jeevanandam M, Ramias L, Schiller WR. Altered plasma free amino acid levels in obese traumatized man. *Metabolism.* 1991;40:385–390.
7. Jeevanandam M, Young DH, Schiller WR. Obesity and the metabolic response to severe multiple trauma in man. *J Clin Invest.* 1991;87:262–269.
8. Ford ES, Giles WH, Dietz WH. Prevalence of the metabolic syndrome among US adults. *JAMA.* 2002;287:356–359.
9. *Third Report of the National Cholesterol Education Program (NCEP) Expert Panel on Detection, Evaluation, and Treatment of High Blood Cholesterol in Adults (Adult Treatment Panel III) (Final Report).* National Heart, Lung, and Blood Institute, National Institutes of Health, Publication #NIH 02;5215. Bethesda, MD: National Heart, Lung, and Blood Institute, National Institutes of Health; 2002.
10. Lemieux I, Pascot A, Couillard C, et al. Hypertriglyceridemic waist: a marker of the atherogenic metabolic triad in men? *Circulation.* 2000;102:179–184.
11. Lakka HM, Laaksonen DE, Lakka TE, et al. The metabolic syndrome and total and cardiovascular disease mortality in middle-aged men. *JAMA.* 2002; 288:2709–2716.
12. Haffner S, Taegtmeyer H. Epidemic obesity and the metabolic syndrome. *Circulation.* 2003;108:1541–1545.
13. Mattison R, Jensen M. The adipocyte as an endocrine cell. *Curr Opin Endocrin Diab.* 2003;10:317–321.
14. Bray GA. Risks of obesity. *Endocrinol Metab Clin N Am.* 2003;32:787–804.
15. Dixon JB, Dixon ME, O'Brien PE. Depression in association with severe obesity: changes with weight loss. *Arch Intern Med.* 2003;163:2058–2065.
16. Kushner RF, Roth JL. Assessment of the obese patient. *Endocrinol Metab Clin N Am.* 2003;32:915–933.
17. Bray G. Pathophysiology of obesity. *Am J Clin Nutr.* 1992;55:488S–494S.
18. National Heart, Lung, and Blood Institute. Clinical Guidelines on the Identification, Evaluation, and Treatment of Overweight and Obesity in Adults. The evidence report. *Obes Res.* 1998;6(suppl 2):51S–210S.
19. Fujioka S, Matsuzawa Y, Tokunaga K, et al. Contribution of intra-abdominal fat accumulation to the impairment of glucose and lipid metabolism in human obesity. *Metabolism.* 1987;36:54–59.
20. National Heart, Lung, and Blood Institute, and North American Association for the Study of Obesity. *Practical Guide to the Identification, Evaluation, and Treatment of Overweight and Obesity in Adults.* Publication #NIH 00-4084. Bethesda, MD: National Institutes of Health; 2000.
21. Gray D, Bray G, Bauer M, et al. Skinfold thickness measurements in obese subjects. *Am J Clin Nutr.* 1990;51:571–577.
22. Kokkoris P, Pi-Sunyer FX. Obesity and endocrine disease. *Endocrinol Metab Clin N Am.* 2003;32:895–914.
23. Dickerson R, Rosato E, Mullen J. Net protein anabolism with hypocaloric parenteral nutrition in obese stressed patients. *Am J Clin Nutr.* 1986;44;747–755.
24. Choban PS, Burge JC, Scales D, Flancbaum L. Hypoenergetic nutrition support in hospitalized obese patients: a simplified method for clinical application. *Am J Clin Nutr.* 1997;66:546–550.
25. Amato P, Keating K, Quercia R, et al. Formulaic methods of estimating calorie requirements in mechanically ventilated obese patients: a reappraisal. *Nutr Clin Pract.* 1995;10:229–232.
26. Verga S, Buscemi S, Caimi G. Resting energy expenditure and body composition in morbidly obese, obese, and control subjects. *Acta Diabetol.* 1994;31:47–51.
27. Frankenfield DC, Rose WA, Smith JS, et al. Validation of several established equations for resting metabolic rate in obese and nonobese people. *J Am Diet Assoc.* 2003;103:1152–1159.
28. Barak N, Wall-Alonso E, Cheng A, et al. Use of bioelectrical impedance analysis to predict energy expenditure of hospitalized patients receiving nutrition support. *J Parenter Enteral Nutr.* 2003;27:43–46.
29. Shikora S, Muskat P. Protein-sparing modified fast total parenteral nutrition formulation for a critically ill morbidly obese patient. *Nutrition.* 1994; 10:155–158.
30. Liu KJ, Cho MJ, Atten MJ, et al. Hypocaloric parenteral nutrition support in elderly obese patients. *Am Surg.* 2000;66:394–400.
31. Hopkins B. Assessment of nutritional status. In: Gottschlich M, Matarese L, Shronts E, eds. *Nutrition Support Dietetics Core Curriculum.* 2nd ed. Silver Spring, MD: American Society for Parenteral and Enteral Nutrition; 1993.
32. Ireton-Jones C. Obesity. In: Gottschlich M, Matarese L, Shronts E, eds. *Nutrition Support Dietetics Core Curriculum.* 2nd ed. Silver Spring, MD: American Society for Parenteral and Enteral Nutrition; 1993.
33. Ireton-Jones C, Francis C. Obesity: nutrition support practice and application to critical care. *Nutr Clin Pract.* 1995;10:144–149.
34. Institute of Medicine. *Dietary Reference Intakes for Energy, Carbohydrate, Fiber, Fat, Fatty Acids, Cholesterol, Protein, and Amino Acids.* Washington, DC: National Academy of Sciences; 2003.
35. National Task Force on the Prevention and Treatment of Obesity. Very low-caloric diets. *JAMA.* 1993;270:967–974.
36. Weinsier RL, Wilson LJ, Lee J. Medically safe rate of weight loss for the treatment of obesity: a guideline based on risk of gallstone formation. *Am J Med.* 1995;98:115–117.
37. Shiffman ML, Kaplan GD, Brinkman-Kaplan V, Vickers FF. Prophylaxis against gallstone formation with ursodeoxycholic acid in patients participating in a very-low-calorie diet program. *Ann Intern Med.* 1995;122: 899–905.
38. Gastric bypass diet and bariatric surgery for obesity. In: *Manual of Clinical Nutrition Management.* Atlanta, GA: Morrison Management Specialist; 2003:B-10 to B-20.
39. Shikora SA. Enteral feeding tube placement in obese patients: considerations for nutrition support. *Nutr Clin Pract.* 1997;12(suppl):S9–S13.
40. Jefferson P, Ball DR. Central venous access in morbidly obese patients. *Anesth Analg.* 2002;95(3):782.
41. Nutrition management of obesity. In: *Manual of Clinical Dietetics.* 6th ed. Chicago, IL: American Dietetic Association; 2000:621.
42. Matuchansky C, Messing B, Jeejeebhoy K, et al. Cyclical parenteral nutrition support. *Lancet.* 1992;340:588–592.

Margretta R. Seashore, MD, FAAP, FACMG;
Crystal A. Reil, RD, CD-N

29

Inborn Errors of Metabolism

Introduction

Specialized nutrition support is frequently required for patients who have an inborn error of metabolism. These inherited disorders result in abnormal concentrations of certain metabolites, which frequently cause neurologic symptoms. Treatment goals include supporting normal growth and optimizing neurologic development in children, as well as minimizing neurologic compromise in patients of all ages. Nutritional therapy for these patients usually involves following a specific nutrition protocol. In some of these disorders, the intake of certain nutrients such as specific amino acids needs to be limited or supplemented. In addition, specific nutrients such as carnitine may be prescribed. Specialized enteral and parenteral nutrition products may also be necessary to optimize therapy.

I. Nutrition Aspects of the Disorder

A. Intake
1. Treatment for many inborn errors of metabolism involves alterations of dietary intake
    a) By substrate restriction (phenylalanine in phenylketonuria).
    b) By vitamin/cofactor administration (biotin in biotinidase deficiency)
    c) By end-product supplementation (arginine in argininosuccinic acidemia)
2. Problems with intake
    a) Infants and children with many of these diagnoses may have severe neurologic impairment that limits their ability to consume food orally.[1]
    b) Many inborn errors of metabolism are associated with abnormal concentrations of metabolites, which often cause anorexia, nausea, and vomiting, resulting in limited oral nutrition intake.
    c) Most of the specialized formulas that have been developed for patients with inborn errors of metabolism contain elemental amino acids and are not very palatable. Patients tend to demonstrate improved acceptance with these formulas when they are used on a consistent basis since infancy.
3. Some older children with inborn errors of metabolism who are not neurologically impaired may naturally self-restrict specific nutrients from their diets that are likely to cause metabolic aberrations.

B. Absorption
1. In most inborn errors of metabolism, the normal absorption of nutrients is not affected.
2. In lysinuric protein intolerance, there is a defect in the transport of dibasic amino acids (lysine, arginine, and ornithine) not only in the intestine but also in the liver and kidney.[2]

C. Utilization
1. The problem in most inborn errors of metabolism is that there is an enzyme defect that either causes accumulation of a substrate or a toxic metabolite, or prevents production of an essential end product.[1,3]
2. Therapy in these disorders may be an attempt to increase enzyme activity (or even replace the enzyme by transplantation), and in most cases requires some sort of dietary prescription.[1,3]

D. Losses
1. In some inborn errors of metabolism, the metabolites whose concentrations become abnormally increased (such as amino acid metabolites and other organic acids) bind to carnitine and glycine. The resulting acylcarnitines and acylglycines are water soluble and are excreted in the urine without further metabolism.
2. Acylcarnitine lost in the urine frequently leads to a secondary carnitine deficiency. Inborn errors of metabolism where carnitine supplementation is usually given are shown in Table 29-1.[4]

II. Nutritional Alterations Seen with the Disorder

A. Common
1. All inborn errors of metabolism result in abnormal concentrations of certain metabolites; diagnosis of the specific enzyme defect in these conditions is usually made by measuring the concentrations of various metabolites in blood or urine, although in certain conditions specific enzyme analysis is required.
2. Because of the wide range of inborn errors, there are no uniform nutritional alterations seen in these conditions; in those patients with severe neurologic impairment, both under- and overnutrition are possible.

B. Less common
1. As listed in Table 29-1, a number of these conditions result in a secondary carnitine deficiency. Patients with carnitine deficiency can develop a Reye-like syndrome, including hypoglycemia with illness or stress.
2. Several other conditions are associated with hypoglycemia, including glycogen storage disease type I,[5,6] and hereditary fructose intolerance.[7]

III. Focused Assessment

A. History
1. Growth and development of the patient needs to be a major focus of the nutrition history; in most cases, poor growth and delayed neurologic development are the results of late treatment, poor intake, or poor metabolic control.[1,3]

TABLE 29-1. Inborn Errors of Metabolism in Which Carnitine Supplementation is Usually Given

3-Hydroxyisobutyric aciduria
Isovaleric acidemia
Glutaric aciduria type I
Methylmalonic acidemia
Propionic acidemia
Carbamoyl-phosphate synthetase deficiency
Ornithine transcarbamylase deficiency
Citrullinemia
Argininosuccinic aciduria
Argininemia
N-Acetylglutamate synthetase deficiency
Long-, medium-, or short-chain fatty acid oxidation defects

2. In all patients, a detailed summary of nutritional intake needs to be completed. At a minimum, the history should document average caloric and protein intake. For patients with errors in amino acid metabolism, the specific intake of individual amino acids should be calculated.
3. Tolerance of oral nutrition is also an important focus of the history, particularly because some of these patients frequently experience anorexia, nausea, and vomiting.
4. Symptoms suggestive of hypoglycemia should be noted.

B. Physical exam
1. Accurate documentation of the patient's height (length), weight, and head circumference (birth to age 3) is one of the most important parts of the physical examination.
2. Neurologic examination is particularly important in determining not only whether the patient is developmentally normal but also whether there might be factors such as spasticity or chewing or swallowing difficulties that might affect dietary intake or nutritional requirements, or interfere with the development of feeding capabilities.

C. Quality of life
1. Quality of life varies considerably with each diagnosis and also depends on whether the patient was treated early in life with proper metabolic control.
2. Inborn errors of metabolism do not resolve as the patient ages, so dietary treatment should be considered lifelong unless effective alternate therapies are discovered (enzyme replacement, organ transplantation, or gene therapy).
3. The level of care required is an important factor in planning nutrition support for these patients.

IV. Objectives/Goals of Therapy in Infants and Children

A. Support normal growth
B. Minimize neurologic impairment
C. Prevent metabolic crises[8]
1. The primary goal is usually to correct the primary metabolic imbalance, such as by restricting a particular amino acid in an amino acidopathy. Often, medical foods are utilized for such therapy.
2. Occasionally, a substrate is given to provide an alternative metabolic pathway, such as giving glycine and carnitine to children with isovaleric acidemia.
3. Occasionally, a particular substrate of a blocked pathway needs to be given, such as glucose to patients with type I glycogen storage disease.
4. In these patients, it is also possible for certain substances, such as carnitine, to become "conditionally essential" (Table 29-1).
5. Additional vitamins are often useful either to stabilize altered enzymes (thiamine in maple syrup urine disease), to replace deficient cofactors (vitamin B_{12} in methylmalonic aciduria), or to supplement nutrients not released from their apoenzyme (biotin in biotinidase deficiency).

V. Management

A. Special aspects of diet and nutritional supplements
1. In many of these patients, the intake of specific compounds or substances frequently must be limited to optimize metabolic control.[1,7,9]
   a) In many inborn errors of amino acid metabolism, the intake of specific amino acids must be restricted (Table 29-2).
   b) In some inborn errors of carbohydrate metabolism, a particular kind of carbohydrate may need to be limited (Table 29-3).

TABLE 29-2. Inborn Errors of Amino Acid Metabolism that Require Limited Intake of Particular Amino Acids

Inborn error of metabolism	Amino acid that must be limited
Phenylketonuria	Phenylalanine
Maple syrup urine disease (Branched-chain ketoaciduria)	Leucine, isoleucine, valine
Tyrosinemia types I and II	Phenylalanine, tyrosine
Homocystinuria	Methionine
Isovaleric acidemia	Leucine
3-Methylcrotonylglycinuria	Leucine
3-Methylglutaconic aciduria	Leucine
3-Hydroxy-3-methylglutaric aciduria	Leucine
Glutaric aciduria type I	Lycine, tryptophan
2-Ketoadipic aciduria	Lycine, tryptophan
Propionic acidemia	Isoleucine, methionine, threonine,valine
Methylmalonic acidemia	Isoleucine, methionine, threonine,valine

TABLE 29-3. Inborn Errors of Amino Acid Metabolism that Require Limited Intake of Particular Carbohydrates

Inborn error of metabolism	Carbohydrate that must be limited
Galactosemia	Galactose
Hereditary fructose intolerance	Fructose, sorbitol, sucrose
Glycogen storage disease types I and II	Lactose, fructose, sucrose

c) In some inborn errors of metabolism, select nutrients (ie, carbohydrate, fat, or protein) must be restricted in treating the disorder (Table 29-4).

2. For those conditions where specific amino acids need to be restricted (Table 29-2), chemically defined formulations (medical foods) have been developed. For each of these conditions, specific protocols have been developed to optimize the nutrition support;[4,9] these protocols are useful regardless of whether the nutrition is being given orally, enterally, or parenterally.
   a) The basic approach in each of these protocols is to create a nutrition prescription based on the need to limit or supplement a particular substrate or substrates, while meeting total protein, energy, and fluid requirements. In cases where the intake of a particular amino acid is limited, the daily intake of that amino acid may be given in the form of normal table foods. To prevent the development of protein deficiency, additional protein is given in the form of a medical food that does not contain the restricted amino acid(s). Additional calories are provided with a protein-free formula or protein-free foods.
   b) Usually, recommended dietary allowances for protein and energy are utilized in the prescription. However, when medical foods that contain free L-amino acids are used, the total protein requirements frequently exceed the recommended dietary allowances for protein.

TABLE 29-4. Inborn Errors of Metabolism that Require Limited Intake of Carbohydrate, Fat, or Protein

Inborn error of metabolism	Type of nutrient that must be limited
Pyruvate dehydrogenase deficiency	Carbohydrate
3-Hydroxy-3-methylglutaric aciduria	Protein, Fat
Fatty acid oxidation defects	Long-,medium-, or short-chain fatty acids
Urea cycle disorders	Protein
Nonketotic hyperglycinemia	Protein
Lysinuric protein intolerance	Protein

   c) Changes in the nutrition prescription are made at regular intervals based on the infant's or child's growth and development and clinical symptoms as well as metabolic control and nutritional status as assessed by laboratory testing.
   d) For many infants and children with inborn errors of metabolism, the majority of their nutritional needs are met by medical food(s), as only a small amount of normal foods are allowed in accordance with their disease-specific dietary restriction(s).[8]
   e) When preparing medical foods, care must be taken to prevent the Maillard reaction, which involves condensation of amino acids and sugars into an undigestible complex. This reaction is accelerated by heat and gives the formula a yellow to brown color.[7]

3. In the special case of children with glycogen storage disease type I, frequent feedings of carbohydrate are needed to prevent hypoglycemia.[5,6]
   a) During the day, some of the carbohydrate is often given orally as boluses of uncooked cornstarch.
   b) Overnight, hypoglycemia is prevented by either continuing oral boluses of uncooked cornstarch or providing an enteral infusion of glucose polymers at about 8 to 9 mg of carbohydrate per kilogram per minute.[5]

B. Special aspects of enteral nutrition
1. Patients who have severe neurologic impairment, frequent metabolic crises, or intolerance of the medical foods often benefit from enteral feedings; placement of a feeding gastrostomy is usually indicated.
2. For those patients on enteral feedings, the nutrition prescription is similar to what is used for patients on oral nutrition. If a diet restricted in an amino acid(s) is being used, the restricted amino acid(s) is usually supplied via a commercial formula.[10]

C. Special aspects of parenteral nutrition
1. In some patients with inborn errors of metabolism, aggressive nutritional intervention may be important at the time of initial diagnosis or at times of catabolic stress to prevent severe neurologic complications and even death.[11]
2. In many cases, all that is needed is to infuse glucose at high-infusion rates; the concomitant hyperinsulinemia suppresses catabolism and improves metabolic control.
3. In selected circumstances involving inborn errors of amino acid metabolism, specialized parenteral amino acid formulations deficient in one or more amino acids may be useful to optimize the plasma amino acid concentrations.[11]
4. In patients with propionic and methylmalonic acidemia, long-term parenteral nutrition with standard amino acid solutions has also been reported to be effective.[12,14]
5. Use of IV fat emulsion may need to be restricted in patients with a disorder of long-chain fatty acid oxidation or glutaric aciduria type II.[15]

D. Focused monitoring/goals assessment
1. To meet the goals of adequate growth and minimal neurologic impairment, children with inborn errors of metabolism need to have frequent monitoring of their condition; the metabolites that are measured depend on the specific condition and are part of the treatment protocol.
2. Changes in the nutrition prescription need to be made frequently (days to months) depending on the age of the patient, their rate of growth, the inborn error, and the degree of metabolic control.

E. Patient/caregiver education
1. The patient and/or caregiver needs to be fully educated in all aspects of the nutrition prescription; in the case of inborn errors

of amino acid metabolism, detailed lists of the amino acid content of foods are available to aid in meal planning.[4,16]

2. Specific instruction needs to be given about the signs and symptoms of metabolic crises, because early medical/nutritional intervention is critical to prevent long-term sequelae.

REFERENCES

1. Elsas LJ, Acosta PB. Nutrition support of inherited metabolic disease. In: Shils ME, Young VR, eds. *Modern Nutrition in Health and Disease.* 8th ed, Philadelphia, PA: Lea & Febiger; 1994:1147–1206.
2. Scriver C, Beaudet A, Sly W, Valle D. *The Metabolic Basis of Inherited Disease.* 8th Edition ed: McGraw Hill; 2001.
3. Acosta PB. Nutrition support of inborn errors of metabolism. In: Queen PM, Land CE, eds. *Handbook of Pediatric Nutrition.* Gaithersburg, MD: Aspen Publishers; 1993:315–364.
4. Acosta PB, Yannicelli S. *Nutrition Support Protocols.* 4th ed. Columbus, OH: Ross Laboratories; 2001.
5. Schwenk WF, Haymond MW. Optimal rate of enteral glucose administration in children with glycogen storage disease type I. *N Engl J Med.* 1986;314:682–685.
6. Chou JY, Matern D, Mansfield BC, Chen YT. Type I glycogen storage diseases: disorders of the glucose-6-phosphatase complex. *Curr Mol Med.* 2002;2(2):121–143.
7. Bell L, Sherwood WG. Current practices and improved recommendations for treating hereditary fructose intolerance. *J Am Diet Assoc.* 1987;87:721–728.
8. A.S.P.E.N. Board of Directors: Guidelines for the use of parenteral and enteral nutrition in adult and pediatric patients. *J Parenter Enteral Nutr.* 1993:17:1SA–52SA.
9. Mead Johnson Nutritionals. *Dietary Management of Metabolic Disorders.* Evansville, IN: Mead Johnson & Co; 1991.
10. Parini R, Sereni LP. Bagozzi DC, et al. Nasogastric drip feeding as the only treatment of neonatal maple syrup urine disease. *Pediatrics.* 1993;92:280–283.
11. Morton DH, Strauss KA, Robinson DL, Puffenberger EG, Kelley RI. Diagnosis and treatment of maple syrup disease: a study of 36 patients. *Pediatrics.* 2002;109(6):999–1008.
12. Kahler SG, Millington DS, Cederbaum SD, et al. Parenteral nutrition in propionic and methylmalonic acidemia. *J Pediatr.* 1989;115:235–241.
13. Walter JH, Leonard JV, Thompson GN. Halliday D: Parenteral nutrition in propionic acidemia and methylmalonic acidemia. *J Pediatr.* 1990;117:339
14. Kalloghlian A, Gleispach H, Ozand PT. A patient with propionic acidemia managed with continuous insulin infusion and total parenteral nutrition. *J Child Neurol.* 1992;7:88–91.
15. al-Essa MA, Rashed MS, Bakheet SM, Patay ZJ, Ozand PT. Glutaric aciduria type II: observations in seven patients with neonatal- and late-onset disease. *J Perinatol.* 2000;20(2):120–128.
16. Nelson JK, Moxness KE, Jensen MD, Gastineau CF, eds. *Mayo Clinic Diet Manual.* 7th ed. St. Louis, MO: Mosby; 1994:495–545.

Charles J. Foulks, MD, FACP, FACN

30

Chronic Kidney Disease

Introduction

Patients with Chronic Kidney Disease have a wide spectrum of clinical disorders that may affect the provision of adequate nutrition. This chapter focuses on the nutritional support of patients with Chronic Kidney Disease (Stages III–V) and patients who have undergone renal transplantation and have superimposed illnesses. It is now widely accepted by the nephrology community that the term Chronic Kidney Disease (CKD) covers all gradations of renal dysfunction (Table 30-1).

I. Nutritional Assessment of Patients with Chronic Kidney Disease (CKD)

A. History—This assessment requires a detailed history and review of the medical records including past medical and surgical history, history of renal disease and dialysis treatments, medications, and previous and current dietary intake. It is important to document the types and amount of food eaten in the previous 2–4 weeks and the presence of anorexia, nausea, vomiting, diarrhea, or early satiety. The patient's ethnic background and cultural food should be noted.

B. Physical examination

1. Anthropometric measurements are affected by the fluid status of the patient and are often of limited usefulness in patients with renal failure and superimposed illnesses.
   a) Dry body weight (edema-free body weight) should be recorded if known. If not, one can substitute standard or normal body weight, defined as the median body weight of normal Americans of the same age range, height, sex, and skeletal frame size as the patient as determined from the National Health and Nutrition Examination Survey (NHANES) data.[1] In reality, most clinicians either accept the weight given by the family or they estimate the weight.
   b) Height, skeletal frame size (estimated, rarely measured).
   c) Body mass index = body weight/(height)2, expressed in kg/m2.
   d) For patients whose body weight is greater than 120% or less than 90% of standard body weight, nutrients may be prescribed according to the adjusted actual body weight (aBW). The following formula can be used to calculate the adjusted aBW: adjusted aBW (kg) = ((edema-free aBW- nBW) (0.25)) + nBW, where edema-free aBW is the patient's actual body weight minus any estimated excess or deficit in total body water, and nBW is the normal or standard body weight for the patient, as determined from the NHANES data.[2] The NHANES data are not used or referred to by busy clinicians and most use the patient's usual weight (from the patient, the family, or from medical records) instead of the NHANES nBW.
   e) Skinfold measurements (eg, biceps, triceps, or subscapular) may be used to estimate body fat; however, these assessments are not practical in a clinical setting, particularly in patients who may have an abnormal amount of total body water. They are subject to marked inter-observer variability and are of little clinical utility.
2. Change in fluid status is determined by maintaining accurate intake and output records and especially by precisely measuring weight on a daily basis. The astute clinician will also use the physical examination and interval history to help make the diagnosis of volume depletion, hypervolemia, or normovolemia.
3. Subjective global nutritional assessment can give a rapid, reproducible, overall assessment of the protein-calorie nutritional status of the patient.[3] Selective global nutrition assessment uses the following six subjective measurements:
   a) the patient's history of weight loss
   b) incidence of anorexia
   c) vomiting and diarrhea
   d) the clinician's estimate of muscle wasting
   e) edema
   f) loss of subcutaneous fat

   These measures are graded as 1 = severe, 3 = moderate, and 5 = none. A subjective nutrition assessment of the patient is then made as normal, mildly to moderately malnourished, or severely malnourished. This method has been applied to the assessment of CKD patients in a number of studies.[4,5]
4. Visual signs of micronutrient (eg, zinc or iron) or essential fatty acid deficiencies.

C. Biochemical assessment should include:

1. Serum urea nitrogen (SUN; reflecting protein intake and catabolic state), creatinine (reflecting muscle mass), potassium and phosphorus (reflecting the stage of CKD and starvation, especially if the potassium and phosphorus are normal or low), calcium, magnesium, glucose, sodium, chloride, bicarbonate, albumin, transferrin, and prothrombin time (INR; if elevated, reflecting starvation or the absence of intake of green and yellow vegetables).
2. Blood pH, PCO2, and PO2, if a serious acid-base disorder is suspected.

TABLE 30-1. Classification of Chronic Kidney Disease (CKD)

Stage	Description	GFR (mL/min/1.73m²)
1	Kidney damage with normal or increased GFR	≥90
2	Kidney damage with mild decrease in GFR	60–89
3	Moderate decrease in GFR	30–59
4	Severe decrease in GFR	15–29
5	Kidney Failure	<15 (or dialysis)

Chronic kidney disease is defined as kidney damage or GFR < 60 mL/min/1.73 m2 ≥ 3 months. Kidney damage is defined as pathologic abnormalities or markers of damage, including abnormalities in blood or urine tests or imaging studies.
Reprinted from National Kidney Foundation, K/DOQI. Clinical practice guidelines for chronic kidney disease: evaluation, classification, and stratification. *Am J Kidney Dis* 2002;39 (suppl 1):S1-S000 with permission from National Kidney Foundation.

3. Calculated Glomerular Filtration Rate (GFR)—Glomerular filtration rate is a reflection of renal function as derived from clearance tests that measure the rate at which substances are cleared from the plasma by the glomeruli. See Appendix 29-1 for formulas and resources.
4. Urea nitrogen appearance (UNA)—This allows the clinician to estimate net protein degradation. Because urea is the major nitrogenous product of protein metabolism, UNA correlates closely with total nitrogen output. UNA indicates the net rate of protein catabolism (ie, total body degradation minus total body synthesis of proteins and amino acids).
   a) In clinically stable patients, who are in strongly positive or negative protein balance, the UNA will indicate recent protein intake. If both nitrogen intake and total nitrogen appearance, as estimated from the UNA, are known, nitrogen balance can be calculated from the difference between these values.[6]
   b) In patients who are receiving exogenous protein or amino acids by enteral or parenteral routes, the difference between nitrogen intake and UNA provides a measure of the catabolic status of the patient. For patients who are in negative nitrogen balance, the degree to which the total nitrogen appearance, estimated from the UNA, exceeds the nitrogen intake is often a measure of the severity of their underlying illnesses.
   c) UNA can be calculated as follows:

$$\text{UNA}(g/d) = \text{urinary urea nitrogen}(g/d) + \text{change in SUN}(g/d)$$

$$\text{Change in SUN} = (\text{SUN}f - \text{SUN}i) \times ((0.60)(\text{BW})) + (\text{BW}f - \text{BW}i)(\text{SUN}f)$$

   where SUN = serum urea nitrogen (g/L), BW = body weight (kg), i and f = initial and final values for the period of measurement. The Total Body Water is 0.60 × (body weight). This estimate should be adjusted in patients who are edematous or lean.
   d) For patients who are undergoing hemodialysis, the UNA must be calculated during the interdialytic interval and extrapolated to 24 hours, or it may be measured directly or through dialysis kinetic techniques.[2,6] To assess UNA in people undergoing Continuous Veno-Venous Hemofiltration or Hemodialysis (CVVH/CVVHD), the urea in the ultrafiltrate or dialysate must be collected and measured, and this value must be added to urinary urea nitrogen and changes in body urea nitrogen. Practically speaking, the UNA is rarely used clinically. Many nephrologists estimate the degree of catabolism by calculating the rate of rise of the SUN from one day to the next. In general, if the rate of rise of the SUN ≤ 30 mg/dL per day, the stress of the illness is presumed to be mild.
5. Total nitrogen appearance in (g/d) = 1.19 UNA (g/d) + 1.27 g/d, where total nitrogen appearance is the sum of all outputs of nitrogen from the body, including dialysate, urine, and feces, plus the change in body urea nitrogen. This equation was derived from clinically stable CKD patients who were not undergoing hemodialysis or peritoneal dialysis, and its applicability to unstable, stressed CKD patients or acute renal failure (ARF) patients is unknown.[6]
6. Protein equivalent of total nitrogen appearance (PNA in g/d) = total nitrogen appearance (g of nitrogen per day) × 6.25. PNA expresses total nitrogen appearance in terms of the equivalent amount of protein that has been lost or has undergone net catabolism. In previous publications, PNA has been referred to as PCR (protein catabolic rate).

II. Objectives and Goals for Nutrition Support for Patients with Chronic Renal Disease

A. Overall goals for nutritional treatment
   1. To maintain, improve, and, if possible, restore normal body composition of somatic proteins, visceral proteins, and other nutrients as well as normal immune function, wound healing, and host resistance.
   2. To prevent or ameliorate uremic toxicity and other metabolic disorders and to prevent or correct abnormal total body water and serum electrolyte and hydrogen ion disorders.

B. Nutritional support for patients with CKD
   1. The prescription for nutritional support varies according to the patient's nutritional status, degree of catabolism, GFR, and clinical condition. The patient's tolerance for water, minerals, amino acids and protein; the degree of uremic toxicity; and the plans for dialysis or ultrafiltration therapy may heavily influence the prescription for oral, enteral, or parenteral nutrition. Often, patients undergoing long-term peritoneal dialysis are treated with hemodialysis therapy during an acute illness if it is of sufficient magnitude to require nutrition support.
      a) A hospitalized patient with CKD who has little or no protein depletion, a low UNA (eg, 4 to 5 g/d), and SUN < 90 mg/dL; and in whom the health care team is trying to avoid dialysis treatment (eg, awaiting vascular access maturation, acceptance into a dialysis unit); may be treated with 0.5–0.6 g/kg/d of protein (>75% high biologic value) with supplementation of water soluble vitamins and minerals. This is a version of the low protein diet used in the management of the pre-ESRD (end stage renal disease) patient, and as long as energy needs are met and the catabolic stress is modest, this diet will suffice to prevent nutritional injury. If the patient

requires treatment with parenteral nutrition, 20–30 g/d of essential amino acids with appropriate caloric provision can be safely used until dialysis is begun, and can be used for 2–3 weeks. No more than 30–40 g of the nine essential amino acids per day should be given, because larger quantities may cause hazardous amino acid imbalances and precipitate uremic symptoms.[7,8] Although histidine is not an essential amino acid in normal patients, it is an essential amino acid in the CKD patient. Modern essential amino acid formulations contain histidine. When dialysis is initiated, nutrition support with essential amino acids is modified to provide larger amounts of both essential and nonessential amino acids at 1.2–1.3 g/kg nBW/d.

b) For hypercatabolic or severely wasted CKD patients or for patients who are expected to require dialysis in the near future, a higher amino acid or protein intake may be prescribed; however this will hasten the uremic state and will require dialysis to be started early. Generally about 1.2 g/kg/d should be prescribed for patients who will receive intermittent hemodialysis. This is the amount used for stable, ESRD patients although the clinical circumstances may call for an increase in the protein intake > 1.2 g/kg/d. If a CKD patient undergoing hemodialysis is given greater than 1.2 g/kg/d protein, the dialysis schedule must be intensified and daily dialysis should be strongly considered. For individuals receiving CVVH/CVVHD, 1.5 to 2.5 g of protein per kg per day is often prescribed.[9,10] These increased nitrogen loads and the larger volumes of water necessary to provide these nutrients may increase the need for dialysis therapy unless the CVVH/CVVHD is performed efficiently.

2. Energy requirements can be estimated in several ways for patients with renal failure.

a) The Harris-Benedict equation,[11] which estimates the basal energy expenditure (BEE) from the individual's age, sex, weight, and height, can be calculated as follows:

$$\text{Female: BEE} = 655 + (9.6 \times \text{aBW}) + (1.8 \times \text{height}) + (4.7 \times \text{age}),$$

$$\text{Male: BEE} = 66 + (13.7 \times \text{aBW}) + (5 \times \text{height}) + (6.8 \times \text{age})$$

where aBW = edema-free actual body weight (kg) if it is between 90% and 120% of normal (standard) body weight, height = height (cm), and age = age (years). If aBW is <90% or >120% of normal body weight, the adjusted aBW is used (see above).

b) The estimated energy requirement should be increased as needed for stress and then by 25% to adjust for individual variability and physical activity, if any, and to ensure that energy intake is sufficient. The higher energy intakes may increase the efficiency of nitrogen utilization when small quantities of protein or amino acids are provided to the patient. The calculation of energy requirements for ill patients with CKD is energy requirement = estimated BEE + adjustment factor for illness + 25%.

c) As an approximate guide, acutely ill patients with CKD usually require between 30 and 45 kcal/kg of normal or adjusted actual body weight per day. The lower end of this range is recommended for the elderly individuals, non-hypercatabolic obese patients, and patients with higher nitrogen intake (ie, 1.5 to 2.5 g of protein or amino acids per kg per day). The higher end of this range is used for patients who are severely catabolic or who have low nitrogen intakes. Data in non-hypercatabolic animals indicate that a higher energy intake is necessary to maintain nitrogen balance when a low nitrogen diet is given. In general, energy intakes > 45 kcal/kg/d are not recommended because the high energy levels tend to promote hypercapnia, obesity, and fatty liver.[12] In addition, greater energy intakes usually increase the amount of fluid necessary to meet these higher calorie goals.

C. Specific guidelines for parenteral nutrition (PN) for patients with CKD

1. Because most patients with CKD do not tolerate large volumes of water, efforts are made to use more concentrated nutrient solutions. A 70% dextrose (d-glucose) solution is usually used. This solution provides 70 g/dL of d-glucose monohydrate (3.4 kcal/g) or about 63 g of anhydrous glucose so that 70% d-glucose monohydrate provides 2.38 kcal/mL of solution.
2. Amino acids are usually supplied in 8.5%, 10%, or 15% solutions. To provide more concentrated PN solutions, 10% or 15% amino acids are usually employed. However, the 15% amino acid solution is more expensive. A mixture of essential and nonessential amino acids generally provides 3.5 kcal/g. Specialized solutions are available that provide the nine essential amino acids with or without arginine, a mixture of the nine essential amino acids and the nonessential amino acids in a 2:1 ratio, or a high concentration of branched-chain amino acids.
3. Patients receiving PN should be given IV fat emulsions. Fat emulsions are necessary to prevent essential fatty acid deficiency, to reduce the risk of hyperglycemia that is associated with large dextrose loads, and to provide a more normal mixture of fuel substrates. Fat emulsions are available as 10% or 20% emulsions and provide 1.1 and 2.0 kcal/mL, respectively. The 20% emulsion is recommended when fluid restriction is indicated. The phosphorus content of fat emulsions is about 14.8 mmol/L in both the 10% and 20% emulsions. Therefore, using a 20% fat emulsion may be more desirable when phosphorus intake needs to be restricted. Fat emulsions should be incorporated into the dextrose and amino acid solution and infused simultaneously as a "3-in-1" formulation.
4. Mineral and electrolyte composition of the nutritional prescription must be adjusted according to the patient's clinical condition and serum chemistries.

a) Sodium and water intake should be adjusted according to the fluid status of the patient and are often restricted to control edema or hypertension. Most non-edematous patients with CKD can tolerate a daily intake of 1000 to 2000 mg (43 to 87 mEq) of sodium, particularly if they are receiving regular dialysis therapy. Water intake may be limited to the urine output plus 500 mL/d for insensible losses if the patient is normothermic. However, to provide sufficient protein or amino acids and energy, patients receiving nutrition support, particularly those given PN, often are given quantities of water in excess of what they need or can tolerate. Careful attention to the sodium concentration (a measure of water status) or serum osmolality should guide the amount of water that should be administered. The nephrologist must be intimately involved with the development and use of PN.

b) To prevent hyponatremia in patients receiving large water loads, the sodium concentration of the PN solution is usually maintained at about 40 to 50 mEq/L, although higher amounts may be required to maintain a normal osmolality.

c) Potassium intake is limited because of decreased excretion and because hypercatabolism and acidemia may increase the movement of intracellular potassium out of the cell. Potassium intake is often limited to 30 to 50 mEq/d until it has been established that the patient tolerates or requires larger doses of potassium. An alternate is to provide 10–20 mEq of potassium/1000 kcal.

d) Phosphorus intake is restricted to maintain normal or near-normal serum levels. In general, such patients are given 200–300 mg of phosphorus per day. Alternatively, phosphorus can be given as 10–20 mmol for every 1000 kcal delivered.

e) Special attention should be paid to serum potassium and phosphorus at the initiation of PN. The potassium and phosphorus in the PN are often withheld from patients who are hyperkalemic or hyperphosphatemic at the onset of nutrition therapy. Once nutrition support is inaugurated in these individuals, serum potassium and phosphorus concentrations may fall precipitously, particularly if the patient is receiving dialysis therapy. Some patients may present with severe protein-calorie malnutrition and these are the patients who are at the highest risk of the refeeding syndrome in which the patient has depleted potassium and phosphorus stores and the serum values may plummet when dextrose is provided. Patients who are severely malnourished and who are believed to have had poor intake over 2–4 weeks should be considered to be thiamine deficient and thiamine 100 mg should be given intravenously before dextrose is given.

5. Calcium provision in parenteral solutions should provide 10–15 mEq/d for the short term. If the PN is to be required for more than 3–4 weeks, the provision of more calcium (up to 20mEq/d) should be considered, as metabolic bone disease may begin during this time. The provision of calcium in patients with rhabdomyolysis, multiple myeloma, or tumor-lysis syndrome should be minimal and closely regulated. The serum concentration of total calcium should be maintained between 8.5 g/dL and 10 g/dL.

6. Magnesium is usually provided at 10–30 mEq/d. In CKD patients who have undergone cardiac surgery and who require PN, the magnesium level must be measured frequently and maintained in the normal range.

7. Trace minerals probably do not need to be added to PN solutions, with the exception of iron and possibly zinc, unless parenteral nutrition is the sole source of nutrition support for more than 2 weeks. Iron should be avoided in the infected or septic patient. The nutritional requirements for trace minerals have not been established for uremic patients receiving PN. In general, the following trace minerals can be given once weekly if the patient is receiving PN for more than 2 weeks: chromium (10 mcg), copper (1 mg), iodide (75 mcg), manganese (500 mcg), selenium (60 mcg), and zinc (5 mg). However, the need for trace minerals is probably not great if the patient is receiving parenteral blood products.

8. Vitamin requirements have not been well defined for patients with CKD who are receiving nutritional support. Water-soluble vitamins are lost into the dialysate, except for B_{12}, which is protein bound in plasma. These losses as well as a number of drug-nutrient interactions may alter the intestinal absorption, metabolism (eg, vitamin B_6 or 1,25-dihydrocholecalciferol), or actions (eg, folate) of these vitamins.

a) There appears to be an increased need for certain vitamins in patients undergoing dialysis. Patients receiving hemodialysis should receive 10 mg/d of pyridoxine hydrochloride (8.2 mg/d of pyridoxine) to prevent deficiency.[13] No more than 60 to 100 mg/d of ascorbic acid should be given because of the risk of increasing serum oxalate concentrations and precipitating episodes of pseudo-gout when greater ascorbic acid doses are administered.[14] About 1.0 mg of folate is given each day. The recommended daily allowances for the other water-soluble vitamins are given each day.[15]

b) In general, vitamin A supplements should be avoided in CKD patients because serum vitamin A levels are elevated, and small supplements of vitamin A have been reported to cause toxicity.[16] If patients are to receive PN for more than 1 to 2 weeks, small doses of vitamin A may be given (ie, 800 retinol equivalents, which is the recommended daily allowance).

c) Vitamin K (10 mg) should be given weekly to patients. It is generally given intramuscularly. It is particularly important to give vitamin K to patients who are receiving antibiotics that may suppress the intestinal bacteria that produce vitamin K.

d) Although vitamin D is a fat-soluble vitamin and stores should not be depleted during the few days to weeks that most patients receive parenteral nutrition, the turnover of 1,25-dihydroxycholecalciferol is much faster.[17] Therefore, there may be a need for supplementation with this vitamin D analog in patients with CKD who are receiving nutrition support for a prolonged period of time.

D. Specific guidelines for enteral nutrition for patients with CKD.

1. Generally, the guidelines listed for PN can be applied to enteral nutrition support. Specific formulas are available to meet the needs of patients during the different phases of renal failure. Enteral products vary in the amount of electrolytes, vitamins, and minerals provided.

a) It is often difficult to meet the individual's energy requirement or limited protein need and to restrict the necessary electrolytes at the same time. Because of these specific nutritional constraints engendered by renal failure, specialized formulations for patients with CKD have been developed. For example, a calorie-dense formula is necessary to meet the patient's energy needs under the constraints of limited water tolerance. Most commercial formulas for patients with renal failure provide appropriate vitamins and minerals and 1.5 to 2.0 kcal/mL, with generally about 6% to 20% of calories derived from protein or amino acids.

b) Protein sources in renal-specific formulas are variable. Some formulas provide the nine essential amino acids (Amin-Aid, McGaw Laboratories). Others provide high-quality protein (Nepro, Suplena, Ross Products). Essential amino acid formulas may be used for short periods of time (no more than 2 to 3 weeks) to prevent or delay the use of dialysis therapy as described above. These essential amino acid preparations are indicated only for short-term use because the total essential amino acid intake must be limited to marginal quantities, ie, 0.30 to 0.50 g/kg/d and a total of no more than 30 to 40 g/d. Also, Amin-Aid does not provide vitamins and essential minerals; these must be added separately. Most enteral formulas provide approximately 30% of calories from fat. Specialty formulas for renal disease such as Nepro and Suplena (Ross Products) provide approximately 40% of calories from fat, as they are limited in carbohydrate and protein content, respectively. Formulas with a lower fat content may be beneficial if malabsorption is present. However, it may be difficult to meet the patient's calorie and fluid prescription with these preparations.

c) Enteral formulas vary in sodium and potassium content. Standard 1.0-kcal/mL formulas generally supply 500 to 1000 mg/L of sodium and 1000 to 2000 mg/L of potassium; 2.0-kcal/mL formulas provide similar amounts of sodium and potassium. However, patients generally require less of these formulas to meet their energy needs; hence, their total sodium and potassium intake may be less. Most CKD patients can tolerate 1000 to 2000 mg/d (43 to 87 mEq/d) of sodium and 1100 to 1950 mg/d (30 to 50 mEq/d) of potassium. Potassium may be increased to 2700 mg/d (about 70 mEq/d) if well tolerated, or reduced if the serum potassium increases.

d) Phosphorus intake from enteral formulas should be limited to 10–20 mEq per 1000 kcal or lower if the patient is hyperphosphatemic. Magnesium intake should be approximately 10 mEq/d and should be carefully monitored especially in cardiac surgery patients or those with active or unstable ischemic heart disease.

III. Nutritional Support for Renal Transplant Patients

A. Nutritional therapy for renal transplant patients varies according to the different stages in the clinical course of the patient.

1. Patients who are immediately post-transplantation may require about 1.3 to 1.5 g/kg/d of protein because of the high doses of prednisone administered and the catabolic stress of surgery. If patients have a very high UNA, they may receive protein up to 2.0 g/kg/d. For patients who develop ARF or who have delayed graft function in the transplanted kidney, these higher protein intakes increase the need for hemodialysis therapy. When the dose of prednisone is reduced to <30 mg/d, protein intake can be decreased.
2. Later in the clinical course after renal transplantation, when a rejection or an acute reaction supervenes and the prednisone dose is increased, protein or amino acid intake may again be increased.
3. Renal transplant recipients who have diminished GFR but do not have acute rejection and who are not on high doses of prednisone may be prescribed 0.60 g of protein per kg per day. This intake should maintain good nutrition and may retard the rate of progression of renal failure.[18]
4. Although renal transplant patients often increase their body fat after transplantation and hence may benefit from calorie restriction, during an acute rejection reaction their energy needs are similar to stressed ARF patients (30 to 45 kcal/kg). Although most transplant patients and many surgeons advocate an unlimited diet, it is prudent to recommend, at the least, an American Heart Associate (AHA) Step 1 diet with the RDI for protein intake of 0.75 g/kg/d. If the transplant patient has a GFR using the Modification of Diet in Renal Disease (MDRD) GFR formula (see Appendix 29-1) that is less than 60 mL/min/1.73 m^2 bsa, protein restriction to 0.6 g/kg aBW should be prescribed.
5. Plasma glucose levels may be elevated because of glucocorticoid therapy. Under these circumstances, carbohydrate intake should be limited to about 60% of calories and, to the extent possible, should be complex. Patients who develop diabetes mellitus should be placed on a diet appropriate for their weight and an exercise program, and their blood glucose should be tightly controlled with the goal for the Hemoglobin A1c in the normal range.
6. Renal transplant patients also tend to have increased serum triglyceride and cholesterol concentrations.[19] Lipids should be limited to <30% of calories and should be limited to 2 to 3 times per week if triglyceride levels are markedly elevated. Again, the use of the AHA diets are recommended and if the LDL cholesterol cannot be controlled < 100 mg/dL, use of an HMG co-A reductase inhibitor is indicated. The lipid levels should be controlled for secondary, not primary, prevention guidelines.
7. Sodium and potassium generally do not need to be restricted after the transplant unless the patient is hypertensive; has renal, heart, or liver failure; or is retaining sodium and water due to other causes.
8. When catabolic stress supervenes, renal transplant recipients are given essentially the same nutrition support as acutely ill patients who do not have renal failure and who are receiving glucocorticoid therapy. If acutely ill renal transplant recipients also have renal failure, their nutrition support is similar to that of non-transplanted CKD patients who have superimposed stress.

IV. Intradialytic Parenteral Nutrition (IDPN)

A. Intradialytic parenteral nutrition is not commonly used in hospitalized ESRD patients with acute superimposed illnesses, because the day-to-day nutritional needs rarely can be met by nutrients infused during the dialysis period alone. However, intradialytic parenteral nutrition may be useful to provide extra nutrients during dialysis in patients in whom oral or enteral intake is sub-optimal, because infused water and electrolytes can be easily removed during these times. These conditions rarely occur clinically. The one clinical setting in which IDPN might be helpful is in the patient with ischemic bowel who cannot meet nutrient needs with oral intake. In this instance the IDPN may provide the supplemental nutrition that the patient requires.

1. Amino acids, glucose, and lipids may be delivered IV during hemodialysis treatment. The mixture is infused into the venous drip chamber. For patients receiving oral or enteral nutrition support, intradialytic parenteral nutrition offers an opportunity to provide additional nutrients to augment the oral or enteral nutrition without the need to catheterize a central vein.
2. Standard mixtures of essential and nonessential amino acids without added electrolytes are generally used. Amino acid solutions of 8.5% or 10% and dextrose monohydrate concentrations of 50% to 70% are generally mixed together; 10% or 20% lipid emulsions may also be used. The nutrient concentrations of the solutions selected are determined by the patient's requirements and tolerance for water and sodium.
3. The nutrients are usually given in a 750- to 1000-mL solution that is infused throughout the hemodialysis treatment.
4. On the other hand, nutrition support can be readily administered during CVVH or CVVHD. Patients receive these renal replacement therapies virtually continuously and therefore are easily able to handle the nutritional load. The PN prescription during CVVH/CVVHD is described above. The PN solutions can be infused into the blood line that is post-dialyzer or CVVH/CVVHD filter to decrease the need for central line placement. However, a risk of this procedure is that if the CVVH/CVVHD is suddenly discontinued, the patient may have no central vein access to continue receiving PN.

V. Monitoring Patients Receiving Nutritional Support

A. At the onset of nutritional support (ie, for about the first week)

1. Daily: complete blood count, serum sodium, potassium, chloride, bicarbonate, urea, creatinine, glucose, phosphorus, calcium, magnesium, and blood gases (measurement of blood gases is not always indicated)
2. Daily: water intake and output, accurate body weights
3. Once or twice weekly: UNA

B. During weeks 2 to 4

1. Every other day or twice weekly: serum sodium, potassium, chloride, bicarbonate, urea, creatinine, glucose, body weight

2. Once or twice weekly: calcium, phosphorus, magnesium, complete blood count
3. Weekly: serum albumin, transferrin

VI. Complications of Nutrition Support

A. Complications of PN. (For a complete review of complications, see PN Management chapter). One of the most common complications of PN in patients with CKD is hyperglycemia. This complication occurs because patients often receive large doses of dextrose to meet their calorie needs, and they frequently have glucose intolerance. Increased serum glucose concentrations have been implicated as a cause of impaired leukocyte function, which can suppress wound healing. Serum glucose should be monitored closely; insulin should be provided in the PN solution to maintain serum glucose within the normal range.

B. Complications of enteral nutritional support in patients with CKD. (For a complete review of complications, see EN management chapter.)
   1. Because the electrolyte composition of enteral formulas cannot be manipulated as easily as with PN solutions, it may be difficult to maintain serum electrolytes within the normal range with enteral formulas.
   2. It also is often difficult to maintain water balance with enteral formulas, because large volumes of formula are often required to meet energy needs. At times, enteral formulas must be diluted with water and occasionally fortified with salt.
   3. The complications that are common to all patients receiving enteral nutrition such as diarrhea, aspiration, and mechanical problems with pumps and tubing are also common in patients with ARF and CKD.

(Renal disease chapters in first edition contributed by Christie Amble, Joel Kopple, Robert Wolk, Rowena Stokowski, and Peter Yorgin)

REFERENCES

1. National Center for Health Statistics. *DHHS publication (PHS)87-1688.* Washington, DC: National Center for Health Statistics, U.S. Public Health Service; 1987.
2. Kopple JD, Jones MR, Keshaviah PR, et al. A proposed glossary for dialysis kinetics. *Am J Kidney Dis.* 1995;26:963–981.
3. Detsky AS, McLaughlin JR, Baker JP, et al. What is subjective global assessment of nutrition status. *J Parenter Enteral Nutr.* 1987;11:8–13.
4. Cianciaruso B, Brunori G, Kopple JD, et al. Cross-sectional comparison of malnutrition in continuous ambulatory peritoneal dialysis and hemodialysis patients. *Am J Kidney Dis.* 1995;26:475–486.
5. Young GA, Kopple JD, Lindhom B, et al. Nutritional assessment of continuous ambulatory peritoneal dialysis patients: An international study. *Am J Kidney Dis.* 1991;17:462–471.
6. Goa XL, Kopple JD. Relationship between dietary protein, urea nitrogen appearance (UNA) and total nitrogen appearance (TNA) in patients with chronic renal failure (CKD) [abstract]. *J Am Soc Nephrol.* 1995;5:491.
7. Najjar MF, Rowland M. *Anthropometric Reference Data and Prevalence of Overweight, United States, 1976–1980.* Hyattsville, Md: U.S. Dept. of Health and Human Services, Public Health Service, National Center for Health Statistics; 1987.
8. Nakasaki H, Katayama T, Yokoyama S, et al. Complications of parenteral nutrition composed of essential amino acids and histidine in adults with renal failure. *J Parenter Enteral Nutr.* 1993;17:86–90.
9. Chima CS, Meyer L, Hummell AC, et al. Protein catabolic rate in patients with acute renal failure on continuous arteriovenous hemofiltration and total parenteral nutrition. *J Am Soc Nephrol.* 1993;3(8):1516–1521.
10. Bellomo R, Mansfield D, Rumble S, et al. A comparison of conventional dialytic therapy and acute continuous hemodiafiltration in the management of acute renal failure in the critically ill. *Renal Failure.* 1993;15:595–602.
11. Harris JA, Benedict FG. *A Biometric Study of Basal Metabolism in Men.* Publication 279. Washington, DC: Carnegie Institute; 1919.
12. Askanazi J, Rosenbaum SH, Hyman AL, et al. Respiratory changes induced by large glucose loads of total parenteral nutrition. *J Am Med Assoc.* 1980; 243:1444–1447.
13. Kopple JD, Mercurio K, Blumenkrantz MJ, et al. Daily requirement for pyridoxine supplements in chronic renal failure. *Kidney Int.* 1981;19:694–704.
14. Pru C, Eaton J, Kjellstrand C. Vitamin C intoxication and hyperoxalemia in chronic hemodialysis patients. *Nephron.* 1985;39:112–116.
15. National Research Council. *Recommended Dietary Allowances.* 10th ed. Washington, DC: National Academy Press; 1989.
16. Gleghorn EE, Eisenberg LD, Hack S, et al. Observations of vitamin A toxicity in three patients with renal failure receiving parenteral alimentation. *Am J Clin Nutr.* 1986;44:107–112.
17. Audran M, Kumar R. The physiology and pathophysiology of vitamin D. *Mayo Clin Proc.* 1985;60:851–866.
18. Nelson J, Beauregard H, Gelinas M, et al. Lipoprotein abnormalities in renal transplant recipients with chronic vascular rejection. *Transplant Proc.* 1992;24:366.
19. Dimeny E, Fellstrom B, Larsson E, et al. Lipoprotein abnormalities in renal transplant recipients. *Clin Nephrol.* 1982;18:306.

SUGGESTED WEB SITE REFERENCE

1. National Kidney Foundation Kidney Disease Outcomes Quality Initiative. Available at: http://www.kidney.org/professionals/kdoqi/index.cfm. Accessed October 2, 2004.

APPENDIX

30-1

Calculated Glomerular Filtration Rate (GFR)

The estimations of GFR from serum creatinine concentration or from formulas that rely on age, sex, weight, and serum creatinine are imprecise and may over- or underestimate the actual GFR. Several formulas exist but they are flawed because they were developed in normal, healthy persons aged 18–65; they use too few variables; and they ignore the influences of sex and ethnicity. The National Kidney Disease Education Program, a joint program between the NIH and the Kidney Disease Outcomes Quality Initiative of the National Kidney Foundation, has proposed using the estimation formula developed by the Modification of Diet in Renal Disease study (MDRD). This equation has been validated in a large cohort of patients with kidney disease, has been proven superior to other regression formulas, and does not rely upon weight. The results from this formula are already normalized to a 1.73-m^2 body surface area. The simple and extended formulas have exponents that are in fractions and are negative. Therefore, because of the complicated math, it is most practical to use a GFR calculator found on the web such as: http://www.nkdep.nih.gov/GFR-cal-adult.html (this site also has a calculator for children), http://medcalc3000.com/GFREstimator.htm, or http://www.nephron.com/cgi-bin/MDRD-GFR.cgi (this site has the Cockcroft-Gault formula, the extended MDRD formula, and a formula for pediatrics). These equations can be downloaded into a PDA or placed on a computer desktop as a shortcut to the web site.

David Frankenfield, MS, RD

31

Pregnancy

Introduction

Nutrition support plays a role in almost every phase of the life cycle. For the pregnant woman and her fetus, nutrition support can be lifesaving. For the practitioner, nutrition support of the pregnant woman can be intimidating, partly because the need for nutrition support in pregnancy is rare (limiting experience), and partly because few scientific data exist on which to base provision of care. This chapter will outline the standard for enteral and parenteral feeding during pregnancy.

I. Background. Optimal outcome in pregnancy is dependent upon good maternal nutrition.[1] Poor maternal nutrition can lead to intrauterine growth retardation, low-birth-weight babies, and increased prenatal morbidity and mortality.[2,3] If the mother cannot maintain adequate oral nutritional intake because of disease or other conditions, intake can be ensured by use of tube feeding or parenteral nutrition. Nearly all of the literature regarding nutrition support during pregnancy is anecdotal, consisting of case reports.[4–7] Thus, principles and practices for nutrition support during pregnancy are very much experience based and extrapolated from normal diet in pregnancy and nutrition support practices in nonpregnant people.

II. Nutritional Aspects of Pregnancy

A. Intake. In normal pregnancy there are few conditions which seriously decrease nutrient intake. Nausea may occur because of gastric atony, which is consistent with generalized relaxation of smooth muscles during pregnancy. Severe nausea or vomiting impairs nutrient intake, sometimes severely. However, the nausea of pregnancy is not usually a major impediment to nutrition intake. In one study, more than half of pregnant women reported an obvious increase in appetite and thirst[8] beginning in the first trimester. However, nutrient intake generally increases even without an increase in appetite.[9] Greater intake and reduced ability to consume large meals (because of early fullness) as pregnancy progresses may cause a change in dietary habits, with more frequent but smaller meals being consumed.

   Obviously, preexisting impediments to nutrient intake would remain problems during pregnancy, and in fact the related nutrient deficits might be exacerbated, since nutrient requirements in pregnancy are somewhat higher than normal. Impediments to intake need not be physical or disease related. Poor dietary habits exist in various segments of the population because of a lack of resources or education, or cultural or other pressures to avoid certain foods. The most common condition that might seriously impair nutrient intake is hyperemesis gravidarum.

B. Absorption. Nutrient absorption is not adversely affected during normal pregnancy, but preexisting conditions that impair absorption may remain and lead to malnutrition because increased demand for nutrient intake is imposed upon an already limited ability to digest and absorb nutrients. On the other hand, there is anecdotal evidence for improved absorption during pregnancy among women with normally impaired absorption. One such case was described by Montgomery and Pincus in 1955.[10] A woman with 3 feet of duodenum and jejunum who passed two to four soft stools per day containing significant undigested fat and meat fibers plus undigested vegetable matter began to pass only one, more formed stool per day upon becoming pregnant. Microscopic examination of the fecal material appeared to show less undigested food than that found in prepregnancy fecal material. The patient consumed 4000 to 5000 kcal/d and gained 14 pounds during pregnancy, delivering a 6-pound infant. Two more successful pregnancies followed, and in each case the patient's postpartum bowel function returned to that occurring before the first pregnancy.

C. Utilization. Pregnancy is an anabolic state. An average of 925 g of protein and 3825 g of fat accumulate in the mother and fetus.[11] Oxygen consumption increases steadily through pregnancy, starting with a 5% increase in the first 10 weeks, then increasing by approximately 7%, 11%, and 15% in each subsequent 10-week period. These increases must be thought of as general values, as there is great interindividual variability in actual measurements in oxygen consumption, especially in the last 10 weeks.[12] Eighty percent of the increase in oxygen consumption is for maternal tissue metabolism and work (cardiac output, respiration, uterus muscles, breast, and kidney).[11] The remaining 20% is for the fetus.

   Additional macronutrient intake is needed to meet increased energy requirements and to provide substrate for tissue growth. The increase in oxygen consumption of pregnancy represents oxidative macronutrient use and accounts for only about 40% of the increase in total macronutrient requirements. The remaining 60% of macronutrient requirement increase is used for tissue growth.[11]

D. Losses. Nutrient losses during pregnancy are not different from those in nonpregnancy. In fact, certain nutrient losses are reduced. For example, iron is normally absorbed from the gastrointestinal tract in proportion to the level of deficiency in the body. Because iron requirements during pregnancy are elevated, a greater percentage of dietary iron is absorbed (ie, less is lost).[13] Furthermore, menstruation ceases, eliminating another source of iron loss.

III. Nutritional Alterations in Pregnancy

A. Common. Calorie and protein requirements are elevated in pregnancy. As discussed Section II.C, calorie requirements are elevated for both increased fuel utilization (oxygen consumption) and tissue growth. The average increase in calorie requirement is 300 kcal/d, although the caloric requirement through pregnancy increases from the first to the third trimester.[14] Calorie intake should be adjusted up or down to achieve weight gain goals (Table 31-1).[15] Protein intake should be increased by about 10 to 15 g/d above the recommended dietary allowance or should be sufficient to achieve positive nitrogen balance. As with calories, the increase in protein requirement is greater later in pregnancy.

Requirements for micronutrients, with some exceptions, are elevated during pregnancy (Table 31-2).[14,16] Both fetal growth and development and growth of maternal tissues (placenta, uterus, breast, blood tissue) must be supported. Hypoalbuminemia (mean total decline of 1 g/dL) is common in pregnancy and represents a dilution of blood volume.[17] For similar reasons, hemoglobin falls in the first and second trimesters of pregnancy but then rises in the third trimester.

Alterations in glucose homeostasis can occur, with fasting hypoglycemia and postprandial hyperglycemia. Serum triglycerides and cholesterol levels are generally elevated during pregnancy.[18]

B. Less common. Disease states may add further demands for nutrients and alter the efficiency of nutrient utilization during pregnancy.[19] Accidental or surgical trauma, infection, sepsis, or other diseases eliciting a systemic inflammatory response can increase body catabolism and metabolic rate. Fetal requirements must still be met during times of metabolic stress. Nitrogen balance is difficult to achieve in metabolically stressed patients on bed rest. Protein intake should not exceed 2.0 g/kg.[20] See disease-specific chapters in this volume for the requirements of each disease state.

Malnutrition also alters nutritional needs above the alterations seen with normal pregnancy. Underweight women are encouraged to gain slightly more weight than normal-weight women, and obese women are encouraged to gain slightly less (Table 31-1).[21]

IV. Focused Assessment[22,23]

A. History. Numerous factors can influence fetal growth rate.[14] Fetal growth rate is an important parameter, since birth weight is an important indicator of pregnancy outcome.[17] Factors predicting low fetal growth rates include maternal cigarette smoking, nutrient intake and dietary habits, weight prior to becoming pregnant, number of previous pregnancies, and maternal history of low-birth-weight babies. Each of these factors, in addition to weight history, should be ascertained during the workup.[14]

B. Physical examination. Prepregnancy body weight and weight gain during pregnancy are critical determinants of fetal growth rate and pregnancy outcome.[2] Therefore, prepregnancy weight in relation to height (percentage of ideal body weight or body mass index) is an important physical finding (Table 31-1).[21] Consistency in methods and equipment is necessary in making these measurements, since the change over time is important to monitor, and alterations in methods or equipment may mask changes in true body weight. Certain overt vitamin and protein deficiencies can be detected upon physical examination. The signs of such deficiencies are the same as in nonpregnant women.

TABLE 31-1. Weight Goals for Pregnant Women Based on Prepregnancy Weight[15]

Body mass index*	Percentage of ideal weight	Weight gain (kg)
<19.8	<90	12.5–18.0
19.8–26	90–120	11.5–18.0
>26	>120	7.0–11.5

*Body mass index calculated as weight/height^2 with height in meters and weight in kilograms.

V. Objectives and Goals of Therapy.

The goal of nutrition support during pregnancy is the delivery of a normal-weight, healthy child. To that end, macronutrient and micronutrient intake must be adequate to achieve weight gain goals[24] and to ensure adequate substrate and cofactors for development of fetal organ systems. To meet the goal of a successful pregnancy, the nutrition plan should help the pregnant woman consume enough energy and protein to gain the appropriate amount of weight and to achieve a positive nitrogen balance. Adequate and safe vitamin and mineral supplementation should be provided. If nonvolitional nutrition support (tube feeding or parenteral feeding) is necessary, the goal is to meet the calorie, protein, and micronutrient needs while avoiding complications associated with the nutrient delivery method (mechanical, physiologic, or infectious complications).

VI. Management

A. Special aspects of diet and nutritional supplements. In normal pregnancy, unless there are physiologic, economic, social, or cultural restrictions on intake, the pregnant woman can normally regulate nutrient intake without much conscious effort.[9] If impinging factors do exist, they must be identified and circumvented to ensure adequate intake.

In underweight or obese women, women with concurrent disease states, or women with impaired intake, more than usual care must be taken in diet planning and monitoring. Plans for increasing nutrient intake (eg, use of calorie-dense foods, more frequent meals, vitamin and mineral supplements) should be individualized based on what is causing the impaired intake.[19]

Potential nutrition problems are most appropriately identified by eliciting from the woman her dietary patterns (food history, food frequency questionnaires, interview questions about special problems or conditions that might affect diet adequacy). This approach to identifying nutrition problems and the need for intervention is preferable to biochemical testing (except for hemoglobin and hematocrit levels).[9] Multivitamins are recommended for women who do not normally consume an adequate diet or who are in high-risk categories (multiple fetuses, smoking, ethanol or other drug abuse, chronic disease). If the diet is adequate and the woman does not fit into a high-risk category, micronutrient supplementation is not considered necessary by the Food and Nutrition Board of the National Academy of Sciences (one exception is for iron, the requirements for which the board believes cannot reasonably be met by diet alone).[21] Folate intake appears to be a critical factor during the development of the neural tube.[25] The need for folate is most critical during the first month of fetal development, when many women are still unaware

TABLE 31-2. Micronutrient Requirements in Pregnancy (Dietary Reference Intakes)[14,16]

Nutrient	Nonpregnancy requirement	Pregnancy requirement	Percentage of nonpregnancy requirement
Vitamin A (mcg)	700	770	110
Vitamin D (mcg)	5	5	100
Vitamin E (mg alpha-TE)	15	15	100
Vitamin K (mcg)	90	90	100
Vitamin C (mg)	75	85	113
Pyridoxine (mg)	1.3	1.9	146
Thiamine (mg)	1.1	1.4	127
Riboflavin (mg)	1.1	1.4	127
Niacin (NE)	14	18	128
Folate (mcg)	400	600	150
Cobalamin (mcg)	2.4	2.6	108
Calcium (mg)	1000	1000	100
Phosphorus (mg)	700	700	100
Magnesium (mg)	320	350	109
Zinc (mg)	8	11	138
Iodine (mcg)	150	220	147
Selenium (mcg)	55	60	109
Iron (mg)	18	27	150

NE, niacin equivalents; TE = tocopherol equivalents
Adapted with permission from Food and Nutrition Board, Institute of Medicine, National Academy of Sciences. Dietary Reference Intakes: Recommended Intakes for Individuals. www.nap.edu. 2004.
Accessed Aug. 21, 2004.

of their pregnancy. Routine, early use of folate supplements therefore seems reasonable. Some medications, such as anticonvulsants, alter nutrition requirements. For that reason, the American College of Gynecology recommends that pregnant women taking anticonvulsants supplement their diet with 4 mg per day of folic acid. Micronutrient supplements, when prescribed, should be taken between meals or at bedtime, to promote absorption.[21]

B. Special aspects of enteral nutrition

1. Indications. Indications for tube feeding in pregnant women are the same as those for nonpregnant people. Women who are unable to eat adequately but have a functional gastrointestinal tract are candidates for tube feeding. Nutrient requirements will be based on needs during pregnancy plus needs for specific disease states if present. Use of tube feeding per se does not alter nutrient requirements or utilization.

   One special indication for tube feeding during pregnancy is hyperemesis gravidarum. This condition often resolves after the first trimester, and in previously well-nourished women it may not require intervention. An intermediate step before the use of tube feeding is oral supplementation and intensive nutrition counseling.[19] Antiemetics and promotility agents are also important interventions for patients with hyperemesis. If tube feedings are necessary, continuous feeding offers the best chance for success.[19] As always, both the benefits and risks of tube feeding should be considered. Tube feedings should be initiated slowly and advanced slowly as tolerated. Oral intake should be eliminated until tolerance to the tube feeding is established (so as not to confuse food intolerance with tube feeding intolerance). Oral feeding should be reintroduced slowly, to tolerance.

2. Access. Nasogastric tubes are indicated if the stomach is functional, and nasojejunal tubes are indicated if the stomach is dysfunctional. For endoscopic nasojejunal tube placement, the woman should not be exposed to sedatives that might injure the fetus, and if radiation exposure is necessary for tube placement, special care must be taken to avoid exposing the fetus.

3. Regimen. Certain conditions, such as hyperemesis gravidarum or diabetes, or use of small-bowel feeding tubes may require a continuous rather than an intermittent feeding schedule to ensure adequate tolerance. Often, 24-hour continuous feeding is best tolerated; however, intermittent feedings (cyclic nocturnal; or for gastric tubes, bolus or gravity drip) allow the woman greater freedom of movement and independence. The feeding schedules

should not sacrifice intake for the sake of greater independence, however.

4. Duration. Initiation and termination of tube feedings can occur at any time during pregnancy. A fair attempt at oral feeding should first be made before tube feeding is initiated, and the cause of oral feeding failure should be resolved before the termination of tube feeding.
5. Formulas. In most cases, a polymeric tube feeding is sufficient. In patients with a preexisting disease such as Crohn's disease, digestion and/or absorption impairment may necessitate elemental or peptide-based feedings. Feedings containing dietary fiber are desirable to minimize the chance of developing constipation. The tube feeding should provide adequate calorie, protein, and micronutrient support for the stage of pregnancy (micronutrient limitations may be overcome by use of supplements). Free water can be added as flushes or boluses.
6. Monitoring. Maternal weight gain and fetal growth are the most important factors in assessing the adequacy of tube feeding. It is important to differentiate weight gain due to fluid retention from other weight gain, especially with preeclampsia. Actual feeding volume infused (to identify underfeeding or overfeeding) and the presence of an inflammatory response (to identify possible hypermetabolism) may be helpful in determining why weight gain or nitrogen balance goals are not being achieved. Biochemical testing for nutritional adequacy can be limited to nitrogen balance, hemoglobin, and hematocrit checks. Nitrogen balance is not usually monitored in this population; however, values should be positive with provision of adequate protein. Table 31-3 provides laboratory values used to assess anemia in pregnant women. Hyperglycemia is a risk factor for fetal macrosomia and death. Therefore, women with glucose intolerance should be identified and their blood glucose concentration monitored, with insulin coverage to maintain blood glucose levels below 120 mg/dL. Metabolic monitoring (labs, fluid balance) and tolerance to feeding should follow the guidelines set forth in Chapter 5. Indirect calorimetry is sometimes performed during pregnancy when nonvolitional feedings are used or if appropriate weight gain is not being achieved. If indirect calorimetry is performed, it must be recognized that the results will reflect only the energy requirement for fuel utilization, not the substrate requirement for tissue accumulation.
7. Objectives. The goals of tube feeding during pregnancy are to achieve appropriate weight gain, to achieve positive nitrogen balance, and to provide safe and adequate micronutrient therapy. In addition, complications associated with tube feeding should be avoided by timely monitoring and intervention.

TABLE 31-3. Assessment of Anemia in Pregnancy

	First trimester	Second trimester	Third trimester
Hemoglobin (g/dL)	11	10.5	11
Hematocrit (%)*	33	32	33
Iron deficiency	<Ferritin 20 mcg/L with hemoglobin >10.5 g/dL		
Iron deficiency anemia	<Ferritin 12–20 mcg/L with low hemoglobin		

*CDC criteria for anemia in children and childbearing-aged women. MMWR. 1980;38:400–404.

C. Special aspects of parenteral nutrition

1. Indications. Parenteral nutrition should be considered only if all attempts at oral and tube feeding have failed and the woman is or is becoming malnourished. Parenteral nutrition is the most expensive and risky form of nutrition support, but it can be lifesaving when the gastrointestinal tract is dysfunctional. Higher rates of complications during the use of parenteral nutrition have been reported in pregnant women.[26,27] Women with hyperemesis gravidarum will often continue to have symptoms of nausea and retching even with parenteral nutrition. Parenteral nutrition is not a treatment but can support the fetus and mother until enteral feeding can be reinstituted.
2. Access. For short-term use, either central venous or peripherally inserted central catheters are acceptable. Single- or multiple-lumen catheters can be used. For long-term use, surgically inserted or implanted single- or multiple-lumen catheters are available. Peripheral parenteral nutrition generally is not indicated for greater than 2 weeks because it cannot provide enough calories and there is a risk of phlebitis. If the gut is dysfunctional and all requirements must be met parenterally, peripheral solutions may not be adequate because of limitations on solution osmolality, while if supplementation of oral intake is all that is required, tube feeding is more appropriate, since the gut is functional. Peripheral parenteral nutrition solutions usually are more dilute (higher volume), with a higher percentage of fat emulsion, than central parenteral nutrition. For these reasons, peripheral solutions often are not ideal for pregnant women.
3. Regimen. Parenteral nutrition must always be administered by infusion pump. Parenteral nutrition can be infused continuously over 12 to 24 hrs/d. One common infusion method is to infuse nocturnally over 12 hours to allow freedom of movement and independence from the pump during the day. Keeping mean blood glucose concentrations below 100 mg/dL during parenteral nutrition has been reported to lead to good pregnancy outcome, including a decreased incidence of macrosomia and neonatal hypoglycemia.[28] Women with glucose intolerance need longer cycles (16 hours) with cautious taper down. Blood glucose concentration should be monitored midcycle and 1 hour postinfusion.
4. Duration. Parenteral nutrition is generally not indicated during the first trimester for several reasons:
   a) Nutrient requirements during the first trimester generally are not much higher than normal requirements.
   b) The woman can usually support the early phase of pregnancy from endogenous nutrients and minimal exogenous intake.
   c) Many early feeding problems (eg, hyperemesis gravidarum) resolve by the end of the first trimester. If there is significant weight loss or malnutrition and gut dysfunction, then total parenteral nutrition may be considered during the first trimester. During the second and third trimesters, parenteral nutrition should not be used if duration of therapy is anticipated to be less than 1 week. Once initiated, parenteral nutrition can be maintained indefinitely if proper access and care of the access device is achieved.
5. Formulas. With parenteral nutrition, carbohydrate, lipid, protein, electrolytes, vitamins, and minerals are each added to the mixture separately (ie, parenteral nutrition is completely modular). This allows full flexibility in designing the regimen. Glucose intake generally is limited to 5 mg/kg/min (7 g/kg/d) or less.[19] Standard

amino acid solutions with a balance of essential and nonessential amino acids should be used.[19] Solutions high in branched-chain amino acids, sometimes used in liver disease and sepsis, have not been tested for possible teratogenic effects (per package insert). Lipids should make up no more than 30% of total calories to limit possible hypertriglyceridemia and immune dysfunction. Minimal essential fatty acid intake should be 4.5% of total calories.[29] Both linolenic and linoleic acids should be provided; all commercially available lipid emulsions contain both types of fatty acids.

Micronutrients infused parenterally are not subject to the sometimes inefficient enteral absorption process and so have much greater bioavailability than micronutrients fed enterally. Therefore, the requirements for micronutrients in parenteral nutrition are sometimes lower than in enteral nutrition. The composition of parenteral micronutrient preparations may meet or exceed the recommended allowances for some micronutrients. Therefore, standard intravenous multivitamin and trace mineral preparations may provide adequate micronutrient intake during pregnancy (Table 31-4), with the following exceptions:

a) Folate is sometimes supplemented (1 mg/d), even though the content in most standard parenteral multivitamin preparations meets the recommended dietary allowance for pregnancy.
b) Vitamin K is not contained in all multivitamin preparations and therefore must sometimes be supplemented (1 mg/d). It must be kept in mind that there is Vitamin K activity in intravenous fat emulsions, reducing or negating the need for supplementation of Vitamin K.[30,31]
c) For long-term parenteral nutrition, iron may be supplemented. There are several methods of iron supplementation. A weekly dose of 25 mg intramuscularly meets iron requirements but may

TABLE 31-4. Vitamin and Mineral Requirements in Pregnancy Compared With Standard Multivitamin and Trace Element Parenteral Preparations*

Nutrient	Pregnancy requirement**	Standard parenteral content***
Vitamin A	770 mcg	3300 international units
Vitamin D	5 mcg	200 international units
Vitamin E	15 mg alpha-TE	10 international units
Vitamin C (mg)	90	200
Vitamin K (mcg)	90	150
Thiamine (mg)	1.4	6
Riboflavin (mg)	1.4	3.6
Pyridoxine (mg)	1.9	6
Niacin (NE)	18	40
Pantothenic acid (mg)	6	15
Biotin (mcg)	30	60
Folate (mcg)	600	600
Cyanocobalamin (mcg)	2.6	5
Zinc (mg)	11	2.5–5****
Copper (mg)	1.0	0.3–0.3****
Manganese (mg)	2.0	0.6–1****
Selenium (mcg)	60	20–60****

NE, niacin equivalents; TE, tocopherol equivalents

* Check specific manufacturer's labeling for parenteral vitamin, mineral, and trace element doses.

** Food and Nutrition Board, Institute of Medicine, National Academy of Sciences. Dietary Reference Intakes: Recommended Intakes for Individuals. www.nap.edu. 2004. Accessed Aug. 21, 2004.

*** US Department of Health and Human Services. Parenteral multivitamin products. *Fed Regist.* 2000;65:21200–21201.

**** Task Force for the Revision of Safe Practices for Parenteral Nutrition. Safe practices for parenteral nutrition. *J Parenter Enteral Nutr.* 2004;28:S39–S70.

be uncomfortable for the patient. Some clinicians provide low-dose iron dextran in the parenteral solution when a fat emulsion free base solution is used and test doses are properly administered.[32] It is always best to provide iron supplements orally if possible.

d) Iodine may be supplemented if parenteral nutrition is required for longer than 2 weeks, as currently available trace element preparations do not contain it.

e) Calcium, phosphorus, and magnesium are not contained in any multiple–trace element preparations and thus need to be supplemented.

Unlike micronutrient requirements, dextrose, lipid, and amino acid requirements during parenteral nutrition are equivalent to those provided by the enteral route, because enteral absorption of these macronutrients is approximately 98% (ie, there is very little difference in the bioavailability of macronutrients delivered parenterally versus enterally).

6. Monitoring. Monitoring of parenteral nutrition is similar to that for tube feeding. See Chapter 8 for specific monitoring methods during parenteral nutrition. Monitoring serum glucose and triglyceride levels is particularly important during pregnancy.
7. Objectives. The goals during parenteral nutrition are the same as those in oral or tube feeding: appropriate weight gain, positive nitrogen balance, safe and adequate micronutrient intake, and avoidance of complications associated with the therapy.

REFERENCES

1. Kramer MS. Intrauterine growth and gestational duration determinants. *Pediatrics.* 1987;80:502.
2. Van den Berg BJ. Maternal variables affecting fetal growth. *Am J Clin Nutr.* 1981;34:722–726.
3. Naeve RL. Weight gain and the outcome of pregnancy. *Am J Obstet Gynecol.* 1979;135:3–9.
4. Breen KJ, McDonald IA, Panelli D, et al. Planned pregnancy in a patient who was receiving home parenteral nutrition. *Med J Aust.* 1987;146:215.
5. Mughal MM, Shaffer JL, Turner M, et al. Nutritional management of pregnancy in patients on home parenteral nutrition. *Br J Obstet Gynaecol.* 1987;94:44.
6. Tresadern JC, Falconer GF, Turnberg LA, et al. Maintenance of pregnancy in a home parenteral nutrition patient. *J Parenter Enteral Nutr.* 1984;8:199.
7. Badgett T, Feingold M. Total parenteral nutrition in pregnancy: case review and guidelines for calculating requirements. *J Matern Fetal Med.* 1997;6:215.
8. Taggart N. Food habits in pregnancy. *Proc Nutr Soc.* 1961;20:35.
9. Hytten FE. The alimentary system. In: Hytten FE, Chamberlain G, eds. *Clinical Physiology in Obstetrics.* Oxford, UK: Blackwell Scientific Publications; 1980:147–162.
10. Montgomery TL, Pincus IJ. A nutritional problem in pregnancy resulting from extensive resection of the small bowel: case report. *Am J Obstet Gynecol.* 1955;69(4):865–868.
11. Hytten FE. Nutrition. In: Hytten FE, Chamberlain G, eds. *Clinical Physiology in Obstetrics.* Oxford, UK: Blackwell Scientific Publications; 1980:147–162.
12. Goldberg GR, Prentic AM, Coward WA, et al. Longitudinal assessment of energy expenditure in pregnancy by the doubly labeled water method. *Am J Clin Nutr.* 1993;57:494–505.
13. Svanberg B. Absorption of iron in pregnancy. *Acta Obstet Gynecol Scand.* 1975;48(suppl):69.
14. Food and Nutrition Board, Institute of Medicine, National Academy of Sciences. Dietary Reference Intakes: Recommended Intakes for Individuals. www.nap.edu. Accessed Aug. 21, 2004.
15. Abrams B. Weight gain and energy intake during pregnancy. *Clin Obstet Gynecol.* 1994;37:515.
16. Wada L, King JC. Trace element nutrition during pregnancy. *Clin Obstet Gynecol.* 1994;37:574.
17. Robertson EG, Cheyne GA. Plasma biochemistry in relation to oedema of pregnancy. *J Obstet Gynaecol Br Commonw.* 1972;79:769–776.
18. MacBurney M, Wilmore DW. Parenteral nutrition in pregnancy. In: Rombeau J, Caldwell M, eds. *Parenteral Nutrition.* 2nd ed. Philadelphia, PA: WB Saunders; 1992.
19. Greig PD, Elwyn DH, Askanazi J, et al. Parenteral nutrition in septic patients: effect of increasing intake. *Am J Clin Nutr.* 1987;46:1040–1047.
20. National Academy of Sciences. *Nutrition During Pregnancy.* Washington, DC: National Academy Press; 1990.
21. Hamaoui E, Hamaoui M. Nutritional assessment and support during pregnancy. *Gastroenterol Clin North Am.* 1998;27:89.
22. Suitor CW. Nutritional assessment of the pregnant woman. *Clin Obstet Gynecol.* 1994;37:501.
23. Dawes MG, Grudzinskas JG. Patterns of maternal weight gain in pregnancy. *Br J Obstet Gynaecol.* 1991;98:195–201.
24. Czeizel AE, Dudas I. Prevention of the first occurrence of neural tube defects by periconceptual vitamin supplementation. *N Engl J Med.* 1992;327: 1832–1835.
25. Russo-Stieglitz KE, Levine AB, Wagner BA, et al. Pregnancy outcome in patients requiring parenteral nutrition. *J Matern Fetal Med.* 1999;8:164.
26. Caruso A, DeCarolis S, Ferrazzani S, et al. Pregnancy outcome and total parenteral nutrition in malnourished women. *Fetal Diagn Ther.* 1998;13:136.
27. Kitzmiller JL. Intensified glucose monitoring in gestational diabetes. *Clin Diabetes.* 1995;13:110.
28. Crawford MA. Estimation of essential fatty acid requirements in pregnancy and lactation. *Prog Food Nutr Sci.* 1980;4:75–80.
29. Camilo ME, Jatoi A, O'Brien M, et al. Bioavailability of phylloquinone from an intravenous lipid emulsion. *Am J Clin Nutr.* 1998;67:716.
30. Duerksen DR, Papineau N. The prevalence of coagulation abnormalities in hospitalized patients receiving lipid-based parenteral nutrition. *J Parenter Enteral Nutr.* 2004;28:30.
31. MacBurney M, Matarese LE. Pregnancy. In: Matarese LE, Gottschlich MM, eds. *Contemporary Nutrition Support Practice.* 2nd ed. Philadelphia, PA: Saunders; 2003:337–356.

SUGGESTED READINGS

Gardner DK. Parenteral nutrition in pregnancy. *Nutr Clin Pract.* 2000;15: 63–64.

Wagner BA, Worthington P, Russo-Stieglitz KE, Levine AB, Armenti VT. Nutritional management of hyperemesis gravidarum. *Nutr Clin Pract.* 2000;15:65–76.

J. Scott Whittaker, BSc, MD;
Laura Sware, RD; Lori Hards, BSc, RD

32

Anorexia Nervosa

Introduction

Anorexia nervosa is a psychiatric condition that is observed predominantly, but not exclusively, in girls and young women and is characterized by restriction of food intake in what has been termed the "relentless pursuit of thinness." Males represent about 5 to 10 percent of anorexia nervosa patients. Patients with anorexia nervosa are generally subclassified into "restricting type" and "binge-eating/purging type." Patients in the latter group, in addition to restricting food intake, partake in bouts of bingeing and vomiting, and they tend to have a poorer prognosis. Unlike most other patients in developed countries with wasting disorders, patients with anorexia have no underlying physical problem with food intake or absorption. Hence, the patients' physical and biochemical abnormalities are almost entirely attributable to starving or vomiting or to the use of emetics, laxatives, or diuretics. This chapter will discuss the nature of anorexia nervosa, with special emphasis on nutritional consequences, nutritional assessment, and approach to therapy.

I. Nutritional Aspects of the Disorder

A. Intake
1. By definition, patients with anorexia nervosa have decreased food intake. There is a wide variation among these patients in quantity and quality of food eaten as well as in the frequency of meals. Generalizations from studies therefore must be tempered with knowledge of the individual patient.
2. Recent studies have shown that compared with controls, patients with restrictive anorexia nervosa eat proportionally fewer of their calories as fat.[1] Proportionally more calories are eaten as carbohydrate, with about the usual or a higher proportion of calories taken as protein. Up to one half of patients with anorexia nervosa practice vegetarianism.[2,3] Furthermore, because total food intake is decreased, there often are absolute decreases in micronutrient intake.[4] Many patients with anorexia nervosa supplement their diet with multivitamin preparations, and the tendency to relative increases in intake of vegetables usually allows vitamin requirements to be met. Intake of trace elements, particularly zinc and copper, is more likely to be decreased.[2]

B. Absorption
1. Nutrient absorption is expected to be normal in patients with anorexia. However, in some patients, oral glucose results in no appreciable rise in plasma glucose, while intravenous glucose results in the normal expected rise in plasma glucose.[5] The proposed explanation is that glucose absorption is delayed as a result of decreased intestinal motility. The plasma glucose response to oral glucose returns to normal with renutrition.
2. There have been isolated reports of an association between anorexia and inflammatory bowel disease, including Crohn's disease.[6–8] Crohn's disease may be associated with nutrient malabsorption if there is extensive small-bowel disease or if small-bowel resections have resulted in a short bowel.

C. Utilization. Most nutrients appear to be absorbed and metabolized normally, but serum carotene levels are elevated, leading to suggestions of decreased hepatic metabolism; however, studies have not found altered metabolism of carotene.[9]

D. Losses. Vomiting and the use of purgatives, laxatives, and diuretics in some patients lead to losses of water and various electrolytes, including sodium, chloride, potassium, magnesium, hydrogen ion (with vomiting), and bicarbonate (with diarrhea).

E. Nutrient requirements
1. Metabolic rates in malnourished phase of anorexia nervosa are lower than predicted by the Harris-Benedict equation,[10,11] but no single simple formula is available. A reasonable average resting energy expenditure in a moderately malnourished patient is about 70% of the predicted value, but different studies have found a wide range of values.[12] This initial low resting rate is of limited importance, because refeeding quickly leads to increases in metabolic rates to levels very similar to those predicted by the Harris-Benedict equation.[13]
2. Adipose tissue in the body contains about 8 kcal per gram of tissue; hence, restoration of body fat theoretically requires ingestion of about 3600 kcal per pound of fat (8000 kcal/kg) exclusive of the thermic effect of food and energy required to produce the supporting connective tissue. Lean body mass contains less stored energy but needs relatively more energy to build. Studies have shown that to increase the weight of patients with anorexia nervosa by 1 kg, about 5000 to 7500 kcal above maintenance needs is required.[13] Care must be taken in these patients to avoid rapid weight increases with large calorie loads because of the potential risk of "refeeding syndrome."
3. The term *refeeding syndrome* has been used to describe the metabolic complications observed in malnourished patients when nutrition support is initiated, including hypophosphatemia,[14–19] hypokalemia,[20] and hypomagnesia[20,21] as well as cardiovascular, pulmonary, and hepatic compromise.[14]
4. Protein restitution in patients with anorexia nervosa is relatively easily accomplished when a complete diet is given, as would be predicted with a protein-calorie malnourished state.[22]

II. Nutritional Alterations Seen With the Disorder

A. Nutrition changes are listed in Table 32-1. For the most part, clinically detectable vitamin deficiencies are exceedingly rare, but abnormalities in enzymatic function, indicating subclinical deficiency, are not rare. The clinically notable changes that occur with anorexia nervosa include protein-calorie malnutrition, which is universal, increases in serum carotene concentrations, and possible zinc deficiency as well as osteoporosis.

B. Zinc metabolism in patients with anorexia nervosa has been of considerable interest because of the known effects of zinc deficiency in reducing or altering taste acuity and decreasing food intake. In some studies, decreased quantities of zinc in plasma have been found, although there is little correlation between plasma levels and total body zinc. Controlled trials of zinc supplementation have shown inconsistent results, with one report showing improvement in the rate of restoration of body mass index,[40] whereas older reports found no difference in nutritional parameters.

C. Bone density consistently has been found to be depressed in patients with anorexia nervosa; bone biopsies are consistent with osteoporosis.[41] There are several possible explanations for the changes observed in female patients, including retarded bone maturation, low estrogen status, and elevated levels of plasma cortisol.[41,42] Although there is no doubt that calcium intake is depressed in these patients, calcium supplementation alone does not reverse the changes. There have been rare reports of osteomalacia in anorexia nervosa.[24,25]

TABLE 32-1. Nutritional Deficiencies in Anorexia Nervosa

Nutrient	Prevalence of deficiency
Macronutrients	
Muscle wasting	Universal
Adipose tissue depletion	Universal
Micronutrients	
Fat-soluble vitamins	
Vitamin A	Levels tend to be high[23]
Vitamin D	Rare; 2 case reports of osteomalacia[24,25]
Vitamin E	Biochemical[23,26]
Vitamin K	None (1 case in bulimia nervosa)[27]
Water-soluble vitamins	
Thiamine	Biochemical[28]
Riboflavin	Biochemical[29,30]
Niacin	Rare; 2 case reports of pellagra[31–33]
Pyridoxine	Biochemical[29]
Folate	Biochemical[34]
Vitamin B12	Rare; 2 case reports[35,36]
Vitamin C	Rare; 3 case reports of scurvy[37–39]
Trace elements	
Zinc	Serum levels usually normal but may be low; decreased urinary excretion is common; taste sensation is normal; supplementation may be helpful[40]
Other nutrients	
Calcium	Intake is decreased; serum levels are normal; osteoporosis is common[41–43]

III. Focused Assessment

A. History

1. There are two aspects that need careful attention: psychiatric and medical. This discussion focuses on the medical aspects, which comprise malnutrition and its consequences as well as other behaviors that influence the physical condition of the patient, particularly vomiting and the use of emetics, diuretics, and laxatives.
   a) Weight. A detailed weight history should include current weight, premorbid weight (most useful in adults who had acquired a stable height and weight), highest and lowest (adult) weights, and, in women, the weight at which amenorrhea or oligomenorrhea occurred. The current weight is more properly part of the physical examination, because self-reported weights are frequently inaccurate or unknown to the patient.
   b) Weight control. The way the patient has lost weight is important. This history, when accurately obtained, allows characterization of patients into "restricting" and "binge-eating/purging" classes. The diet history should be carefully obtained, with attention to types and amounts of foods eaten, frequency of eating, and duration of the dieting pattern. Involvement in organized groups of dieters as well as use of ancillary diet aids such as liquid protein drinks and vitamin supplements should be determined.
2. Beliefs about food should be determined, including the patient's feelings about food allergies and intolerances.
3. When bingeing has been a feature of the illness, the frequency and duration of episodes as well as the food or foods usually consumed should be determined.
4. It is necessary to inquire about purging behaviors, including vomiting and methods of inducing vomiting. Vomiting occurs in approximately a third of patients, though it is less common in restricting patients[44] than in binge-eating/purging patients, up to 80% of whom may vomit.[45] Whether the patient uses emetics such as ipecac must be determined because these substances can lead to cardiac myonecrosis and death.[46,47] Laxative and diuretic use is extremely common in patients with anorexia nervosa, especially those who also have bulimia. Often, in the case of laxatives, tens or even hundreds of tablets are taken. The laxatives used are most frequently the stimulant type, such as phenolphthalein. These substances may lead to profound fluid and electrolyte disturbances. It should be determined whether the patient has a history of this behavior (ie, hospital admission for volume depletion or hypokalemia).
5. Exercise behavior, including type and duration, must be determined. Aerobics and running are frequently used as methods of weight loss.

B. Physical examination

1. A detailed physical examination is clearly essential, because nutrition assessment is best done by looking at the patient. The importance of physical examination and careful, detailed history taking as opposed to other measures is highlighted by the term "subjective global assessment."[48] For example, patients with anorexia nervosa usually have normal concentrations of serum albumin; hence, traditional objective measures may be misleading.

a) Body measurements. All patients should have their height and weight checked, and body build should be estimated. Body mass index and percentage of ideal body weight should be calculated. Anthropometric measures such as skinfold thicknesses and midarm muscle circumference are sometimes used.

b) Physical findings. General examination includes attention to muscle mass and subcutaneous tissue stores as well as the presence of edema, which is not common in patients with anorexia nervosa before refeeding. Thinning of scalp hair and the presence of lanugo hair may be evident, and occasionally the yellow appearance of carotenemia may be noticed (with normal sclerae).[49] The skin is often dry, nails are brittle, and there may be acrocyanosis and cold extremities.[49] Pulse rate and blood pressure are often quite low.[50]

2. When vomiting is a feature of the illness, there may be parotid enlargement, thickening of the dorsal aspects of the fingers of the hand used to induce vomiting (Russell's sign), and erosion of the enamel of the lingual aspects of the upper teeth. Petechiae are seen less often but may involve the sclerae, face, and palate.
3. Medical complications, including volume depletion, may occur in those who are vomiting or abusing laxatives or diuretics. Electrolyte disturbances may lead to weakness and dysrhythmias,[51] but physical findings are usually absent.

C. Laboratory tests

1. Hematologic changes are common and include anemia, neutropenia, and occasionally thrombocytopenia.[52] Anemia, observed in up to 30% of patients, is usually normochromic and normocytic and is only rarely due to iron deficiency.[53] Neutropenia secondary to bone marrow hypoplasia occurs in up to 50% of patients and appears to be attributable to the generalized malnutrition rather than to a specific nutrient abnormality.[52,54] In particular, folic acid and vitamin B_{12} levels are almost always normal.
2. Electrolyte disturbances include hyponatremia, hypochloremia, hypokalemia (severe [ie, <2.6] in about 5% of patients), and metabolic alkalosis.[55] These changes almost inevitably result from vomiting or from laxative and diuretic use. Occasionally, water intoxication may be the cause of hyponatremia.[56,57] Urea concentrations may be elevated in about one quarter of patients.
3. Electrocardiographic abnormalities occur in most patients, perhaps 60% to 70%.[58,59] The changes include sinus bradycardia, low-amplitude QRS complexes, and nonspecific changes in ST and T waves. Hypokalemia may result in the presence of U waves. Prolongation of the QT interval (ie, QT interval greater than 0.44 seconds) is a very worrisome finding and may be associated with sudden death.[60]

IV. Objectives and Goals of Therapy.

The short-term and long-term goals of therapy may be at odds with each other at times.

A. The short-term goals are readily apparent: treatment of complications of the condition, some of which may be life-threatening, and restoration of nutritional status to the premorbid state.

B. One of the long-term goals is to restore a normal body image so that normal nutritional status can be maintained.

V. Management

A. Patients with anorexia nervosa have essentially a normal gastrointestinal tract, with perhaps the exception of some dysmotility with profound malnutrition.[61] Hence, complete reversal of metabolic and nutritional abnormalities can be anticipated with successful therapy. The psychiatric portion of therapy is not addressed here but obviously is critical as well.

B. Short-term intervention for fluid and electrolyte abnormalities, other complications, profound malnutrition, or rapid weight loss necessitates hospital admission. There are no well-defined guidelines for degree of weight loss requiring rapid intervention, but previous studies on starvation have suggested that a decrease of 30% in a previous healthy weight should lead to consideration for hospitalization[62,63]; a decrease of 40% constitutes strong grounds for hospitalization. Many workers in the field are concerned that even a 25% reduction in body weight from a previous healthy weight may lead to cognitive impairment, with serious difficulties in intervention on an outpatient basis. However, there appear to be no data to allow a firm recommendation.

C. There is no other area of nutritional intervention in which a multidisciplinary approach to the patient is more important. Psychiatrists, internists, pediatricians, nutritionists, pharmacists, and nurses are all critical parts of the treatment team because of the multifaceted problems faced by the anorexia nervosa patient.

D. Two decisions must be made about the weight restoration program.

1. The actual target must be agreed upon, including which parameter will be taken as the measure. Often, this is body weight or body mass index, but some have suggested anthropometric measures such as body fat.[64] All these measures have confounding problems, including weight gain via edema and high inter- and intraobserver errors with measurements of skinfold thickness.
2. The actual goal weight or other value must be decided. In the case of target weight, the decision must take into account premorbid weight, if a reliable number is determinable, as well as published "ideal weight," which is a poor term to use in this field of medicine. The amount of recent weight loss has a bearing on target weight. The target weight should include an acceptable weight for discharge from the hospital for inpatients as well as a long-term goal weight.

E. Much of the approach taken by centers that focus on treatment of patients with anorexia nervosa is based on local preferences and biases as well as past experience. There is a paucity of studies evaluating the different modes and nuances of therapy on outcome; therefore, programmatic development has been largely anecdotal, often borrowed from larger centers that have described their approaches in a number of publications. There have also been changes in the recommendations for hospital admission.

1. In the classic treatise of Toronto-based Garfinkel and Garner[65] published in 1982, there was an attitude that favored hospital admission. They believed that it was usually warranted to admit the anorexic patient to hospital. The Toronto Programme for Eating Disorders has seen a steady decline in the percentage of patients admitted as inpatients, however.
2. In support of the outpatient approach is a study that showed no difference in outcome between inpatient and outpatient treatments after 1 year, although there were methodological problems with randomization.[66] Counter to this trend is the financial incentive for private facilities to favor hospital admission.

F. Special aspects of diet and nutritional supplements

1. Outpatient treatment

a) Weight restoration in patients not requiring hospitalization is generally believed to be optimally achieved by consumption of a normal diet, with avoidance of "artificial" means of nutrition support such as liquid supplements or tube feeding. Because these patients tend to be initially better nourished than their inpatient counterparts, a slower rate of weight gain is generally accepted.

b) There are two types of outpatients: those followed by a psychiatrist and his or her team in a private setting, and those admitted to day-treatment programs.

c) In the total outpatient setting, as in the day care and inpatient settings, a dietitian or nutritionist is frequently the person who prescribes the dietary education and counseling and recommends caloric goals and other nutrient intake. In some centers, an internist or pediatrician is actively involved in this aspect.

d) Discussion about the types and quantities of foods eaten is an important part of dietary counseling. Patients should be permitted to avoid only a limited number of foods; an important goal is to widen food choices. There can be no hard guidelines for caloric intake, but frequent follow-up (weekly, biweekly, or monthly) is essential to determine whether goal intakes and weights or other nutrition assessment goals are being met. It is necessary to intervene early if there are shortfalls. Because these patients are usually consuming very little when initially assessed and because of the dangers of rapid weight gain and edema, the initial recommended caloric intake generally should be quite low—1000 to 1500 kcal/d. Weekly increments of about 250 to 500 kcal/d[12] up to a level that results in a weekly weight gain of 1 kg (2 lb) are recommended. The absolute number of calories needed to accomplish this varies widely, depending on basal needs and levels of exercise.

e) The downside to a total outpatient approach is that eating patterns cannot be observed, and other activities such as bingeing and purging cannot be monitored.

f) Day-treatment programs use approaches similar to the total outpatient approach but allow for closer monitoring of food intake, provision and observation of one or two meals, and provision of a wider variety of food types. Group counseling is usually a part of this process. The efficacy of each component of these programs has not been determined.

2. Inpatient treatment

a) Inpatient medical and nutritional treatment often has different phases. Initially, stabilization of an ill patient involves bed rest, fluid and electrolyte (especially potassium and phosphorus and occasionally magnesium) repletion, and administration of micronutrients before formal nutritional repletion.

b) Blood tests are done immediately on admission, as indicated in Table 32-2; an electrocardiogram should be done if there are electrolyte disturbances or signs or symptoms of possible cardiac origin. Laboratory values that should be monitored over the first week include phosphorous, potassium, magnesium, glucose, and urinary electrolytes. Phosphorus requirements during repletion are greater than those provided in a standard diet or with enteral feeding. The need for extra phosphorus is determined by monitoring levels in serum.

c) Refeeding either is undertaken immediately or, occasionally, is delayed for 24 hours, at which point monitoring becomes very important. Refeeding can lead to alterations in serum phosphorus and potassium concentrations, peripheral edema, dysrhythmias, congestive heart failure, and gastric retention, the latter especially if tube feeding is instituted. To avoid refeeding syndrome, electrolyte abnormalities should be looked for and corrected before nutrition support is initiated, whether by the oral, enteral, or parenteral route. Circulatory volume should be restored slowly; pulse rate and fluid intake and output should be monitored. Refeeding is begun slowly by providing ~20 to 25 kcal per kg of body weight or ~1000 to 1500 kcal/d to start, and calorie increases should be modest during the first week.[12]

TABLE 32-2. Monitoring of Inpatients

Initial	Follow-up
Hemoglobin, white blood cell, and platelet counts	Weekly unless abnormal
Sodium, potassium, chloride, HCO_3	Daily for 3 days, then every 3 days until stable
Calcium, magnesium, phosphorus	Daily for 3 days, then every 3 days
Creatinine	Daily for 3 days, then every 3 days
Glucose	Daily for 3 days, then every 3 days
Prothrombin time or INR	None if normal
B12, folate levels	None
Electrocardiogram	If abnormal (other than bradycardia)
Bone density if depressed	Annually

INR, international normalized ratio

d) There are no simple measures to determine subclinical deficiencies of many vitamins. Multivitamin supplementation is prescribed as vitamins will be needed once anabolism is stimulated. Trace element requirements during refeeding in most cases should be no different from those recommended for the general population, with the exception of zinc, which some authors recommend should be supplemented at perhaps 15 mg of elemental zinc per day.[40]

e) Oral intake of a balanced diet is recommended, with some patients using liquid polymeric supplements. The use of these supplements is controversial. In the severely malnourished patient, cognitive function may be impaired, or patient's energy level or desire to cooperate may be impaired, and enteral nutrition may be recommended, starting at the same levels as one would use for oral refeeding.

G. Special aspects of enteral nutrition

1. Enteral feeding remains a controversial topic in anorexia nervosa, with respect to both indications and the ethics of placing a tube in an uncooperative or unwilling patient.

2. In very malnourished patients, tube feeding appears to be essential for restoring body mass because these patients may be incapable of restoring body mass on their own. The unusual complication of gastric retention may occur; monitoring patient complaints and abdominal size and taking an abdominal film in selected patients should help avoid the very rare complication of gastric rupture. The other difference in this population is that the patient may waste the formula by running the tube into the toilet, the sink, or a container. Whenever the weight response to the feeding appears to be inappropriate, the possibility of wastage should be considered.

H. Special aspects of parenteral nutrition

1. Only very few patients require parenteral nutrition. Indications in this setting include severe gastric retention or some unrelated but important gastrointestinal problems, such as bowel obstruction from adhesions or Crohn's disease. In cases of gastric retention

where vomiting is not an issue, a postpyloric nasoenteric tube should be considered before parenteral nutrition is instituted. Rarely, patients who may be completely unwilling to take a nasogastric tube for feeding may be willing to have a central venous catheter placed. Concerns remain about the possibility of these patients tampering with the intravenous tubing, with the potentially lethal complications of infection or air embolus.

2. Furthermore, with parenteral nutrition there is a tendency to push calories perhaps more than with tube feeding, with potentially disastrous complications of cardiac or pulmonary decompensation or hypophosphatemia[14] (although phosphorus levels in current regimens usually are adequate to prevent the latter).

I. Focused monitoring and goals assessment
   1. Although nutritional replenishment is one of the main goals of therapy, patients frequently have very mixed and often very negative feelings about replenishment.
      a) Weighing and other anthropometric measures have to be performed to monitor one aspect of efficacy, but these weigh-ins may be very disturbing to the patient and should be carried out with a minimum of fanfare. It may be useful to have the patient's back to the scales to deemphasize this aspect of monitoring.
      b) Because the long-term focus is on altered behavior and attitudes (ie, psychological aspects), it is reasonable to deemphasize short-term renutrition goals.
      c) Problems arise when nutrition goals are not being met and there is a need to determine why, because then an unavoidable discussion of weight becomes the central focus.
   2. The behavioral aspects of eating that need to be changed from the morbid state include normalization of energy intake, expansion of food types, normalization of the rate and frequency of eating, elimination of bulimic activities, and socialization of eating. These activities can be monitored by mealtime observation of the patient, which unfortunately represents deviation from a normal setting.
   3. Monitoring for clinical complications such as refeeding edema, gastric retention, and cardiac complaints should be done at least daily. Blood work should be done as outlined in Table 32-2.

J. Education of patients and caregivers
   1. Nutrition counseling is a key component of therapy of the patient with anorexia nervosa. However, there has been no formal assessment of its efficacy.
   2. Many of the educational aspects of therapy are less nutrition related than behaviorial. Many patients with anorexia nervosa are highly intelligent and motivated and should be encouraged to become knowledgeable about nutrition, including the effects of starvation.

REFERENCES

1. Fernstrom MH, Weltzin TE, Neuberger S, Srinivasagam N, Kaye WH. Twenty-four-hour food intake in patients with anorexia nervosa and in healthy control subjects. *Biol Psychiatry.* 1994;36(10):696–702.
2. Bakan R, Birmingham CL, Aeberhardt L, Goldner EM. Dietary zinc intake of vegetarian and nonvegetarian patients with anorexia nervosa. *Int J Eat Disord.* 1993;13(2):229–233.
3. O'Connor MA, Touyz SW, Dunn SM, Beumont PJ. Vegetarianism in anorexia nervosa? A review of 116 consecutive cases. *Med J Aust.* 1987;147(11–12): 540–542.
4. Hadigan CM, Anderson EJ, Miller KK, et al. Assessment of macronutrient and micronutrient intake in women with anorexia nervosa. *Int J Eat Disord.* 2000;28(3):284–292.
5. Nozaki T, Tamai H, Matsubayashi S, Komaki G, Kobayashi N, Nakagawa T. Insulin response to intravenous glucose in patients with anorexia nervosa showing low insulin response to oral glucose. *J Clin Endocrinol Metab.* 1994;79(1):217–222.
6. Bayle FJ, Bouvard MP. Anorexia nervosa and Crohn's disease dual diagnosis: a case study. *Eur Psychiatry.* 2003;18(8):421–422.
7. Gryboski JD. Eating disorders in inflammatory bowel disease. *Am J Gastroenterol.* 1993;88(2):293–296.
8. Mallett P, Murch S. Anorexia nervosa complicating inflammatory bowel disease. *Arch Dis Child.* 1990;65(3):298–300.
9. Rock CL, Swendseid ME. Plasma carotenoid levels in anorexia nervosa and in obese patients. *Methods Enzymol.* 1993;214:116–123.
10. Schebendach J, Golden NH, Jacobson MS, et al. Indirect calorimetry in the nutritional management of eating disorders. *Int J Eat Disord.* 1995;17(1): 59–66.
11. de Zwaan M, Aslam Z, Mitchell JE. Research on energy expenditure in individuals with eating disorders: a review. *Int J Eat Disord.* 2002;32(2): 127–134.
12. Rock CL, Curran-Celentano J. Nutritional disorder of anorexia nervosa: a review. *Int J Eat Disord.* 1994;15(2):187–203.
13. Krahn DD, Rock C, Dechert RE, Nairn KK, Hasse SA. Changes in resting energy expenditure and body composition in anorexia nervosa patients during refeeding. *J Am Diet Assoc.* 1993;93(4):434–438.
14. Huang YL, Fang CT, Tseng MC, Lee YJ, Lee MB. Life-threatening refeeding syndrome in a severely malnourished anorexia nervosa patient. *J Formos Med Assoc.* 2001;100(5):343–346.
15. Haglin L. Hypophosphataemia in anorexia nervosa. *Postgrad Med J.* 2001; 77(907):305–311.
16. Fisher M, Simpser E, Schneider M. Hypophosphatemia secondary to oral refeeding in anorexia nervosa. *Int J Eat Disord.* 2000;28(2):181–187.
17. Cariem AK, Lemmer ER, Adams MG, Winter TA, O'Keefe SJ. Severe hypophosphataemia in anorexia nervosa. *Postgrad Med J.* 1994;70(829): 825–827.
18. Winston AP, Wells FE. Hypophosphatemia following self-treatment for anorexia nervosa. *Int J Eat Disord.* 2002;32(2):245–248.
19. Marinella MA. The refeeding syndrome and hypophosphatemia. *Nutr Rev.* 2003;61(9):320–323.
20. Crook MA, Hally V, Panteli JV. The importance of the refeeding syndrome. *Nutrition.* 2001;17(7–8):632–637.
21. Fonseca V, Havard CW. Electrolyte disturbances and cardiac failure with hypomagnesaemia in anorexia nervosa. *Br Med J (Clin Res Ed).* 1985;291 (6510):1680–1682.
22. Russell JD, Mira M, Allen BJ, et al. Protein repletion and treatment in anorexia nervosa [see comment]. *Am J Clin Nutr.* 1994;59(1):98–102.
23. Langan SM, Farrell PM. Vitamin E, vitamin A and essential fatty acid status of patients hospitalized for anorexia nervosa. *Am J Clin Nutr.* 1985; 41(5):1054–1060.
24. Verbruggen LA, Bruyland M, Shahabpour M. Osteomalacia in a patient with anorexia nervosa. *J Rheumatol.* 1993;20(3):512–517.
25. Oliveri B, Gomez Acotto C, Mautalen C. Osteomalacia in a patient with severe anorexia nervosa. *Rev Rhum Engl Ed.* 1999;66(10):505–508.
26. Moyano D, Sierra C, Brandi N, et al. Antioxidant status in anorexia nervosa. *Int J Eat Disord.* 1999;25(1):99–103.
27. Niiya K, Kitagawa T, Fujishita M, et al. Bulimia nervosa complicated by deficiency of vitamin K–dependent coagulation factors. *JAMA.* 1983;250(6): 792–793.
28. Winston AP, Jamieson CP, Madira W, Gatward NM, Palmer RL. Prevalence of thiamin deficiency in anorexia nervosa. *Int J Eat Disord.* 2000;28(4): 451–454.
29. Rock CL, Vasantharajan S. Vitamin status of eating disorder patients: relationship to clinical indices and effect of treatment. *Int J Eat Disord.* 1995; 18(3):257–262.
30. Van Binsbergen CJ, Odink J, Van den Berg H, Koppeschaar H, Coelingh Bennink HJ. Nutritional status in anorexia nervosa: clinical chemistry, vitamins, iron and zinc. *Eur J Clin Nutr.* 1988;42(11):929–937.
31. Judd LE, Poskitt BL. Pellagra in a patient with an eating disorder. *Br J Dermatol.* 1991;125(1):71–72.
32. Rapaport MJ. Pellagra in a patient with anorexia nervosa. *Arch Dermatol.* 1985;121(2):255–257.
33. Prousky JE. Pellagra may be a rare secondary complication of anorexia nervosa: a systematic review of the literature. *Altern Med Rev.* 2003;8(2): 180–185.

34. Moyano D, Vilaseca MA, Artuch R, Valls C, Lambruschini N. Plasma total-homocysteine in anorexia nervosa. *Eur J Clin Nutr.* 1998;52(3):172–175.
35. Kam T, Birmingham CL, Goldner EM. Polyglandular autoimmune syndrome and anorexia nervosa. *Int J Eat Disord.* 1994;16(1):101–103.
36. Patchell RA, Fellows HA, Humphries LL. Neurologic complications of anorexia nervosa. *Acta Neurol Scand.* 1994;89(2):111–116.
37. George GC, Zabow T, Beumont PJ. Letter: scurvy in anorexia nervosa. *S Afr Med J.* 1975;49(35):1420.
38. Woodruff PW, Morton J, Russell GF. Neuromyopathic complications in a patient with anorexia nervosa and vitamin C deficiency. *Int J Eat Disord.* 1994;16(2):205–209.
39. Christopher K, Tammaro D, Wing EJ. Early scurvy complicating anorexia nervosa. *South Med J.* 2002;95(9):1065–1066.
40. Birmingham CL, Goldner EM, Bakan R. Controlled trial of zinc supplementation in anorexia nervosa. *Int J Eat Disord.* 1994;15(3):251–255.
41. Mehler PS. Osteoporosis in anorexia nervosa: prevention and treatment. *Int J Eat Disord.* 2003;33(2):113–126.
42. Rigotti NA, Nussbaum SR, Herzog DB, Neer RM. Osteoporosis in women with anorexia nervosa. *New Engl J Med.* 1984;311(25):1601–1606.
43. Golden NH. Osteopenia and osteoporosis in anorexia nervosa. *Adolesc Med.* 2003;14(1):97–108.
44. Keel PK, Fichter M, Quadflieg N, et al. Application of a latent class analysis to empirically define eating disorder phenotypes. *Arch Gen Psychiatry.* 2004;61(2):192–200.
45. Mazzeo SE, Espelage DL, Sherman R, Thompson R. Trends in eating disorder symptomatology in an outpatient clinic: 1988–1998. *Eat Behav.* 2003;4(2):211–220.
46. Ho PC, Dweik R, Cohen MC. Rapidly reversible cardiomyopathy associated with chronic ipecac ingestion. *Clin Cardiol.* 1998;21(10):780–783.
47. Friedman AG, Seime RJ, Roberts T, Fremouw WJ. Ipecac abuse: a serious complication in bulimia. *Gen Hosp Psychiatry.* 1987;9(3):225–228.
48. Detsky AS, McLaughlin JR, Baker JP, et al. What is subjective global assessment of nutritional status? *J Parenter Enteral Nutr.* 1987;11(1):8–13.
49. Strumia R, Varotti E, Manzato E, Gualandi M. Skin signs in anorexia nervosa. *Dermatology.* 2001;203(4):314–317.
50. Mont L, Castro J, Herreros B, et al. Reversibility of cardiac abnormalities in adolescents with anorexia nervosa after weight recovery. *J Am Acad Child Adolesc Psychiatry.* 2003;42(7):808–813.
51. Mehler PS, Krantz M. Anorexia nervosa medical issues. *J Womens Health (Larchmt).* 2003;12(4):331–340.
52. Devuyst O, Lambert M, Rodhain J, Lefebvre C, Coche E. Haematological changes and infectious complications in anorexia nervosa: a case-control study. *Q J Med.* 1993;86(12):791–799.
53. Kennedy A, Kohn M, Lammi A, Clarke S. Iron status and haematological changes in adolescent female inpatients with anorexia nervosa. *J Paediatr Child Health.* 2004;40(8):430–432.
54. Abella E, Feliu E, Granada I, et al. Bone marrow changes in anorexia nervosa are correlated with the amount of weight loss and not with other clinical findings. *Am J Clin Pathol.* 2002;118(4):582–588.
55. Schutte M, Mehler P. Metabolic abnormalities in eating disorders. In: Mehler P, Anderson A, eds. *Eating Disorders: A Guide to Medical Care and Complications.* Baltimore, MD: Johns Hopkins University Press; 2000:76–85.
56. Santonastaso P, Sala A, Favaro A. Water intoxication in anorexia nervosa: a case report. *Int J Eat Disord.* 1998;24(4):439–442.
57. Cuesta MJ, Juan JA, Peralta V. Secondary seizures from water intoxication in anorexia nervosa. *Gen Hosp Psychiatry.* 1992;14(3):212–213.
58. Panagiotopoulos C, McCrindle BW, Hick K, Katzman DK. Electrocardiographic findings in adolescents with eating disorders. *Pediatrics.* 2000;105(5):1100–1105.
59. Vanderdonckt O, Lambert M, Montero MC, Boland B, Brohet C. The 12-lead electrocardiogram in anorexia nervosa: a report of 2 cases followed by a retrospective study. *J Electrocardiol.* 2001;34(3):233–242.
60. Moss A, Schwartz P. Sudden death and the idiopathic long Q-T syndrome. *Am J Med.* 1979;66(1):6–7.
61. Kamal N, Chami T, Andersen A, Rosell FA, Schuster MM, Whitehead WE. Delayed gastrointestinal transit times in anorexia nervosa and bulimia nervosa. *Gastroenterology.* 1991;101(5):1320–1324.
62. Cahill GF Jr. Starvation in man. *N Engl J Med.* 1970;282(12):668–675.
63. Cahill GF Jr. Survival in starvation. *Am J Clin Nutr.* 1998;68(1):1–2.
64. Goldner E, Birmingham C. Anorexia nervosa: methods of treatment. In: Alexander L, Lumsden B, eds. *Understanding Eating Disorders.* Washington, DC: Taylor & Francis International; 1994:135–158.
65. Garfinkel P, Garner D. *Anorexia Nervosa: A Multidimensional Perspective.* New York, NY: Brunner/Mazel; 1982.
66. Crisp AH, Norton K, Gowers S, et al. A controlled study of the effect of therapies aimed at adolescent and family psychopathology in anorexia nervosa. *Br J Psychiatry.* 1991;159:325–333.

SECTION EDITOR
Charles Mueller, PhD, RD, CNSD

VI

Site Related and Ethical Issues

Denise Baird Schwartz, MS, RD, FADA, CNSD;
Caroline M. Apovian, MD, FACN

33

Acute Care Organizations

Introduction

Nutrition support in acute care organizations requires an understanding of the processes, personnel, tools, communication systems, and regulatory agencies that form the nutrition support care structure. Identifying patients at risk and providing specialized nutrition therapy in a safe and effective manner is the goal of nutrition and nutrition support departments and committees. The concept of the nutrition support team, an interdisciplinary collaboration among nurses, pharmacists, physicians, and dietitians, is explained and reimbursement issues are outlined.

I. Integrating Nutrition Support in Acute Care Organizations

A. Process (first row in Table 33-1)
1. Identification of nutrition status
   a) Screening process to identify level of care, and high risk versus low risk patients
   b) Designates timing of initial nutrition assessment by dietitian/dietetic technician and follow-up frequency
   c) Determination of a patient's current nutrition status via diet therapy, anthropometric data, biochemical data, and clinical signs when available
   d) Determination of a patient's nutrient requirements
   e) Goals to identify/apply early nutrition therapies for patients at risk for malnutrition
2. Nutrition therapy implementation
   a) Appropriate patient selection, including nutrition support team consultation/evaluation for specialized nutrition support
   b) Correct composition and route of nutrition delivery
3. Nutrition therapy monitoring
   a) Monitoring done by nutrition support team or appropriate individuals as set forth in the institution's policies and procedures
   b) Management of treatment, and type and amount of nutrients infused
   c) Achievement of documented goals
   d) Provide a pharmaceutical approach with achievement of targeted nutrient goals[1]
   e) Eliminate difference between prescribed versus actually administered amounts of formula/solutions[1]
   f) Goal-centered for improved patient outcome

B. Health care team members (second row in Table 33-1)
1. Registered Dietetic Technician—Provides patient nutrition screening and basic level assessments of patients at low risk for nutrition deficits[2,3]
2. Registered Dietitian—Provides nutrition assessment, develops medical nutrition therapy (MNT) care plan, and monitors goal achievement[3,4]
3. Physician—Provides leadership, coordinating medical practice with nutrition support in conjunction with other team members[5]
4. Registered Nurse—Intravenous site maintenance, parenteral and enteral nutrient delivery, and nasogastric and small bowel feeding tube placement[6]
5. Registered Pharmacist—Focuses on parenteral nutrition compounding, preventing electrolyte derangements and drug-nutrient interaction[7]
6. Registered Nurse Epidemiologist—Documents infection rate related to central line access and ventilator-associated pneumonia rate
7. Respiratory Therapist—Participates in ventilator weaning and assaying metabolic rates to optimize nutrient delivery[3]
8. Physical Therapist—Provides appropriate exercises as clinical status warrants to increase muscle mass in conjunction with nutrition support intervention[3]
9. Speech Pathologist—Assesses ability to resume safe swallow when transitioning from nutrition support and in recommendations for nutrient delivery options when dysphagia present
10. Social Worker—Provides psychological support and addresses social issues and financial concerns related to nutrition support[3]
11. Case Manager—Participates in evaluating situations where the appropriate cost effectiveness of interventions for specialized nutrition support might be enhanced and optimum patient placement based on medical needs
12. Ethics Committee Member—Assists in development of ethical guidelines when feeding may or may not be in patient's best interest
13. Patient Involvement in Healthcare—Patient/caregivers involved whenever appropriate and possible in discussions and decisions about their treatment; essential when long-term nutrition intervention is likely

C. Tools/equipment (third row in Table 33-1)
1. Computerized data management system
2. Patient's chart
3. Enteral and parenteral nutrition protocols
4. Enteral and parenteral equipment/pumps
5. Enteral formulas and parenteral solutions
6. Patient education forms and materials
7. Parenteral nutrition compounding equipment
8. Metabolic cart

D. Information communication (fourth row in Table 33-1)
1. Computer information system

TABLE 33-1. Nutrition Support—Who Owns the Process?

Process	Identification nutrition status		Nutrition therapy implementation		Nutrition therapy monitoring
	Nutrition screening	Nutrition assessment	Enteral nutrition (EN)	Parenteral nutrition (PN)	Enteral and parenteral nutrition
Health Care Team Members	DTR, RD MD referrals	RD	MD order	MD order	MD orders changes to alimentation
			RD determines nutrient adequacy	RD determines nutrient adequacy	RD recommendations to meet nutrient needs to achieve documented goals to improve outcomes based on changing parameters
	RN triggers		RN administers EN	RN administers PN	RN determines GI tolerance to EN and PN IV site management
				PharmD compounds PN	PharmD monitors PN compounding and electrolytes Epidemiologist monitors central line infection rates Respiratory Therapist performs metabolic rates Speech Pathologist monitors transition to oral diet Case Manager coordinates transfer to home on nutrition therapy
Tools/ Equipment	Laboratory		Feeding Tubes Protocol Equipment—pumps[a] Enteral feeding bags[b] Enteral formulas[c] Education Form—Enteral Nutrition	Parenteral Nutrition Protocol Parenteral Nutrition Orders Equipment—pumps[a] Feeding bags[b] Parenteral bags, IV tubing[b] Education Form—Parenteral Nutrition	
Information Communication	Progress/notes/interdisciplinary documentation		Progress notes/ interdisciplinary documentation	Progress notes/ interdisciplinary documentation	Progress notes interdisciplinary documentation Weekly multidisciplinary rounds Medical Committees[d]
Regulations/ Recommendations		JCAHO State law A.S.P.E.N.	JCAHO A.S.P.E.N. HACCP	JCAHO A.S.P.E.N. CDC	JCAHO A.S.P.E.N.
Assess/Improving Performance		Quarterly Level of care evaluation Monthly peer reviews	Monthly RD peer reviews	Annual Parenteral Nutrition Utilization Study Monthly RD peer reviews	Annual Parenteral Nutrition Utilization Study Nutrition Management of Ventialtor Dependent Patients IOP Monthly RD peer reviews

a. Biomedical Engineering
b. Central Supply
c. Nutrition Services
d. Nutrition and Metabolic Committee, ICU Committee, Pharmacy and Therapeutic Committee

September 2003 Denise Schwartz, MS, RD, FADA, CNSD
Nutrition Support Coordinator, Providence Health System, San Fernando Valley Service Area, Burbank, CA

2. Progress notes/interdisciplinary charting
3. Multidisciplinary rounds
4. Medical committees
5. Hospital-wide continuing medical education programs
6. Department education programs

E. Regulations/recommendations (fifth row in Table 33-1)
1. Intent of regulations and recommendations—To provide clear guidelines on what is supposed to be optimum nutrition support
2. Joint Commission on Accreditation of Healthcare Organizations (JCAHO)[8]
   a) The hospital defines in writing the data and information gathered during assessment and reassessment.
   b) The hospital defines in writing the time frame(s) for conducting the initial assessment(s).
   c) Patients are reassessed as needed.
   d) Development of a plan for care, treatment, and services is individualized and appropriate to the patient's needs, strengths, limitations, and goals.
   e) Care, treatment, and services are provided in an interdisciplinary, collaborative manner.
   f) The hospital has a process for preparing and/or distributing food and nutrition products as appropriate to the care, treatment, and services provided.
   g) The patient receives education and training specific to the patient's needs and as appropriate to the care, treatment, and services provided.
   h) The hospital collects data to monitor its performance.
   i) Data are systematically aggregated and analyzed.
   j) Undesirable patterns or trends in performance are analyzed.
   k) Processes for identifying and managing sentinel events are defined and implemented.
   l) Information from data analysis is used to make changes that improve performance and patient safety and reduce the risk of sentinel events.
   m) An ongoing, proactive program for identifying and reducing adverse events and safety risks to patients is defined and implemented.
   n) Competence to perform job responsibilities is assessed, demonstrated, and maintained.
3. State regulations[9]
   a) Provides for licensing and certification of health facilities
   b) Competency validation for patient care personnel
   c) Designates nutrition care integration in patient care plan, documentation in medical record, and transfer of information at discharge to ensure continuity of nutrition care
4. American Society for Parenteral and Enteral Nutrition (A.S.P.E.N.)
   a) Standards for Specialized Nutrition Support: Adult Hospitalized Patients[6]
      (1) Organization defines interdisciplinary nutrition support process, requires policies and procedures and performance improvement component
      (2) Nutrition care process includes nutrition screening and nutrition assessment
      (3) Development of nutrition care plan includes defined objectives, interdisciplinary approach, goals and expectations, selection of nutrition therapy route, and formula selection
      (4) Implementation includes ordering process, nutrition support access, formulation preparation, additives, packaging and labeling, administration of specialized nutrition support formulations, and sentinel event management
      (5) Monitoring and re-evaluating nutrition care plan includes defining parameters and frequency of monitoring, procedures and re-evaluation of nutrition care plan
      (6) Transition of therapy involves assuring adequacy of intake, continuity of care, and termination of nutrition therapy
   b) Standards for Hospitalized Pediatric Patients[10]
      (1) Criteria established for identification of pediatric patients who are nutritionally-at-risk
      (2) Use of subjective and/or objective criteria specific to pediatrics; appropriate growth charts shall be used
      (3) Nutrition assessment and reassessment shall be performed by or under supervision of a registered dietitian with pediatric experience or by a pediatric nutrition care specialist within a time frame specified by institutional policy
      (4) Development of nutrition care plan using interdisciplinary approach, with documentation of goals of nutrition therapy, discharge planning, route selection of nutrition therapy, and patient/care giver education
      (5) Implementation of nutrition care should commence following assessment and development of a nutrition care plan with a defined ordering process minimizing risks to the patient
      (6) Patient monitored for therapeutic and adverse effects and clinical changes that may influence nutrition therapy using protocols specific to pediatric patients involving physical assessment, biochemical indices, and nutrition therapy tolerance
      (7) Transitional and discontinuation of nutrition therapy shall be addressed
5. Centers for Disease Control (CDC) guidelines pertaining to nutrition support[11]
   a) Guidelines for the prevention of intravascular catheter-related infections
   b) Designates hang time for parenteral solutions
   c) Indicates timeliness for replacement of administration sets

F. Assess/improving performance (sixth row in Table 33-1)
1. Goal
   a) Better define the patient populations requiring specialized nutrition support
   b) Focus on areas where improvement is required
   c) Monitor and evaluate quality of care provided
   d) Pursue opportunities to improve patient care
   e) Identify and correct problems to save costs
   f) Implement cost containment for product selection, standardization, and management efforts
2. Peer review—to enhance performance of each clinician based on identified standards agreed on by the group of clinicians
3. Parenteral and enteral utilization analysis—to determine if appropriate patient selection for nutrition therapy occurs and impact on patient outcomes
4. Sterility testing of parenteral nutrition solutions—to maintain safe compounding practice for parenteral solutions
5. Medication safety variance reports
   a) Identify frequency of occurrence of problems with enteral and parenteral nutrition therapy and drug-nutrient interaction
   b) Develop a mechanism to prevent problem reoccurrence
6. Sentinel event
   a) Unexpected occurrence involving death or serious physical or psychological injury, or risk thereof
   b) Conducts a timely, thorough, and credible root cause analysis; developing an action plan designed to implement improvements

to reduce risk; implementing the improvements; and monitoring the effectiveness of those improvements

7. Improving organization performance applied to specific nutrition support processes[12–14]
   a) Important for identifying processes that need to be changed to improve the outcome[15]
   b) Provides an awareness of need and how to improve practice and assess performance[15]
   c) Used as a means of identifying success

II. Nutrition Support Organizational Structure

A. Nutrition support team
1. Functions and goals
   a) Defined as a group of healthcare professionals who in their daily activities manage patients who require either enteral or parenteral nutrition[13]
   b) Provides optimum nutrition support practice to improve patient outcomes, defined as decreased intensive care unit (ICU) days, decreased hospital days, and decreased morbidity and mortality[3,16,17]
   c) Promotes cohesive patient management with a collaborative approach to patient care[18]
   d) Achieves recognition and integration as a primary clinical service
   e) Acts as a consultation service
   f) Provides continuity of care for patients being discharged home on nutrition support
   g) Decreases both the variance in practice and cost of nutrition support[18,19]
2. Key characteristics of a successful nutrition support team[3,20]
   a) Motivated, committed, and persistent team members
   b) Attention to team welfare and high quality working relationships
   c) Good communication both internally among team members and with other professional patient care providers
   d) Shared team vision
   e) Robust clinical audit program
   f) Integrates the expertise of each individual team member
   g) Awareness of each member's particular knowledge, skills, and attitudes towards nutrition support practice
   h) Strategizes for sharing success
   i) Members keep abreast of the literature and current practice, attend professional meetings, and network
3. Role of nutrition support team members
   a) Physician
      (1) Leadership role on the collaborative nutrition support team[5]
      (2) Reviews the completed nutrition assessment and approves the therapeutic plan as the decision-making leader
      (3) Responsible for medical direction of team overseeing patient care activities[3]
      (4) Familiar with all aspects of nutrition care from screening, assessment, care plan development, implementation, monitoring, and reassessment, to therapy termination[5]
      (5) Effective collaborator, leading, working with, and accepting direction from team members representing other disciplines[5]
      (6) Evaluates the pathophysiology and expected clinical course
      (7) Ensures that the nutrition support goals, route of delivery, and formula selected are clinically appropriate[5]
      (8) Focuses on the anticipated medical and surgical plan and how nutrition support measures are beneficial
      (9) May place central venous catheter
      (10) Participates in the administrative responsibilities to make certain the team has the appropriate multidisciplinary focus, that policies and procedures are in place, and that education programs are implemented
      (11) Participates in education of medical staff and students in matters related to nutrition assessment, care plan, and treatment of patients
      (12) Ensures appropriate medical documentation related to malnutrition, and enteral and parenteral nutrition
   b) Dietitian
      (1) Acts as patient's primary advocate for all aspects of nutrition care[21]
      (2) Acts as a liaison with other in-patient dietitians in matters related to specialized nutrition support
      (3) Provides initial and periodic assessments of nutrient intake and nutrition status, including the diagnostic recommendation for various classifications of malnutrition[3,4,22,23]
      (4) Anticipates the effect of procedures, treatments, therapies and psychosocial issues on the patient's nutrition status[21]
      (5) Advises colleagues of altered or potential nutrition deficiencies[22]
      (6) Documents nutrition care plans for the application of medical nutrition therapy for high nutrition risk or nutritionally compromised patients[4]
      (7) Translates clinical nutrition concepts into simple language for the patient with acceptable strategies for implementing nutritional change[22]
      (8) Maintains current knowledge of developments in product specifications, technology, and clinical practice[22]
      (9) Participates in the design, implementation, and monitoring of nutrition therapies, including oral, enteral and parenteral, and transition at discharge[3,4,22,23]
      (10) Writes orders for enteral and parenteral nutrition as delineated by clinical privileges of the institution[3]
      (11) May place enteral feeding tubes preceded by specialized training, demonstrated competency, and delineated institution clinical privileges[3]
      (12) Oversees enteral nutrition compounding based on safety/quality standards
      (13) Provides appropriate nutrition education for healthcare professionals, students, and patients and their families and caregivers[3,4,22]
      (14) Participates in patient-focused quality assurance process with well-controlled projects, highlights good practice, and identifies where sub-optimal practice needs change to improve clinical effectiveness Collaborates with team physician(s) in proper medical record documentation related to both treatment and diagnosis allowing for appropriate coding and reimbursement[21]
      (15) Participates in ethical deliberations for withdrawing nutrition support and selecting palliative alternatives[4,21,24]
      (16) Participates in research studies and quality assurance process[4,21]
   c) Nurse
      (1) Primary liaison with unit nursing staff, may provide direct patient care, consultation with nurses and other healthcare professionals[25,26]

(2) Educates patients and caregivers, students, colleagues, and the public[25,26]
(3) Assesses ability of patient/caregiver to safely perform tasks related to nutrition therapy
(4) Principle resource on implementation of administration of feeding formulations and management of access devices, and vascular access expert[3,25]
(5) May place peripherally inserted central catheter lines (PICC) preceded by specialized training, demonstrated competency, and delineated institution clinical privileges[27]
(6) Facilitates discharge planning, and educates patient and family in techniques of home nutrition support prior to discharge[3]
(7) Participates in research activities and administrative functions[25,26]
(8) Conducts educational and quality assurance programs on administration of parenteral and enteral formulas and central venous access or feeding tube care[3]

d) Pharmacist
(1) Oversees compounding of parenteral nutrition based on safety/quality standards[28,29]
(2) Uses acceptable standard ranges for parenteral nutrition solutions to prevent potential problems with compatibility and stability[3,28,29]
(3) Ensures that the nutrition care plan includes the route and composition of formulation, pharmacological adjuncts to nutrition support, and nutrient delivery system[7,29]
(4) Uses expertise to evaluate nutrient-nutrient, drug-nutrient, and drug-disease interactions; drug doses; and drug-induced feeding intolerance[3,30]
(5) Helps teach home nutrition support techniques to patients and their families prior to discharge[3,7]
(6) Participates in surveillance and management of therapy-associated complications, and delivery of cost-effective care[7]

4. Credentialing team members in nutrition support
a) Physician
(1) Licensed physician or Doctor of Osteopathy certified through the National Board of Nutrition Support Certification as a Certified Nutrition Support Physician (CNSP) and/or American Board of Physician Nutrition Specialists certified[5] Recommended that candidates taking the CNSP examination for certification have at least two years of experience beyond residency training in administration and monitoring of patients receiving parenteral and enteral nutrition

b) Dietitian[3]
(1) Registered dietitian certified through National Board of Nutrition Support Certification as a Certified Nutrition Support Dietitian (CNSD)
(2) Recommended that candidates taking examination have at least two years of experience in parenteral and enteral nutrition

c) Nurse
(1) Registered nurse certified through National Board of Nutrition Support Certification as a Certified Nutrition Support Nurse (CNSN)
(2) Recommended that candidates taking examination have at least two years of experience in parenteral and enteral nutrition

d) Pharmacist[31]
(1) Pharmacist certified through the Board of Pharmaceutical Specialties (BPS), designated as a Board Certified Nutrition Support Pharmacist (BCNSP)
(2) Certification through BPS is a credential granted to pharmacists who have demonstrated a level of competence in nutrition support that exceeds minimum requirements for licensure
(3) Certification is granted on the basis of successful completion of eligibility criteria and includes passing a written examination, and in some cases, an experimental component

B. Nutrition support committee
1. Functions and goals
a) Defined as a formalized committee of individuals to address institutional issues for patients receiving enteral or parenteral nutrition
b) To provide, facilitate, and disseminate information on optimum nutrition support practice to improve patient outcomes
c) Standardizes ordering, preparation, and administration of nutrition support so that infection rate, glucose tolerance, fluid and electrolyte imbalances, and acid-base disturbances are reduced[30]
d) Develops nutrition regimens and education and monitoring protocols
e) Ensures early recognition/documentation of malnutrition and high quality performance in nutrition therapy
f) Reinforces the importance of medical nutrition therapy in the overall treatment and achievement of positive outcomes for patients
g) Supports high quality, cost-effective patient care by overseeing product/device selection, standardization, and management as this relates to enteral/parenteral and metabolic monitoring
h) Develops policies and procedures for safe practice and effective risk management, and enhances quality of care as well as legal protection
i) Develops clear guidelines for the instigation and selection of appropriate route of nutrition intervention
j) Identifies compelling rationale for choosing enteral over parenteral nutrition support with functional gastrointestinal tracts[18]
k) Promotes timeliness of nutrition intervention, so that severe nutrition depletion is avoided[18]
l) Produces proof of effectiveness of nutrition therapies
m) Provides mechanism for education, research, and quality management
n) Provides documentation of practice and outcomes
o) Develops effective methods to spread new practices widely throughout the organization[30]

2. Role of committee members
a) Physician—effectively understands and manages the array of policies and procedures, finance, and quality improvement issues confronted by nutrition support intervention[5]
b) Dietitian
(1) Develops policies and procedures and standards of practice to ensure optimal nutrition support through nutrition screening, nutrition assessment, and development of a medical nutrition therapy (MNT) care plan, its implementation, monitoring and reassessment, and transition or termination of nutrition care as appropriate[4]
(2) Provides transitional elements to all modalities of alimentation, oral to enteral to parenteral[4]
(3) Obtains institutional clinical privileges for order-writing in the medical record with or without physician co-signature,

for nutrition support interventions and monitoring within institutional governance of medical policy and procedure. Clinical privileges may also encompass specific skills such as feeding tube insertion and metabolic rate measurement.[3,32,33]

c) Nurse
   (1) Participates in the development and review of nutrition organizational policies and procedures for specialized support[26]
   (2) Supports nursing in the development of policies related to administration of enteral/parenteral nutrition and issues related to patient care
   (3) Develops protocols for central and peripheral line monitoring[26]
   (4) May obtain clinical privileges for placement of peripherally inserted central catheters preceded by specialized training, demonstrated competency, and delineated institution clinical privileges[27]
   (5) Keeps database for line infections

d) Pharmacist
   (1) Develops policies and procedures for parenteral nutrition, addressing labeling, compounding, formulas, stability, and filtration[28,29]
   (2) Maintains quality monitors regarding effectiveness of parenteral nutrition
   (3) Determines implications of Food and Drug Administration's amendment on regulations on aluminum in large and small volume parenterals used in parenteral nutrition[34]
   (4) Develops policies on the safe use and guidelines for use of extemporaneously prepared lipid emulsion syringes[29,34]
   (5) Develops safe infusion dosing of macronutrients (protein, fat, and carbohydrate), as well as electrolytes and medications in enteral and parenteral nutrition with minimum and maximum dosages[29,34]

e) Administrator—focuses on financial aspects of nutrition support therapy in conjunction with other healthcare team members to provide cost effective nutrition while improving patient outcomes.

3. Committee reporting structure examples
   a) Chair of Nutrition Support Committee reports to Pharmacy and Therapeutics Committee or directly to Patient Care Committee and then this committee reports to the Executive Committee.
   b) Sub-committee on Specialized Nutrition Support reports to the Nutrition Advisory Board, which reports to the Medical Board. Directors of Nutrition Support Services report to Medical Directors of various services and these Medical Directors then report to the Chief Medical Officer.
4. Communicating committee actions and recommendations
   a) Each committee member responsible for dissemination of policies and procedures and recommendations of Nutrition Support Committee to their respective disciplines
   b) Development of tools and education of hospital staff and other health care providers on nutrition support policies and procedures coordinated by Nutrition Support Committee members

C. Factors influencing existence and structure of nutrition support team[3]
   1. Institution size
   2. Age-specific needs: adults, pediatrics, and neonates
   3. Internal structure/decision making process
   4. University affiliation and academic role of institution
   5. Local case mix
   6. Objectives of hospital/conflicting priorities
   7. Staff availability/changes/shortages
   8. Profit versus nonprofit
   9. Competition for scarce healthcare resources
   10. Local practice and comparison to published data
   11. Dynamic health care environment issues, affecting all patient care and health care providers
   12. Previously recognized clinical issues with the treatment of patients requiring enteral or parenteral nutrition

III. Controlling costs of nutrition support

A. Nutrition Support Team/Committee can result in improved cost efficacy as documented by data in the literature[3]
B. Reducing complications with optimum nutrition support delivery[3]
C. Accurately determining appropriate parenteral and enteral nutrition candidates[3,35]
D. Reducing laboratory tests for monitoring parenteral and enteral nutrition[3]
E. Preventing overfeeding[3]
F. Decreasing duration of nutrition support[3]
G. Standardizing enteral and parenteral nutrition protocols
H. Reducing use of expensive, non-standardized parenteral nutrition formulations[3]
I. Preventing waste of formulas[3]
J. Formal infection control practices reducing catheter related sepsis[35]
K. Encouraging appropriate use of enteral nutrition rather than parenteral nutrition[35]
L. Achieving economics of scale through standardization of solutions and devices
M. Preventing inappropriate use of parenteral nutrition[3]
N. Performing cost analysis of supplies and solutions[3]
O. Cost versus charges
P. Cost-effectiveness outcomes[15]

IV. Reimbursement Issues

A. Reimbursement for nutrition support service consultation
   1. Physician nutrition support service billing
   2. Initial consult
   3. Follow-up consults (concurrent care)
   4. Institution coding for malnutrition diagnosis and for enteral/parenteral treatment in association with specified diagnosis
   5. Billing for metabolic monitoring
B. Reimbursement for acute care nutrition support[36]
   1. Medicare—parenteral and enteral nutrition (PEN) covered under both parts of Medicare when "medically necessary"
      a) Part A—inpatient hospital care, skilled nursing care, home care nursing visits, hospice care
      b) Part B—nonhospital costs such as physician services, medical supplies, and equipment
   2. Diagnosis-Related Grouping (DRG) system—payments to hospitals under Medicare Part A made pursuant to predetermined specific rates according to patients' primary diagnoses, PEN covered as part of the hospital stay
      a) Malnutrition and other nutrition diagnoses qualify as co-morbidities or complications.
      b) Co-morbidity—condition that existed at the time of hospital admission that causes at least one extra day of hospitalization
      c) Complication—arises during the hospital stay

   d) Co-morbidity and complications result in higher reimbursement through DRGs
3. Medicaid—administered and funded jointly by the states and the federal government. There is great diversity in programs, but Medicaid programs for PEN coverage in general mimic the Medicare coverage program.
4. International Classification of Diseases (ICD)-9-CM classifies morbidity and mortality information based on the official version of the World Health Organization's 9th Revision. The ICD-9-CM is recommended for use in all clinical settings but is required for reporting diagnoses and diseases to all U.S. Public Health Service and Health Care Financing Administration programs. The ICD-9-CM is used for DRG coding of co-morbidities and conditions. The following are relevant ICD-9-CM codes.[37]
   a) 99.15—Parenteral infusion of concentrated nutritional substances
   b) 96.6—Enteral infusion of concentrated nutritional substances
   c) 260.0—Kwashiorkor
   d) 261.0—Marasmus
   e) 262.0—Other severe protein-calorie malnutrition: nutritional edema without dyspigmentation of skin and hair
   f) 263.0—Malnutrition of moderate degree
   g) 263.1—Malnutrition of mild degree
   h) 263.8—Other protein-calorie malnutrition
   i) 263.9—Unspecified protein-calorie malnutrition

REFERENCES

1. Jonkers CF, Prins F, Van Kempen A, Tepaske R, Sauerwein HP. Towards implementation of optimum and better clinical nutrition support. *Clinical Nutrition.* 2001;20(4):361–366.
2. Arena J, Walters P. Do you know what a dietetic technician can do? A focus on clinical technicians. *J Am Diet Assoc.* 1997;97(suppl 2):S139–S141.
3. Colaizzo-Ana T. The evolution of nutrition support services. In: Matarese LE, Gottschlich mM, eds. *Contemporary Nutrition Support Practice.* 2nd ed. Philadelphia, Pa: Saunders; 2003:1–13.
4. A.S.P.E.N. Board of Directors. Standards of practice for nutrition support dietitian. *Nutr Clin Prac.* 2000;15:53–59.
5. A.S.P.E.N. Board of Directors. Standards of practice for nutrition support physician. *Nutr Clin Prac.* 2003;18:270–275.
6. A.S.P.E.N. Board of Directors and Task Force. Standards for specialized nutrition support: adult hospitalized patients. *Nutr Clin Prac.* 2002;17:384–391.
7. A.S.P.E.N. Board of Directors. Standards of practice for nutrition support pharmacist. *Nutr Clin Prac.* 1999;14:275–281.
8. Joint Commission on Accreditation of Healthcare Organizations. *Hospital Accreditation Standards.* Oakbrook Terrace; IL: Joint Commission on Accreditation of Healthcare Organizations; 2004:333–384.
9. Barclays Official California Code of Regulations. *Title 22. Social Security Division 5. Licensing and Certification of Health Facilities. Home Health Agencies Clinics and Referral Agencies.* San Francisco, CA: Barclays Law Publishers; 1999:759–773.
10. A.S.P.E.N. Board of Directors. Standards of practice for hospitalized pediatric patients. *Nutr Clin Prac* 1996;11:217–228.
11. Centers for Disease Control. Guidelines for the prevention of intravascular catheter-related infections. *MMWR.* 2002;51(RR10):1–26.
12. Schwartz DB. Enhanced enteral and parenteral nutrition practice and outcomes in an intensive care unit with a hospital-wide performance improvement process. *J Am Diet Assoc.* 1996;96:484–489.
13. Winkler MF, Hedberg A. Quality and performance improvement. In: Matarese LE, Gottschlich MM, eds. *Contemporary Nutrition Support Practice.* 2nd ed. Philadelphia, PA: Saunders; 2003:616–624.
14. Marian M, Stieber M. Quality performance improvement, indicators, and standards. In: Gottschlich MM, ed. *The Science and Practice of Nutrition Support A Case-Based Core Curriculum.* Dubuque, IA: Kendall/Hunt Publishing Company; 2002:757–776.
15. August DA, Thorn D, Gannon J. Outcomes research. In: Gottschlich MM, ed. *The Science and Practice of Nutrition Support: A Case-Based Core Curriculum.* Dubuque, IA: Kendall/Hunt Publishing Company; 2002:777–792.
16. Senkal M, Dormann A, Stehle P, Shang E, Suchner U. Survey on structure and performance of nutrition-support teams in Germany. *Clinical Nutrition.* 2002;21(4):329–335.
17. DeJonghe B, Appere-De-Vechi C, Fournier M, et al. A prospective survey of nutritional support practices in intensive care units: what is prescribed? What is delivered: *Crit Care Med.* 2001;29:8–12.
18. Bowman LC, Williams R, Sanders M, Ringwald-Smith K, Baker D, Gajjar A. Algorithm for nutritional support experience of the metabolic and infusion support service of St. Jude Children's Research Hospital. *Int J Cancer Supplement.* 1998;11:76–80.
19. Maurer J, Weinbaum F, Turner J, et al. Reducing the inappropriate use of parenteral nutrition in acute care teaching hospital. *J Parent Ent Nutr.* 1996;20: 272–274.
20. Howard P. Organizational aspect of starting and running an effective nutrition support service. *Clinical Nutrition.* 2001;20(4):367–374.
21. Mueller C, Shronts EP. Position of The American Dietetic Association: the role of registered dietitians in enteral and parenteral nutrition support. *J Am Diet Assoc.* 1997;97(3):302–304.
22. Howard P, Jonkers-Schuitema CF, Kyle U. The role of the nutritional support dietitian in Europe. *Clinical Nutrition.* 1999;18(6):379–383.
23. Schwartz DB. History and evolution of a successful certification program in nutrition support: the CNSD experience. *J Am Diet Assoc.* 2003;103(6): 736–741.
24. Maillet JO, Potter RL, Heller L. Position of the American Dietetic Association: ethical and legal issues in nutrition, hydration, and feeding. *J Am Diet Assoc.* 2002,102(5).716–726.
25. Guenter P, Curtas S, Murphy L, Orr M. The impact of nursing practice on the history and effectiveness of total parenteral nutrition. *J Parent Ent Nutr.* 2004;28(1):54–59.
26. A.S.P.E.N. Board of Directors. Standards of practice for nutrition support nurse. *Nutr Clin Prac.* 2001;16:56–62.
27. Vanek WV. The ins and outs of venous access: part II. *Nutr Clin Prac.* 2002; 17:142–155.
28. O'Neal BC, Schneider PJ, Pedersen CA, Mirtallo JM. Compliance with safe practices for preparing parenteral nutrition formulations. *Am J Health-Syst Pharm.* 2002;59:264–269.
29. National Advisory Group on Standards and Practice Guidelines for Parenteral Nutrition. Safe practices for parenteral nutrition formulations. *J Parent Enter Nutr.* 1998;22(2):49–66.
30. Schneider PJ, Bothe A, Bisognago M. Improving the nutrition process: assuring that more patients receive optimal nutrition support. *Nutr Clin Prac.* 1999;14:221–226.
31. Ebiasah RP, Schneider PJ, Pedersen CA, Mirtallo JM. Evaluation of board certification in nutrition support pharmacy. *J Parent Enter Nutr.* 2002; 26(4):230–247.
32. Silver HJ, Wellman NS. Nutrition diagnosing and order writing: value for practitioners, quality for clients. *J Am Diet Assoc.* 2003;103(11):1470–1472.
33. Mueller CM, Colaizzo-Anas T, Shronts EP, Gaines JA. Order writing for parenteral nutrition by registered dietitians. *J Am Diet Assoc.* 1996;96:764–768.
34. Driscoll DF. Compounding TPN admixtures: then and now. *J Parent Ent Nutr.* 2003;27(6):433–438.
35. Payne-James J. Cost-effectiveness of nutrition support teams. Are they necessary? *Nutrition.* 1997;13(10): 928–930.
36. Centers for Medicare & Medicaid Services. Chapter 3: Inpatient Hospital Billing. In: *Medicare Claims Processing Manual.* Rev. 221. Baltimore, MD: Centers for Medicare & Medicaid Services; 2003.
37. *International Classification of Disease-9-CM.* Department of Health and Human Services, Centers for Disease Control and Prevention, Epidemiology Program Office, Division of Public Health Surveillance and Informatics. June 5, 2003.

Mary Ellen Posthauer, RD, CD, LD;
Gretchen Robinson, MS, RD, LD, FADA

34

Long-Term Care Facilities

Introduction

Nutrition support practice in long-term care (LTC) facilities resembles nutrition support practice among other adult populations. This chapter focuses on special considerations for the mostly elderly residents in these facilities. Notable among these differences are the mandated assessment and care plan systems set forth by the Centers for Medicare and Medicaid Services (CMS). These systems not only direct care and monitor facility practice but also direct reimbursement for care, including nutrition support.

I. Background.

The provision of nutrition is a key component of the care provided to residents in LTC facilities. The decision to provide enteral or parenteral nutrition to residents requires careful consideration of the therapies' potential benefits and risks. Practitioners should understand mandated care guidelines for LTC facilities as well as professional good practice standards to achieve optimal outcomes for residents.

A. Demographics of aging and malnutrition in aging. Health care trends indicate that the number of US individuals 85 years and older will increase to 18 million by 2050.[1] During the same period, the number of people over 85 with moderate or severe dementia will increase from 1.4 million to 6.3 million.[2] The incidence of LTC placement increases with age: 31% of those who are severely impaired and between the ages of 65 and 70 reside in LTC facilities, compared to 61% of those age 85 and older. There were 1,465,000 people in LTC facilities in 1997 nationally, approximately 4% of the older population.[3] In 1997, 46% of the LTC population was aged 85 or older, compared to 33% aged 75 to 84, 13% aged 65 to 74, and 8.5% under age 65.[4]

B. Definition of LTC. The US Senate Special Committee on Aging described LTC as follows: LTC "differs from other types of health care in that the goal of long-term care is not to cure an illness, but to allow an individual to attain and maintain an optimal level of functioning. Long-term care encompasses a wide array of medical, social, personal and supportive and specialized housing services needed by individuals who have lost some capacity for self-care because of a chronic illness or disabling condition."[5]

C. Role of nutrition support in LTC. Available data indicate that advancing age brings physiological changes: reduction in lean body mass, decline in bone density, increase in total body fat, and decrease in total body water. These changes affect an individual's nutrition requirements independent of disease or rehabilitation.[6] Nutritional interventions include liberalizing therapeutic diets, using nutritional supplements, using specialized feeding utensils and instruments to facilitate oral intake, and providing nutrition support. The use of enteral nutrition in elderly residents has increased significantly since 1990, with an estimated 10% of today's LTC facility residents receiving enteral nutrition through percutaneous endoscopic gastrostomy devices.[7] Approximately one third of residents in LTC facilities who have advanced dementia have their nutritional requirements met by enteral nutrition.[8] Most receive enteral nutrition because of dementia related to chronic neurologic impairment or, to a lesser extent, cancer.[9–11]

D. Residents' rights: to feed or not to feed? Residents' rights are paramount in the decision to feed or not to feed. All professionals should be able to assist residents and their families in the decision about whether to use nutrition support at the end of life or in conditions of terminal disease, including end-stage dementia. Advance directives are the primary tools for documenting a resident's preferences regarding nutrition support. A resident can change these directives if the resident is still competent at the time a decision is being made about tube feeding.[12] In the absence of advance directives, professionals should be prepared to provide expert guidance to families and accommodate the resident's known beliefs, including ethnic and cultural values, and best interests.[6,13]
   1. Advance directives. Advance directives enable residents to document in advance preferences regarding treatment and care, including end-of-life wishes. Two common forms of advance directives are a living will and a durable power of attorney for health care.
      a) A living will states a person's choices regarding future medical care decisions, including the use of artificial life support and nutrition support.
      b) A durable power of attorney for health care enables a resident to appoint another individual to make all decisions regarding health care, including choice of provider, medical treatment, and end-of-life care.

E. Professional staff. The great majority of LTC facilities do not have formal nutrition support teams or services. An interdisciplinary team of health professionals provides nutrition support. Residents and their families are involved as much as possible in care and treatment decisions.[14,15]
   1. Physicians
      a) Maintain overall responsibility for residents' care.
      b) Diagnose disease conditions and alterations in metabolism; confirm malnutrition.
      c) Evaluate the residents' nutrition needs in relation to the clinical profile.
      d) Prescribe all diets and nutrition support interventions.

e) Prescribe, review, and modify medication regimes to adjust for possible side effects contributing to eating problems.
f) Consult with family/caregivers to determine residents' wishes regarding nutrition support.

2. Physician's assistants
   a) Evaluate the clinical status, including the nutritional status, of residents in the absence of or in collaboration with the physician.
   b) Collaborate with the other team members (ie, nurse, speech pathologists, dietitian).
   c) Prescribe diets and nutrition support regimens as needed.
3. Nurses
   a) Provide direct resident care
   b) Administer nutrition support and manage the care of nutrition support access devices.
   c) Serve as primary liaison with nursing staff, certified nursing assistants, and other team members.
   d) Inform physician and family/caregivers of any condition changes (ie, weight loss, falls, pressure ulcers, medication change, mental status).
4. Occupational and/or physical therapists
   a) Assess residents' potential for eating rehabilitation.
   b) Introduce compensatory techniques to minimize the effects of sensory-perceptual problems that affect eating performance.
   c) Use specialized seating and orthoses to facilitate the postural control and coordination necessary for eating.
   d) Provide adaptive tableware and utensils to assist with self-feeding.
   e) Devise adaptations and environmental controls to facilitate independent self-feeding.
   f) Recommend eating and feeding techniques to promote the residents' abilities to self-feed.
   g) Provide or recommend active and passive range-of-motion exercises and coordination and strength-building exercises to facilitate functional self-feeding.
   h) Evaluate the impact of cognitive impairments on eating and self-feeding ability and address cognitive issues to ensure that safe feeding practices are followed.
   i) Recommend seating devices (eg, wheelchair arm supports and wedge cushions) to ensure the safety of clients during eating and transfer from wheelchair to dining chair.
5. Speech pathologists
   a) Perform dysphagia/swallowing evaluations.
   b) Provide retraining in swallowing; design and supervise exercises to strengthen facial muscles, increase range of motion of the lips and control of the tongue, and facilitate safe oral and pharyngeal phase swallowing.
   c) Evaluate the resident's ability to eat and drink by mouth and ensure proper positioning and techniques necessary for safe swallowing.
   d) Assess ability to resume safe swallowing when transitioning from nutrition support and recommend nutrient delivery options when dysphagia is present.
6. Social workers
   a) Function as the residents' advocate in all aspects of care.
   b) Assist residents and families in articulating wishes regarding nutritional interventions.
   c) Educate families about residents' conditions and prognoses.
   d) Initiate advance directives at admission and review them with families and caregivers as conditions change.
   e) Provide psychological support and address social and financial concerns.
7. Pharmacists
   a) Review medications for adverse effects on nutritional status.
   b) Compound parenteral nutrition and monitor solution stability and safety.
   c) Participate in surveillance and management of therapy, including associated complications and delivery of cost-effective care.
8. Dietitians
   a) Are the primary advocates for all aspects of residents' nutritional care.
   b) Provide initial and periodic assessment of nutrient intake and nutrition status.
   c) Are the professionals primarily responsible for the design, implementation, and monitoring of nutritional interventions.
   d) Anticipate the effect of procedures, treatments, therapies, and psychosocial issues on the residents' nutrition status.
   e) Advise colleagues of altered nutritional status or potential nutrition deficiencies.
   f) Document nutrition assessment and nutrition care plans.
9. Others. A number of additional personnel (eg, certified nursing assistants, dietary technicians and assistants, and other food service personnel) also have a role in nutritional care, although the role can vary from one facility to another. Their duties range from delivering trays and supplements to assisting with meals and feeding.

II. Nutrition Care Process.

Wherever relevant, Standards for Nutrition Support for Adult Residents of Long-Term Care Facilities[16] should be used in tandem with the following section on the nutrition care process.

A. Nutrition assessment. In general, as the elderly age, their caloric intake declines[17] and they become increasingly frail. Frailty is distinguished by weakness, immobility, and weight loss caused or exacerbated by inadequate nutrition. Frailty occurs frequently in older residents with moderate to advanced dementia. It is not known whether it is a result of the aging process, malnutrition, or both.
   1. Residents usually have comorbid conditions such as dementia, Parkinson's disease, cerebrovascular accident, congestive heart failure and cardiovascular disease, chronic obstructive pulmonary disease, diabetes, and rheumatoid arthritis and osteoarthritis. In many cases, these conditions lead to increased levels of circulating cytokines, which can subtly alter normal metabolism and immunity. One effect of increased systemic cytokines is decreased serum albumin, which has long been used as an indicator of nutritional status. In fact, it is much more useful as an indicator of morbidity.[18,19]
   2. Elements of assessment
      a) Weight[16]
         (1) Determine whether resident is nutritionally at risk
            (a) Involuntary loss or gain of ≥10% of usual body weight within 6 months
            (b) Or involuntary loss or gain of ≥5% of usual body weight in 1 month
            (c) Or a weight 20% over or under ideal body weight
         (2) Determine possible causes of weight change
            (a) Review for clinical signs, symptoms, and causes of malnutrition.
            (b) Review for increased nutrient needs.
            (c) Review lab tests indicating undernutrition.
            (d) Review clinical conditions that may cause unintended weight loss.

(e) Review medications that cause anorexia, altered taste, and psychosocial needs.

b) Food/fluid intake/adequacy

(1) The estimated adequate fluid requirement per 24 hours is 1 mL fluid per kcal, 30 mL per kg, minimum 1500 mL per day regardless of weight. Requirements are adjusted as needed for cardiac, pulmonary, and renal restrictions.[20]

(2) The estimated adequate energy requirement per 24 hours is basal metabolic rate (as estimated by the Harris-Benedict equation[21]) × 1.3 (unspecified factor for activity and/or stress[22,23]).

(3) The estimated adequate protein requirement per 24 hours is 1 g per kg, and up to 1.5 g per kg for healing pressure ulcers or surgical wounds.[24]

(4) Elderly residents are more likely than younger adults to be deficient in vitamins D, B_{12}, folate, and riboflavin. See Chapter 2 for the dietary reference intakes.

(5) Obtain diet history, food allergies/intolerances, food preferences, and cultural concerns.

(6) Observe intake during meals.

(7) Determine possible causes of dehydration and identify appropriate interventions.

(8) Review advance directives, verifying with residents and family their wishes regarding nutrition support.

c) Drug-nutrient interactions

(1) Review medical record for current medications.

(2) Evaluate nutritional implications of current medications.

d) Serum laboratory concentrations. Laboratory assays can be prudently used to confirm suspected nutrition-related problems (organ dysfunction, nutrient deficiencies) identified by clinical diagnosis, observation, history, and physical examination. The use of hepatic proteins and total cholesterol to measure nutritional status is controversial. In general, they are more useful as prognostic indicators.[18,19]

e) Physical and mental function relevant to oral intake[25]

(1) Evaluate functional abilities during meals.

(a) Identify need for use of adaptive devices.

(b) Identify need for special positioning devices.

(c) Identify physical and/or verbal cues resident needs to initiate and continue with meal.

(2) Evaluate oral status.

(a) Perform complete oral cavity assessment.

(b) Review need for mechanically altered diet.

(3) Evaluate for signs and symptoms of dysphagia.

(4) Evaluate for communication barriers (vision, speech, hearing, cognition status).

f) Pressure ulcers. Poor nutritional status is a risk factor for development of pressure ulcers, but attempts to prevent the occurrence of pressure ulcers by nutritional intervention have produced equivocal outcomes. This may be due to the difficulty in meeting daily requirements as well as the lack of definitive data on the nutritional requirements of wound healing. Attention should focus on adequate nutrition up to 35 kcal/kg/day and 1.5 g protein/kg/day. Adequate micronutrient provision with special attention to vitamin A, B vitamins, vitamin C, zinc, manganese, copper, and selenium may also be helpful.[26]

B. Oral diet interventions

1. Liberalized diet for older adults in LTC. The American Dietetic Association maintains that the quality of life and nutritional status of older residents in LTC facilities may be enhanced by a liberalized diet. This diet refers to the withholding of restrictive nutrition prescriptions such as those used for renal and cardiovascular abnormalities. The purpose of liberalizing restrictive diets is to promote intake and improve quality of life in anorexic residents who might otherwise be uninterested in therapeutic diets.[27]

2. Restorative dining.[25] Restorative dining refers to improving or maintaining a resident's ability to eat independently, rehabilitating residents who cannot eat independently to a level where they require minimal assistance, or enabling the caregiver to provide assistance to residents who cannot eat entirely independently.

3. Self-help devices/utensils.[25] Utensils modified to compensate for residents' inability to use standard utensils can facilitate adequate oral intake. Posture, food consistency, and table height should be addressed before adaptive equipment and utensils are considered. Two principal considerations in selecting modified utensils are (1) the device should address the problem that interferes with the resident's eating ability; and (2) the device should be acceptable to the resident. There are various utensils and devices to aid in eating:

a) Lightweight utensils

b) Plate guard/scoop dish/inner-lip plate

c) Nonslip matting

d) Rocker knife/roller knife

e) Utensil with built-up, angled, or bent handles

f) Wrist support/splint

g) Wide handles on thermal mugs

h) Suction-based tableware

i) Long, bendable straw and holder

j) Covered mug with lid

k) Nosey cut-out tumbler

l) Dysphagia cup

4. Oral supplements. Nutritional supplements can be initiated when oral intake is determined to be inadequate. Most supplements are commercially available liquid formulations. Evidence suggests that supplements can improve outcomes in elderly residents with hip fractures,[28] pressure ulcers,[29] or chest infections.[30] One recent study indicated that providing supplements 60 minutes before a meal increases total caloric intake.[31]

a) Standard liquid supplements (2 cal/mL), lactose-free

b) Concentrated liquid supplements (2 cal/mL), lactose-free

c) Juice-based formulas with minimal fat

d) High-calorie puddings, cookies, and energy bars

C. Nutrition support (enteral and parenteral nutrition)

1. Enteral nutrition. See Chapter 5 for enteral nutrition management in general adult populations.

a) Candidates. Enteral nutrition (tube feeding) is used in residents of LTC facilities for the same reasons it is used in adult populations: inadequate oral intake. Most residents requiring enteral nutrition have sustained neurologic injury such as stroke or head trauma, or have degenerative neurologic conditions such as Alzheimer's disease, end-stage dementia, or Parkinson's disease.[32–34] Residents' wishes regarding enteral nutrition should be factored into decisions about whether to use enteral nutrition, as should specific achievable goals for an individual resident.[35]

b) Access. Enteral nutrition access is based on the physiology of the gastrointestinal tract and the anticipated length of time enteral support will be needed. Enterostomy devices placed either surgically or percutaneously are the most common access routes in LTC facility residents and are recommended when enteral nutrition is anticipated to be required for greater than 30 days. Of these, percutaneous endoscopic gastrostomies predominate.[9] For short-term enteral nutrition (less than 4 weeks), nasoenteric tubes are used.[6]

c) Administration. Enteral feeding is administered continuously, intermittently, or by gravity.
   (1) Continuous administration is given at a slow, continuous rate via a pump over 16 to 24 hours per day. This is the preferred method when enteral nutrition is initiated; the resident has not been fed for 3 or more days; or the resident is unstable and at risk for aspiration.
   (2) Cyclic administration is continuous feeding for a specified period of time (ie, 8–16 hours) in amounts to meet estimated nutritional needs, usually via a pump. This method is used when progressing to oral feedings and for residents unable to tolerate intermittent or bolus feedings. Cyclic feedings promote resident mobility, allowing participation in rehabilitation and other activities.
   (3) Intermittent administration delivered via slow gravity drip, pump, or intermittent bags. Usually, 250 to 500 mL of formula is delivered over 60 to 75 minutes 5 to 8 times per day as needed to meet estimated nutritional needs. The schedule simulates the meal pattern and allows more freedom of activity between meals. This type of feeding is contraindicated in residents at high risk of aspiration.
   (4) Bolus administration of 200 to 400 mL over 20 to 30 minutes 3 to 5 times per day, usually administrated by a 60-mL syringe or gravity.

d) Formulas
   (1) Polymeric formulas are composed of isolated sources of protein, carbohydrate, and fat in high-molecular form. These formulas usually have a low osmolality (300–500 mOsm/kg) and are lactose-free; some are supplemented with fiber. They usually contain 1 kcal/mL, although some are concentrated up to 2 kcal/kg for residents requiring fluid restriction.
   (2) Monomeric or elemental formulas contain hydrolyzed macronutrients and are lactose-free. They are more expensive than polymeric formulas and should be used for residents with maldigestion or malabsorption.
   (3) Modular nutrients are individually packaged macronutrients (protein, carbohydrate, fat) that are usually used to supplement standard formulas in varying amounts to meet individual nutritional requirements.
   (4) Disease-specific formulas are modified in one or more nutrients for certain disease states. Most of these formulas are more expensive, so their potential benefit to residents should be evaluated before they are used.

e) Drug-nutrient interactions. See Chapter 9. Medications may be administered via enterostomy tube.[36,37]
   (1) Flush the feeding tube with water prior to medication administration, between medications, and after the last medication to reduce clogging of the tube.
   (2) Never add medications directly to enteral formulas or administer them through the same port of the feeding tube when the feeding is being infused.
   (3) Use liquid forms of medications whenever possible. Check the dosage, since many liquid forms are intended for pediatric use.
      (a) Dilute liquid medications with at least 30 mL of water.
      (b) Many liquid medications have high osmolalities (>1000 mOsm/kg). Administration of hyperosmolar products through the feeding tube may result in diarrhea, cramping, abdominal distention, and vomiting.
   (4) Consult the pharmacy for questions regarding drug/enteral formula administration compatibility.

f) Monitoring guidelines. Monitoring guidelines for stable residents of LTC facilities are variable, depending on individual resident morbidity. For less stable residents or those requiring parenteral nutrition (see Section II.C.2), monitoring may be more frequent.[38] The following are suggested monitoring parameters for enteral nutrition[37]:
   (1) Serum albumin, electrolytes, blood urea nitrogen (BUN)/creatinine, magnesium, phosphorus, calcium, complete blood cell count, glucose—every 6 months
   (2) Weight—monthly or as needed
   (3) Intake and output—daily
   (4) Bowel function—daily
   (5) Patency of tube—daily
   (6) Residual check—prior to each feeding

g) Common complications
   (1) Diarrhea
   (2) Constipation
   (3) Nausea and vomiting
   (4) Abdominal distension, bloating, cramping, and gas
   (5) Aspiration
   (6) Clogged tube

h) Transition from enteral nutrition to oral intake[39]
   (1) The speech pathologist evaluates the resident's readiness for an oral diet.
   (2) The dietitian and the speech pathologist consider modifications in the oral diet to maximize intake.
   (3) Daily food/fluid intake is monitored.
   (4) Adding a nighttime enteral nutrition cycle is considered.
   (5) Resident weight is monitored frequently.
   (6) Enteral nutrition is stopped when oral intake is adequate.

2. Parenteral nutrition. See Chapters 7 and 8 for parenteral nutrition ordering and management. Anecdotally, parenteral nutrition is rarely used in LTC settings, possibly because of risk (of sepsis and other complications), inability to prepare solutions at the facility, lack expertise in management, and cost. Perhaps the decision to initiate parenteral nutrition in elderly residents is less likely to favor starting the therapy because clinicians, residents, and surrogates perceive (correctly) that the risks of parenteral nutrition can outweigh the potential benefits to residents at the end of their lives. The use of peripheral parenteral nutrition as opposed to central parenteral nutrition is discouraged in LTC because short-term nutrition support is unlikely to benefit residents[6] and the fragility of skin in the elderly complicates venous access.[24]

   a) Parenteral nutrition should be considered for LTC facility residents who have gastrointestinal dysfunction (similar to general adult populations) such as occurs with diffuse peritonitis, intestinal obstruction, intractable vomiting, paralytic ileus, intractable diarrhea, gastrointestinal ischemia, and short-gut syndrome.[6]
   b) Access for LTC facility residents is provided by permanent devices such as an implanted port or a subcutaneously tunneled (Hickman) catheter.[40] Peripherally inserted central catheters (PICCs) are also used for venous access greater than 1 month, although not usually more than several months. Appropriately trained nurses can place PICCs, although fragile peripheral vessels in the elderly may complicate the use of these devices.
   c) Parenteral nutrition monitoring is generally more frequent than enteral nutrition monitoring. The following are suggested general parameters[16]:
      (1) Physical assessment

(2) Clinical status
(3) Actual nutrient intake
(4) Fluid balance
(5) Weight
(6) Assessment of major organ function
(7) Visual inspection of access devices and site
(8) Temperature and signs and symptoms of infection
(9) Serum chemistries, including complete blood cell count

d) Transitional Feeding-Total parenteral nutrition is discontinued when adequate oral intake or enteral nutrition has been established. See Section II.C.1.h for a discussion of the transition to oral intake.

III. Mandated Care and Regulation

A. Resident Assessment Instrument (RAI). RAI is an interdisciplinary care system mandated by the CMS that sets forth a program designed to assess all aspects of clinical status and to facilitate problem identification, clinical interventions, and care plans for LTC facility residents. The components of RAI are the Minimum Data Set (MDS), Resident Assessment Protocols (RAPs), and triggers.[41]
1. The MDS is a form containing a range of clinical and functional status attributes that provide the foundation for the comprehensive assessment of residents of LTC facilities. The oral/nutritional status sections contain categories for oral problems; height and weight; weight change; nutritional problems; nutritional attributes, including oral, parenteral, and enteral interventions; and parenteral or enteral intake.
2. RAPs are problem-oriented frameworks for organizing MDS data; they form the basis for individualized care planning. There are 18 RAPs focused on social, medical, and psychological problems. Specific nutrition RAPs include nutritional status, feeding tubes, and dehydration and fluid maintenance.
3. Triggers are links between the MDS and RAPs. They identify RAPs that can be applied from MDS data. Examples of nutrition triggers are weight loss; taste alterations; parenteral/intravenous feedings; tube feedings; mechanically altered diets; incomplete meal consumption (leaving 25% of food uneaten); pressure ulcers; syringe feeding; and therapeutic diet.
4. Utilization guidelines explain how to use the RAI care system. These guidelines are available on the Internet in the RAI User's Manual.[41]

B. RAI timelines[41]
1. Initially, upon admission to facility
2. Quarterly, with each care plan review
3. With each significant change in condition
4. Upon readmission
5. Annually

C. Care plan[41]
1. Care plans are to be completed within 7 days of completing the RAI.
2. Care plans must include measurable objectives and time frames and describe services that are to be furnished.
3. Care plans are revised on an ongoing basis and reflect changes in residents' clinical status and care.

D. CMS Quality Indicator. The MDS is also used to evaluate the quality of care a facility provides. There are 24 quality indicators among the numerous clinical assessment entities in the MDS. These indicators compose the Facility Quality Indicator Profile. This profile helps identify possible areas for quality improvement within a facility.[41]

E. Data Assessment Verification Project (DAVE). DAVE is a program funded by CMS to monitor and improve the care provided to residents of LTC facilities. The MDS provides the data for the program to monitor the quality of care, to report to the public on the quality of care, and to determine Medicare payments. DAVE also evaluates the MDS in order to improve the accuracy of the data that the MDS generates.[42]

F. Joint Commission on Accreditation of Healthcare Organizations (JCAHO).[38] The 2004 JCAHO accreditation processes emphasize continuous standards compliance, with a focus on encouraging health care organizations to continuously use the standards to achieve and maintain excellent operations systems.
1. Tracer methodology. The tracer system is an evaluation process conducted by the JCAHO during on-site surveys that traces the care residents receive in a facility. The surveyor randomly selects active files and traces residents throughout the organization. The surveyor may pull closed charts if a standards compliance issue is identified to determine whether the problem is part of a pattern or an isolated case. Surveyors also interview staff members involved in the care of residents.
2. JCAHO LTC standards relevant to enteral and parenteral nutrition
   a) Residents are involved in decisions about care, treatment, and services provided.
   b) Residents have the right to refuse care, treatment, and services in accordance with laws and regulations.
   c) The organization addresses the wishes of residents relating to end-of-life decisions.
   d) Residents—and, when appropriate, their families—are informed about the outcomes of care, treatment, and services, including unanticipated outcomes.
   e) The organization defines in writing the time frame for conducting initial (nutritional) assessments.
   f) Initial (nutritional) assessments are performed as defined by the organization.
   g) Residents are reassessed as needed.
   h) Development of a plan of care, treatment, and services is individualized and appropriate to the resident's needs, strengths, limitations, and goals.
   i) The organization provides care, treatment, and services for each resident according to the plan for care, treatment, and services.
   j) Care, treatment, and services are provided in an interdisciplinary, collaborative manner.
   k) The organization coordinates the care, treatment, and services provided to a resident as part of the plan for care, treatment, and services and makes sure that they are consistent with the organization's overall scope of care, treatment, and services.
   l) Comfort and dignity are optimized during end-of life care.
   m) The effects of medication(s) on residents are monitored.
   n) The organization designs infection control programs to reduce the risks of acquired or transmitted infections.
   o) The organization collects data to monitor its performance.
   p) The organization provides staff and licensed independent practitioners in an adequate number and mix that are consistent with the organization's staffing plan.
   q) The organization has a complete and accurate clinical record for every individual assessed or treated.
   r) Clinical record documentation includes at least quarterly notations regarding the provision of and response to nutrition care services.

G. State regulations
1. License and certify LTC facilities.

2. Validate competencies for personnel involved in resident care.
3. Designate nutrition care integration in the patient care plan, documentation in the medical record, and transfer of information at discharge to ensure the continuity of nutrition care.

H. State licensure. All LTC facilities are governed by state licensure, usually under the health department. State surveyors conduct unannounced annual surveys. The state licensure boards are also responsible for investigating all complaints that are logged to their department about any issue in an LTC facility that involves the quality of care, the environment, or staffing issues. The majority of state licensure laws are derived from federal regulations.

I. Hazard Analysis Critical Control Points (HACCP).[36,43] HACCP is a program based on historical data about the causes of food spoilage and illness. It focuses on a systematic, thorough plan covering step-by-step operations, procedures, and control measures designed to reduce the risk of food-borne disease. When problems are detected, prompt action should be taken to correct them. HACCP points of concern relevant to enteral nutrition include improper handling, holding, and administration of enteral formulas.

IV. Reimbursement

A. Medicare. CMS is the federal agency responsible for the administration of Medicare and Medicaid. Medicare is the health care insurance program for people age 65 or older, some people under age 65 with disabilities, and people with end-stage renal disease. Medicare is administered in two parts: Part A (hospitalization) and Part B (medical insurance). Part B has provisions for parenteral and enteral nutrition, but nutrition support in LTC facilities is nominally covered as a per diem charge under the prospective payment system using the resource utilization groups (RUGs) system. RUGs determines the amount of required care and thus determines (prospectively) the payment required to cover the care of LTC facility residents.

1. The MDS determines a resident's RUG classification.
2. Tube-fed residents fall into one of two RUGs categories: special care and clinically complex. Parenteral nutrition falls into the extensive service category. Categories are determined by activity of daily living scores and the specific mix of clinical conditions.
3. LTC facilities are reimbursed at a higher rate if they are able to classify residents in the enteral nutrition categories. This fact may present a financial gain to facilities that is not entirely justified, because published evidence on the effectiveness of enteral nutrition in LTC populations is poor,[44,45] and residents with advanced dementia receiving enteral nutrition may use less nursing time than residents who are fed by hand.[46] At least in theory, the DAVE project monitors LTC facilities' match between reimbursement and actual resident acuity.

B. Medicaid. Medicaid comprises individual state insurance programs. Most states include nutrition support reimbursement as part of per diem rates for nursing home care, although beneficiaries must be enrolled in Medicare Part B to receive coverage for nutrition support.

1. The Medicaid per diem reimbursement rate varies among states.
   a) As with the Medicare system, residents are placed in the special care category, which provides higher reimbursement for enteral nutrition.
   b) Not all states use the RUGs classification system; some use reimbursement schemes that lead to higher payment for enteral nutrition (ie, Massachusetts uses "predetermined management," assigning tube-fed residents 135 minutes and hand-fed residents 45 minutes[47]).
   c) Residents enrolled in Medicare Part B can collect allowable charges for parenteral and enteral nutrition.

C. Medicare Part B reimbursement guidelines for nutrition support

1. Enteral
   a) Requirements
      (1) Permanence of condition (3 months is considered permanent)
      (2) Qualifying diagnosis and functional impairment precluding oral intake
      (3) Acceptable calorie, protein, and fluid requirements
         (a) Residents who are stable, healthy, and sedentary should receive 25 kcal/kg/day. Active residents with comorbidities under active treatment should receive 30 to 35 kcal/kg/day.
         (b) Suggested protein requirements are 1.0 to 1.5 g/kg/day.
         (c) Suggested fluid requirements are 30 to 35 cc/kg/day.
   b) Product justification
      (1) Category 1 (semisynthetic intact protein or protein isolates) or Category 2 (calorie-dense formulas) provides complete nutrition and is considered appropriate for most residents without metabolic stress or significant compromises in gastrointestinal, pulmonary, renal, liver, or immune function. Standard products provide 1.0 to 2.0 kcal/mL.
      (2) Specialty products and formulas (Categories 3–6) must be justified with documentation supporting medical necessity and evidence that a general-purpose product was used unsuccessfully in the past or the trial of a general-purpose product would put the resident's well-being or survival at risk.
      (3) Blenderized foods given via an enteral tube are not covered by Medicare.
   c) Equipment and supplies
      (1) Gravity or bolus feedings must be tried and cause a documented complication before a pump is considered medically necessary.
      (2) Medicare will not pay for a pump to prevent complications.
      (3) One feeding supply kit corresponding with the method of administration may be issued daily.
      (4) Medicare allows for one gastrostomy or jejunostomy tube or three nasogastric tubes every 90 days.
2. Parenteral nutrition
   a) Permanence of the condition (3 months is considered permanent) is a requirement.
   b) Parenteral nutrition is covered for a resident with the ability to obtain partial nutrition from oral intake or a combination of oral/enteral/parenteral intake as long as the following conditions are met:
      (1) The resident's gastrointestinal tract is permanently unresponsive to standard medical management (ie, continuous enteral nutrition via pump is not tolerated).
      (2) The resident is unable to maintain weight and strength (10% weight loss over 3 months and serum albumin <3.4 g/dL).
   c) Other requirements
      (1) A range of 20 to 35 kcal/kg/day; a physician must document caloric requirements outside this range.
      (2) The physician must document a medical necessity for protein requirement outside the range of 0.8 to 1.5 g/kg/day; dextrose concentration less than 10%; or fat emulsion use greater than 15 units of a 20% solution or 30 units of a 10% solution per month.

(3) There must be documentation of medical necessity for special parenteral solutions, for instance, essential amino acid solutions.

d) Equipment and supplies

(1) Infusion pumps are covered for parenteral nutrition.

(2) One supply kit and one administration kit is covered each day parenteral nutrition is administered.

REFERENCES

1. US Census Bureau. *Statistical Abstract of the United States; 1999.* Washington, DC: US Census Bureau; 1999.
2. US Department of Health and Human Services. *The Characteristics of Long-Term Care Users.* Rockville, MD: Agency for Healthcare Research and Quality; 2000.
3. Gabrel CS. *Characteristics of Elderly Nursing Home Current Residents and Discharges: Data from the 1997 National Nursing Home Survey.* Advance Data from Vital and Health Statistics, No 312. Hyattsville, MD: National Center for Health Statistics; 2000.
4. National Center for Health Statistics. *Health, United States, 2000.* Hyattsville, MD; 2000.
5. Special Committee on Aging, United States Senate. *Developments in Aging; 1997 and 1998.* Vol 1. Report 106-229. Washington, DC: 2000.
6. A.S.P.E.N. Board of Directors. Guidelines for the use of parenteral and enteral nutrition in adults and pediatric patients. *J Parenter Enteral Nutr.* 2002;26(suppl):15SA–59SA.
7. Mitchell SL, Kiely DK, Lipsitz LA. The risk factors and impact on survival of feeding tube placement in nursing home residents with severe cognitive impairment. *Arch Intern Med.* 1997;157(3):327–332.
8. Mitchell SL, Teno JM, Roy J, et al. Clinical and organizational factors associated with feeding tube use among nursing home residents with advanced cognitive impairment. *JAMA.* 2003;290(1):73–80.
9. Grant MD, Rudberg MA, Brody JA. Gastrostomy placement and mortality among hospitalized Medicare beneficiaries. *JAMA.* 1998;279(24):1973–1976.
10. Light VL, Siezak FA, Porter JA, Gerson LW, McCord G. Predictive factors for early mortality after percutaneous endoscopic gastrostomy. *Gastrointest Endosc.* 1995;42(4):330–335.
11. Taylor CA, Larson DE, Ballard DJ, et al. Predictors of outcome after percutaneous endoscopic gastrostomy: a community-based study. *Mayo Clin Proc.* 1992;67(11):1042–1049.
12. Morrison RS, Olson E, Mertz K, Meier DE. The inaccessibility of advance directive on transfer from ambulatory to acute care settings. *JAMA.* 1995; 274:478–482.
13. Position of the American Dietetic Association. Ethical and legal issues in nutrition, hydration, and feeding. *J Am Diet Assoc.* 2002;102:716–726.
14. Consultant Dietitians in Health Care Facilities. *Nutrition Management and Restorative Dining for Older Adults.* Chicago, IL: American Dietetic Association; 2001:19–20.
15. A.S.P.E.N. Board of Directors. Standards of practice for nutrition support pharmacists. *Nutr Clin Pract.* 1999;14:275–281.
16. A.S.P.E.N. Board of Directors. Standards for nutrition support for adult residents of long-term care facilities. *Nutr Clin Pract.* 1997;12:284–293.
17. Anonymous. Daily dietary fat and total food energy intakes: Third National Health and Nutrition Examination Survey, phase III: 1988–1991. *MMWR.* 1994;43:116–125.
18. Reuban DB, Cheh Al, Harris TB, et al. Peripheral blood markers of inflammation predict mortality and functional decline in high-functioning community-dwelling older persons. *J Am Geriatr Soc.* 2002;50:638–644.
19. Erchler WB, Keller ET. Age-associated increased interleukin-6 gene expression, late-life diseases and frailty. *Ann Rev Med.* 2000;51:245–270.
20. Chernoff R. Thirst and fluid requirements. *Nutr Rev.* 1994;52:S3–S5.
21. Harris JA, Benedict FG. *A Biometric Study of Basal Metabolism in Man.* Publication No 279. Washington, DC: Carnegie Institute of Washington; 1919.
22. Taffe DR, Thompson J, Butterfield G, Marcus R. Accuracy of equations to predict basal metabolic rate in older women. *J Am Diet Assoc.* 1995;95: 1389–1392.
23. Henderson CT, Trumbore LS, Mobarhan S, Benya R, Miles TP. Prolonged tube feeding in long-term care: nutritional status and clinical outcomes. *J Am Coll Nutr.* 1992;11:309–325.
24. Johnston RE, Chernoff R. Geriatrics. In: Matarese LE, Gottschlich MM, eds. *Contemporary Nutrition Support Practice.* 2nd ed. Philadelphia, PA: Saunders; 2003:376–383.
25. Robinson G, Leif BJ. *Nutrition Management and Restorative Dining for Older Adults.* Chicago, IL: Consultant Dietitians in Health Care Facilities/American Dietetic Association; 2001:117–119.
26. Mathus-Vliegen EM. Old age, malnutrition, and pressure sores: an ill-fated alliance. *J Gerontol A Biol Sci Med Sci.* 2004;59:355–360.
27. American Dietetic Association. Position statement: liberalized diets for older adults in long term care. *J Am Diet Assoc.* 2002;102:1316–1323.
28. Delmi M, Rapin CH, Bengoa JM, et al. Dietary supplementation in elderly patients with fractured neck of the femur. *Lancet.* 1990:335:1013–1016.
29. Breslow RA, Hallfrisch J, Guy DG, et al. The importance of dietary protein in healing pressure ulcers. *J Am Geriatr Soc.* 1993;41:357–362.
30. Woo J, Ho SC, Mak YT, et al. Nutritional status of elderly patients during recovery from chest infection and the role of nutritional supplementation assessed by a prospective randomized single blind trial. *Age Ageing.* 1994;23:40–48.
31. Wilson MM, Purushothaman R, Morley JE. Effect of liquid dietary supplements on energy intake in the elderly. *Am J Clin Nutr.* 2002;75(5):944–947.
32. Morley JE, Silver AJ. Nutritional issues in nursing home care. *Ann Intern Med.* 1995;123:850–858.
33. Posthauer ME, Russell C. Ensuring optimal nutrition in long-term care. *Nutr Clin Pract.* 1997;12:247–255.
34. Peck AP, Cohen CE, Mulvihill MN. Long-term feeding of aged demented nursing home patients. *J Am Geriatr Soc.* 1990;38:1195–1198.
35. Mueller C, Gilbride J, Nestle M. Enteral nutrition support in elderly residents of long-term care facilities. Controversies and practical solutions. *Top Clin Nutr.* 2003;18:13–20.
36. *Enteral Therapy Policy and Procedure Manual for Assisted Living, Home Care, Nursing Facilities.* Alexandria, VA: American Society of Consultant Pharmacists; 1999.
37. Avoiding drug-nutrient interactions in enteral nutrition. *Nutrition and the M.D.* 2003;29:7–8.
38. *Comprehensive Accreditation Manual for Long Term Care.* Oakbrook Terrace, IL: JCAHO; 2004.
39. Dorner B. *Diet Manual, A Comprehensive Resource and Guide.* Akron, OH: Becky Dorner and Associates; 2002:210–217.
40. Ireton-Jones C. Enteral and parenteral nutrition. In: Robinson G, Leif BJ. *Nutrition Management and Restorative Dining for Older Adults.* Chicago, IL: Consultant Dietitians in Health Care Facilities/American Dietetic Association; 2001:363–388.
41. *MDS 2.0 RAI User's Manual.* Marblehead, MA: HCPro; 2003.
42. Data Assessment and Verification Project. June 20, 2003. Available at: http://www.cms.hss.gov/providers/psc/DAVE/background.asp. Accessed August 26, 2004.
43. Dentinger B, Faucher KJ, Ostrom SM, Schmidl MK. Controlling bacterial contamination of an enteral formula through use of a unique closed system: contamination, enteral formulas, system. *Nutrition.* 1995;11:747–750.
44. Finucane TE, Christmas C, Travis K. Tube feeding in patients with advanced dementia. A review of the evidence. *JAMA.* 1999;282:1365–1370.
45. Gilluk MR. Rethinking the role of tube feeding in patients with advanced dementia. *N Engl J Med.* 2000;342:206–210.
46. Callahan CM, Buchanan NN, Slump TE. Health care costs associated with percutaneous endoscopic gastrostomy among older adults in a defined community. *J Am Geriatric Soc.* 2001;49:1525–1529.
47. Mitchell SL. Financial incentives for placing feeding tubes in nursing home residents with advanced dementia. *J Am Geriatr Soc.* 2003;51:129–131.

Debra S. Kovacevich, RN, MPH;
Marsha E. Orr, RN, MS

35

Considerations for Home Nutrition Support

Introduction

Home nutrition support (HNS) is the provision of nutrients and any necessary adjuvant agents to patients by administration into the intestine or stomach or by intravenous infusion for the purpose of improving or maintaining a patient's nutritional status in the home care environment.[1] There are few differences between the indications for home and acute care specialized nutrition; however, nutritional formulas and solutions, access devices, administration schedules, and the frequency and intensity of laboratory and clinical monitoring can differ substantially. Additionally, home care organizations and hospitals are accredited using distinct standards, so there are different standards of care for home care and hospital services. Ideally, the concept of the nutrition support team—interdisciplinary collaboration among nurses, pharmacists, physicians, and dietitians—endures in both settings. The goal of care is to provide individualized, compassionate, appropriate, cost-effective, safe, and effective HNS.

I. Identification of Candidates for HNS.

Patients should be thoroughly evaluated prior to the initiation of HNS therapy to ensure the best possible outcome.

A. Candidates include patients who are unable to maintain nutritional status by oral intake alone.
B. The patient's medical condition must be stable enough to allow for safe discharge to an alternative care site (ie, nursing home, intermediate care facility, infusion center, or home).
C. Patients and caregivers should understand and accept the risks and responsibilities for home nutrition therapy.
   1. Patients and caregivers should understand the following:
      a) The rationale for and the risks, benefits, and responsibilities of HNS
      b) Therapeutic expectations, including immediate and long-term goals, and the anticipated length of therapy
      c) The cost of therapy, insurance coverage, and the patients' and caregivers' financial responsibilities
   2. Patients and caregivers should be willing and able to perform HNS procedures and agree to the therapy.
D. Adequate professional support must be available to implement therapy, provide care, and monitor therapy.
   1. An interdisciplinary approach by qualified health care professionals is necessary to ensure that all aspects of care are addressed throughout the duration of therapy.
      a) An interdisciplinary nutrition care plan must be developed.
      b) Only authorized individuals can prescribe or order nutrition therapies.
      c) Responsibilities for nutrition support functions (preparation, storage, distribution, administration, monitoring) must be defined and assigned to appropriate individuals.
   2. There must be appropriate involvement of patients, family members, caregivers, clergy, and others in decisions about nutrition support, which may include initiating, continuing, withholding, or withdrawing nutrition support.
   3. The home environment must allow for safe storage, preparation, and administration of therapy.
      a) Storage areas must be available to protect the equipment and solutions from damage and contamination; they must be located out of the reach of children and pets.
      b) A clean environment is required for preparing solutions and equipment.
   4. A home infusion provider for nutrition and medical products, services, and other necessary supplies must be available.[2]
      a) The provider must prepare, deliver, and store nutrient solutions under proper conditions in a safe, accurate, and timely manner.
      b) Changes in nutrition support must be accommodated in a timely manner.
      c) Ongoing monitoring of the patient for is required safety, effectiveness, and appropriateness of nutrition support.

II. Formulation of a Discharge Plan.

Prior to the initiation of home therapy, an interdisciplinary team should develop and document a comprehensive plan for nutrition support. A thorough reassessment must be undertaken of the nutrition support plan, because patients' needs and requirements will change as they move from hospital to home. All the patients' home care needs have to be addressed by including relevant health care professionals prior to hospital discharge. Often, it is more difficult to initiate services once the patient is home; this may result in delays of needed services such as physical therapy and social work.

A. Definition of the individual's nutrition goals
   1. Short- and long-term goals need to be developed with the patient, the caregivers, and health care professionals involved in the care of the patient.
   2. The duration of therapy anticipated must be discussed with the patient and caregivers.

B. Development of a patient-specific nutrient prescription
1. Calculate macronutrient requirements to meet nutritional goals.
a) Determine the desired proportion of calories from carbohydrates, protein, and fat.
b) Address the need for specialized formulas.
c) Adjust the nutrient prescription for impairments in organ function (eg, reduced amount of protein for renal failure).
2. Determine the amounts of vitamins, trace elements, and minerals to be added to the nutrition formulation. Patients who received less than daily infusions of parenteral or enteral solutions or who are transitioning to an oral diet may need supplemental oral vitamins and minerals to meet recommended dietary reference intakes.
3. Calculate the patient's total daily fluid needs, including losses from the gastrointestinal (GI) tract.
4. Order appropriate levels of electrolytes to maintain normal serum concentrations. The prescription must be appropriate for organ dysfunction or large GI losses.
5. Evaluate serum glucose levels to determine the need for insulin or adjustment in the nutrients provided. Instruct patients and caregivers on how to monitor glucose levels and adjust insulin dosages to maintain acceptable levels.

C. Selection of the appropriate route of administration for parenteral and enteral nutrition
1. The parenteral route should be used only when the GI tract does not allow adequate absorption or transport of sufficient nutrients to maintain appropriate weight or growth and to support life.
2. The enteral route is indicated in patients with a functional GI tract who are malnourished or are at risk for malnutrition from not eating and in whom oral feedings are inadequate to maintain nutrition status. It is also indicated in patients who will not, should not, or cannot eat adequately to maintain their nutrient stores.[3]

D. Selection of the appropriate access device to allow for safe administration of specialized nutrition in the home setting. The patient should be involved in selecting the type of access device, including its location. If two access locations will provide equally acceptable access, the patient should be allowed to choose between them.
1. Enteral access should be placed in a location accessible to the patient and caregivers so that they can connect or disconnect tubing, change dressings, and observe for signs and symptoms of infection. The device should be properly secured to prevent inadvertent dislodgment. The site for the enteral route may be the stomach or the small intestine. Feeding into the stomach (eg, nasogastric, gastrostomy access) is the preferred route and is indicated when there is impairment in the ability to swallow or obstruction between the mouth and stomach and the patient is not at increased risk for aspiration. Feeding into the small intestine (eg, nasointestinal, jejunostomy access) is indicated when there is delayed gastric emptying, an obstructive upper-intestinal-tract tumor, other severe disease, or an increased risk of aspiration.
a) Long-term enteral access devices include gastrostomy tubes, percutaneous endoscopic gastrostomy tubes, jejunostomy tubes, low-profile gastrostomy and jejunostomy devices, and combined gastric decompression and jejunostomy feeding tubes.
b) Low-profile or skin-level enteral feeding devices are used more frequently in home care for the very old (eg, a confused geriatric patient) or the very young (eg, an active pediatric patient).
c) Nasointestinal or nasojejunal tubes are not frequently used in home care because they are irritating, leading to sinusitis, otitis, hoarseness, vocal cord paralysis, nasal septum necrosis, and nasopharyngeal ulcers. Additionally, they are uncomfortable and less stable, must be regularly replaced, and are prone to clogging.
d) To the extent possible, patients should be involved in the decision about the type of enteral access device selected.
(1) Nasally placed tubes add psychosocial stress but may be needed initially to demonstrate tube feeding tolerance. These types of feeding tubes should be replaced as soon as possible.
(2) Low-profile devices placed through a mature gastrostomy are less obtrusive than gastrostomy tubes and should be considered.
(3) Preplacement markings for gastric and jejunostomy tubes allow for self-care and may decrease complications.[4]
2. Parenteral access should be in a location that is visible and easy for the patient and caregivers to reach to connect or disconnect intravenous tubing, change dressings, and observe for signs and symptoms of infection.
a) Standard long-term central venous access devices include implanted and tunneled catheters.
b) Peripherally inserted central catheters (PICCs) are generally used for intermediate-term therapy.
c) The tip of central venous access catheters should be located in the superior vena cava adjacent to the right atrium.[5]
d) Peripheral catheters <8 inches in length should not be used in the home care setting for the administration of parenteral nutrition due to the increase risk of phlebitis and infiltration.
e) Peripheral catheters (midlines) are used for short-term therapy (<7 days) and when the final dextrose concentration of the solution/emulsion is less than 10% and/or the final osmolarity is less than 900 mOsm.[5]
f) To the extent possible, patients should be involved in the decision about the type of central venous access device selected.
(1) The type of catheter required should be based on the length of therapy, the frequency of infusions, and caregiver/patient ability.
(2) Central venous access devices are available with single, double, or triple lumens. Many patients may require multiple intravenous infusions for therapies such as antibiotics or chemotherapy. Catheters with the smallest number of lumens that can still meet all the intravenous therapy needs of the patient and medication dosing intervals should be used to minimize the risk of infection and decrease time and cost for catheter care.
(3) Advantages and disadvantages of each type of catheter should be thoroughly discussed with the patient.
(a) Implanted ports may be desirable for cosmetic reasons or for patients who are frequently on and off therapy. Adolescents may prefer an implanted port, as it is not visible to their peers once the needle is removed. The port is ideal for individuals who swim, as the needle may be removed prior to going into the pool. Many individuals do not prefer an implanted port due to the weekly or daily needle stick and risk of extravasation. Some patients apply a topical anesthetic 30 to 60 minutes prior to needle insertion to decrease the pain.
(b) PICCs may not be suitable for patients who need to change their own dressing due to a lack of visiting nurse services. An extension tube usually needs to be added so the patient can flush and connect parenteral nutrition

solutions. Whenever possible, the patient's nondominant arm should be used for catheter insertion.

E. Development of a schedule for the infusion of parenteral and/or enteral nutrition therapy that takes into account the patient's nutritional and fluid needs and lifestyle
   1. The infusion schedule must be appropriate for the therapy and manageable for the patient and caregivers.
   2. "Cycled" infusions are typically administered at night to allow for independence during the day.
   3. Cycling of infusions should be started prior to discharge to assess patient tolerance. It is preferable for the goal infusion rate to be achieved prior to discharge. Goal infusion rates are usually 10 to 12 hours per night based on the amount of dextrose in the solution, glucose levels, and fluid tolerance. To avoid hyperglycemic episodes and minimize the use of insulin, the dextrose infusion rate should be calculated at the peak rate of infusion and not exceed 14 mg/kg/min in pediatrics, 17 mg/kg/min in infants, and 12 mg/kg/min in adults.
   4. Infants, children, and adults with glucose intolerance may not be able to be cycled or off therapy for long periods. Cycle schedules should be decreased by 1 to 2 hours per day.
   5. It may not be necessary to taper parenteral nutrition solutions up and down based on the amount of dextrose in the solution. However, because ambulatory infusion devices can gradually increase and decrease the solution without the patient having to reprogram the pump on a nightly basis, it is prudent to use a tapering schedule. Usual taper-up and taper-down times are 1 or 2 hours. Tapering may be particularly important for pediatric patients.
   6. The acceptable range for glucose levels has not been determined in the home care population. However, research in other settings suggests that levels should be maintained at <110 mg/dL.[6] For diabetics, the goal should be attaining a glucose level between 100 and 200 mg/dL while minimizing the incidence of hypoglycemia.[7]
   7. In some carefully selected circumstances, determined by the physician, the patient and caregivers, and the home care organization, parenteral nutrition may be initiated in the home (started, advanced, and cycled without being administered in the hospital prior to discharge). This option should be considered only when an assessment confirms that the benefits greatly outweigh the risks.[1] General criteria for home initiation include but are not limited to the following:
      a) The patient is clinically stable. High-risk patients who may not be candidates include patients at risk for refeeding syndrome; infants; intravenous drug abusers; and patients with poorly controlled diabetes, fluid and electrolyte disorders, and major organ failure.[1] Patients with these conditions may require more frequent monitoring than can be accomplished in the home.
      b) The patient and caregivers have previous experience with parenteral nutrition or infusion therapy.
      c) The patient and caregivers learn readily and are willing and able to perform the additional monitoring to ensure the safety of home initiation.
      d) The patient and caregivers are able to recognize complications of therapy and how to troubleshoot or notify medical personnel.
      e) The patient is able to receive a home formula in which the dextrose concentration is gradually increased over several days (typically starting with 150–200 g/day and increasing by no more than 100 g/day to the final concentration).
      f) The patient's blood sugar is carefully monitored by capillary blood testing or serum glucose levels drawn no less than daily.
      g) It is possible to do frequent laboratory monitoring during advancement of the home formula's dextrose concentration and total volume, and the laboratory monitoring includes electrolytes, calcium, phosphorus, magnesium, and glucose.
      h) The patient's insurance provider covers visiting nurse services to assist with monitoring and education.
      i) The home care nurses and pharmacists carefully assess the patient for potential adverse reactions no less than daily during home initiation of parenteral nutrition.

F. Establishment of appropriate preparation and administration techniques for the patient and caregivers
   1. Home parenteral nutrition is prepared in the infusion pharmacy under a laminar flow hood using appropriate sterile compounding processes (US Pharmacopeia).[8] Home additives are limited to pharmaceuticals, such as multivitamins, that lose potency once exposed to light or are unstable for the standard length of storage of home parenteral nutrition solutions/emulsions.
      a) Home additives to parenteral solutions typically include multivitamins, H_2 blockers, and insulin. The compatibility of all additives must be verified by a pharmacist before the additive is administered at home.
      b) Commercially prepared home enteral solutions are preferable to powdered solutions that must be reconstituted in the home setting.
      c) Home additives to enteral solutions may include modular nutrients, water, or selected medications. Clean technique must be used to prepare enteral solutions in the home.
      d) Home parenteral solutions must be maintained at appropriate temperature during transport to the patient's home. Patients and caregivers must be taught the proper storage and temperature conditions for keeping parenteral nutrition in the home.
      e) Parenteral nutrition solutions should be labeled with instructions for use and beyond-use dating (see Chapter 7 for specific labeling recommendations).
      f) Enteral nutrition formulas must be stored and maintained in an area that does not exceed the manufacturer's recommended temperature ranges for storage (avoiding excessive heat or freezing).
      g) Once cans or containers of enteral nutrition formulas are opened in the home, the remaining formula should be used within 24 to 48 hours according to manufacturer's recommendations.
      h) Patients and caregivers should be taught to carefully examine containers/bags of parenteral and enteral nutrition for evidence of damage, leaks, discoloration, odor, separation, contamination, or beyond-use dating.
   2. Techniques for administering enteral and parenteral therapy must be appropriate and safe.
      a) An infusion pump must be used to administer parenteral nutrition solutions. Volumetric or peristaltic pumps with free flow protection are recommended for administration of parenteral nutrition.
      b) Enteral feeding into the small intestine is best tolerated when infused slowly via enteral pump. Pump-assisted feedings may be administered continuously or cycled over a shorter time according to patient tolerance. Gastric feedings may be delivered by pump, by gravity drip, or by using a syringe and administering each feeding over 30 to 60 minutes or according to patient tolerance.
   3. The home care organization must have a process for routine maintenance and for emergency repair and replacement of infusion equipment. It may be necessary to have a replacement infusion

pump available in the home if the patient is unable to tolerate being off the infusion until a delivery can be made.

4. A plan for the care, repair, or replacement of the enteral or parenteral access device should be developed as part of the home care plan or as part of the home care organization's policies and procedures to address the following:
    a) Procedures for emergency repairs and replacement of the access device
    b) Procedures for preventing and managing occlusion
    c) Procedures for site care and dressing changes to prevent infections

G. An interdisciplinary plan for monitoring home nutrition therapy should be established to ensure positive nutritional, psychological, and metabolic outcomes.[9] Through monitoring, the incidence of complications can be minimized and the nutritional status of the patient can be optimized.
1. Specific monitoring parameters and the frequency of monitoring depend on the therapy, the severity of illness, and the presence of diseases that require more frequent monitoring.
2. In addition to monitoring nutritional parameters, mechanical, infectious, metabolic, GI, hepatic, renal, bone, and growth indices in children should be followed at established intervals.
    a) Vitamin and mineral studies should be obtained for patients on long-term therapy.
    b) The use of long-term (home) parenteral nutrition has been associated with the development of metabolic bone disease (MBD). Usually asymptomatic, bone pain and fracture may occur with minimal trauma. Elevated urinary calcium and increases in serum concentrations of calcium, phosphorus, and alkaline phosphatase may be present. Osteoporosis and osteomalacia have both been linked to parenteral nutrition-associated MBD. The causes of MBD are poorly understood and include MBD predating parenteral nutrition (such as can occur with inflammatory bowel disease), excess dietary protein, aluminum contamination (of parenteral solutions), metabolic acidosis (associated with amino acid metabolism), and abnormalities in vitamin D metabolism (associated with parenteral nutrition).[10] Recently, a group of investigators noted that the current incidence of MBD in patients receiving long-term parenteral nutrition is not significantly larger than the incidence in sex-matched healthy subjects. Furthermore, MBD is probably related primarily to the underlying reason for which parenteral nutrition was indicated.[11]
    c) Laboratory monitoring for home enteral nutrition patients is poorly described and is not perceived to be as important as for home parenteral nutrition patients. However, laboratory tests of electrolytes, renal function, glucose, calcium, magnesium, phosphorus, and albumin should be done, especially during times of tube feeding intolerance.
3. The patient and caregivers should be included in the development of the plan for monitoring, including frequency of nursing visits, laboratory work, and office visits. Appropriate transportation must be available (or arranged).
4. The patient and caregivers must be able and willing to take an active role in monitoring the patient's response to nutrition therapy. Monitoring may include intake (oral, tube, parenteral); output, when indicated (urine, stool, and other body fluids); body weight; temperature; medication (type, amount, and timing); blood glucose (if needed); and changes in the appearance or function of the access site, unusual sensations during or after administration of the nutrition formula, pain (new, increased intensity, changed), bleeding, or inability to administer solutions. The patient and caregivers should be taught parameters to report adverse effects to the appropriate member of the health care team.

H. The goals and progress toward them should be regularly evaluated. As feasible, the patient is transitioned from one feeding modality to another to promote progression toward an enteral or oral diet, with the goal to discontinue nutrition support if possible.
1. Calorie counts should be obtained prior to tapering enteral or parenteral therapy to an oral diet or when transitioning to enteral from parenteral nutrition.
2. Nutrition infusions may be tapered in a variety of ways. Patients who are able to maintain their hydration status may wish to decrease the number of infusions per week to give themselves a "holiday." Another method may be to begin decreasing the total amount of calories provided per day by enteral or parenteral nutrition. Patients should be instructed to take an oral multivitamin with minerals during the transition phase.
3. Enteral or parenteral nutrition should not be discontinued until at least 75% of the patient's nutritional requirements have been obtained via the alternate source, tolerance has been demonstrated, and the patient is either gaining or maintaining weight according to goals.
4. Children on parenteral and/or enteral nutrition may display an oral aversion to food and may require behavioral interventions.

I. For patients who will receive lifetime therapy, goals and outcomes may focus on maintaining an adequate nutritional status. For children, goals and outcomes may focus on adequate growth and development.

III. Coordination of the Referral for HNS.

Safe and effective HNS requires a comprehensive, well-executed, interdisciplinary discharge plan that includes the patient's physician, the hospital health care team, the home care team, and the patient, and family/caregivers. The plan should be developed before discharge.

A. Selection of a home care provider may depend upon contractual agreements between the patient's insurance provider and home care agencies. However, hospital staff that has the responsibility for discharge planning must ensure that the home care provider is able to safely provide HNS services. Markers of high-quality agencies include the following:
1. Accreditation by a national accreditation body, such as the Joint Commission for Accreditation of Healthcare Organizations (JCAHO), the Accreditation Commission for Healthcare (ACHC), or the Community Health Accreditation Program (CHAP)
2. Staff who have expertise in specialized nutrition as evidenced by national certification or documented experience, competency, and continuing education about HNS
3. Specific protocols, pathways, or procedures for HNS
4. Adherence to standards of practice developed by national and state organizations
5. Twenty-four-hour availability of services

B. The hospital team and the home care provider must work collaboratively to ensure that the patient is adequately prepared for discharge. Discharge planning includes
1. Supplies and equipment determined, ordered, and delivered to the patient's home
2. Development and documentation of an administration schedule, nutrient prescription, type of infusion pump, additional medications, and materials for access site care
3. Development and documentation of goals of care, frequency of monitoring, methods of communication between the hospi-

tal team and all members of the home care team, and physician follow-up

4. Definition of nursing services prior to discharge, including the frequency of visits, monitoring guidelines, and required blood work

IV. Education and Training of Patients and Caregivers

The goals of education are to provide the patient and caregivers with knowledge and skills that facilitate appropriate involvement in self-care, decision making, and successful outcomes for nutrition support. Training should be well designed and individualized to meet learning needs.

A. Education is individualized and provided by an interdisciplinary staff in a coordinated and consistent fashion.
   1. Training should be individualized according to the patient's and caregivers' assessed needs, abilities, and readiness to learn.
   2. Training should be provided by qualified interdisciplinary staff who have appropriate education, specialized training, and experience in HNS.
   3. There must be written policies and procedures coordinating the education process so that information provided to the patient and caregivers is consistent.
   4. Educational materials (written information or other educational devices) should be provided.
   5. Ongoing patient and caregiver training should be provided during care.
      a) Ongoing education has been shown to have a positive impact upon patient outcomes, specifically catheter related infection.[12–14]
      b) Patients and families often display deterioration of sterile technique over time, and reeducation sessions help to improve compliance.
   6. Education interventions ideally address the emotional response to specialized nutrition support.[12]

B. The patient and caregivers need to receive education and demonstrate competence in preparing and administering nutrients.
   1. Parenteral nutrition patients and their caregivers must receive training and demonstrate competence in storage and inspection of solutions and containers, response to beyond-use dating, aseptic procedures for solution admixing and administration, issues of compatibility/stability of solutions, an infusion method/schedule, use and maintenance of equipment, and disposal of used equipment.
   2. Enteral nutrition patients and their caregivers need to receive training and demonstrate competence in storage and inspection of formula, response to expiration dates, clean technique for formula preparation and administration, issues of stability, product hang time, infusion method/schedule, cleaning and reuse of supplies, use and maintenance of equipment, and disposal of used equipment and supplies.

C. The patient and caregivers must receive education and demonstrate competence in access care. The patient and caregivers must receive training and demonstrate competence in aseptic technique for parenteral access and clean technique for enteral access to maintain the access device and its site, infection prevention, connecting and disconnecting to and from the access device, medication administration, and postinfusion flushing to prevent obstruction.

D. The patient and caregivers must receive education and demonstrate competence in recognition of and appropriate response to complications.
   1. Intolerance to the therapy, such as GI or metabolic therapy, and intolerance resulting from the disease process or from drug-nutrient interactions
   2. Mechanical complications such as catheter or tube occlusion, leakage, breakage, or dislodgment and equipment malfunction or breakage
   3. Localized (access site) or systemic infection
   4. Relevant drug-drug, drug-nutrient, and nutrient-nutrient interactions; side effects; infusion solution or formula stability issues; and precipitation
   5. Monitoring parameters should be given to the patient/caregiver so they know when and whom to contact should complications occur.

E. The patient and caregivers should receive education about the need for medical services to evaluate the ongoing effectiveness of HNS.
   1. In-home evaluation by home health professionals as needed.
   2. Routine (and nonroutine) physician evaluation.
   3. The patient and caregivers(s) should receive periodic reassessment and retraining as needed.
   4. The patient can be discharged when services are no longer required or when services can no longer be provided safely in the home or by the home care provider.

V. Reimbursement for HNS

A. HNS is covered by federal (Medicare) and state (Medicaid) health care programs when specific criteria are met.[15,16]
   1. Parenteral nutrition is covered under the prosthetic device act of Medicare, which requires an "artificial gut" (intravenous delivery) and "permanency" (at least 90 days of therapy). The patient must have documented evidence of inability to tolerate feeding through the enteral route (malabsorption, obstruction, resection, maldigestion).
      a) There is less than 5 feet of small bowel beyond the ligament of Treitz.
      b) GI losses exceed 50% of an oral intake of 2.5 to 3 L/day, and urine output is less than 1 L/day.
      c) Bowel rest is required for at least 90 days, and 20 to 35 kcal/kg/day is prescribed for a patient with specified conditions.
      d) Many other aspects of parenteral nutrition require specific justification, such as calorie levels <20 kcal/day or >35 kcal/day, protein >1.5 g/day or <0.8 g/day, and lipids >15 units of 20% or >30 units of 10% per month. When these criteria are not adequately documented, payment is denied or delayed.
   2. Enteral nutrition is also covered under the prosthetic device act, where the enteral feeding tube becomes the "artificial gut" and the permanency requirement must still be met. The patient must have disease of the small intestine such that digestion or absorption of an oral diet is insufficient to maintain weight and strength.
   3. Documentation must include information about why the patient's needs cannot be met by oral nutrition. Enteral nutrition formulas are divided into specific "categories." Aside from the standard formulas in Category I, formulas in all other categories require specific documentation to support their use.
      a) B4150; Category I: semisynthetic intact protein/protein isolates
      b) B4151; Category I: natural intact protein/protein isolates
      c) B4152; Category II: intact protein/protein isolates (calorically dense)
      d) B4153; Category III: hydrolyzed protein/amino acids
      e) B4154; Category IV: defined formula for special metabolic need
      f) B4155; Category V: modular components
      g) B4156; Category VI: standardized nutrients

B. State-funded programs (Medicaid, Medi-Cal, TennCare) develop state-specific criteria for coverage of specialized nutrition. Because these plans vary widely, they are not covered in detail here.
C. Managed care and private insurance coverage of specialized nutrition also varies widely. Often, managed care plans "contract" with home care providers for therapy-specific or per diem rates that may include supplies, pharmacy services, and nursing services. Other plans use Medicare criteria for coverage.
D. A major concern with long-term HNS is exceeding the lifetime maximum for insurance coverage. This is a special concern for infants and young children who are expected to require HNS for extended periods of time or their lifetimes.

VI. HNS Outcomes.

For patients, their caregivers, health care professionals, and health care payers, it is critical to determine the outcomes and psychosocial implications of such an expensive therapy. The study of health-related quality of life in the fields of home enteral and parenteral nutrition is still in its infancy. Yet it is an important aspect of providing care to enhance patient experiences.

A. Currently, there is no national outcome reporting system specifically for HNS. Most home care organizations incorporate outcome measures into their quality improvement processes; however, these data are proprietary. Although Medicare has incorporated outcome measurements for home care through its OASIS system, parenteral and enteral nutrition has not been reported separately.
B. Data compiled by the former Health Care Financing Administration (now Centers for Medicare and Medicaid Services) and Blue Cross/ Blue Shield of South Carolina during 1986 to 1993, and the North American HPEN Patient Registry (no longer active), was used to provide HNS outcome reports during the late 1990s.[17–19]
C. Other outcome data have been reported from programs in large medical centers.[20,21]
D. During the past decade, outcome reports from outside the United States have been published.[22–25]
E. Outcome reports for specific age-related or disease-related cohorts, such as children, patients with AIDS, and patients with cancer, have also been published.[26–29] Factors influencing patient outcome on home parenteral nutrition include the following:
    1. Patients with Crohn's disease, ischemic bowel, or a congenital disorder have an 87%, 84%, and 80% 3-year survival, respectively. Patients with motility disorder (pseudo-obstruction), radiation enteritis, or chronic adhesive disease have a 62%, 58%, and 40% 3-year survival, respectively. Patients with advanced cancer usually do not survive past 4 months, with only 20% surviving their first year on home parenteral nutrition.[30]
    2. Bowel anatomy may influence survival. Patients with bowel obstruction on home parenteral nutrition have a risk of death 2.5 times higher than that of non obstructed patients.[31] Permanent intestinal failure is likely if the small bowel is <100 cm in adults and <50 cm in children. The presence of in-continuity of terminal ileum or colon enhances weaning off home parenteral nutrition and survival.
    3. The mortality rate of Crohn's patients is significantly lower in large programs than in small programs.
    4. Patients dependent on opiates and sedatives have increased sepsis rates and require more hospital admissions.[28]
    5. Quality of life tends to be higher in younger patients, long-term patients, and patients with a high self-esteem, good family support, and the ability to return to work or school.
    6. Quality of life tends to be poorer in patients who are elderly, single, poor, or unemployed; those addicted to narcotics; and those who are early in their therapy.
    7. Affiliation with a national support group significantly increases quality of life, lowers depression scores, and lowers the incidence of catheter-related infections.[32,33] The major national support organization for home nutrition patients is the Oley Foundation (www.oley.org). Local chapters are available in many regions of the United States. Its purpose is to enrich the quality of life and functional status of persons requiring HNS therapies, build a "community" among those facing a lifetime of nutrition support, improve the quality of life for families challenged with this therapy, and promote the availability of information and opportunities for home parenteral and enteral nutrition families.
F. The most common complications of home parenteral nutrition are
    1. Catheter-related infection and sepsis
    2. Fluid and electrolyte disturbances
    3. Liver or bone disease
G. Most deaths during home parenteral and enteral treatment are from the underlying disease.[34,35]
H. Outcome data on home enteral nutrition patients are very limited, and outcomes may be due to the patient's underlying disease state. Common disease groups include patients with neurological dysfunction, upper GI cancers, anorexia, failure to thrive, swallowing disorders, cerebrovascular accidents, and neuromuscular disorders.
    1. At 1 year, between 45% and 60% of patients with varying diseases had died. The actual number of patients who were able to transition to oral intake ranged between 19% and 30%.
    2. Quality of life scores are lower in home enteral nutrition patients than the normal control group, which may be due to significant medical disabilities in the home enteral nutrition group.[36]
    3. Children on home enteral nutrition are able to gain weight, increase muscle strength, and increase overall muscle mass.[37,38]
I. The most common complications of home enteral nutrition are
    1. GI complications
    2. Tube displacement, occlusions, or leaking
    3. Dehydration

VII. Accreditation of Home Care and HNS.

Accreditation by national organizations provides an organization with an objective performance evaluation of its customer care, measured against national standards. It may also serve to meet certain Medicare certification requirements, expedite third-party payments, and favorably influence managed care contract decisions.

A. Three organizations currently provide accreditation for home care organizations:
    1. JCAHO
    2. ACHC
    3. CHAP
B. Each organization has developed standards against which the home care agency is measured. Although the standards differ, all three organizations examine areas such as staff education and competency, patient safety, infection control, quality improvement, compliance with law and regulation, confidentiality and privacy, fiscal management, equipment management, and quality of care.

(Home care material from the 1st edition was contributed by Jennifer K. Nelson, Jay Mirtallo, and Nancy J. Evans-Stoner)

REFERENCES

1. A.S.P.E.N. Board of Directors. Standards for home nutrition support. *Nutr Clin Pract.* 1999;14:151–162.

2. Ireton-Jones C, DeLegge MH, Epperson LA, et al. Management of the home parenteral nutrition patient. *Nutr Clin Pract.* 2003;18:310–317.
3. A.S.P.E.N. Board of Directors and the Clinical Guidelines Task Force. Guidelines for the use of parenteral and enteral nutrition in adult and pediatric patients. *J Parenter Enteral Nutr.* 2002;26:1SA–138SA.
4. Hanlon MD. Preplacement marking for optimal gastrostomy and jejunostomy tube site locations to decrease complications and promote self-care. *Nutr Clin Pract.* 1998;13:167–171.
5. Task Force for the Revision of Safe Practices for Parenteral Nutrition. Safe practices for parenteral nutrition. *J Parenter Enteral Nutr.* 2004;28: S39–S70.
6. Van den Berghe G, Wouthers P, Weekers F, et al. Intensive insulin therapy in critically ill patients. *N Engl J Med.* 2001;345:1359–1367.
7. Hirsch IB, Paauw DS, Brunzell J. Inpatient management of adults with diabetes. *Diabetes Care.* 1995;18;870–878.
8. USP General Information Chapter: pharmaceutical compounding–sterile preparations. Rockville, MD: United States Pharmacopeial Convention; 2003.
9. Vanderhoff JA, Young RJ. Overview of considerations for the pediatric patient receiving home parenteral and enteral nutrition. *Nutr Clin Pract.* 2003;18:221–226.
10. Seidner DL, Licata A. Parenteral nutrition–associated metabolic bone disease: pathophysiology, evaluation, and treatment. *Nutr Clin Pract.* 2000;15: 163–170.
11. Haderslev KV, Tjellesen L, Haderslev PH, Staun M. Assessment of the longitudinal changes in bone mineral density in patients receiving home parenteral nutrition. *J Parenter Enteral Nutr.* 2004;28:289–294.
12. Smith CE, Curtas S, Kleinbeck SV, et al. Clinical trial of interactive and videotaped educational interventions reduce infection, reactive depression, and rehospitalizations for sepsis in patients on home parenteral nutrition. *J Parenter Enteral Nutr.* 2003;27:137–145.
13. Silver HJ, Wellman NS. Family caregiver training is needed to improve outcomes for older adults using home care technologies. *J Am Diet Assoc.* 2002;102:831–836.
14. Silver HJ, Wellman NS, Glaindo-Ciocon D, et al. Family caregivers of older adults on home enteral nutrition have multiple unmet task-related training needs and low overall preparedness for caregiving. *J Am Diet Assoc.* 2004; 104:43–50.
15. DMERC Region D Supplier Manual, Chapter 9, PEN-1 through PEN-6, 2001. Available at: http://www.cms.hhs.gov/suppliers/dmepos/default.asp Accessed August 19,2004.
16. DMERC Region D Supplier Manual, ENT (L11568) Enteral Nutrition, 2002. Available at http:www.cms.hhs.gov/manuals/14_car/3b3300.asp Accessed December 28, 2004.
17. Howard L, Ament M, Fleming CR, Shike M, Steiger E. Current use and clinical outcome of home parenteral and enteral nutrition therapies in the United States. *Gastroenterology.* 1995;109:355–365.
18. Williams DM. The current state of home nutrition support in the United States. *Nutrition.* 1998;14:416–419.
19. Howard L, Malone M. Clinical outcome of geriatric patients in the United States receiving home parenteral and enteral nutrition. *Am J Clin Nutr.* 1997;99:1364–1370.
20. Scolapio JS, Fleming CR, Kelly DG, et al. Survival of home parenteral nutrition-treated patients: 20 years of experience at the Mayo Clinic. *Mayo Clin Proc.* 1999;74:217–222.
21. Knafelz D, Bambarara M, Diamanit A, et al. Complications of home parenteral nutrition in a large pediatric series. *Transplant Proc.* 2003;35: 3050–3051.
22. Ksiazyk J, Lyszkowska M, Kierkus J, et al. Home parenteral nutrition in children: the Polish experience. *J Pediatr Gastroenterol Nutr.* 1999;28: 152–156.
23. Bakker H, Bozzetti F, Staun M, et al. Home parenteral nutrition in adults: a European multicentre survey in 1997. ESPEN-Home Artificial Nutrition Working Group. *Clin Nutr.* 1999;18:135–140.
24. Moreno JM, Gomis P, Valero MA, et al. Home parenteral nutrition. A six-year combined program (adult and pediatric patients). *Med Clin (Barc).* 2000;29:617–618.
25. Engstron I, Bjornestam B, Finkel Y. Psychological distress associated with home parenteral nutrition in Swedish children, adolescents, and their parents: preliminary results. *J Pediatr Gastroenterol Nutr.* 2003;37:246–250.
26. Kang A, Zamora SA, Scott B, et al. Catch-up growth in children treated with home enteral nutrition. *Pediatrics.* 1998;102:951–955.
27. Ireton-Jones CS, Stiller DL. Evaluation of outcomes for patients with AIDS receiving home total parenteral nutrition. *Nutrition.* 1998;14:731–735.
28. Richards DM, Scott NA, Shaffer JL, et al. Opiate and sedative dependence predicts a poor outcome for patients receiving home parenteral nutrition. *J Parenter Enteral Nutr.* 1997;21:336–338.
29. Howard L. Home parenteral and enteral nutrition in cancer patients. *Cancer.* 1993;72(suppl):3531–3541.
30. North American Home Parenteral and Enteral Nutrition Patient Registry. *Annual Report With Outcome Profiles 1985–1992.* Albany, NY: Oley Foundation; 1994.
31. Messing B, Lemann M, Landais P, et al. Prognosis of patients with non-malignant chronic intestinal failure receiving long-term parenteral nutrition. *Gastroenterology.* 1995;108:1005–1010.
32. Smith CE. Quality of life in long-term total parenteral nutrition patients and their family caregivers. *J Parenter Enteral Nutr.* 1993;17:501–506.
33. Smith CE, Curtas S, Werkowitch M, et al. Home parenteral nutrition: does affiliation with a national support and educational organization improve patient outcomes? *J Parenter Enteral Nutr.* 2002;26:159–163.
34. Silver HJ, Wellman NS, Arnold DJ, et al. Older adults receiving home enteral nutrition: enteral regimen, provider involvement, and health care outcomes. *J Parenter Enteral Nutr.* 2004;28:92–98.
35. Light VL, Slezak FA, Porter JA, et al. Predictive factors for early mortality after percutaneous endoscopic gastrostomy. *Gastrointest Endosc.* 1995;42: 330–334.
36. Schneider SM, Pouget I, Staccini P, et al. Quality of life in long-term home enteral nutrition patients. *Clin Nutr.* 2000;91:25–28.
37. Steinkamp G, von der Hardt H. Improvement of nutritional status and lung function after long-term nocturnal gastrostomy feedings in cystic fibrosis. *J Pediatr.* 1994;124:244–248.
38. Kang A, Zamera SA, Scott B, et al. Catch-up growth in children treated with home enteral nutrition. *Pediatrics.* 1998;102:951–955.

SUGGESTED READINGS

Candusso M, Faraguna D, Sperli D, et al. Outcome and quality of life in paediatric home parenteral nutrition. *Curr Opin Clin Nutr Metab Care.* 2002;5: 309–314.

Davis JH. Total parenteral nutrition (TPN) at home: prototype high-tech home care nursing. *Gastroenterol Nurs.* 1996;19:207–209.

Goff K. Cost and cost-benefit of enteral nutrition. *Gastrointest Endosc Clin North Am.* 1998;8:733–744.

Jeppesen PB, Langholz E, Mortensen PB. Quality of life in patients receiving home parenteral nutrition. *Gut.* 1999;44:844–852.

Moreno Villares JM. The practice of home artificial nutrition in Europe. *Nutr Hosp.* 2004;19:59–67.

Pironi L, Paganelli F, Mosconi P, et al. The SF-36 instrument for the follow-up of health-related quality-of-life assessment of patients undergoing home parenteral nutrition for benign disease. *Transplant Proc.* 2004;3:255–258.

Reimund JM, Duclos B, Cuby C, et al. Home parenteral nutrition: clinical and laboratory analysis of initial experience (1994–1997). *Ann Nutr Metab.* 1999;43:329–338.

Julie O'Sullivan Maillet, PhD, RD, FADA

36

Ethics

Introduction

The purpose of this chapter is to provide guidance to clinicians in ethical issues that are relevant to nutrition support. Ethics are defined and placed in the context of patient care. Significant legal decisions are discussed, as are specific attributes of patients that influence their care, such as clinical status, stage of life, cultural tradition, and religion. Finally, practical considerations for ethical deliberations related to nutrition support are offered.

I. Background

A. Ethics is the study of morals.
   1. Ethics are standards of conduct or codes of conduct.
   2. Ethics is the part of philosophy that deals with morals.
   3. Morality defines how people ought to behave toward one another.
   4. The goal of moral behavior is to protect the values cherished by society.
   5. The values include quality of life, liberty, and freedom.
   6. Ethical dilemmas occur when ethical principles conflict.
   7. Conflicts are often between two rights or between a right and a duty. For example, the individual has the right to choose, and society has the duty to protect individuals.

B. Ethical principles of autonomy, beneficence, nonmaleficence, and justice apply to all health professionals.
   1. Autonomy is the right of individuals to make their own decisions.
   2. Beneficence is doing the right thing for the patient.
   3. Nonmaleficence is doing no harm ; it is balancing helping the patient through care as opposed to hurting them.
   4. Justice is acting fairly—providing similar treatment to patients in similar situations.

C. There are three major ethical theories represented by three philosophers: the utilitarian view (Mills), the deontological view (Kant), and the virtues view (Aristotle).
   1. The utilitarian view is that ethical decisions are a balance of positive values over negative values for all involved, so consequences matter.
   2. The deontological view is that acts can be inherently right or wrong independent of consequences.
   3. The virtues view involves the use of various virtues—integrity, respect, compassion, and the character of the patient—to guide care.

II. Ethical Issues in Patient Care

A. Within American bioethics, the patient's right to self-determination is the guiding principle.
   1. Patients and families face a difficult process when ethical issues supersede medical issues. The health care team should help the patient and family understand their options.
   2. Food and fluids are essential for life. There are strong cultural and philosophical issues that distinguish feeding issues from other medical care issues.

B. Patients need to be informed and deemed competent when they make their treatment choices. Competence is having an adequate decision-making capacity. Generally, a patient is considered to be able to make an informed decision if he or she responds appropriately, the decision is authentic, and the decision is voluntary.
   1. Advance directives can aid in explaining the patients' wishes. The two most common forms of advance directives are the living will and durable power of attorney (see Section III.D).
   2. Substitute decision makers may serve for the patient in some states when the patient cannot make a decision.

C. Generally, the individual's right takes precedence over the health care providers' view, with the following exceptions:
   1. Providers have the right to determine the medical futility of a treatment and need not offer or provide a futile treatment.
   2. When the individual's view is unknown, a surrogate decision maker is consulted. When the surrogate decision maker disagrees with the provider, the court generally supports feeding.

D. Distinguishing between obligatory and optional patient care involves examining the positive and negative consequences of the action.
   1. Will the action prolong life or prolong death?
   2. Will the action provide comfort or prolong suffering?
   3. How will the action provide a benefit and/or burden to the patient?

E. The use of an ethics team for consultation is highly encouraged in complex decision-making situations.
   1. The complexity and irreversibly of stopping feeding mandates that the health care team, the patient, and the family participate in decisions.
   2. If disagreement occurs, ethics committees or consultants should be contacted.

III. Key Legal and Regulatory Decisions Influencing Patient Care and Feeding

A. In the case of *In re Quinlan* in 1976, the US Supreme Court ruled that patients have the right to terminate medical care, because the individual has the right of autonomy.[1]

B. In the case of Nancy Beth Cruzan in 1991, the US Supreme Court ruled that nutrition and hydration are considered medical care and thereby can be terminated on the wishes of the patient. The ruling also dictated that states have the right to determine what constitutes "clear and convincing evidence" of the patient's wishes.[2]

C. In cases where a child has become incompetent or never was competent and is permanently unconscious, the courts have honored the parental decision.[3]

D. The Patient Self-Determination Act, effective 1991,[4] encourages the use of advanced directives, including a living will and durable power of attorney, as evidence of the patient's choice.
   1. A living will is a written legal document that states the care a patient would want at a time when the patient is incapable of making health care decisions.
   2. A person with durable power of health care is appointed by the patient to make health care decisions when that patient is not capable of making decisions. States vary in their acceptance of orally identified durable powers of attorney.
   3. The Patient Self-Determination Act has been only somewhat effective. The use of living wills and health care durable power of attorney is still low and inconsistent.[5] Health professionals need to continue to advocate the use of these tools to improve patient care.

E. Helga Wanglie was an elderly stroke patient who was unconscious. Her physician wanted to discontinue her enteral nutrition, stating that it was medically inappropriate. Her husband disagreed, and in 1991 the Minnesota court (*In re Helga Wanglie*) held that the spouse was the best decision maker.[6] The patient remained on enteral nutrition to the end of life.

F. *Finn v the Commonwealth of Virginia,* 1998[7], ruled that discontinuing enteral nutrition for a severely brain-damaged individual upon that individual's previously stated wishes was permissible, because natural progress of dying rather than removal of feeding was the cause of death.

G. In the 1992 Baby K case, a court ruled that an infant with anencephaly should receive life support, including nutrition and hydration, if the parents requested. The issue of futility was not clearly addressed.[8]

H. On October 21, 2003, the Florida legislature empowered the governor of Florida to reinstate enteral nutrition to Terri Schiavo, a chronically disabled woman, despite a court order allowing the discontinuation.[9] Her husband states that she did not "want tubes," but her family disagrees. Terri has no advance directive. The case continues.

I. In 1993, Robert Wendland suffered brain damage in an accident, but he is not permanently unconscious. In 1995, his wife tried to stop enteral nutrition, saying that her husband would not want to live under these circumstances. His mother disagreed. In 2001, the California Supreme Court ruled that the enteral nutrition could not be stopped because the patient's wishes were not known.[10,11]

IV. Ethical Issues Regarding Feeding Patients

A. Food and fluids may be optional or obligatory, depending on the situation.
   1. Food and fluids are obligatory when they improve the patient's health status or well-being. Thus, for acutely ill patients, feeding is obligatory. Food and fluids are also obligatory in chronic care to improve health status, such as in diabetes or wound healing.
   2. Artificially provided food and fluids are optional and provided on the basis of individual patient preference for terminally ill and permanently unconscious patients (see Section IV.C).
   3. Withdrawal of food and fluids in other cases may be optional or obligatory depending on the situation and the intent. For example, it is obligatory to orally feed the elderly, but it is not obligatory to provide enteral nutrition to the elderly unless doing so will improve the medical outcome, with variation based on patient preference.
   4. There is no ethical distinction between withholding food and withholding fluids. Withdrawal of food and withdrawal of fluids should be considered equal unless the patient or family wishes to distinguish them.
   5. Although there is no ethical distinction between withholding and withdrawing treatment, in practice is it more emotionally difficult to withdraw. Because of this, there may be a temptation not to initiate a treatment that may ultimately require discontinuation. However, it is ethically more appropriate to initiate a treatment with potential benefit and later discontinue it if the benefit is not realized than to withhold it to avoid this difficult situation.

B. The route of feeding will influence the feeding choices.
   1. Oral feeding should be encouraged whenever possible, with the emphasis on patient wishes and the physical and emotional enjoyment of food. Therapeutic diets should be reevaluated for outcome and discontinued when a positive outcome cannot reasonably be expected.
   2. If oral intake is decreasing, nutrition supplements may be encouraged to increase intake and reduce symptoms of malnutrition or prevent hunger. The emphasis is on patient comfort, both physiological and emotional.
   3. The potential benefits of intravenous hydration and enteral or parenteral nutrition should be weighed against the burdens of artificial feeding. Self-determination is the guiding principle; therefore, using the level of intervention preferred by the patient is generally recommended. However, it is essential that the health professional provide the facts about risk, benefit, and expected outcome to promote an "informed" patient decision. If conflicts occur, the use of an ethics committee or consultant is recommended.
   4. Institutions should have protocols on the provision and termination of enteral and parenteral nutrition.

C. Patients' health status will influence feeding choices.
   1. Acutely ill patients should be fed when medically stable based on the best feeding choices for each patient.
   2. Chronically ill patients should be fed based on best nutritional practices and patient willingness to follow that advice. If a patient refuses the optimal diet after clear education, discussion should be documented, but in most cases patients' right of determination predominates.
   3. Advance directives should guide feeding decisions for patients in a persistent vegetative state (PVS). The Multi-Society Task Force on PVS defines PVS as "a vegetative state present one month after traumatic or nontraumatic brain injury or lasting for at least one month in patients with degenerative or metabolic disorders or developmental malformations."[12] Others define "persistent" as extending to 1 to 3 years. While society has agreed that care may be stopped for patients in a PVS, the requirement to honor the patient's wishes in relation to the issue of futility is still in an early stage and is evolving.
   4. Patients with advanced dementia in the United States receive enteral nutrition more frequently than those in other countries. Several authors have reviewed the literature and have not found evidence that enteral nutrition prolongs survival, reduces pressure sores, or improves function.[13–16] Their recommendations are to have the least restrictive environment, to allow patients to select their foods, and to encourage hand feeding rather than enteral nutrition. If enteral nutrition is initiated, goals for the intervention should be established and monitored. If the goals are not being met, the enteral nutrition may be stopped.

5. Terminally ill patients often lose their appetite and reduce their consumption of food and fluids. In a study of 31 terminally ill cancer patients,[17] the patients were given fluids and food as requested. Despite low intakes, hunger was low to nonexistent. Ice chips and lip moisturizer reduced thirst and dry mouth. There is growing evidence that the patients do not suffer and may benefit from reduced hydration. Feeding decisions[18] should maximize enjoyment of food, minimize symptoms, and continually be reassessed to maximize responses to patient needs when palliative care is the goal.[19]
6. Feeding nonpermanently unconscious but disabled patients is currently being debated in the courts (see Sections III.H and III.I). Both cases illustrate the importance of an advanced directive.

D. Patient stage of life also influences feeding choices.
   1. For newborns
      a) The American Academy of Pediatrics says that the neonatologist/pediatrician must advocate for the best for the infant; this beneficence overrides parental autonomy.
      b) Communication among practitioners, parents, and ethical services before delivery is encouraged.
      c) Consent for treatment should be obtained before medical treatment of the infant; otherwise, a battery charge is possible.
      d) Parental decisions can be overruled by court order.
      e) The initial "Baby Doe" law from the 1980s requiring that aggressive treatment be provided with or without parental consent was invalidated in 1986, with the Supreme Court reiterating the rule of consent. The Baby Doe law should not be viewed as requiring feeding, however.
      f) In most cases, informed parental decisions should be used.[20]
   2. For children
      a) The guidelines of the American Academy of Pediatrics consider feeding the standard of care unless otherwise indicated by the parents.
      b) When parents disagree on feeding, the decision is generally to support the parent maintaining feeding.
      c) The assent (not consent) of minors who are old enough to participate in treatment decision making is strongly encouraged by the American Academy of Pediatrics.[21]
   3. For geriatric patients
      a) An alert elderly individual should be treated as any other adult would be.
      b) A cognitively impaired elder often has a substitute decision maker. Unfortunately, in a Boston/Ottawa study, these decision makers often did not know whether the patient had an advance directive or what the elder's enteral nutrition wishes were.[22]
      c) When there is disagreement among surrogate decision makers, feeding should be favored.

E. Culture, religion, and values will influence feeding choices.
   1. Many environmental factors influence decisions, including cultural and religious beliefs and personal and family experiences, philosophies, and values. Although within American bioethics, autonomy and self-determination are guiding principles (see Section II), diverse cultural differences exist, and good cross-cultural understanding and communication are important to quality care.[23] Religion and culture are neither independent nor homogeneous; there are wide variations in family and personal beliefs within each. Much of what we discuss in bioethics is based on a European-American model. Yet within many Asian communities, families insist that the patient, especially an elderly patient, not be told the prognosis or be burdened with decisions. To combine normal practice and respect cultural preferences, the health care professional might ask the patient who should receive the medical information, thus allowing the patient "informed refusal" through a surrogate. This preference should be documented. Kagawa-Singer suggests that cultural influence be ascertained through questions related to the mnemonic ABCDE:
      Attitudes of patients and families within their culture
      Beliefs, such as religious beliefs and traditions
      Content, such as personal history, including economics, emigration, and role of food in the family
      Decision-making style within the family and culture
      Environment, such as interpreters of culture or language[23]

      Being aware of and sensitive to cultural differences—without stereotyping—is essential to providing good care.
   2. Health care providers must be comfortable discussing religious and spiritual issues, particularly end-of-life issues, with patients. Religious beliefs come up in many discussions of resuscitation or termination of feeding. Care must be given to elicit concerns but not impose beliefs or try to resolve spiritual issues that are beyond the health care provider's expertise.[24] The religious premises discussed below offer general frames of reference for ethical deliberation on feeding issues.
   3. The US Catholic Church[25] stated in 1999 that the presumption should be to feed and provide fluids, but that there is a subjective element that should be guided by the patient's family and the health care professional. This guidance should include weighing the benefit and burden to the patient. In early 2004, the Pope stated that feeding was required: "I should like particularly to underline how the administration of water and food, even when provided by artificial means, always represents a *natural means* of preserving life, not a *medical act*. Its use, furthermore, should be considered, in principle, *ordinary* and *proportionate*, and as such morally obligatory, insofar as and until it is seen to have attained its proper finality, which in the present case consists in providing nourishment to the patient and alleviation of his suffering."[26] He concluded by saying that one should "guard jealously the principle according to which the true task of medicine is 'to cure if possible, always to care.' " The interpretation of this statement will evolve within the Church. It is substantively different from the 1992[27] and 1999[25] American National Conference of Catholic Bishops statements that focused on moral obligation, stating that if medical care had no benefit, it could not be obligatory but should not be considered automatically indicated. The conferences recognized that the patient, family, and health care professionals generally can best decide the benefits and burdens for each individual.[25,27]
   4. Many Protestant churches[28] have rejected the concept of prolonging life at all costs, saying that artificial feeding that prolongs dying is different from artificial feeding that enhances quality of life.
   5. Within Judaism, the concept of continuing treatment (feeding) once it is initiated is prevalent. Orthodox groups are the most insistent and Reform groups less insistent that feeding not be stopped once it is started. The question of the need to initiate treatment is controversial.[29,30] Feeding decisions are often postponed until making them becomes medically essential.
   6. Within Islam, sanctity of life is important, but "maintaining a terminal patient on artificial life support for a prolonged period in a vegetative state is not encouraged," and advanced directives are encouraged.[31]

V. Key Considerations to Frame Ethical Deliberations

A. Know the ethical positions of professional associations as well as state laws and institutional policies.

1. Professional associations
   a) The American Medical Association recommends that patient preferences prevail on forgoing "life-sustaining treatment," defined as "any treatment that serves to prolong life without reversing the underlying medical condition."[32] This includes artificial nutrition and hydration.
   b) The American Nurses Association distinguishes between food and water orally administered and artificial nutrition and hydration, stating that use of the latter should be justified. If artificial nutrition is forgone, comfort care should continue.[33]
   c) The American Dietetic Association recommends that the patient be at the center of the issue and that the health care team develop criteria for nutrition and hydration.[19]
   d) The American College of Physicians recommends honoring "voluntary refusal of hydration."[34]
   e) The American Academy of Pediatrics[35] includes enteral nutrition and intravenous feeding as part of life support that may be discontinued. More recently, in discussing palliative care states, the academy stated that the family opinion is key.[36]
2. State laws. The use of surrogate decision makers is dependent on state law. The health care team should work closely with these decision makers to act based on patient preference. If patient preference is not known, the team should act based on the best interests of the patient.[32]
3. Institutional policies
   a) Institutions should have policies on administering and removing artificial nutrition and hydration.
   b) Staff and patients should be aware of these policies.

B. When in doubt, consult with the ethics team.

C. Use several frameworks to assist in deliberations.

1. The wanted-warranted question
   a) If what is requested by the patient or family is also warranted by evidence, there is no dilemma. Ethical dilemmas occur when there is a conflict between different principles and different value systems.
   b) The question of sustaining life versus prolonging dying is important. Health care professionals are obligated to sustain life but not to prolong dying. The concept of intent is important here.
2. A patient-centered focus
   a) Identify the ethical question.
   b) Define the context of the situation.
   c) Identify family/patient issues: values, living wills, and substitute decision making.
   d) Review law and policies.
   e) Search for options.
   f) Choose and explain options.[19]
3. Consideration of the goals of health care
   a) Maximize health by curing or minimizing conditions/disorders.
   b) Minimize suffering by reducing symptoms.
   c) Balance the two and see if you feel good about the decision.

REFERENCES

1. *In re Quinlan,* 70 NJ 10,355, A2d 647, *cert denied sub nom, Garger v New Jersey,* 429 US 922 (1976).
2. *Nancy Beth Cruzan, by Her Parents and Co-Guardians, Lester L. Cruzan, et ux. Petitioners v Director, Missouri Department of Health, et al.* Supreme Court Docket number 88:1503. Argued: December 6, 1989: Decided June 25, 1990.
3. Nelson LJ, Rushton CH, Cranford RE, Nelson RM, Glover JJ, Truog RD. Forgoing medically provided nutrition and hydration in pediatric patients. *J Law Med Ethics.* 1995;23(1):33–46.
4. White M, Fletcher J. The Patient Self-Determination Act. *JAMA.* 1991;266 (3):410–412.
5. Kass-Bartelmes BL, Hughes R. Advance care planning: preferences for care at the end of life. *Research in Action,* Issue 12. Agency for Healthcare Research and Quality. Available at: http://www.ahrq.gov/research/endliferia/endria.htm. Accessed August 9, 2004.
6. *In re Helga Wanglie,* Fourth Judicial District (Dist. Ct. Div.) PX-91-283. Minnesota, Hennepin County.
7. *James S. Gilmore II v Michele Finn; Michele P. Finn v James S. Gilmore III,* 259 Va 448; 527 SE2d 426; 200 Va Lexis 52 (2000).
8. Annas G. Asking the courts to set the standard of emergency care—the case of baby K. *New Engl J Med.* 1994;330(21):1542–1545.
9. Bandow D. How much is Terri Schiavo's life worth? April 12, 2004. Available at: http://www.terrisfight.org/. Accessed May 1, 2004.
10. Reynolds D. CA high court says wife can't stop disabled husband's food, water. *Inclusion Daily Express,* August 9, 2001. Available at http://www.ragged-edge-mag.com/drn/drn080901wendland.htm. Accessed May 1, 2004.
11. Lo B, Dornbrand L, Wolf L, Groman M. The Wendland case—withdrawing life support from incompetent patients who are not terminally ill. *N Engl J Med.* 2002;346(19):1489–1493.
12. The Multi-Society Task Force on PVS. Medical aspects of the persistent vegetative state. *New Engl J Med.* 1994;330:1499–1506.
13. Finucane T, Christmas C, Travis K. Tube feeding in patients with advanced dementia. *JAMA.* 1999;282:1365–1370.
14. McCann R. Lack of evidence about tube feeding—food for thought. *JAMA.* 1999;282:1380–1381.
15. Gillick M. Rethinking the role of tube feeding in patients with advanced dementia. *N Engl J Med.* 2000;342:206–209.
16. Sheiman S. Tube feeding the demented nursing home resident. *J Am Geriatr Soc.* 1996;44:1268–1270.
17. Winter SM. Terminal nutrition: framing the debate for the withdrawal of nutritional support in terminally ill patients. *Am J Med.* 2000;109:723–741.
18. Emanuel LL, von Gunten CF, Ferris FD. *The Education for Physicians End-of-Life Care.* Chicago, IL:Institute of Ethics, American Medical Association; 1999.
19. Maillet JD, Potter RL, Heller L. Position of the American Dietetic Association: ethical and legal issues in nutrition, hydration and feeding. *J Am Diet Assoc.* 2002;102:716–726.
20. Pinkerton JV, Finnerty JJ, Lombardo PA, Rorty MV, Chapple H, Boyle RJ. Parental rights at the birth of a near-viable infant: conflicting perspectives. *Am J Obstet Gynecol.* 1997;177(2):283–290.
21. American Academy of Pediatrics, Committee on Bioethics. Informed consent, parental permission and assent in pediatric practice. *Pediatrics.* 1995;95:317.
22. Mitchell S, Berkowitz R, Lawson F, Lipsitz L. A cross-national survey of tube-feeding decisions in cognitively impaired older persons. *J Am Geriatr Soc.* 2000;48:391–397.
23. Kagawa-Singer M, Blackhall L. Negotiating cross-cultural issues at the end of life. *JAMA.* 2001;286(23):2993–3001.
24. Lo B, Ruston D, Kates L. Discussing religious and spiritual issues at the end of life. *JAMA.* 2002;287(6):749–755.
25. National Conference of Catholic Bishops Committee for Pro-Life Activities. Nutrition and hydration: moral and pastoral reflections. *J Contemp Health Law Policy.* 1999;15:455–477.
26. Pope John Paul. Address of John Paul II to the Participants in the International Congress on "Life-Sustaining Treatments and Vegetative State: Scientific Advances and Ethical Dilemmas." March 20, 2004. Available at: http://www.terrisfight.org/. Accessed May 1, 2004.
27. National Conference of Catholic Bishops, Committee for Pro-Life Activities. Nutrition and hydration: moral and pastoral reflections. *Catholic News.* April 1992:18–20.
28. Frederick HD. On dying and dying well: spiritual and moral aspects. *J Soc Med.* 1977;70:75–81.
29. Dorff E. A Jewish approach to end-state medical care. *Conserv Jud.* 1991;43:3–51.
30. Gillick M. Artificial nutrition and hydration in the patient with advanced dementia: is withholding treatment compatible with traditional Judaism? *Ethics.* 2001;27:12–15.

31. Athar S. Information for health care providers when dealing with a Muslim patient. Islamic Medical Association of North America. Available at: http://www.islam-usa.com/e40.html. Accessed May 1, 2004.
32. American Medical Association. Withholding or withdrawing life-prolonging medical treatment. Updated June 1996. Available at: http://www.ama-assn.org/apps/pf_new/pf_online. Accessed April 19, 2004.
33. American Nurses Association. Position statement—forgoing nutrition and hydration. Effective date: April 2, 1992. Available at: http://www.ana.org. Accessed April 19, 2004.
34. Quill T, Byock IR. Responding to intractable terminal suffering: the terminal sedation and voluntary refusal of food and fluids: position paper. *Intern Med.* 2000;132:408–414.
35. American Academy of Pediatrics, Committee on Bioethics. Guidelines for forgoing life-sustaining medical treatment. *Pediatrics.* 1994;93:532–536.
36. American Academy of Pediatrics, Committee on Bioethics and Committee on Hospital Care. Palliative care for children. *Pediatrics.* 2000;106:351–357.

Index

H

Q

R

S